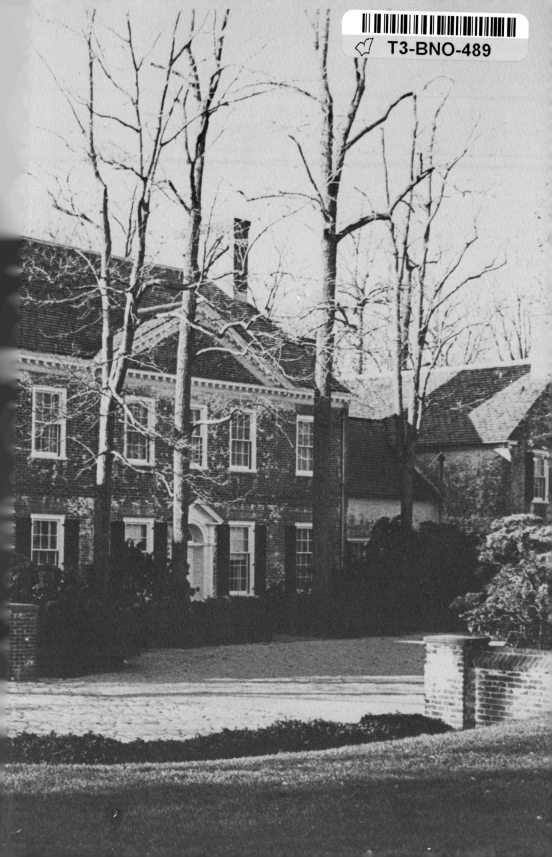

Nitrosamines and
Human Cancer

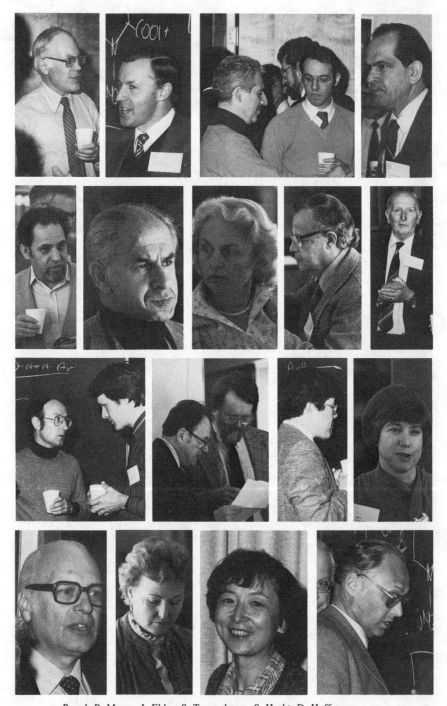

Row 1: P. Magee; J. Elder; S. Tannenbaum, S. Hecht; D. Hoffmann.
Row 2: D. Fine; J. Weisburger; R. Kimbrough; P. Grasso; C. Walters.
Row 3: R. Montesano, R. Peto; A. Pegg, C. Harris; C. Yang; L. Anderson.
Row 4: P. Reed; R. Hicks; L. Fong; H. Bartsch.

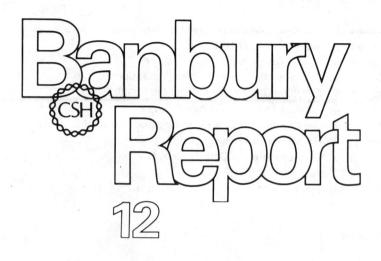

Nitrosamines and Human Cancer

Edited by

PETER N. MAGEE
Fels Research Institute
Temple University School of Medicine

COLD SPRING HARBOR LABORATORY
1982

BANBURY REPORT SERIES

Banbury Report 1: Assessing Chemical Mutagens
Banbury Report 2: Mammalian Cell Mutagenesis
Banbury Report 3: A Safe Cigarette?
Banbury Report 4: Cancer Incidence in Defined Populations
Banbury Report 5: Ethylene Dichloride: A Potential Health Risk?
Banbury Report 6: Product Labeling and Health Risks
Banbury Report 7: Gastrointestinal Cancer: Endogenous Factors
Banbury Report 8: Hormones and Breast Cancer
Banbury Report 9: Quantification of Occupational Cancer
Banbury Report 10: Patenting of Life Forms
Banbury Report 11: Environmental Factors in Human Growth and Development

Banbury Report 12
Nitrosamines and Human Cancer

Printed in the United States of America

Cover and book design by Emily Harste

Library of Congress Cataloging in Publication Data

Main entry under title:

Nitrosamines and human cancer.
(Banbury report, ISSN 0198-0068 ; 12)
Bibliography: p.
Includes index.
1. Nitrosoamines–Toxicology.
2. Carcinogenesis. I. Magee, Peter N.
II. Series. [DNLM: 1. Nitrosamines–Congresses.
2. Neoplasms–Chemically induced–Congresses.
3. Dose-response relationship, Drug–Congresses. W3 BA19 v.12 / QA 202 N732 1982]
RC268.7.N59N58 1982 616.99'4071 82-12952
ISBN 0-87969-211-1

Acknowledgments

This meeting on the possible role of nitrosamines in human cancer would not have been possible without the encouragement of James D. Watson, the Director of Cold Spring Harbor Laboratory, and the enthusiasm of Victor K. McElheny, the former Director of Banbury Center. The meeting and production costs of this book were supported by funds from the National Cancer Institute (Grant 1 R13 CA31384-01 NSS).

The editor is most impressed by the great speed and efficiency with which Lynda Moran, the Banbury editor, and Joanne DeOliveira, the Banbury editorial assistant, proceeded with the preparation of this book. I also wish to acknowledge my gratitude to Beatrice Toliver, administrative assistant at Banbury Center, and Helen Bleil, my secretary, for making the meeting arrangements flow so smoothly.

PARTICIPANTS

Lucy M. Anderson, Sloan-Kettering Institute for Cancer Research

Michael C. Archer, Department of Medical Biophysics, University of Toronto, Canada

Herman N. Autrup, Laboratory of Human Carcinogenesis, National Cancer Institute

Klaus D. Brunnemann, Naylor Dana Institute for Disease Prevention, American Health Foundation

Helmut Bartsch, Programme of Environmental Carcinogens and Host Factors, International Agency for Research on Cancer, Lyon, France

André Castonguay, Naylor Dana Institute for Disease Prevention, American Health Foundation

Brian C. Challis, Department of Chemistry, Imperial College of Science and Technology, London, England

Allan H. Conney, Department of Biochemistry and Drug Metabolism, Research Division, Hoffmann-La Roche Inc.

Pelayo Correa, Department of Pathology, Louisiana State University Medical Center

Graham J. Durant, SmithKline & French Research Limited, Hertfordshire, England

James B. Elder, Department of Surgery, University of Manchester, England

David H. Fine, New England Institute for Life Sciences

Wolfgang E. Fleig, Zentrum für Innere Medezin der Universität Ulm, Ulm-Donau, Federal Republic of Germany

Louise Yuk-ying Fong, Department of Biochemistry, University of Hong Kong, Hong Kong

William A. Garland, Research Division, Hoffmann-La Roche Inc.

Stanley Goldfarb, Department of Pathology and Laboratory Medicine, University of Wisconsin School of Medicine

Charles T. Gombar, Fels Research Institute, Temple University School of Medicine

Paul Grasso, BP Group Occupational Health Centre, Middlesex, England

George W. Harrington, Department of Chemistry, Temple University

Curtis C. Harris, Laboratory of Human Carcinogenesis, National Cancer Institute

Philip E. Hartman, Department of Biology, The Johns Hopkins University

Stephen S. Hecht, Naylor Dana Institute for Disease Prevention, American Health Foundation

R. Marian Hicks, The School of Pathology, Middlesex Hospital Medical School, London, England

Dietrich Hoffmann, Naylor Dana Institute for Disease Prevention, American Health Foundation

David E. Jensen, Fels Research Institute, Temple University School of Medicine

Renate D. Kimbrough, Center for Environmental Health, Centers for Disease Control

William Lijinsky, Chemical Carcinogenesis Program, Frederick Cancer Research Facility, National Cancer Institute

Peter N. Magee, Fels Research Institute, Temple University School of Medicine

Christopher J. Michejda, Chemical Carcinogenesis Program, Frederick Cancer Research Facility, National Cancer Institute

George E. Milo, Department of Physiological Chemistry, Ohio State University Comprehensive Cancer Center

Sidney S. Mirvish, Eppley Institute for Research in Cancer and Allied Diseases, University of Nebraska Medical Center

Ruggero Montesano, Programme of Mechanisms of Carcinogenesis Division of Chemical and Biological Carcinogenesis, International Agency for Research on Cancer, Lyon, France

Ismail Parsa, Department of Pathology, State University of New York, Downstate Medical Center

Anthony E. Pegg, Department of Physiology and Specialized Cancer Research Center, Pennsylvania State University, College of Medicine

Richard Peto, Clinical Trial Service Unit, Radcliffe Infirmary, University of Oxford, England

Rudolf Preussmann, Institute of Toxicology and Chemotherapy, German Cancer Research Center, Heidelberg, Germany

Peter I. Reed, Berkshire Area Health Authority-East District, Wexham Park Hospital, Berkshire, England

Nrisinha P. Sen, Health Protection Branch-Health and Welfare Canada, Ottawa, Canada

Ronald C. Shank, Department of Community and Environmental Medicine, California College of Medicine, University of California at Irvine

Michael L. Simenhoff, Division of Nephrology, Jefferson Medical College, Thomas Jefferson University

Peter F. Swann, Courtauld Institute of Biochemistry, Middlesex Hospital Medical School, London, England

Steven R. Tannenbaum, Department of Nutrition and Food Science, Massachusetts Institute of Technology

Clifford L. Walters, Biochemistry Section, Leatherhead Research Association, Leatherhead,Surrey, England

John H. Weisburger, Vice President for Research, Naylor Dana Institute for Disease Prevention, American Health Foundation

Chung S. Yang, College of Medicine and Dentistry of New Jersey, New Jersey Medical School

INTRODUCTION

PETER N. MAGEE
Fels Research Institute
Temple University School of Medicine
Philadelphia, Pennsylvania 19140

Since the discovery of the carcinogenic action of dimethylnitrosamine (NDMA) by the author and the late Dr. John M. Barnes in 1956, well over a hundred nitrosamines and other N-nitroso compounds have been found to be carcinogenic in experimental animals. A recent compilation has listed 39 different susceptible animal species, including monkeys, among mammals, as well as birds, fish and amphibia. The compounds show a remarkable degree of organ specificity which varies with their chemical structures and tumors have been induced in most organs of rodents and other species by the administration of different nitroso compounds under varying experimental conditions. Other biological actions which have been found for these compounds include toxicity and cytotoxicity, mutagenicity, teratogenicity. Some cytotoxic nitrosourea derivatives have also been used in cancer chemotherapy. N-nitroso compounds are thus very useful agents for studies of the pathology and biochemistry of chemical carcinogenesis and they have been, and continue to be, used extensively for this purpose in laboratories throughout the world.

Nitrosamines and other N-nitroso compounds are formed by nitrosation of a variety of secondary and tertiary amino compounds and their presence has been detected in various environmental situations including some foods and beverages and in the atmosphere. In addition carcinogenic nitrosamines can be formed in the body by the nitrosation of various amines. Conditions favorable for such nitrosation reactions are found in the acidic conditions of the mammalian stomach when nitrites are present, derived from saliva and from certain foods, particularly those to which they have been added as preservatives.

In an essay on nitrosamines published in 1974, John Barnes made the following statement (Barnes, 1974).

"While the identification of dozens of chemical carcinogens will certainly make it possible to eliminate some from particularly dangerous environments such as certain occupations, it seems unlikely that it will help to control much of the disease as seen in the general population. Preoccupation with the occurrence and behavior of minute amounts of nitrosamines in the human environment will probably divert skills from more profitable studies of the behavior of nitrosamines in experimental systems.

Any patient reader who has reached the end may well decide that this is an essay that matches Dr. Johnson's definition. If it leaves the reader with the impression that nitrosamines have a much greater potential as research tools than they have as health hazards, it will have served its purpose."

This Banbury Conference was planned to bring together a group of scientists with common interests in the possible role of nitrosamines in the causation of human cancer and to encourage them to present and discuss their research findings. It was hoped that the large amount of new information that would thus be collected in one volume would permit the reader to re-evaluate the conclusions of Barnes concerning the possible relationships of nitrosamines to human cancer.

REFERENCES

Barnes, J. M. 1974. Nitrosamines. *Essays in Toxicology* 5:1.

CONTENTS

SESSION 7: DOSE RESPONSE RELATIONSHIPS IN NITROSAMINE
               CARCINOGENESIS

SESSION I:

EVIDENCE SUGGESTING THAT HUMANS ARE SUSCEPTIBLE TO CARCINOGENESIS BY *N*-NITROSO COMPOUNDS

In Vitro Transformation of
Cultured Human Diploid Fibroblasts

GEORGE E. MILO AND RONALD W. TREWYN
Department of Physiological Chemistry and
Comprehensive Cancer Center
The Ohio State University
Columbus, Ohio 43210

The carcinogenicity of nitrosamines and nitrosamides was reported to be dependent upon the alkylation of macromolecules following the breakdown of the nitroso compounds (Loveless 1969). In mammalian rodent systems, a carcinogenic event occurred following methylation of the DNA (Magee and Hultin 1962; Magee and Farber 1962). Loveless (1969) suggested that the O^6 position of DNA-guanine is quantitatively alkylated by N-nitroso compounds. Gerchman and Ludlum (1973) suggested that methylated-O^6 guanine is read not as a guanine but adenine, therefore a misspelling occurs at a critical site in the DNA with a subsequent carcinogenic response. Subsequently, Goth and Rajewsky (1974) indicated that the persistence of this error was the most important step in the carcinogenesis process and that the alkylation must persist until the DNA replicates semiconservatively and the daughter cells receive this aberrant DNA.

In human cells treated with a carcinogen (Milo et al. 1978a,b) we recognized that damage to DNA by these agents was repaired quickly by error-free repair systems (Milo and Hart 1976). Over the years attempts to reproducibly transform randomly proliferating human diploid cell populations has met with failure. However, we describe a program for the induction of carcinogenesis in vitro with human diploid fibroblasts using nitroso compounds as the instruments to deliver a carcinogenic insult. The biological endpoint measuring the carcinogenic insult will be an expression of anchorage-independent growth, cellular invasiveness and neoplasia in a xenogeneic host.

METHODS

Chemicals

The chemicals of interest for this study are dimethylnitrosamine, (NDMA, $CH_3N(NO)CH_3$); diethylnitrosamine (NDEA, $CH_3CH_2N(NO)CH_3$); N-methyl-N'-Nitro-N-nitrosoquanidine (MNNG); ethylnitrosourea (ENU, $C_2H_5N(NO)-CONH_2$); and methylnitrosourea (MNU, $CH_3N(NO)CONH_2$). These chemicals were furnished by the NCI Chemical Repository DCCP-NCI for this study sponsored by the National Cancer Institute. The modulators were obtained from commercial sources: insulin (Sigma Chemical, St. Louis, MO), phorbol myristate acetate, (Consolidated Midland Corp., Brewster, NY) and anthralin, (Sigma Chemical Co., St. Louis, MO).

Cell Cultures

Neonatal foreskin fibroblast cell populations were prepared as described previously, (Riegner et al. 1976; Oldham et al. 1980). Briefly, the fibroblasts were separated immediately from the mixed culture by selective detachment from the epithelial cells attached to a plastic substratum. The fibroblast cultures were passaged routinely using 0.1% trypsin and the subsequent cultures were maintained on Eagles-minimum essential medium (MEM) prepared with Hanks' balanced salt solution, 25.0mM HEPES buffer (GIBCO, Grand Island, NY) at pH 7.2. Additional supplements were added as needed (Riegner et al. 1976). The cultures were incubated in an atmosphere of 4% CO_2-enriched air atmosphere at 37°C.

Transformation Procedure

Toxicity Protocol

The transformation procedure is broken down into two distinct operational procedures: the cytotoxicity evaluation of each suspect carcinogen and the transformation protocol. Each chemical regardless of its structural similarity must be evaluated for its cytotoxic effects. Foreskin fibroblasts were isolated from the tissue (Oldham et al. 1980; Allred et al. 1982) and seeded at the first passage at 40 cells/cm^2 in MEM supplemented with growth additives, (Milo and DiPaolo 1978) Complete Media V (CMV), and incubated at 37° in a 4% carbon dioxide-enriched air environment and 10% FBS. The chemicals of interest are added to the populations for a 16-hour period at different concentrations of the chemical. The experimental medium was removed and replaced with MEM supplemented with 20% FBS, (Milo and DiPaolo 1980; Oldham et al. 1980). Two weeks later the cultures were fixed in 10% phosphate-buffered formalin and were stained with hematoxylin and eosin, and enumerated manually or on a differential image optical analyzer (Gavino et al. 1982). The data is expressed as relative colony forming efficiency i.e., the number of colonies 10 cells in size or larger that formed within 21 days of concluding treatment divided by the number of colonies that formed in the untreated populations X 100.

Transformation Protocol

The concentrations of the compound of interest found to give an effective cytotoxic dose of 50%, 25% or noncytotoxic dose on cells at 40 cells/cm^2 were used as the concentrations of choice to initiate the transformation process. We run every treatment in triplicate (i.e., on 3 different cultures derived from an initial culture prior to population doubling [PDL] 6). The randomly logarithmically growing cultures at 5000 cells/cm^2 are seeded into a Dulbecco's Modified MEM minus arginine and glutamine and supplemented with dialyzed-FBS for 16 hours. The 2-hour-initiated thymidine radiolabeling index decreases from 18-23% to 0.1% to 0% in that time, (Milo and DiPaolo 1980; Oldham et al. 1980). At that time the cells are released from the G$_1$ block by the readdition of CMV-10% FBS containing 2mM glutamine and 1mM arginine plus either modulator 10U/ml insulin 0.1µg/ml anthralin or 5 $\times$ 10^{-7}M PMA. Ten hours following release from the G$_1$ block the cells exhibit S phase entry. The carcinogens of interest were added and left on for 12 hours. At the conclusion of the treatment the experimental medium was removed and replaced with CMV supplemented with 10% FBS. The cells were allowed to recover for 2 days and then were split 1:2 into CMV containing 2x vitamins, 8x nonessential amino acids and 20% FBS, hereafter referred to as 8x medium. When these treated cultures reached 80% to 90% confluent density they were serially passaged 1:10 into 8x medium until PDL-20.

Characterization of Transformed Cells:

Anchorage Independent Growth

The carcinogen populations at PDL 20 were seeded at 50,000 cells in 2ml of 0.33% agar, (in a 25cm^2 well) prepared in Dulbecco's LoCal medium (Biolabs, Northbrook, IL) supplemented with additives, (Milo et al. 1981c) and 20% FBS. This cell suspension was layered over 5ml of a 2% agar base prepared in RPMI 1629 medium (GIBCO) plus additives, (Milo et al. 1981a,c). The seeded cultures were not disturbed for 1 week and were subsequently observed on a weekly basis for 3-4 weeks. Cultures were scored as positive when colonies of > 50 cells were observed. Colonies were removed and reestablished in culture. After attachment and growth to ~20% density the cells were trypsinized and reseeded to distribute evenly over the substratum.

Cellular Invasiveness

The carcinogen-treated population that formed colonies in soft agar were reestablished in culture and subsequently evaluated for tumor potential, (Noguchi et al. 1978; Milo et al. 1981c), using chick embryonic skin (CES) in vitro. The CES organ culture was modified to optimize sensitivity to the transformed cells and frequency of success for a rapid assay for cellular neoplasia. Eggs were incubated for 9-10 days in a humidifed egg incubator. The embryos were removed from the eggs, the skins separated from the dorsal part of the embryo and placed on an agar base containing 10 parts of 1% agar in Earle's balanced salt solution, 4 parts FBS, and 4 parts chick embryo extract. The treated cells,

250,000 in number contained in $0.04\mu l$ of MEM, were added to the CES organ culture. These cultures were incubated in a humidified incubator at $37°C$ in a 4% CO_2 enriched air atmosphere. On day 4 the skins were removed and fixed in Bouin's solution. The stained $5\mu M$ sections on slides were examined by light microscopy (Milo et al. 1981a).

Tumor Growth in Nude Mice

Treated populations that exhibited anchorage independent growth were evaluated in 6 week old nude mice (Sprague-Dawley). The mice were irradiated with 137CS source at 450 RAD whole body irradiation 48 hours prior to sub-cutaneous injection of 5×10^6 cells. Six weeks later the tumors were counted and the incidence of tumor formation recorded (Milo et al. 1981a).

RESULTS

The cell population treated with the individual compounds included herein were treated at equivalent cytotoxic doses to transform the human foreskin fibroblasts. It has been found that treatment regimens for transformation protocols were more reliable when the populations at risk to the suspect carcinogenic agent were treated at $ED_{10,25 \text{ or } 50}$ toxic doses or noncytotoxic equivalent doses rather than chemical equivalent doses. In all experiments where toxic values exceeded the ED_{50} values the incidence of transformation as measured by anchorage independent growth and cellular invasiveness tended to drop to zero (control values). Once the toxicity of these compounds has been evaluated then the toxicity of the modulators has to be determined. All modulators were used at ED_0 doses, i.e. a noncytotoxic dose. The problem one was faced with in these comparisons were the integrated effects that the modulators have on cell permeability. This was why we used these modulators on the cells at exceedingly low concentrations to elicit the proper response without interfering with the cytotoxic dose of the carcinogens of interest (Table 1).

Table 1
Cytotoxicity of Nitrosamine Derivatives Determined on Human Foreskin Fibroblasts In Vitro

Chemical Compound	Cytotoxic Effect ED 50 in 4 $(\mu g/ml)$
NDMA	0.001
NDEA	0.01
MNU	29.0
ENU	44.0
MNNG	0.1

These concentrations represent the cytotoxic dose that yielded a 50% inhibition of the relative cloning efficiency. (Data from Allred et al. 1982).

Early Stage

Treated populations responded to the carcinogenic insult in a different predictable manner than populations just responding to toxic insults. First, for example, populations responding to toxic levels of modulators while exhibiting selective changes in plasma membrane permeability, did not exhibit altered lectin agglutination profiles as seen by populations responding to a carcinogenic insult.

Once carcinogen-treated populations exhibited these features they were serially passaged for PDL 20 before seeding in soft agar.

Transitional Stage

Using the growth medium we described under transformation protocol (Material and Methods section), the optimum time for seeding the treated populations in soft agar was 20 PDL following treatment with the carcinogen. Second, it was interesting to note that at this PDL; NDMA-, NDEA-, and MNNG-treated populations exhibited anchorage independent growth while ENU- and MNU-treated populations did not exhibit this feature. NDMA induced colony formation in soft agar of 13 colonies/10^5 cells; NDEA, 8 colonies/10^5 cells and MNNG, 1 colony/10^5 cells. The colonies 50 cells in size or larger were removed and reseeded in flasks. At a 80% preconfluent density the cells were seeded onto CES and 4 days later evaluated (Table 2). The treated populations that exhibited anchorage independent growth also exhibited cellular invasiveness.

Table 2

Evaluation of Different Nitrosamine-Treated Cell Populations for Anchorage-Independent Growth, Cellular Invasiveness, and Tumor Incidence

Chemical compound	Cytotoxic effect (ED 50 μg/ml)[a]	Cellular invasiveness[b]	Anchorage-independent growth[c]	Tumor incidence[d]
NDMA	0.001	+	13	2/6
NDEA	0.01	+	8	3/8
MNU	29.0	−	0	N.D.
ENU	44.0	−	0	N.D.
MNNG	0.1	+	1	3/5

[a]Represents the cytotoxic dose that yielded a 50% inhibition of the relative cloning efficiency.

[b]A positive response indicates that out of 6 CES organ cultures one or more sections upon examination by the pathologist exhibited cellular invasiveness.

[c]Colonies 50 cells or more in size were scored as positive when counted 21 days post-seeding in the soft agar overlayer. Each 25 cm² well was seeded with 50,000 cells, (Methods section).

[d]The numerator represents the number of positive takes (tumors) over the number of mice injected with 5 × 10^6 treated cells. (Methods section).

Late Stage

At this time the different treated populations were injected in nude mice and the incidence of tumor formation noted. Injected NDMA-treated cells elicited an incidence of tumor formation in 2 out of 6 mice; NDEA-treated cells 3 out of 8 mice and MNNG treated cells 3 out of 5 mice. The tumors were examined by histopathology and interpreted to be undifferentiated mesenchymal tumors. The cellular tumors evaluated from the CES were described as simulated firbosarcomas. This definition was used because the pathologist was describing cellular invasion into CES, an organ culture, in vitro. The two interpretations are not incompatible.

DISCUSSION

The data here were presented to illustrate the sequencing that can optimize the program of human foreskin fibroblast response to a carcinogenic insult in vitro. These compounds that were evaluated for their carcinogenic potential appear to require cell proliferation for the fixation of the carcinogen damage. Once the insult is fixed, a program of selective expression of the initiated cells occurs over a protracted time period, PDL 20, followed by anchorage independent growth of the transformed cells.

A similar selection pressure is also expressed by the cell population prior to carcinogen treatment, i.e. cells passaged in culture > 10 PDL are refractory to a carcinogenic insult (Sutherland, et al. 1980; Milo et al. 1981c; Zimmerman and Little et al. 1981). These observations are not unusual in themselves, for example, we have seen the same refractoriness exhibited by human foreskin populations to feline sarcoma virus-directed transformations in vitro (Milo et al. 1981b) at high PDL. These vector-directed transformations also exhibit multistage (early, transitional, and late stage of expression of carcinogenesis) carcinogenesis exhibited by the nitrosamine-transformed cell populations. An interesting feature of the chemical carcinogen-induced transformation of human cells as seen by Silinskas et al. (1981) was that they used a different medium to culture their cells in soft agar and observe colony formation around 8-13 PDL following carcinogen treatment rather than PDL 20. Zimmerman and Little (1981), and Sutherland et al. (1980) observed also that cells treated at PDL > 10 were refractory to the carcinogenic insult. Recently, Tejwani et al. (1982) demonstrated that DNA-adducts formed by benzo[a] pyrene (B[a]P) or B[a]P 9,10-ene diol epoxide anti form of B[a]P in susceptible populations were qualitatively similar to the principal adduct formed in the refractory cells i.e. B[a]P 9,10-ene diol epoxide-deoxyguanosine adduct.

It is our contention that optimum sensitivity occurs in S-phase to the carcinogen insult and that the response can be amplified by the addition of modulators (Milo and DiPaolo 1980). These events are followed by the persistence of the adducts during the critical point of the fixation of the carcinogenic insult immediately prior to and during the early phase of replication of DNA in S-phase. These events are followed by a selection process for the early stage of carcinogenesis, i.e., altered lectin agglutination profiles (Milo et al. 1981c) and expression of the early transformed phenocopy.

As pointed out by Zimmerman and Little (1981) and reported by Kapp and Painter (1979) the rate of scheduled DNA synthesis in human cells is proportional to the number of functional replicons in S at a given time. They also point out that repair of DNA damage is not extensive over the treatment period.

Following from this we hold the cells in G_1 block prior to S-phase entry in the presence of the exogenously supplied modulators which may amplify the number of replication sites and expose carcinogenic site(s) that would otherwise be masked. It may not require a permanent change in a molecular event such as that described or such as deficient DNA repair synthesis or persistence of damage, but it may require a change in events of the replicon similar to that seen in normal differentiation patterns. As we presently know, human nasopharyngeal carcinomas tumors are exceedingly difficult to grow in vitro. They purportedly differentiate in culture and produce keratin and enter an amitotic stage, (R. Glaser, pers. comm.). Milo et al. (1981a) showed that carcinogen-initiated keratinocytes when seeded directly into soft agar produce colonies. They express anchorage-independent growth. However, when carcinogen-initiated keratinocytes are transferred to culture conditions following carcinogen treatment they tend to differentiate and proceed into an amitotic stage. It is possible that there is a program for carcinogenesis in human cells that when followed rigorously can lead to a reproducible expression of a carcinogenic event. This program is comprised of a sequence of events that must occur prior to expression, i.e. activation, selective adduct formation, error-prone repair, protein modulation. These events are then followed by a program of events leading to a transformed phenocopy exhibiting anchorage-independent growth, cellular invasiveness and neoplasia.

ACKNOWLEDGMENT

We would like to acknowledge Drs. Stephen Weisbrode and John Donahoe for their assistance in interpreting the tumors excised from the nude mice and the cellular invasiveness of the CES. We would like also to acknowledge the assistance of Mrs. Inge Noyes and Jeff Gerard for their technical assistance. This work was supported in part by AFOSR F 49620-80 and AFOSR-80-0283.

REFERENCES

Allred, L., J. Oldham, G. Milo, O. Kinding, and C. Capen. 1982. Multiparametric evaluation of the toxic responses of normal human cells treated in vitro with different classes of environmental toxicants. *J. Toxicol. Environ. Health* **10**:143.

Gavino, V., G. Milo, and D. Cornwell. 1982. Analysis for the automated estimation of clonal growth and its application to the growth of smooth muscle cells. *Cell and Tissue Kinetics* **15**:225.

Gerchman, L. and D. Ludlum. 1973. The properties of 0^6-methylguanine in template for RNA polymerase. *Biochim. Biophys. Acta* **308**:310.

Goth, R., and M. Rajewsky. 1974. Molecular and cellular mechanisms associated with pulse-carcinogenesis in the rat nervous system by ethylnitrosourea: ethylation of nucleic acids and elimination rates of ethylated bases from the DNA of different tissues. *Z. Krebsforsch* **82**:37.

Kapp, L. and R. Painter. 1979. DNA fork displacement rates in synchronous aneuploid and diploid mammalian cells. *Biochim. Biophys. Acta* **562**:222.

Loveless, A. 1969. Possible relevance of 0^6-alkylation of deoxyguanosine to the mutagenicity and carcinogenicity of nitrosamines and nitrosamides. *Nature* **233**:206.

Magee, P.N. and E. Farber. 1962. Toxic liver injury and carcinogenesis. Methylation of rat liver nucleic acids by dimethylnitrosamine *in vivo. Biochem J.* **83**:114.

Magee, P. and T. Hultin. 1962. Toxic liver injury and carcinogenesis. Methylation of proteins of rat liver slices by dimethylnitrosamine *in vitro. Biochem J.* **83**:106.

Milo, G. and R. Hart. 1976. Age related alterations in plasma membrane glycoprotein content and scheduled or unscheduled DNA synthesis. *Arch. Biochem. Biophys.* **17**:110.

Milo, G., and J. DiPaolo. 1978. Neoplastic transformation of human diploid cells in vitro after chemical carcinogen treatment. *Nature* **275**:130.

_____. 1980. Presenitization of human cells with extrinsic signals to induce chemical carcinogenesis. *Int. J. of Cancer* **26**:805.

Milo, G., J. Blakeslee, R. Hart, and D. Yohn. 1978a. Chemical carcinogen alteration of SV-40 virus induced transformation of normal human cell populations. *Chem. Biol. Interact* **22**:185.

Milo, G., J. Blakeslee, D. Yohn, and J. DiPaolo. 1978b. Biochemical activation of AHH activity, cellular distribution of polynuclear hydrocarbon. *Cancer Res.* **38**:1638.

Milo, G., I. Noyes, J. Donahoe, and S. Weisbrode. 1981a. Neoplastic transformation of human epithelial cells in vitro after exposure to chemical carcinogens. *Cancer Res.* **41**:5096.

Milo, G., R. Olsen, S. Weisbrode, and J. McCloskey. 1981b. Feline sarcoma virus induced in vitro progression from premalignant to neoplastic transformation of human diploid cells. *In Vitro* **16**:813.

Milo, G., J. Oldham, R. Zimmerman, G. Hatch, and S. Weisbrode. 1981c. Characterization of human cells transformed by chemical and physical carcinogens, *in vitro. In Vitro* **17**:719.

Noguchi, P., J. Johnson, R. O'Donnell, and J. Petriciani. 1978. Chick embryonic skin as a rapid organ culture assay for cellular neoplasia. *Science* **199**:980.

Oldham, J., L. Allred, G. Milo, O. Kinding, and C. Capen. 1980. The toxicological evaluation of the mycotoxins T-2 and T-2 tetrol using normal human fibroblasts *in vitro. Toxicol. Appl. Pharmacol.* **52**:159.

Riegner, D., T. McMichael, J. Berno, and G. Milo. 1976. Processing of human tissue to establish primary cultures *in vitro.* Tissue Culture Assoc. Lab. Manual (Rockville, MD) **2**:273.

Silinskas, K., S. Kateley, J. Tower, V. Maher, and J. McCormick. 1981. Induction of anchorage-independent growth in human fibroblasts by propane sultone. *Cancer Res.* **41**:1620.

Sutherland, B., J. Arnino, J. Delihas, A. Shih, and R. Oliver. 1980. Ultraviolet light-induced transformation of human cells to anchorage-independent growth. *Cancer Res.* **40**:1934.

Tejwani, R., A. Jeffrey, and G. Milo. 1982. Benzo[a]pyrene diol epoxide DNA adduct formation in transformable and non-transformable human foreskin fibroblast cells *in vitro*. *Carcinogenesis* **3**:(in press).

Zimmerman, R., and J. Little. 1981. Starvation for arginine and glutamine sensitizes human diploid cells to the transforming effects of N-acetoxy-2-acetylamino fluorene. *Carcinogenesis* **2**:1303.

COMMENTS

CONNEY: I have heard of human cells that were transformed in vitro by chemicals, that by all criteria in vitro are transformed cells, but when they are put into nude mice, they start to grow and form a nodule, and then the nodule regresses. There is really something different about this cell. It may be a quasimalignant cell. Have you seen these results?

MILÓ: No! Not after a 4-week interval has elapsed—before tumors are counted.

CONNEY: Is there something in the environment of a so-called quasimalignant cell that can cause that cell to revert back to normal?

MILO: What is the normal phenotype that a cell should regress back towards to be described as a "normal" cell? Tumor material taken from soft-tissue tumors of humans behaves in a nude mouse system in a similar manner as that described for *in vitro* transformed cells.

PREUSSMANN: I was astonished at the vast differences in the cytotoxicity of your compounds. The nitrosoureas were less cytotoxic and the nitrosamines were very cytotoxic. You would expect the reverse order, because nitrosoureas are used in cancer chemotherapy as cytotoxic agents. Could it be that the solutions that you used in your experiments deteriorated after you used it? Those are unstable compounds. Have you any explanation for that?

HICKS: We would confirm the same observation in bladder cells. We cannot kill human bladder cells in culture with MNU.

MICHEJDA: MNNG in human fibroblasts is extremely cytotoxic. MNNG was also rather noncytotoxic in this experiment.

TANNENBAUM: Your effective concentration of NDMA is 1 ng/ml. per milliliter. Many people have done experiments with NDMA in a variety of cells. Usually they are up in millimolar concentrations before they begin to get effect. Has anyone characterized anything about the enzymology of these?

MILO: We are working on it right now.

PREUSSMANN: Could your solution of nitrosourea have been degraded after you put it into your cells?

MILO: Chromatically speaking we know that what we put on does not degrade. NDMA or NDEA also appears to be stable when evaluated by HPLC.

GOLDFARB: Is there really any evidence that we are seeing real invasion or infiltration by these tumor cells into the skin?

MILO: If this occurs you occasionally will see necrosis. The suppression phenomenon can be seen by virtue of the fact that what will happen is that the epidermal type of cells, when they are put on the CES, will have this kind of feature. You will see compression all through the CES when the cells are layered on the skin. When you see invasion, what is seen when subsequently thick slices are taken is shown in the accompanying figure:

Compression of Cells (bolus)

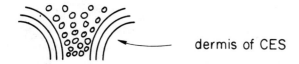

dermis of CES

Invasion of CES

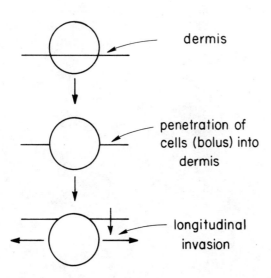

dermis

penetration of cells (bolus) into dermis

longitudinal invasion

When the slides are positive you will see the cells growing down into the CES, and longitudinally under the dermal layer of CES. So we take sequential slices in this area to try to address the problem that you are talking about.

NDMA-Induced Transformation

Proliferation of ductal epithelium with papillary projections was noted in more than two-thirds of explants examined in the second week of culture. Atypical epithelium became noticeable in the 6th culture week. By the 12th culture week morphologically malignant cells were noted forming irregular glandular structures which emerged from the explant surfaces in sheets and islands of pleomorphic cells (Fig. 2).

In Vivo Growth

All nude mice inoculated with cells derived from NDMA-treated explants developed multiple subcutaneous nodules (0.5-4 cm) within 8 weeks (Fig. 3). Tumor nodules in those mice with subcutaneous inoculation in the ventral aspect of their trunks were noticeable early, invaded the abdominal wall and produced ascites in 50% (4/8) of mice within 4 weeks after injection. Histologically, the tumors ranged from undifferentiated to papillary ductal carcinomas.

Distribution Of ^{14}C-Methyl

Autoradiographic sections from explants cultured in the presence of ^{14}C-methyl NDMA for 6 hours revealed a random pattern of distribution of grains over nuclei

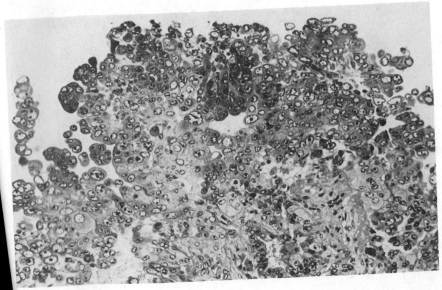

Figure 2
Pancreas explant cultured in the presence of NDMA for 12 wk showing malignant transformation.

Transformation of Human Organ Cultures by Nitrosamines

ISMAIL PARSA AND KHALID M. H. BUTT
State University of New York
Downstate Medical Center
Brooklyn, New York 11203

Existing evidence suggests that environmental chemicals, and in particular nitrosamines and nitroso compounds, are possible factors involved in the development of human pancreatic carcinoma. This is supported in part by the effects of these compounds in experimental pancreatic carcinogenesis in rodents (Druckrey et al. 1968; Bücheler and Thomas 1971; Pour et al. 1974; Reddy and Rao 1975) and in organ cultures of rat embryonic pancreas (Parsa and Marsh 1976). The reported target cells and species specificity of some of these compounds may merely reflect variations in latency period for carcinogenesis in a given organ and immunogenetic status of the species. An in vitro model of pancreatic carcinogenesis using adult human pancreas explants was reported previously (Parsa et al. 1981). In this model all cell types demonstrated at least a limited ability to proliferate. This report describes the effects of nitrosamines on pancreatic cells and transformation of pancreatic cells by nitrosamines.

MATERIALS AND METHODS

Human Pancreas

Human pancreas including tail and a portion of body was obtained from cadaveric donors with no pancreatic disease, ages 10-56 years. The warm ischemia time varied from 5-15 minutes. Upon removal, pancreases were cooled and kept at 0-5° for up to 4 hours before being cultured. Explants of 1 mm thickness were prepared containing a portion of the main duct and 4-5 mm of its surrounding parenchyma including ductules, acini, and occasional endocrine islets.

Organ Culture

Explants were placed on a strip (4x10 mm) of Millipore filter and floated on 10 ml of prewarmed (37°C) medium in a roller tube. A chemically defined medium (Parsa et al. 1970) was used to which 10 mg per liter of ascorbic acid and 8 mg/liter of bovine pancreas crystalline insulin were added. The roller tubes were incubated at 37°C in an atmosphere of 10% CO_2 in air saturated with water vapor and rotated at 0.5 rpm. The medium was changed daily during the first 4 days and twice a week thereafter. Explants were cultured in the presence or absence of nitrosamines for up to 12 weeks.

Nitrosamines

At the initiation of culture and twice a week thereafter nitrosodimethylamine (NDMA), 20 μg/ml, or N-nitroso-bis(2-hydroxypropyl)amine (BHP), 5 μg/ml, or N-nitroso-bis(oxopropyl)amine (BOP), 0.2 μg/ml was added to the medium.

Microscopic Preparation

Cultured explants were fixed in Bouin's fluid, embedded in paraffin, and cut at 2-4 μm thickness. Sections were stained with hematoxylin and eosin.

Autoradiography

Explants cultured for 6 hours in the presence of 20 μg/ml of ^{14}C-methyl NDMA (15 mC/m mole) were incubated further in medium without NDMA for 0, 12, 24, 48, 72, and 96 hours, were harvested and processed for autoradiography. The procedure was previously described by Parsa et al. (1969). The exposure time was 2 weeks and sections were stained with methyl green and thionin.

In Vivo Inoculation

Cell suspensions (5×10^6 cells) prepared from 12-week-old NDMA-treated explants were injected subcutaneously in the dorsal or ventral aspects of the thorax of 4-8-week-old nude mice, and tumor growths were dissected and processed for morphological examination.

RESULTS

At the initiation of culture all pancreases revealed well preserved acini, ducts, and islets. There was considerable variation in the degree of necrosis, proliferation, and morphological alterations in untreated and nitrosamine-treated explants.

Untreated (Control) Explants

The control explants showed proliferation of columnar epithelium of duct, producing focal papillary projections on the surface in 30% of the within 3 weeks of culture. This was followed by progressive degeneratio weeks 4, 5, and 6. Secondary and smaller ducts and ductules revealed epithelial proliferation with occasional mitoses during the first 2 weeks. cell necrosis was extensive but centroacinar cells appeared well preserved the first 4 weeks and showed occasional mitotic figures. Explants cultur 12 weeks or more showed degeneration and necrosis of all cell types.

BHP and BOP Effects

Explants treated with BOP or BHP showed similar alterations. Necrosis of aci structures was a prevalent feature. The extent of proliferation in duc epithelium was minimal during the first 2 weeks. Degeneration and necrosis all cell types proceeded similarly to that of untreated explants. In about 20 (7/40) of the explants examined between 10 and 12 weeks of culture ther were occasional small to medium sized ductal structures with numerous mitotic figures (Fig. 1) and a few foci of ductal hyperplasia.

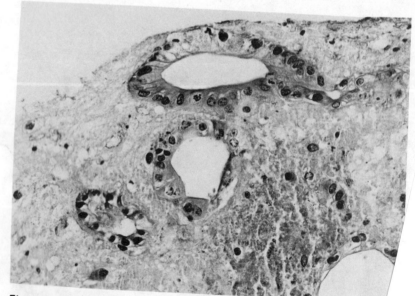

Figure 1
Pancreas explant cultured in the presence of BOP for 12 wk showing multip figures in the ductal epithelium.

Transformation of
Human Organ Cultures by
Nitrosamines

ISMAIL PARSA AND KHALID M. H. BUTT
State University of New York
Downstate Medical Center
Brooklyn, New York 11203

Existing evidence suggests that environmental chemicals, and in particular nitrosamines and nitroso compounds, are possible factors involved in the development of human pancreatic carcinoma. This is supported in part by the effects of these compounds in experimental pancreatic carcinogenesis in rodents (Druckrey et al. 1968; Bücheler and Thomas 1971; Pour et al. 1974; Reddy and Rao 1975) and in organ cultures of rat embryonic pancreas (Parsa and Marsh 1976). The reported target cells and species specificity of some of these compounds may merely reflect variations in latency period for carcinogenesis in a given organ and immunogenetic status of the species. An in vitro model of pancreatic carcinogenesis using adult human pancreas explants was reported previously (Parsa et al. 1981). In this model all cell types demonstrated at least a limited ability to proliferate. This report describes the effects of nitrosamines on pancreatic cells and transformation of pancreatic cells by nitrosamines.

MATERIALS AND METHODS

Human Pancreas

Human pancreas including tail and a portion of body was obtained from cadaveric donors with no pancreatic disease, ages 10-56 years. The warm ischemia time varied from 5-15 minutes. Upon removal, pancreases were cooled and kept at 0-5° for up to 4 hours before being cultured. Explants of 1 mm thickness were prepared containing a portion of the main duct and 4-5 mm of its surrounding parenchyma including ductules, acini, and occasional endocrine islets.

Organ Culture

Explants were placed on a strip (4x10 mm) of Millipore filter and floated on 10 ml of prewarmed (37°C) medium in a roller tube. A chemically defined medium (Parsa et al. 1970) was used to which 10 mg per liter of ascorbic acid and 8 mg/liter of bovine pancreas crystalline insulin were added. The roller tubes were incubated at $37°C$ in an atmosphere of 10% CO_2 in air saturated with water vapor and rotated at 0.5 rpm. The medium was changed daily during the first 4 days and twice a week thereafter. Explants were cultured in the presence or absence of nitrosamines for up to 12 weeks.

Nitrosamines

At the initiation of culture and twice a week thereafter nitrosodimethylamine (NDMA), 20 μg/ml, or N-nitroso-bis(2-hydroxypropyl)amine (BHP), 5 μg/ml, or N-nitroso-bis(oxopropyl)amine (BOP), 0.2 μg/ml was added to the medium.

Microscopic Preparation

Cultured explants were fixed in Bouin's fluid, embedded in paraffin, and cut at 2-4 μm thickness. Sections were stained with hematoxylin and eosin.

Autoradiography

Explants cultured for 6 hours in the presence of 20 μg/ml of ^{14}C-methyl NDMA (15 mC/m mole) were incubated further in medium without NDMA for 0, 12, 24, 48, 72, and 96 hours, were harvested and processed for autoradiography. The procedure was previously described by Parsa et al. (1969). The exposure time was 2 weeks and sections were stained with methyl green and thionin.

In Vivo Inoculation

Cell suspensions (5×10^6 cells) prepared from 12-week-old NDMA-treated explants were injected subcutaneously in the dorsal or ventral aspects of the thorax of 4-8-week-old nude mice, and tumor growths were dissected and processed for morphological examination.

RESULTS

At the initiation of culture all pancreases revealed well preserved acini, ducts, and islets. There was considerable variation in the degree of necrosis, proliferation, and morphological alterations in untreated and nitrosamine-treated explants.

Untreated (Control) Explants

The control explants showed proliferation of columnar epithelium of the main duct, producing focal papillary projections on the surface in 30% of the explants within 3 weeks of culture. This was followed by progressive degeneration during weeks 4, 5, and 6. Secondary and smaller ducts and ductules revealed minimal epithelial proliferation with occasional mitoses during the first 2 weeks. Acinar cell necrosis was extensive but centroacinar cells appeared well preserved during the first 4 weeks and showed occasional mitotic figures. Explants cultured for 12 weeks or more showed degeneration and necrosis of all cell types.

BHP and BOP Effects

Explants treated with BOP or BHP showed similar alterations. Necrosis of acinar structures was a prevalent feature. The extent of proliferation in ductal epithelium was minimal during the first 2 weeks. Degeneration and necrosis of all cell types proceeded similarly to that of untreated explants. In about 20% (7/40) of the explants examined between 10 and 12 weeks of culture there were occasional small to medium sized ductal structures with numerous mitotic figures (Fig. 1) and a few foci of ductal hyperplasia.

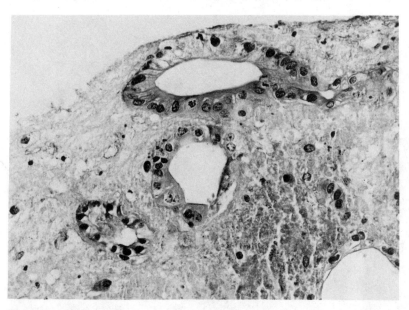

Figure 1
Pancreas explant cultured in the presence of BOP for 12 wk showing multiple mitotic figures in the ductal epithelium.

NDMA-Induced Transformation

Proliferation of ductal epithelium with papillary projections was noted in more than two-thirds of explants examined in the second week of culture. Atypical epithelium became noticeable in the 6th culture week. By the 12th culture week morphologically malignant cells were noted forming irregular glandular structures which emerged from the explant surfaces in sheets and islands of pleomorphic cells (Fig. 2).

In Vivo Growth

All nude mice inoculated with cells derived from NDMA-treated explants developed multiple subcutaneous nodules (0.5-4 cm) within 8 weeks (Fig. 3). Tumor nodules in those mice with subcutaneous inoculation in the ventral aspect of their trunks were noticeable early, invaded the abdominal wall and produced ascites in 50% (4/8) of mice within 4 weeks after injection. Histologically, the tumors ranged from undifferentiated to papillary ductal carcinomas.

Distribution Of ^{14}C-Methyl

Autoradiographic sections from explants cultured in the presence of ^{14}C-methyl NDMA for 6 hours revealed a random pattern of distribution of grains over nuclei

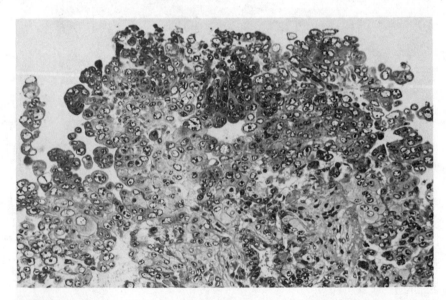

Figure 2
Pancreas explant cultured in the presence of NDMA for 12 wk showing malignant transformation.

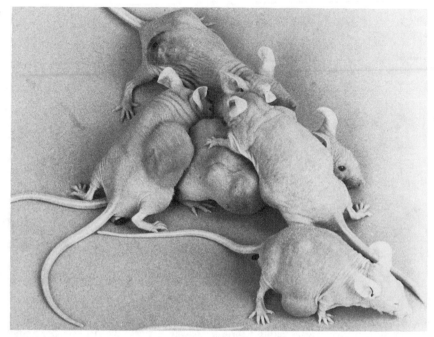

Figure 3
Tumor growth in nude mice, 8 wk after inoculation with NDMA-transformed cells.

and cytoplasm of all cell types except endocrine islets with an average of 15.2 grains/cell (Fig. 4). Labeled explants (6 hours) cultured further for 36 hours in medium without NDMA showed about 80% reduction in the average number of grains/cell (2.9). The grains appeared to be concentrated over certain nuclei, each with an average number of grains of 13.3. Most of the nuclei with grains appeared to belong to cells devoid of zymogen granules (Fig. 5). Further incubation of labeled explants in unlabeled medium for up to 72 hours showed even further reduction of grains per cell to 0.2, most of which were located over few nuclei (5.1 grains/nuclei) (Fig. 6). Labeled explants cultured for up to 96 hours in unlabeled medium showed fewer grains overall with an average of 0.12 grains/cell concentrated over few nuclei (2.8 grains per nuclei).

DISCUSSION

The organ culture model appears to detect differences in carcinogenic potency and the time of latency for tumorogenicity of BHP, BOP, and NDMA in human pancreas explants. The human pancreas cell in vitro is able to metabolize BHP and NDMA and be transformed into carcinoma. The transformation of these

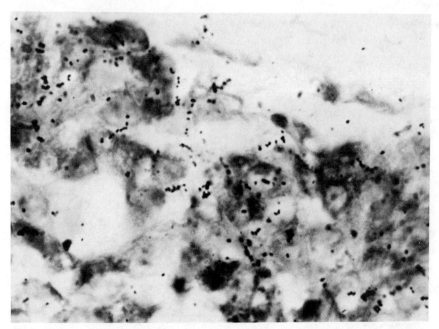

Figure 4
Autoradiograph from explant cultured for 6 hours with ^{14}C-labeled NDMA demonstrating random distribution of nuclear and cytoplasmic grains.

cells by BHP and BOP into biologically malignant cells is yet to be tested. Pancreas cells transformed by NDMA were malignant, demonstrating invasive growth in nude mice. The presence of 20 μg/ml NDMA in the culture medium produces more extensive acinar cell necrosis than is seen in untreated explants. Concomitant increases in proliferation of ductal and centroacinar cells may represent a step in carcinogenic effects of NDMA or a regenerative response to necrosis. The selective presence of ^{14}C-methyl labels in certain nuclei 3-4 days after a 6-hour exposure to labeled-NDMA supports the first possibility, i.e. certain cells are selectively affected by the carcinogen and thus acquire the ability to proliferate as progenitor cells of cancer and eventually give rise to carcinoma.

Under favorable conditions NDMA is extensively produced in human stomach. It is rapidly metabolized by liver and is reported to be present in low concentrations in the blood of healthy individuals. Assuming that NDMA and its metabolites are important in induction of pancreatic carcinoma in vivo, a considerable increase in the reported levels is required to achieve an effective concentration comparable to the in vitro system. This can hypothetically be achieved either by enhanced concentration of NDMA by the acinar cell after absorption from the blood supply, followed by excretion into the pancreatic juice, with its maximum effect on the ductal epithelium; or, by attaining the necessary strength in the gallbladder which may then affect the ductal cells via bile reflux. In the absence of liver disease the latter mechanism may not be effective since NDMA is rapidly deactivated by the normal liver. The proclivity of the acinar tissue in a given individual to concentrate NDMA and its metabolites to an effective level may play an important role in the induction of carcinoma.

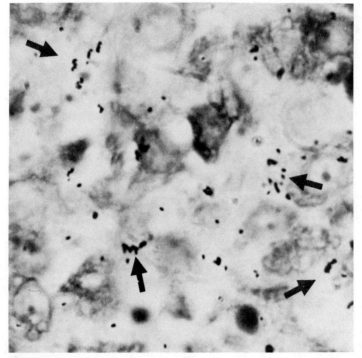

Figure 5
Autoradiograph from explant labeled as in Fig. 4, and cultured further for 36 hr in the absence of labeled-NDMA, showing selective localization of grains over certain nuclei.

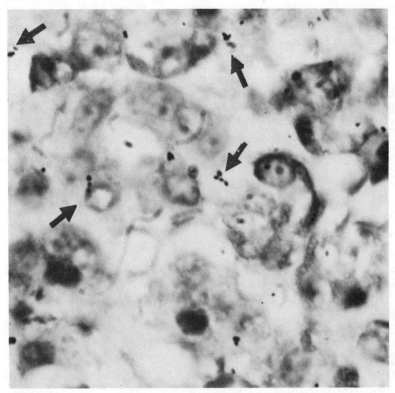

Figure 6
Autoradiograph from explant labeled as in Fig. 4 and cultured in the absence of labeled NDMA for 72 hr, showing reduction in the number of grains with selective localization.

ACKNOWLEDGMENTS

This study was supported in part by the NCI Grant # 1RO1 CA3035401 and 2 R26 CA22682.

REFERENCES

Bücheler, J. and C. Thomas. 1971. Experimentell Erzeugte Drusenmangen-tumoren bei Meershweinchen und Ratte. *Beitr. Pathol.* **142**:194.

Druckrey, H., S. Ivankovic, J. Bücheler, R. Preussmann, and S.C. Thomas. 1968. Erzeugung von Magen-und Pancreas-Krebs beim Meerschweinchen durch Methylnitroso-harnstoff und-uerthan. *Z. Krebsforsch.* **71**:167.

Parsa, I., W.H. Marsh, and P.J. Fitzgerald. 1969. Pancreatic acinar cell differentiation. *Am. J. Pathol.* **57**:489.

_____. 1970. Chemically defined medium for organ culture differentiation of rat pancreas anlage. *Exp. Cell Res.* **59**:171.

Parsa, I. and W.H. Marsh. 1976. An in vitro model of pancreatic carcinoma. *Am. J. Pathol.* **84**:469.

Parsa, I., W.H. Marsh, A.L. Sutton, and K.M. Butt. 1981. Effects of dimethylnitrosamine on organ-cultured adult human pancreas. *Am. J. Pathol.* **102**:403.

Pour, P., F.W. Kruger, A. Cardesa, J. Althoff, and U. Mohr. 1974. Tumorigenicity of methyl-N-propylnitrosamine in Syrian golden hamsters. *J. Natl. Cancer Inst.* **52**:457.

Reddy, J.K. and M.S. Rao. 1975. Pancreatic adenocarcinoma in inbred guinea pigs induced by N-methyl-N-nitrosourea. *Cancer Res.* **35**:2269.

COMMENTS

MIRVISH: Have you ever studied the acute effects, the acute toxic effects, of these nitrosamines in your pancreas?

PARSA: Before we arrived at the dose of 20 μg/ml we had tried a range of doses. Even at 20 μg they are very cytotoxic. But it gives an adequate amount of living tissue and induces enough proliferation so that the induction or transformation is attainable.

KIMBROUGH: If you reduce the dose to a level where no cytotoxicity is seen, do you still get proliferation?

PARSA: For 12 weeks, no. Degeneration and necrosis occurs in the culture but we don't see the trophic effect which has been described for microorganisms in this system.

FLEIG: Could you report some data about the exact occurrence of tumors compared to the controls?

PARSA: There is no tumor developing in control, at least as far as 12 weeks into the experiment, or implantation of untreated tissue in the nude mice. About 30 or 40% of the NDMA-treated for 12 weeks shows both morphologically malignant.

MAGEE: Would the tissue processing remove all the unchanged NDMA?

PARSA: The tissue is washed as carefully as we can wash it. Then it is fixed, put through alcohol to dehydrate it, and then embedded in paraffin. After all this treatment there is too much residual radioactivity there to be just contaminant. In other words, empty spaces between the cells do not show silver grains. That indicates that they are in the cell, whether they are in adduct form or not.

MONTESANO: Dr. Milo and Dr. Parsa, have you data on the cytogenetics of the cells in culture at the time they are injected into the animals and, in the tumors that develop in the nude mice—either the karyotype or the ploidy?

MILO: The untreated cells and treated cells are virtually diploid. We are now attempting to do the karyology on the tumor cells that have gone through anchorage-independent growth and cellular invasiveness to see what the correlations are between those cells and the cells that we are transforming. To date, they appear nearly diploid.

MONTESANO: When you put in cells to culture from tumors, are they still diploid?

MILO: They are pseudodiploid and have translocations.

Pathological Changes
in Human Beings Acutely Poisoned
by Dimethylnitrosamine

RENATE D. KIMBROUGH
Center for Environmental Health
Centers for Disease Control
Atlanta, Georgia 30333

In September 1978 a sudden outbreak of illness occurred among members of an extended family in Omaha, Nebraska (Cooper and Kimbrough 1980). The total number of family members involved was 10; of these, five became ill and two ultimately died (Fig. 1). The United States Centers for Disease Control were at first contacted for assistance because it was thought that the disease had an infectious etiology.

Investigation of the outbreak established that illness was associated with the consumption of lemonade. It was ultimately determined that the lemonade had intentionally been laced with toxic concentrations of dimethylnitrosamine (NDMA). It is the purpose of this paper to describe the clinical and morphological findings in the patients.

SEQUENCE OF EVENTS

The members of the family which were together on the day they became ill were from three households. They consisted of the parents of two married and one unmarried sister. One of the married sisters had one child (patient 1), an 11-month-old boy; the other married sister had two children, a 2½-year-old girl (patient 3) and a 4-month-old baby boy. The unmarried sister, who was pregnant at the time, lived with the sister that had the two children. The parents, the sister (patient 5) with the 11-month-old child, and her husband (patient 4) visited the other sister (daughter) and her husband (patient 2) on Sunday, September 10, 1978. The parents, while at their daughter's house, drank coffee. The sister (patient 5), her husband (patient 4), and their 11-month-old child (patient 1) all drank lemonade, as did the husband (patient 2) of the other sister, and his 2½-year-old daughter (patient 3). The pregnant unmarried sister took one gulp of the lemonade and spit it out, because she thought it tasted funny. She did not become ill. The sister in whose house she lived then discarded the lemonade. She did not drink any lemonade because she does not like lemonade. It was not possible at the time of our investigation to determine

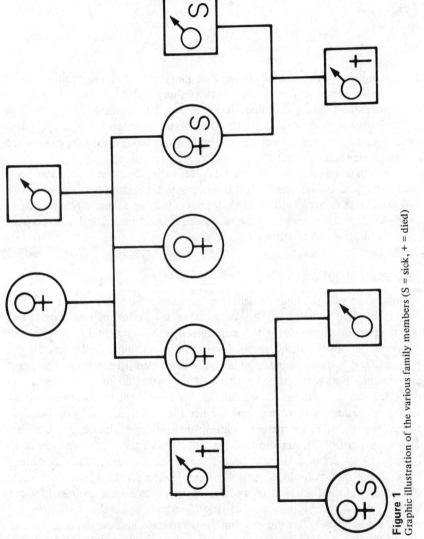

Figure 1
Graphic illustration of the various family members (S = sick, + = died)

when the lemonade was actually prepared, but it may have been prepared and stored in the refrigerator 2 days earlier.

CLINICAL ILLNESS

All five patients within a few hours after consuming the lemonade developed nausea, vomiting, and abdominal pain. The gastrointestinal illness persisted for several days. The two patients that ultimately died developed generalized bleeding within 3 days of onset of illness. These two patients had multiple bruises, epitaxis, and cerebral hemorrhage.

Laboratory tests done on all patients showed abnormalities which were essentially confined to the liver and the platelets. The serum glutamic pyruvic transaminase (SGPT) and serum glutamic oxalic transaminase (SGOT) were elevated, cholesterol was low (72 mg/dl) in one patient and all patients had slight to severe thrombocytopenia (Table 1). Patient 1 and 2 became comatose and died 4 and 5 days after onset of illness, respectively. The other three patients gradually improved and were discharged from the hospital 3 weeks (patient 3), 4 days (patient 4), and 16 days (patient 5) after onset of illness.

AUTOPSY FINDINGS

Patient 1 (11-month-old male)

The gross observations consisted primarily of petechial and larger hemorrhages into the lungs, gastrointestinal tract, and over both hemispheres of the brain. In addition focal atelectases, congestion, and edema were also noted in the lungs (Fig. 2). The liver weighed 350 g, had a friable surface and a granular appearance. Microscopic examination of the liver showed only a few intact hepatocytes immediately adjacent to the portal triads. Most of the other hepatocytes throughout the liver lobules were necrotic and the sinusoids were filled with red blood cells. Occasional polymorphonuclear leukocytes were also noted. The stroma of the liver appeared to be intact. However, the central veins had lost their endothelial lining cells. The bile ducts were unaffected.

The spleen showed some autolysis and congestion. Many lymphocytes were degenerated with very pyknotic nuclei. The lymphocytes were absent from the malpighian corpuscles and reticulum cells were observed in their place. The lymph nodes appeared vacuolated under low power with many empty spaces. Some of the lymphocytes were either clumped or had very pyknotic nuclei. The lungs showed areas of hemorrhage and congestion. In some areas acute inflammatory cells were observed in the alveoli in addition to numerous macrophages. The bronchi and trachea were normal. The inflammatory infiltrates in the lungs were consistent with an early acute bronchopneumonia. Sections from the heart, gastrointestinal tract, pancreas, and kidneys were normal. Section of bone marrow showed normal cellularity with a slightly

Table 1
Main positive laboratory test results in all patients

	Thrombocytes (mm³)	Hemoglobin (g/dl)	White blood cells (mm³)	SGOT (I.U./l)	SGPT (I.U./l)	Alkaline phosphatase (I.U./l)	Lactic dehydrogenase (I.U./l)	Bilirubin total/direct (mg/dl)
Patient 1	19,000	11	4,400		6,520	850		7.4/3
Patient 2	6,000	14, 11	11,000	910-1208	1,700	326	396	
Patient 3	13,000-21,000	11	6,500	702-1550	522	113	395	1
Patient 4	120,000	14.6	5,700-7,200	125		49-68	109; 165	
Patient 5	116,000 later 12,000	13.6	6,500	85; 138; 258				
Normal values	150,000-300,000	13-14	5,000-10,000	5-18	4-24	79-258	56-194	0.1-1.1/0-0.2

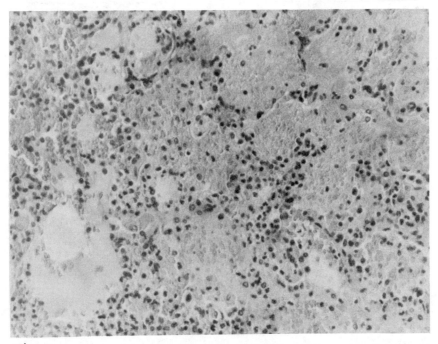

Figure 2
Section of lung from patient 1. Note alveoli filled with red blood cells and in some areas the complete destruction of the alveolar walls (H + E × 100).

increased number of megakaryocytes. The megakaryocytes had normal morphology. Slides from other organs were not available for review.

Patient 2 (24-year-old male)

In this patient the gross observations that were made were again either related to the general bleeding tendency or the effects on the liver. There was marked cerebral edema and subarachnoid hemorrhage in the right side of the brain. The heart showed myocardial and endocardial areas of hemorrhage. The lungs, diaphragm, and stomach showed many petechial hemorrhages. In addition, the bases of both lungs were atelectatic. The liver had a nutmeg appearance and was extremely congested. Microscopic examination showed that the trachea, bladder, adrenals, pancreas, and skin were normal. The bone marrow showed normal cellularity with a normal number of megakaryocytes (Fig. 3). The kidneys were congested and the renal tubules contained red blood cells. The epithelium of the gastrointestinal tract was intact but in many areas aggregates of red blood cells were seen in the mucosa. The cerebral hemorrhage and cerebral edema were

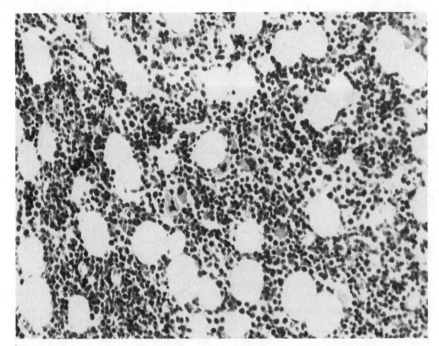

Figure 3
Section of bone marrow from patient 2. Note normal cellularity and numerous megakaryocytes (H + E × 100)

evident microscopically as well. The lymphocytes in lymph nodes and spleen were normal in this case. However, in the spleen occasional clusters of foamy or vacuolated cells were noted. Slight bile stasis was noted in the liver. The hepatocytes in the periphery of the lobules had vacuolated cytoplasm in some instances but were otherwise intact. The hepatocytes in the center of the lobules were either completely necrotic or in various stages of degeneration. The normal appearing stroma in this area contained many cell remnants. In addition, numerous inflammatory cells were seen (Fig. 4). Loss of endothelium of the vascular walls of the central veins was again noted. In many areas of the liver, congestion and hemorrhage were prominent in the central zones. The heart showed congestion and focal endocardial and myocardial hemorrhages. The alveoli of the lungs in many areas were filled with macrophages which contained a brown pigment (Fig. 5). In other areas inflammatory cells predominated. Purulent material indicative of acute focal bronchopneumonia was noted in some sections. These acute inflammatory infiltrates were present in areas where the alveolar walls appeared to be completely necrotic.

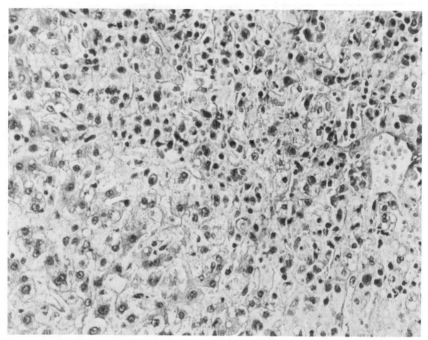

Figure 4
Section of liver from patient 2. Note degenerated parenchymal cells surrounding central veins, inflammatory cells. Hepatocytes in the periphery appear intact. The wall of the central vein has lost most endothelial cells.

Patient 3 (2½-year-old girl)

This child developed an enlarged spleen and liver and had persistent hepato-splenomegaly and elevated liver enzymes. A liver biopsy was therefore obtained 3 months after onset of illness. The microscopic findings were consistent with chronic active hepatitis. No tissue specimens were obtained on the other two patients. The other 5 members of the family had normal liver function tests and normal platelet counts. The one sister who was pregnant at the time delivered a normal term infant.

DISCUSSION

Initially poisoning was not suspected as the cause of illness. When it was determined that all patients had become ill a few hours after ingesting lemonade the possibility of someone having intentionally laced the lemonade with a poisonous substance was considered. Because of the thrombocytopenia and the liver damage, an alkylating agent was suggested as the possible cause of the

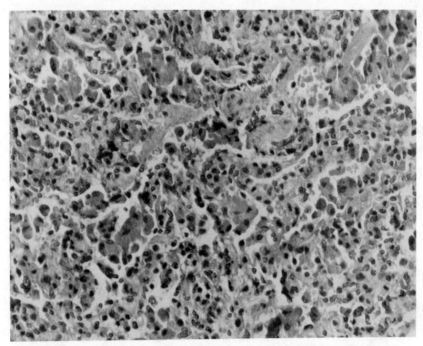

Figure 5
Section of lung from patient 2. Alveoli are filled with fibrin, desquamated cells and occasional inflammatory cells and red blood cells.

illness. With the help of the police it was then established that an acquaintance of this family was working as a biologist at the Eppeley Institute in Omaha, Nebraska. This person had been a boyfriend of Patient 2's wife and had recently been released from the State Penitentiary after having been convicted of shooting at the family in 1975. It was eventually established that NDMA had been added to the lemonade and that the NDMA caused methylation of guanine in the liver of patient 2 (Herron and Shank 1979; Cooper and Kimbrough 1980). The toxic effects of NDMA were primarily confined to the liver and the platelets. The primary interest in NDMA has always centered around its carcinogenic effects and little information is available on its acute toxic effects. Among the nitrosamines, NDMA is one of the most toxic compounds. The oral LD_{50} in rats is 27-41 mg/kg body weight (Heath and Magee 1962). Typically in animals after a lethal dose, acute effects develop within 1-2 days and death occurs within one week. NDMA causes hepatic centrolobular necrosis in several animal species. In animals a slight effect on the lungs has also been observed. The lung lesions have primarily consisted of areas of hemorrhage. When rats, dogs, and mice were exposed to toxic concentrations of NDMA vapors, they developed anorexia, polydypsia, and diarrhea. This was most pronounced in the dogs. The dogs also had elevated rectal temperatures. In dogs, stools became bloody and prothrombin time was prolonged in some of them. A general bleeding tendency was observed in the dogs. At autopsy free blood was found in the peritoneal cavity, gastrointestinal tract, abdominal tissues, lymphatic tissues, and the liver. The liver showed controlobular necrosis. Bleeding was also noticed in rats and mice (Jacobson et al. 1955).

A few cases of acute human poisoning by NDMA have been reported in the literature. Freund (1937) described illness in two workers who were engaged in NDMA production. They developed headaches, backache, abdominal cramps, nausea, anorexia, weakness, drowsiness, and giddiness. After repeated NDMA exposure one of the workers developed ascites, jaundice. He quit his job, but continued to be easily fatigued for many months. The other worker developed an acute episode of illness after dropping a flask of NDMA and cleaning it up. Six days after this exposure he developed pain in his upper abdomen, abdominal cramps, and abdominal distention and also became jaundiced. This patient died about 8 weeks after onset of his illness. At autopsy subpericardial hemorrhages and superficial hemorrhages throughout the entire mucosal surface of the small bowel were noted. The left lower lobe of the lungs was firm and dark red and small hemorrhages were seen in the bronchi and trachea. The spleen was extremely soft. On microscopic examination most organs were normal except for a scarcity of germ centers in the lymph nodes. Congestion, edema, and hemorrhage was observed in some of the other organs. The main pathology was confined to the liver. Diffuse degeneration of the parenchyma with focal and diffuse areas of necrosis were noted. The necrotic areas were infiltrated by round cells and phagocytes. Multiple periportal hemorrhages and intense regenerative proliferation were also observed. Hamilton and Hardy (1949) also mentioned two cases of poisoning among workers. In addition, liver cirrhosis was noted in two men working in a research laboratory. They had been exposed to NDMA for several months when the first case was uncovered (Barnes and Magee 1954).

The findings made on the patients reported about in this paper and a review of the literature describing the acute and subacute toxic effects of NDMA in animals and humans suggest that they are quite similar. Liver damage and diffuse bleeding have been reported in a number of species including humans. In none of the poisoning episodes or the experimental animal studies was the blood-clotting mechanism studied in detail, and platelet counts are not reported in any of the papers. Since the bone marrows of the various patients reported here had a normal or increased number of megakaryocytes, decreased platelet production was apparently not the cause of the low platelet counts. It is possible that the platelets were destroyed because of an autoimmune reaction similar to a mechanism observed in idiopathic thrombocytopenic purpura. It is also of interest that the endothelial cells had disappeared from the lining of some blood vessels, particularly the central veins of the liver. It is therefore possible that the platelets accumulated at the site of tissue injury (Cotran 1965). However, it is difficult to envision that this would be the sole reason for the low platelet counts. It is more plausible to assume that the platelet membrane is altered by NDMA with the result that the platelets become susceptible to rapid destruction in the spleen and other parts of the reticuloendothelial system. Further studies are needed to elucidate these findings. It is also important to determine whether such effects would occur at other than potentially lethal dosage levels. The patients in this episode showed some morphological changes in the lungs following NDMA exposure. Similar findings have been made in animal studies. It can therefore be concluded that the acute toxic effects of NDMA in humans are compatible with those observed in animals.

REFERENCES

Barnes, J.M. and P.N. Magee. 1954. Some toxic properties of dimethylnitrosamine. *Brit. J. Ind. Med.* **11**:167.

Cooper, S.W. and R.D. Kimbrough. 1980. Acute dimethylnitrosamine poisoning outbreak. *J. Forensic Sci.* **25**:874.

Cotran, R.S. 1965. The delayed and prolonged vascular leakage in inflammation. II. An electron microscopic study of the vascular response after thermal injury. *Am. J. Pathol.* **46**:589.

Freund, H.A. 1937. Clinical manifestations in studies in parenchymatous hepatitis. *Ann. Intern. Med.* **10**:1144.

Hamilton, A. and H.L. Hardy. 1949. *Industrial Toxicology* (2nd ed.) p. 311. Paul B. Hoeber Inc., New York.

Heath, D.F. and P.N. Magee. 1962. Toxic properties of dialkylnitrosamines and some related compounds. *Br. J. Ind. Med.* **19**:276.

Herron, D.C. and R.C. Shank. 1979. Quantitative high pressure liquid chromatography analysis of methylated purines in DNA of rats treated with chemical carcinogens. *Anal. Biochem.* **100**:58.

Jacobson, J.H., H.J. Wheelwright, J.H. Clem, and R.N. Shannon. 1955. Studies on the toxicology of N-nitrosodimethylamine vapor. *Am. Med. Assoc. Arch. Ind. Health* **12**:617.

COMMENTS

GOLDFARB: I like your explanation about the intravascular coagulation. Did you consider the possibility of a disseminated intravascular coagulation (DIC), secondary to endothelial necrosis?

KIMBROUGH: That is one possibility, but the observed pathological changes were not typical of a DIC. The other possibility would be that this would represent an autoimmune type reaction, similar to thrombocytopenia purpura which occasionally develops following the administration of drugs, virus infections and things like that.

GOLDFARB: It seems to me it would be rather too soon for that.

LIJINSKY: What dose did these people receive?

KIMBROUGH: It is not known.

LIJINSKY: Couldn't you determine from the anecdotal statements of the family how much they drank? Maybe you know what the concentration was?

KIMBROUGH: The only thing that we could do was to make an association that the people who drank more of the lemonade got sicker than the people that drank less. We do not know how much NDMA was put into the lemonade because it was discarded before we could get to it.

There is a whole lot more to this story. He first tried NDMA on his mother's pets. The other problem was that this case ended up in court. Most of the material that I presented here was actually subpoenaed by the courts, and I served as a witness for the prosecution. The defendant admitted that he had used NDMA, but his confession was taken in such a way that it could not be entered as evidence in court. I never saw his confession, and I don't know whether he ever said actually how much he put into the lemonade. I calculated, based on the rat LD_{50}, that perhaps the child might have gotten something like 300 or 400 mg, and maybe the adult got something like 1.3 g or so.

WEISBURGER: I wonder whether from the fixed sections one could still isolate DNA and get the methylguanine out, either from kidney or liver.

KIMBROUGH: Ron Shank will talke about that.

PEGG: But how do you know that the compound was NDMA, rather than one of the other nitrosamines which could also lead to a methylating agent?

KIMBROUGH: Well, partly because of the defendant's confession. Then the other thing is the pathology that has been reported in people. Of course, I have to admit that for some compounds, there is no information available. I reviewed all the literature. The compound had to fit the following criteria: It had to be a compound that was extremely toxic, and it had to be water soluble in slightly acidic water, namely lemonade. It had to be a chemical that you could not taste, because the people really didn't notice that there was something in the lemonade. By using these criteria in addition to the findings made in our investigation we finally arrived at dimethylnitrosamine.

PEGG: But methylbenzylnitrosamine would work, for example. I am sure Dr. Lijinsky can think of lots of them.

KIMBROUGH: What is the LD_{50} of methylbenzylnitrosamine?

LIJINSKY: It is lower, but it is not very water soluble. It wouldn't do.

Pathological Changes in a Human Subject
Chronically Exposed to Dimethylnitrosamine

WOLFGANG E. FLEIG, ROLF D. FUSSGAENGER,
AND HANS DITSCHUNEIT
Division of Metabolism, Nutrition and Gastroenterology
Department of Internal Medicine
University of Ulm
7900 Ulm, Federal Republic of Germany

N,N-Dimethylnitrosamine (NDMA) is a compound exhibiting both high acute toxicity and chronic effects arising from repeated administration of smaller doses. Freund (1937) was the first to describe acute toxicity in man with fatal outcome following an accident in a chemical laboratory. No carcinogenic action on the liver could be demonstrated following a single administration of a sublethal dose of NDMA to normal adult rats (Magee and Barnes 1959). In contrast, single doses given to animals in a state of liver cell proliferation i.e., to newborn rats or to adults following partial hepatectomy are likely to induce hepatocellular carcinoma (Craddock 1971). Similarly, chronic dietary application of NDMA to rats produces malignant primary hepatic tumors (Magee and Barnes 1956), much like related N-nitroso compounds (Schmaehl and Preussmann 1959). In man, cirrhosis of the liver resulted from a 10-month chronic NDMA exposure (Hamilton and Hardy 1949; Barnes and Magee 1954), but no liver malignancy was observed in these patients. Recent reviews dealing with the toxicity of N-nitroso compounds also do not mention such a case (Magee 1971; Shank 1975).

NDMA is metabolized by the hepatic microsomal mixed function oxidase system in the rat (Magee and Barnes 1967). Therefore, it rapidly disappears within a few hours after ingestion and thereby escapes detection by sensitive methods (Lijinsky et al. 1968; Montesano and Magee 1971). These features suggest the substance as a potent and "low-risk" criminal poison. Here, we report on the pathological findings during the 32-month-long clinical course and at autopsy of a patient chronically exposed to NDMA by her murderous husband.

CLINICAL COURSE

The family history revealed that the father of the patient had died at 52 years of age of a brain tumor, while her mother was 74 years old and suffered from ischemic heart attacks. Her father's sister died at the age of 82 years of adult-onset diabetes. The patient had two children in 1958 and 1963. In 1969, a vaginal hysterectomy was performed due to carcinoma in situ of the cervix. Repeated clinical and histological examinations did not show any abnormalities thereafter.

The 42-year-old woman was admitted to the outpatient clinic in December 1975. She complained about mild fever up to 38°C, sweating, nausea, vomiting, epigastric pain, diarrhea, and intestinal bleeding. Moreover, she suffered from hemorrhagic tracheitis, a sore throat, and excessive salivation. She had lost 5 kg body weight in 6 weeks. She was treated with doxycyclin for 3 weeks, but the fever combined with abdominal pain persisted. Therefore, she was admitted to the hospital.

At this time we observed a slightly reduced general status, a small diffuse enlargement of the thyroid gland and a painful palpation of the upper right and middle left abdomen. Pathological laboratory findings were: enhanced erythrocyte sedimentation rate (ESR) (40/81 mm), slightly increased aminotransferases and γ-glutamyl-transpeptidase (γ-GT) to about 100, 60, and 90 U/l, respectively, and a leukopenia of 2800 leucocytes/μl. Hepatitis B surface antigen (HBsAg) and HBsAK were always negative. X-ray analysis of the gallbladder and the gastrointestinal tract were normal. Liver and spleen scintigraphy showed an inhomogenous structure permitting further evaluation by invasive methods. Transcutaneous hepatic biopsy was interpreted as possibly supporting the initial diagnosis of a viral disease with the liver histology being restored to near normal. Liver tissue was without acute signs of inflammation, but with some irregularity of cell size, which might have indicated an almost completed stage of regeneration after "unspecific hepatitis."

One week following this examination, abdominal pain recurred and ascites developed. Upon puncture, 1200 ml of sterile hemorrhagic protein-poor exudate (28 mg/dl) was obtained. It was decided to further explore intensively any suspicion of a neoplastic process.

Endoscopic retrograde cholecystopancreaticography (ERCP) did not show irregularities. At laparoscopy the liver was smaller than normal, the right lobe showing minimal surface irregularities with local superficial plane retractions. Some areas appeared hyperemic and tended to bleed. Signs of portal hypertension or liver cirrhosis were absent. No evidence was obtained for an abdominal tumor or a peritoneal carcinosis. However, at cavography and azygography a complete obstruction of the vena azygos was observed, indicating some retroperitoneal process.

Therefore, explorative laparotomy was performed. No abdominal, retroperitoneal, or gynecological neoplasia was found. Again, the liver appeared somewhat reduced in size with slightly increased consistency. At microscopy, hepatic structure was virtually normal. At this time we were not aware of any chemical intoxication.

During the further course of the disease from May 1976 until the second admission to the hospital in February 1977, the clinical and laboratory signs for thyreotoxicosis developed (T_4 14μg/dl, free thyroxin equivalent 1.4). Furthermore, a cholestatic syndrome was diagnosed: alkaline phosphatase (AP) 1300 U/l, total/direct bilirubin 165/100 μmol/l, prothrombin time (according to Quick) below 40%, choline esterase 1 kU/l. ESR rose to maximal values of 120/140 mm H_2O with a concomitant rise of IgM to 770 mg/dl. Moreover, the patient developed intractable retrosternal pain, a cavernous hemangioma on one finger, and multiple bleeding of the pharyngeal and nasal mucosa. Hemoglobin fell to 10 g/dl. Hemorrhagic vomiting and massive mucous and saliva secretion induced us to perform an esophagogastroscopy; however, perfect conditions were observed in the upper gastrointestinal tract. (All laboratory data during the clinical course of patient's history and attempted diagnosis are illustrated in Fig. 1.)

She was admitted to the hospital a second time in February 1977, consequent to septic temperatures with nocturnal shivers, deepened jaundice, progressive anemia, and retention of urea and creatinine. Blood cultures suggested an enteric fever, caused by *Salmonella enteritidis* (Gaertner). The Gruber-Widal agglutination titer was positive with a dilution of 1:100, indicating enterobacteria of the D group. The patient developed a hepatic precomatose condition. At physical examination, we found considerable splenomegaly with moderately increased consistency. The liver and the spleen scintigraphy now showed a nearly complete loss of activity over the hepatic area suggesting liver dystrophy. The ERCP at that time likewise showed considerable rarefication of the intrahepatic bile ducts, without extrahepatic obstructions in accordance with the diagnosis of a cholangitis/cholangiolitis.

Again, a laparoscopic inspection of the liver showed progression of liver shrinkage and an extreme splenomegaly (16×8 cm). Histological examination supported the clinical findings only partially. It is noteworthy that there was no cholestasis present at all, indicated by the complete absence of bile pigment depositions. The periportal fields showed distinct enlargement and fibrosis, with inflammatory round cell infiltrations; regenerative nodules and multiple pseudobile duct proliferations with hemosiderin-positive depositions were observed. The picture, at best, was compatible with the diagnosis of some degenerative liver disease together with pericolangitis due to the salmonellosis.

Laboratory findings progressively deteriorated. Multiple petechial and diffuse mucosal and skin bleedings appeared. Hepatic clotting factors were extremely decreased: prothrombin to 57%, factor VII to 21%, factor X to 35% of normal. Moreover, an unexplained Coombs negative hemolytic syndrome developed with macrocytic anemia and intermittent reticulocyte increments up to 100%. Indirect bilirubin rose to 300 μmol/l, lactate dehydrogenase to 800 U/l. Erythrocyte life span was decreased to a mean t1/2 of 8-9 days. Erythrocytes showed marked in vivo hemolysis, and a moderate autohemolysis in vitro (13.4%), which was prevented by adenosine 5'-triphosphate (ATP), but not by glucose. Osmotic resistance was enhanced: it started at 0.45% saline, was 50% with 0.37% saline and complete with 0.1% saline. Methemoglobin was increased

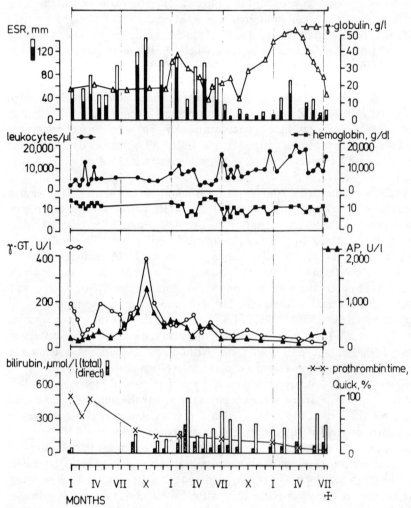

Figure 1
Some significant laboratory data during the clinical course of a patient chronically poisoned by NDMA.

to 1.8 g/dl. With multiple erythrocyte transfusions and substitution of clotting factors, the patient recovered unexpectedly for a couple of weeks.

Incidentally, she was advised not to accept any food or drinks from people outside the hospital. During one of the rare visits of her husband, he offered her a dish of cooked blackberries and inquired later on whether they had agreed with her. This exceptional attention made her suspicious. She remembered the physician's council and arranged a forensic toxicological analysis of this "cup of hemlock." Some days later the mice fed with the blackberry dish had died, whereas control mice fed with a different batch were still alive. As the final result of the chemical analysis, the blackberries contained about 300 mg of NDMA. This was probably the third or fourth dose of equal size, which her husband tried to administer to her.

With this information the puzzling disease became transparent; however, it was too late with regard to the patient's survival. During the following dramatic months the patient had to experience the uncovering of her own assassination and the continuous deterioration of her physical and mental condition. In April 1978, she developed insulin-dependent diabetes mellitus with a K value of 0.3. Basal C peptide levels were very high (6.6-7.0 ng/ml) and did not respond to intravenous or oral glucose. About 100 U/day of Neutral Protamine Hagedorn (NPH) insulin were needed to correct hyperglycemia. In May 1978, the disease was supervened by renal failure, followed by uremic polyserositis with pleural and pericardial exudates. In July 1978, she died of pulmonary edema and cardiac fibrillation in a state of increased potassium of 7.9 mEq/l due to a hemolytic crisis. Of final interest, alpha-fetoprotein was not detected during the entire course of the disease.

PATHOLOGICAL FINDINGS AT AUTOPSY

At autopsy, considerable effusions into all cavities were detected. The liver was markedly reduced in size (710 g, 21 X 14 X 8 cm); the surface was smooth with marginal notches. A spotted gray-brownish color was seen at the sectional plane. Tissue solidity was significantly increased. Histology revealed an abortively regenerating micronodular cirrhosis with pseudolobuli. There were abundant bile duct proliferations within the fibrotic periportal areas. Most interestingly, the cirrhotic lesion appeared to be of primarily periportal type, much in contrast to the centrilobular pattern of necrosis in acute NDMA poisoning in both man and experimental animals (Magee and Barnes 1967). There was no real proof of so-called hyperplastic nodules indicative of preneoplastic changes. Liver parenchyma was reduced to 20% compared to normal organs. Nuclei showed an increased variability in size, and there was an abundance of nuclear glycogen. Most impressively, the whole organ contained tremendous amounts of hemosiderin in powdered, finely, or coarsely grained distribution within parenchymal and nonparenchymal cells. No evidence of inflammatory changes could be found. Draining liver veins were partially obstructed by concentric fibrous layers.

The spleen was 340 g of weight (19 X 10 X 3 cm) with disintegrating structure and a thickened capsule. The white pulp was depleted of lymphocytes, with the stroma predominating at microscopy. Splenic veins were distended and exhibited a thickening of their walls. Iron depositions were minimal.

At the sectional plane, the pancreas was of a gray-brownish color. Functional exocrine and endocrine parenchyma was nearly absent, with its mass exchanged by fibrous tissue. Excretory canaliculi had solidified walls. Remaining parenchymal cells were loaded with iron pigment, much like in the liver.

No significant alterations following chronic NDMA exposure were found in the kidneys. Only discrete changes within the glomeruli could be detected, resembling mesangial extensions and somewhat thickened capillary walls. Besides that, calcareous deposits were seen in the medulla, and discrete degenerative changes of the tubular epithelium were evident.

Massive pulmonary edema was found. Hemosiderin deposits were only sparse. In contrast, significant amounts of hemosiderin were deposited in the myocardium. In addition, foci of necrotic myocardiocytes were seen, and there was distinct evidence of endocardial fibrosis.

Tracheal and gastrointestinal mucosa were littered with intraepithelial bleedings. Stomach and gut were filled with blood most probably arising from multiple gastric and duodenal erosions. Again, significant hemosiderin was present on iron stains.

Impulse cytophotometric analysis of ascitic cellular material did not reveal any atypical DNA pattern. Small portions of tetraploid and octoploid nuclei are compatible with a state of reactive proliferation (K. Goerttler, pers. comm.).

DISCUSSION

This patient's disease was dominated by a chronic degenerative liver failure consequent on repeated NDMA ingestion. Surprisingly, the cirrhotic pattern of this liver does not match the strictly perivenous distribution of necrosis in acute NDMA intoxication. If the repeated acute doses of NDMA had finally led to cirrhosis, one would have expected fibrotic lesions with perivenous bridging. How the clearly periportal cirrhotic bridging in this patient is related to NDMA action remains unclear. There was no evidence of viral disease during the entire course, and hemochromatosis has been excluded, since the biochemical parameters and the pattern of extrahepatic iron deposition did not fulfill the diagnostic criteria. Repeated multiple blood transfusions are also not a sufficient reason for the tremendous iron deposition in several organs, since iron deposits became apparent when the patient had not yet received any blood. Therefore, the "hemosiderosis" might also be a feature attributable to NDMA action.

Another striking feature of the clinical course is the hemolytic anemia, which finally caused the fatal hyperkalemia. Besides that, the pathological changes during the 32-month long clinical course and at autopsy are much like those detected in accidental chronic exposure in man (Barnes and Magee 1954) and in experimental animals chronically exposed to poison by diet (Magee and Barnes 1967). None of the cases in the literature developed hepatic malignancy. This holds true for our patient: no definite evidence of hepatocellular carcinoma or of obvious preneoplastic changes could be detected.

We do not know exactly how much poison had been administered to the patient nor how often it had been administered. However, several lines of evidence suggest multiple, initially smaller, and then larger doses of the poison, which initiated and maintained the liver disease. Knowledge about the toxicity of NDMA primarily arose from animal studies. The acutely lethal dose (LD_{50}) depends on animal species, its weight and the relative size of the liver. It amounts to 40-60 mg/kg body weight in the rat, to 15 mg/kg in the rabbit and to even lower doses in the dog and in man. Lower doses, when chronically administered, lead to liver cirrhosis. In the dog, daily doses of 2 mg/kg, in total 420 mg/kg diethylnitrosamine caused septal fibrosis and slowly progressive cirrhosis, accompanied by ascites and multiple bleeding, comparable to our observations (Schmaehl et al. 1964). Successful induction of a liver carcinoma has been reported in a dog after nearly 2 years of treatment with a total of 565 mg/kg or a mean of 0.8 mg/kg daily (Schmaehl et al. 1964b). In the monkey, oral doses of 2-50 mg/kg daily or a total of 1.4-25.7 g/kg resulted in malignant hepatic tumors (Kelly et al. 1966) after more than 2 years.

In man, acute toxicity has been reported by Freund (1937) from accidental poisoning. Following chronic intoxication, similar to the present case, liver cirrhosis with regenerative nodules has been described (Barnes and Magee 1954). The effective lethal dose could not be determined exactly in any of the cases from the literature. We assume that our patient received less than 1.5 g NDMA in total. This was applied in at least four doses of maximally 250-300 mg each. Thus, through "chronic" or repeated acute toxicity the total amount of 20-25 mg NDMA/kg body weight may have caused this patient's death.

ACKNOWLEDGMENTS

We gratefully acknowledge the successful toxicological analysis of the blackberry dish by Prof. Mittmeyer and his colleagues, Institute of Forensic Medicine, University of Tuebingen. We are also greatly indebted to Prof. D. Schmaehl, Institute of Toxicology and Chemotherapy, German Cancer Research Center, Heidelberg, for his manifold valuable advice during diagnosis and treatment of the patient. Autopsy data were kindly provided by Dr. Meister, Ulm.

REFERENCES

Barnes, J.M. and P.N. Magee. 1954. Some toxic properties of dimethylnitrosamine. *Brit. J. Ind. Med.* **11**:167.

Craddock, V.M. 1971. Liver carcinomas induced in rats by single administration of dimethylnitrosamine after partial hepatectomy. *J. Natl. Cancer Inst.* **47**:889.

Freund, H.A. 1937. Clinical manifestations and studies in parenchymatous hepatitis. *Ann. Intern. Med.* **10**:1144.

Hamilton, A. and H.L. Hardy. 1949. Industrial toxicology. Hoerber, New York.

Kelly, M.G., R.W. O'Hara, R.H. Adamsons, K. Gadekar, C.C. Botkin, W.H. Reese, and W.T. Kerber. 1966. Induction of hepatic cell carcinomas in monkeys with N-nitrosodimethylamine. *J. Natl. Cancer Inst.* **36**:323.

Lijinsky, W., J. Loo, and A.E. Ross. 1968. Mechanism of alkylation of nucleic acids by nitrosodimethylamine. *Nature* 218:1174.

Magee, P.N. 1971. Toxicity of nitrosamines. Their possible human health hazards. *Food Cosmet. Toxicol.* 9:207.

Magee, P.N. and J.M. Barnes. 1956. The production of malignant primary hepatic tumors in rat by feeding dimethylnitrosamine. *Br. J. Cancer* 10:114.

_____. 1959. The experimental production of tumors in the rat by dimethylnitrosamine. *Acta Unio. Contra Cancrum* 15:187.

_____. 1967. Carcinogenic nitroso-compounds. *Adv. Cancer Res.* 10:163.

Montesano, R.M. and P.N. Magee. 1971. Metabolism of nitrosamines by rat and hamster tissue slices in citro. *Proc. Am. Assoc. Cancer Res.* 12:14.

Schmaehl, D. and R. Preussmann. 1959. Cancerogene Wirkung von Dimethylnitrosamin bei Ratten. *Naturwissenschaften* 46:1975.

Schmaehl, D., C. Thomas, and W. Sattler. 1964á. Hepatotoxische und zirrhogene Wirkung von Diaethylnitrosamin bei Hunden. *Drug Res.* 14:73.

Schmaehl, D., C. Thomas, and G. Scheld. 1964b. Cancerogene Wirkung von Diaethylnitrosamin beim Hund. *Naturwissenschaften* 51:466.

Shank, R.C. 1975. Toxicology of N-nitroso compounds. *Toxicol. Appl. Pharmacol.* 31:361.

COMMENTS

WEISBURGER: Do you or Dr. Kimbrough, as part of your routine clinical pathology, have values on cholesterol in the serum, since that is bio-synthesized in liver.

FLEIG: This patient's cholesterol was within the normal range at the beginning of the disease. Later on, as to be expected from progressing liver cirrhosis, it fell to values lower than the lower limit of normal.

KIMBROUGH: It wasn't measured in the child, but in the adult it was very low; it was 72.

GOLDFARB: Isn't the pattern of injury quite unusual in this case, compared to what one might expect? As I understood the way you reconstructed the case from the biopsies to the autopsy, the biopsies originally showed a periportal pattern of injury.

FLEIG: The first biopsies we had didn't show any significant specific change. Our pathologists said it would be compatible with some final stage of hepatitis or toxic event.

GOLDFARB: But did they specify a zonal pattern of injury?

FLEIG: They didn't specify. There were some mononuclear cells in the portal triads, and that was it. There were no necrotic areas.

The first biopsy that showed significant pathological changes was obtained 1 year after the first symptoms had been noted. It showed pathological changes which were accentuated on the periportal tract.

GOLDFARB: This contrasts with Dr. Kimbrough's cases, where the acute necrosis is central zonal. That is what you would generally expect to be the case judging from the rodent experiments. I believe it may be that in this case you are presenting a picture that is complicated by the hemolytic anemia and the transfusions, with a superimposed hemochromatosis. In hemochromatosis, one typically sees a periportal pattern of injury, and you definitely have an organ distribution of hemochromatosis. So it could be that there is a primary liver injury and a hemolytic anemia of some origin which requires many transfusions. The combined effect may then be the original toxic injury plus the superimposed injury of the hemosiderin. This is just a speculation, but I would think that this might explain the unusual distribution of the injury pattern.

FLEIG: We were very much aware of the possibility that this patient was poisoned with NDMA and coincidentally might have suffered from hemo-chromatosis. However, there are many arguments against this. First, there was no laboratory evidence of iron overload at all. In contrast, repeated bone marrow biopsies revealed that iron was even slightly decreased.

Secondly, I definitely disagree with your judging the organ distribu-tion of hemosiderin as typical of hemochromatosis. This is not the typical hemochromatosis pattern. The spleen, for instance, where one would expect considerable amounts of hemosiderin in hemochromatosis patients did not show hemosiderin deposits at all.

Concerning hemolytic anemia and blood transfusions, which ap-proximated 20 liters in this patient, one has to remember that iron de-posits were definitely observed before hemolytic anemia occurred and also before blood transfusions had been given to her. Therefore, these re-markable hemosiderin depositions might in some way be related to the poison itself. This is just a speculation, and nobody knows about possible mechanisms.

GOLDFARB: Perhaps the proper term would be "parenchymal siderosis" superimposed on toxic liver injury, rather than a primary hemochroma-tosis. This is perhaps analogous to the situation in the alcoholic who gets secondary iron deposition.

FLEIG: I agree.

SIMENHOFF: Did you learn from the husband how the nitrosamine was given? Was it administered daily or episodically over a period of time?

FLEIG: It was not chronic poisoning. It was more of a recurrent administra-tion. Therefore, this case is not similar to an experiment where one applies daily doses. The victim received repeated doses of $\sim$ 200-300 mg each with about 5-month intervals.

ELDER: Was there a history of alcohol ingestion before or after the exposure? Did she have any Australia antigen testing and did she have esophageal varices?

FLEIG: She did not have esophageal varices at the time we had the upper GI endoscopy, and I am not aware of esophageal varices being described at autopsy. We have no evidence of any significant alcohol intake in this pa-tient before or during the disease. Australia antigen testing was negative.

GOLDFARB: It seems to me that she probably would have had varices. I think you described a 1600-gm spleen with little hemosiderin in it.

FLEIG: With very little hemosiderin.

GOLDFARB: There is a good possibility that this splenomegaly is secondary to portal hypertension.

MICHEJDA: You described the various pathological changes in most organs, but you didn't say anything about the brain. Were there any brain hemorrhages?

FLEIG: There were no brain hemorrhages, and there was no clinical history of brain hemorrhage. She had one episode of typical hepatic coma.

MICHEJDA: That is interesting because you reported that she probably received 300 mg per shot of the chemical.

FLEIG: A maximum of 300 mg. You must remember that the autopsy of this patient was done about 1 year after the last dose. This is not to be compared with acute poisoning.

KIMBROUGH: Was there evidence of old cerebral hemorrhage in the brain?

FLEIG: No, there was not.

WEISBURGER: In animals I don't recall that we see such pronounced blood thickening problems after nitrosamines administration. I wonder whether you would comment.

FLEIG: We had several conferences with our hematologists before the final diagnosis was made, because this was also a very puzzling hematological disease. There were two distinct problems: one is hemolytic anemia and the other one is the hemorrhagic syndrome. We found that the erythrocyte life span was decreased, that they had a decreased osmotic fragility, increased osmotic resistance, which is compatible with liver cirrhosis. We had a hemolytic anemia of unknown origin. It was Coombs negative, and in vitro hemolysis was not prevented by glucose, but was prevented by ATP addition. So we might deal with some toxic effect on the erythrocyte membrane.

MAGEE: In the first experiment that the late Dr. John Barnes and I reported (1954) the hemorrhagic tendency n the dog was more marked than one notices in the rodents. We never followed this up. I don't know how much other acute toxicity work has been done on dogs, but we found that the hemorrhagic syndrome was much more marked in the dog than we had noted in the rodents.

KIMBROUGH: Jacobson and colleagues (1955) reported this very pronounced hemorrhagic effect. This puzzled me also. Dr. Hardy, now retired, had two workers in the United States. She was very aware of the hemorrhage problem and felt that it had never really been adequately studied.

FLEIG: As I showed you from the clotting factor data, the hemorrhagic syndrome might be, at least in part, related to liver damage, because all the factors that are very decreased are factors of liver origin, whereas factor 8, which presumably arises from the bile ductular cells, was seven times normal.

KIMBROUGH: In the patients that I had, prothrombin time wasn't measured. You had a low prothrombin time, too, didn't you?

FLEIG: Prothrombin time at the final stage was 10% of normal.

BARTSCH: In these poisoning cases, did anybody attempt to measure hemoglobin methylation as a way to estimate exposure?

FLEIG: We didn't measure that.

KIMBROUGH: We only checked it in the liver.

TANNENBAUM: You wouldn't see it 1 year later.

MIRVISH: I just want to point out that I think some of the other nitrosamines in rats, like nitrosopiperidine, also have a high acute toxicity, but there they die from convulsions or something within 5 minutes of injection. Has anybody found an explanation for it?

TANNENBAUM: We have been very curious about methylbenzylnitrosamine in the past, because it is also extremely toxic but it doesn't kill through the liver; it kills by enlarging the whole area of the esophagus to the point where it just closes off the whole area. I think the animal actually dies from asphyxiation. It could be that compounds whose toxicity is not the site of the liver just have completely different mechanisms.

GOLDFARB: I hope that we can get a follow-up, Dr. Kimbrough, on the patients who are still alive following exposure. I also hope that the liver pathology will be reported on those who had toxic liver injury due to NDMA. I think that is a very unique situation.

FLEIG: Dr. Kimbrough, do you know anything about the type of chronic hepatitis found in the patient who eventually recovered?

KIMBROUGH: I did not see the liver biopsy, and I also don't know what the status is. These three patients that survived are being followed by a physician in Omaha. I have not contacted him again.

GARLAND: Dr. Kimbrough, how does the liver necrosis generate upon the NDMA administration? Does it differ from that generated upon an overdose of, let's say, acetaminophen? Is the type of necrosis similar?

KIMBROUGH: Yes, I think it is.

GOLDFARB: I think they are identical. The exact same type of central zone pattern, with necrosis radiating out from the central zones.

KIMBROUGH: We checked and tested for that, and that was negative. Incidentally, I only presented the pathology here, but the work-up that we did to try to prove that this was NDMA was published by Cooper and Kimbrough (1980).

SHANK: Why was NDMA suspected as the toxic agent in the blackberries?

FLEIG: We didn't suspect it, but it was found. First they did the animal studies and then they screened for compounds they suspected. But prior to that they didn't have any idea about the toxin.

MONTESANO: Where did this man get the NDMA?

FLEIG: He was a chemistry teacher, and he bought it.

References

Barnes, J.M. and P.N. Magee. 1954. Some toxic properties of dimethylnitrosamine. *Br. J. Ind. Med.* **11**:167.

Cooper, S.W. and R.D. Kimbrough. 1980. Acute dimethylnitrosamine poisoning outbreak. *J. Forensic Sci.* **25**:874.

Jacobson, J.H., H.J. Wheelwright, J.H. Clem, and R.N. Shannon. 1955. Studies on the toxicity of N-nitrosodimethylamine vapor. *Am. Med. Assoc. Arch. Ind. Health* **12**:617.

SESSION II:

COMPARATIVE METABOLISM AND ALKYLATION REACTIONS

Metabolism of Nitrosamines: Observations on the Effect of Alcohol on Nitrosamine Metabolism and on Human Cancer

PETER F. SWANN
The Courtauld Institute of Biochemistry
Middlesex Hospital Medical School
London, WIP 7PN England

This meeting takes place under the shadow of an important review of the epidemiology of human cancer (Doll and Peto 1981) which concludes that main influences upon cancer are tobacco, diet, and alcohol. It criticizes the experimentalist for failing to explain why they are important, and for failing to suggest a plausible mechanism for their influence. It presents us with a challenge: If we propose a major role for nitrosamines in human cancer we have to reconcile our experiments with the epidemiology.

This is not a balanced review on nitrosamine metabolism. It is focused upon some problems and upon some preliminary experiments with dimethylnitrosamine (NDMA) metabolism which may partly explain the influence of alcohol on the incidence of human cancer.

METABOLISM

General

The nitrosamines are carcinogenic if they can be converted to metabolites which alkylate. The evidence that the alkylation of DNA, in particular the O^6-position of guanine, initiates the cancerous process has been reviewed by Pegg (1977) and Singer (1979) and need not be repeated. Structure-activity relationships, analogy with nitrosoalkylureas, and experiments with esters of nitrosohydroxyalkyl alkylamines have been consistent with the view that the alkylating agent is an alkyldiazonium hydroxide generated after metabolic activation (probably by addition of oxygen) at one of the α-carbon atoms. The structure of the alkylating agent is crucial: Alkylation of the O^6 of guanine depends upon alkylation by an S_N1 mechanism (Lawley 1980). The nitrosamines are good carcinogens because the energy for this is provided by release of nitrogen from the alkylating agent (Moss 1974). Metabolism can take place at other carbons. This metabolism, although it may not activate, can have a profound effect on carcinogenicity by altering the disposition of the nitrosamine.

Since carcinogenesis by nitrosamines depends upon metabolism the cancers, and the organ distribution of them, are a reflection of: 1) the amount of nitrosamine and its distribution in the animal; 2) the ability of each organ to metabolize it to active and inactive compounds; and 3) the inherent susceptibility of each organ to the damage which the nitrosamine produces in its DNA.

The major strategies used to explore the relationship between nitrosamine metabolism and carcinogenesis have been: 1) determination of the structure and amount of altered bases produced in nucleic acids; 2) identification of intermediary metabolites; 3) in vitro metabolism; and 4) study of the effect upon carcinogenic activity of substitution of deuterium for hydrogen at various points in the molecule. For simplicity each of these approaches will be considered separately, but in general they must be combined if they are to be interpreted and applied outside the laboratory.

The Alkylation of DNA

Study of the structure of the reaction products with DNA has given the most valuable insight into the metabolic and chemical changes in the activation of nitrosamines, and measurement of the amount of alkylation has been used to follow the distribution and activation of nitrosamines and also to demonstrate that organs differ in their inherent susceptibility to carcinogenesis.

The nitrosamines are selective in their carcinogenic action and induce tumors in specific organs. The organ specificity depends upon the species. For example, NDMA produces mainly liver and kidney tumors in rats, mainly liver and lung tumors in mice; N-nitroso-2,6-dimethylmorpholine induces tumors of the nose and esophagus of rats (Lijinsky and Taylor 1975), the pancreas of hamsters (Reznik et al. 1978), and the liver of guinea pigs (Rao et al. 1980). It is clear from these few examples that it is not possible to predict the organ specificity of a nitrosamine in one species from our experience in another: in particular the organ specificity in man cannot be predicted with certainty from animal experiments. To translate the animal experiments to man we need to understand the fundamental reason for organ specificity. One of the major contributions of alkylation studies has been to explain organ specificity. Measurement of alkylation has shown that one reason (perhaps the major reason) for organ specificity is the distribution of the nitrosamine and the relative ability of each organ to activate it. A recent example is the demonstration that nitrosobenzylmethylamine induces esophageal cancer because it is metabolized predominantly in that organ (Table 1) (Hodgson et al. 1980). Of equal importance, and even greater theoretical interest, has been the demonstration that a second reason for organ specificity is differences in the inherent susceptibility to carcinogenesis. The best example is brain and liver of the rat. When the DNA of these organs was alkylated to the same extent, tumors were induced in brain but not in liver. Investigation of this difference in susceptibility led Goth and Rajewsky (1974) to the discovery of the difference in the rate of removal of O^6-ethylguanine

Table 1

The Methylation of DNA of the Rat by the Esophageal Carcinogen Nitrosomethylbenzylamine

Site	7-methylguanine	O^6-methylguanine
	(μmoles / mole guanine)	
Esophagus	344	46
Liver	120	4.9
Lung	65	7.7
Forestomach	10	ND
Kidney	3	ND
Stomach	2	ND

Data from Hodgson et al. (1980).

from the DNA of the two organs. This discovery has had a profound influence on our understanding of the mechanism of carcinogenesis—emphasizing both the importance of O^6-alkylation, and of DNA-repair, in the induction of cancer.

The study of changes in inherent susceptibility may be extremely important in other situations. For example the influence of carotenoids on human cancer (Peto et al. 1981) might be the result of an influence of the carotenoid on the production or pharmacokinetics of the carcinogen, or it might be an influence on the susceptibility of the tissue. These two possibilities can be distinguished. In the analogous case where a protein-free diet almost tripled the incidence of kidney tumors induced by a single dose of NDMA (Fig. 1) measurement of the methylation of kidney DNA proved that the change in incidence was entirely the result of the change in pharmacokinetics, and that the diet did not change the susceptibility of the kidney to the carcinogen (Swann et al. 1980).

Further experiments in which alkylation has been used to follow distribution and activation of nitrosamines are discussed below but the concentration upon alkylation of nucleic acids, the consequence of metabolism, has diverted attention from the nature and chemistry of the reactive intermediates. For many years it has been believed that the activation of NDMA proceeds through an initial hydroxylation of one methyl group, then spontaneous decomposition to form monomethylnitrosamine, followed by rearrangement to methyldiazonium hydroxide which would act as a methylating agent with the release of nitrogen. Results with acetoxy-NDMA are consistent with this scheme, which has analogy to the decomposition of nitrosamides.

Until recently it had been assumed that the intermediates were short lived, however NDMA is active in the host-mediated assay (Gabridge and Legator 1969) and cells metabolizing NDMA in culture release a metabolite which can methylate DNA in the culture medium (Umbenhauer and Pegg 1981). The relative stability of a metabolite of NDMA may have a number of important

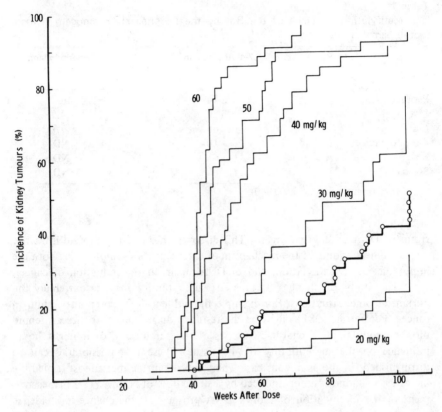

Figure 1

The change in incidence of NDMA-induced kidney tumors in the rat produced by a change from a normal to a protein-free diet. (o————o) indicates incidence produced by a dose of 40 mg/kg in rats on a normal diet. (•————•) indicates incidence produced by the marked doses in rats on a protein-free diet (Reproduced, with permission, from Swann et al. 1980).

consequences (for example, cells which cannot metabolize NDMA may be alkylated as the result of metabolism in adjacent cells), but the most important is that the carcinogenic activity of the nitrosamine depends upon the initial metabolite having sufficient stability to diffuse from the cytoplasm, where it is formed, to the nucleus, where it can react with DNA.

To justify that statement one can compare NDMA with 3,5-diethylcarboxyl-1,4-dihydrocollidine. Like NDMA this dihydrocollidine is metabolized to a methylating agent. The metabolism is mediated by cytochrome P-450. However, the methylating agent derived from the dihydrocollidine reacts immediately with the nitrogen of one of the pyrroles of the haem of the cytochrome. The resultant methylporphyrin is a powerful inhibitor of protohaem ferrolyase, the last enzyme in haem biosynthesis. There is then feed-back induction of 5-aminolaevulinate synthetase, and the induction of hepatic porphyria (De Matteis et al. 1982). By contrast NDMA does not destroy the enzyme which metabolizes it (Heath 1962) presumably because the metabolite diffuses away from the enzyme without reacting.

Recent evidence suggests that this metastable metabolite is the E-stereo-isomer of methyl hydroxymethylnitrosamine. The stability of the metabolites depends upon their stereochemistry. Both carbons, both nitrogens, and the oxygen of NDMA are in the same plane (Klement and Schmidpeter 1968). Thus one methyl group is *cis*, the other *trans*, to the nitroso-oxygen. Similar stereochemistry applies to other nitroso compounds. The energy of activation for rotation around the N-N bond is about 23 kcal/mol so a pure stereoisomer will take several hours to reach equilibrium (Abrahamson et al. 1966). Michejda et al. (1979) have suggested that the methyl *trans* to the nitroso oxygen is preferentially hydroxylated to give the E-stereoisomer of methylhydroxymethyl-nitrosamine. This stereoisomer has been prepared (Mochizuki et al. 1980). It had a t½ at pH 7 (and presumably 20°C) of about 10 seconds (Fig. 2). One would expect the Z-form to be less stable, because it can possibly change directly to methyldiazonium hydroxide by transfer of the hydroxyl-hydrogen to the nitroso-oxygen and extrusion of formaldehyde (Thomson et al. 1977). In 10 seconds a small molecule might diffuse 300 μ (Tipping and Ketterer 1981) which is many times the radius of the hepatocyte, thus in this time the metabolite could diffuse from cytoplasm to nucleus or even from cell to cell.

None of the other postulated metabolites are likely to have the required stability: monomethylnitrosamine is extremely unstable (Müller et al. 1960), and though the more stable *anti* isomer of methyldiazonium hydroxide can be isolated in cold water (Moss 1974) the very low energy of activation suggests that it would decompose very rapidly at 37°C.

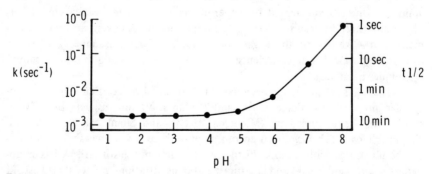

Figure 2
The dependence of the half-life of methylhydroxymethylnitrosamine on pH (Reproduced, with permission, from Mochizuki et al. 1980).

Thus on the basis of this information the hydroxymethylmethylnitros-amine is the critical metastable metabolite. The relative stability of this compound may allow the formation of conjugates, but the very low amount of alkylation of tissues remote from the liver and other organs which can metabolize the nitrosamine (Swann and Magee 1968) suggests that conjugates are not formed in significant quantity.

Isolation of Intermediary Metabolites

Deduction of the metabolic pathways of carcinogens from the identity of intermediary metabolites has been used less with the nitrosamines than with, for example, the polycyclic hydrocarbons. However, the meticulous work of Okada and his colleagues (1975) and Blattmann and Preussmann (1974) has shown that the production of bladder tumours after administration of nitrosodibutylamine (DBN) is the consequence of concentration in the bladder of metabolites of the nitrosamine which were originally produced in the liver. There are many possibilities for the metabolism of complex nitroso compounds and the identification of intermediary metabolites may be essential for an understanding of their carcinogenic action. Among the recent work in this area has been the identification of metabolites of nitrosodipropylamine, nitroso-2-hydroxypropylpropyl-amine, and nitroso-2-oxopropylpropylamine (Leung and Archer 1981) nitroso-methyldodecylamine (Suzuki et al. 1981) and nitrosonornicotine (NNN) (Hecht et al. 1981). Despite the success with DBN it is clear that in general these metabolic studies have to be combined with studies of the structure of the alkylated bases in DNA (Leung and Archer 1981) before a satisfactory understanding can be obtained.

In Vitro Metabolism

The metabolism of nitrosamines cannot be studied in man. Our understanding will have to be built from a general knowledge of the metabolism of nitrosamines in animals augmented by experiments with human tissue samples. It is important that the results from these samples should allow an accurate assessment of the ability of the organ to metabolize the nitrosamine. The results cannot be checked, our confidence is set by the success and failure of similar techniques in animals.

The metabolism of nitrosamines in vitro has been carried out with subcellular preparations, tissue slices, and explants. Various aspects of in vitro studies will be discussed by (Michejda, Hecht, and Shank, all this volume). The problems which have been encountered in these in vitro metabolism studies can be illustrated with NDMA. In the rat, the metabolism of NDMA has an apparent K_m around 70 μM and is saturated at concentrations greater than 120 μM (Heath 1962). The metabolism is closely coupled to the alkylation of nucleic acids (see below). Other pathways of metabolism, denitrosation (Appel et al.

1980) and reduction (Grilli and Prodi 1975), have been postulated, but, although the matter needs further investigation, there is no evidence in the rat of detoxifying pathways of metabolism of NDMA (Heath 1962).

The relatively clear picture in the rat is not reflected in studies with subcellular preparations. These suggest that there are at least three enzymes. Two of these are microsomal: demethylase I (K_m 0.05 mM) and demethylase II (K_m about 120 mM); the third is an enzyme in the post-microsomal supernatant (K_m 0.026 mM) (Kroeger-Koepke et al. 1979; Lai and Arcos 1980). These enzymes have not been purified or fully characterized. The activity of both demethylase I and II is closely coupled to the production of a methylating agent (Lai and Arcos 1980; Jensen et al. 1981). Demethylase II is unlikely to play any role in vivo because its K_m (120 mM) is so much greater than the concentration (0.6 mM) produced by a median lethal dose. Because of the similarity of its K_m to the apparent K_m in vivo it has been suggested that demethylase I is responsible for the metabolism of NDMA in the rat, but there is not yet general agreement with this view.

Part of the metabolism of NDMA is through a pathway which does not produce gaseous nitrogen (Heath 1962; Kroeger-Koepke et al. 1981). This will be discussed by Dr. Michejda, but one important point must be made here. Alkylation by an $S_N 1$ mechanism is essential for the carcinogenic action of the nitroso compounds (Lawley 1980). The energy needed for formation of the carbonium ion for this reaction is provided by the release of molecular nitrogen (Moss 1974). Dr. Kroeger-Koepke's result implies that in vitro part of the NDMA does not produce the methylating metabolite which is necessary for carcinogenesis.

The result suggests that either there are two separate pathways for NDMA metabolism one of which does not produce nitrogen, or that there is only one main pathway with the "loss" of nitrogen occurring as a by-product. If there were two pathways one would expect that the relative reactivity of each pathway would not be the same in all organs, and that an alteration in substrate concentration or the inhibition of one pathway would change the proportion of dose going through the other pathway. However the observations that in the rat the alkylation of nucleic acids is exactly related to dose (Diaz Gomez et al. 1977; Pegg and Perry 1981), and that the amount of DNA-alkylation/mole guanine metabolized is the same in rat liver, rat kidney, and human liver (Montesano and Magee 1970; Swann and McLean 1971); and that inhibitors affect alkylation and metabolism to an equal degree (Swann and McLean 1971), must reinforce Heath's conclusion that there is only one pathway and that the "loss" of nitrogen must occur as a diversion from that pathway. Since the nitrogen of the nitroso group of methylnitrosourea (MNU) is released stoichiometrically any diversion must occur in the metabolic pathway before it reaches the part which is common to both the nitrosamine and nitrosamide.

Studies of the metabolism by subcellular preparations of the complex nitrosamines like NNN (Chen et al. 1979) may be valuable when combined with other studies, but until the problems outlined above have been resolved subcellular preparations cannot be used to assess the ability of human tissues to metabolize nitrosamines. For an accurate assessment slice explants must be used. The rate of metabolism of NDMA by rat liver and kidney slices corresponds closely to the rate in the whole animal. Thus, slices of human tissue which have been used by Montesano and Magee (1970) may be the ideal preparations. Explants growing in tissue culture have also been used, but it is necessary to interpret the results with caution because experiments with rat liver cells suggest that explants may not retain the ability of the intact organ to metabolize the nitrosamine. Rat liver cells lose their ability to metabolize NDMA within a few hours of being taken into culture (Umbenauer and Pegg 1980). They do not regain that ability as they acclimatize to culture conditions.

The Effect of Deuteration

The rationale of experiments with deuterated nitrosamines is that if the metabolic activation of a nitrosamine involves breakage of a C–H bond the rate of that activation will be decreased if the hydrogen is replaced by deuterium. Therefore, it is argued, deuteration of the C–H bonds at which activation takes place will reduce carcinogenic activity.

The decreased carcinogenicity of nitrosomorpholine-3,3,5,5-d_4 and a low dose of dimethylnitrosamine-d_6 (Keefer et al. 1973; Lijinsky et al. 1976) in comparison with their normal counterparts seemed to validate the approach. However, subsequent results have been difficult to interpret. Deuteration did not affect the carcinogenic activity of nitrozazetidine (2,2,4,4-d_4) or larger doses of NDMA (Keefer et al. 1973; Lijinsky and Taylor 1977). Deuteration of the methyl group of nitrosomethylethylamine (methyl-d_3 or ethyl-d_5-methyl-d_3) also did not affect hepatocarcinogenicity, while the deuteration of the ethyl group (ethyl-1-d_2 or ethyl-d_5) increased it. Both compounds deuterated on ethyl-2 (i.e., ethyl-d_5 and ethyl-d_5-methyl-d_3) had a striking change in their organ specificity and produced esophageal tumors. (Lijinsky and Reuber 1980).

This confusion of results possibly reflects an inconsistency in the original conception. Slowing the rate of metabolism will not necessarily alter the carcinogenicity. The carcinogenicity will be affected only if the extent of reaction with the nucleic acids of the target organ is altered. Thus to be effective deuteration has to alter the proportion of carcinogen excreted, metabolized by detoxifying pathways, or the proportion metabolized in nontarget tissues. To be interpreted the carcinogenicity tests need to be augmented by studies or metabolism and disposition.

The Influence of Alcohol on NDMA Metabolism in Rats and Humans

The practical value of the study of metabolism and the use of animal experiments to explain some puzzling observations in man can be illustrated by some recent experiments on the effect of alcohol on NDMA. These studies also show the role of the liver in controlling the disposition of the nitrosamines and in protecting the internal organs from nitrosamines in the diet.

In 1977 Fine et al. showed the transient appearance of NDMA in human blood after a meal of bacon, spinach, tomatoes, and beer. We immediately thought that his report must be incorrect, because from animal experiments we had concluded that this small amount of nitrosamine would be completely metabolized on first pass through the liver (Diaz Gomez et al. 1977). Either we or Fine and his colleagues must be wrong. However we were able to confirm Fine's observation, and extend it by getting positive identification of the nitrosamine from mass spectrometry (P.F. Swann et al. unpubl. results).

Before the significance of these observations in man could be assessed it was necessary to know what rate of synthesis would be required to produce, and maintain, the concentration found in human blood. To this end two simple experiments were carried out in rabbits. The first was to measure the rate of disappearance of $[^{14}C]$ NDMA from the blood after intravenous injection. The nitrosamine (10.5 or 9.6 μg/kg body weight [b.w.]) was injected into the marginal vein of one ear and blood taken at intervals from the other ear. Carrier NDMA was added to the blood, the proteins precipitated with perchloric acid (0.4 N; 1 ml/ml blood) and separated by centrifugation. The $[^{14}C]$ NDMA in the supernatant (200 μl) was separated by HPLC (μ Bondapak – C18, 300 $\times$ 3.9 mm, Waters Instrument Co.) using methanol:H_2O (20:80 vv) as eluant. The radioactivity associated with the carrier NDMA was measured and the amount of $[^{14}C]$ NDMA calculated from the specific activity of the injection solution.

The concentration fell rapidly in the first 3 minutes but after this initial rapid fall, the loss from the blood was exponential with a half-life, in different rabbits, of 10.5, 11, 12, 18.5, and 19 minutes (Fig. 3). Extrapolation gave an average zero-time concentration (C_o) of 0.009 μg/ml blood. On the basis of a simple one compartment model this would suggest an average volume of distribution (V_D) of 1.2 1/kg b.w./min and a clearance rate of 59 ml/kg b.w./min. Measurement of NDMA in the blood during continuous intravenous infusion led to a similar conclusion. During the infusion the concentration in the venous blood rose to a plateau (Fig. 4). When the infusion rate in different rabbits was 0.22, 0.37, or 0.38 μg·kg b.w./min. the plateau concentrations were 3.3, 6.7, and 5.1 μg/1 blood. From this average clearance rate (infusion rate/steady state concentration) was calculated as 65 ml/kg b.w./min.

The liver is the main site of NDMA metabolism and the remarkably close similarity between the clearance rate and the hepatic blood flow in the rabbit (59 ml/min) (Neutze et al. 1968) substantiates the view that at these low concentrations it can metabolize all the nitrosamine passing through it. This would be consistent with our previous experiments with the rat. If this conclusion was correct, why did NDMA appear in the peripheral blood of man after the high nitrate meal? Why was it not stopped by the liver? We believe that the crucial

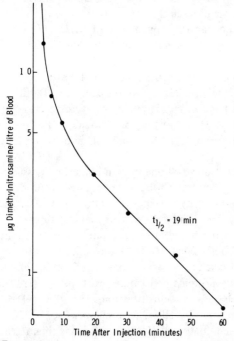

Figure 3

Disappearance of a single intravenous dose of NDMA (10.5 µg/kg) showing half life of NDMA in the rabbit.

aspect is that the meal was taken with beer. Beer is about 5% ethanol. If NDMA (33 µg/kg in 6.7 ml H_2O/kg) is given by stomach tube to the rat there is very little alkylation of kidney DNA because the nitrosamine is removed from the portal blood on first pass through the liver and does not reach the kidney. However, if the same dose is given in 6.7 ml 5% ethanol/kg b.w. which is equivalent to a 70 kg man taking a half-pint of beer, the alkylation of the kidney DNA is increased more than sixfold (Table 2). For this alkylation to take place the nitrosamine must have passed through the liver. The mechanism of this effect of alcohol is not yet known, but it may be a consequence of an inhibition of NDMA metabolism (Phillips et al. 1977; Schwarz et al. 1980).

Alcohol must have a similar effect in man because if NDMA is given in beer the amount appearing in the urine (Eisenbrand et al. 1981) indicates that there is negligible first pass removal; and, the transient increase in the amount of nitrosamine in blood after a high nitrate meal was found only when the meal was taken with beer (Fine et al. 1977) and was not seen when a similar meal was taken without alcohol (Yamamoto et al. 1980; Melikian et al. 1981).

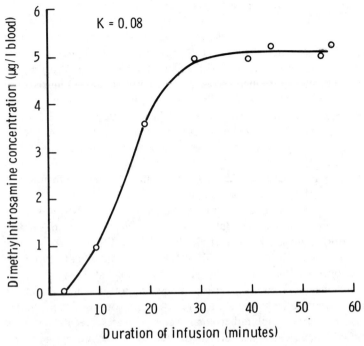

Figure 4
The concentration of NDMA in the blood of a rabbit during continuous infusion of 0.38 μg/kg/min.

Table 2
The Effect of Ethanol on the Alkylation of Rat Liver and Kidney DNA by NDMA[a]

	μmoles 7-methylguanine / mole guanine
LIVER	
NDMA in 1 ml H_2O	8.6
NDMA in 1 ml 5% EtOH	6.9
KIDNEY	
NDMA in 1 ml H_2O	≤0.07
NDMA in 1 ml 5% EtOH	0.48

NDMA in H_2O - - - - Liver : Kidney = 120

NDMA in EtOH - - - - Liver : Kidney = 14

[a]33 μg/kg NDMA, by mouth.

These results in the rat would suggest that if the nitrosamine is taken by mouth with alcohol or another inhibitor of nitrosamine metabolism there will be a marked shift from the production of liver tumors to the production of tumors of other organs. This is indeed observed. The incidence of esophageal tumors induced in rats by nitrosopiperidine (NPIP) and NDEA is increased if they are given in alcoholic solution (Gibel 1967). NDMA given in water induced liver tumors in the mouse, but when given in alcohol induced tumors in the nasal cavity in 36% of the animals (Griciute et al. 1981). Disulphiram, an inhibitor of nitrosamine metabolism, has a similar effect increasing the incidence of nasal tumors produced in rats by NDMA and of esophageal tumors induced by NDEA (Schmähl et al. 1976).

This finding may have considerable significance for man. Ethanol consumption is one of the most important contributing factors for human cancer and is associated with cancers of a number of organs (Tuyns 1979; Rosenberg et al. 1982) notably the esophagus. Yet ethanol, wine, or spirits, are not carcinogenic in laboratory animals (Schmähl et al. 1965, 1976). Ethanol may catalyse nitrosamine formation (Kurechi et al. 1980); and chronic administration increases nitrosamine metabolism (Maling et al. 1975; Garro et al. 1981).

All these may influence the effectiveness of nitrosamines as human carcinogens, but none is likely to have a large effect. By contrast administration of the nitrosamine in ethanol rather than water increases the alkylation of organs, like the kidney, which are normally protected by the liver by the simple matter of facilitating passage of the nitrosamine from the gut to the peripheral circulation. It is this effect which we suggest may be the basis for the influence of ethanol on human cancer, and may provide a link between nitrosamine research and one of the proven aspects of cancer epidemiology.

Esophageal cancer is extremely common in certain areas of the world where there is little consumption of alcohol, notably in parts of China. The cause of these geographical hot spots is not known but the Chinese have assiduously searched for dietary nitrosamines in these areas of their country where esophageal cancer is most prevalent (Li et al. 1980; Yang 1980). It might be valuable if they searched also in the diet for compounds which have the same effect as alcohol, since it is conceivable that the high incidence of tumors is in part the result of the influence of a constituent of the diet on the disposition in vivo of nitrosamines in the diet and synthesized within man himself.

ACKNOWLEDGMENTS

This research was generously supported by the Cancer Research Campaign. I am extremely grateful for the advice and encouragement of Terry Gough, Larry Keefer, Soterios Kyrtopoulos, and Raymond Mace, and to Miss Alison Brough who prepared this manuscript.

REFERENCES

Abrahamson, K.H., P.T. Inglefield, E. Krakower, and L.W. Reeves. 1966. The description and use of a spin-echo spectrometer to study chemical exchange. *Can. J. Chem.* **44**:1685.

Appel, K.E., D. Schrenk, M. Schwarz, B. Mahr, and W. Kunz. 1980. Denitrosation of N-nitrosomorpholine by liver microsomes: possible role of cytochrome P-450. *Cancer Lett.* **9**:13.

Blattmann, L. and R. Preussmann. 1974. Biotransformation von Carcinogenen Dialkylnitrosaminen Weiter Urinmetaboliten von Di-N-butyl- und Di-N-pentyl-nitrosamin. *Z. Krebsforsch.* **81**:75.

Chen, C-H., P.T. Fung, and S.S. Hecht. 1979. Assay for microsomal α-hydroxylation of nitrosonornicotine and determination of the deuterium isotope effect for α-hydroxylation. *Cancer Res.* **39**:5057.

De Matteis, F., A.H. Gibbs, P.B. Farmer, J.H. Lamb, and C. Hollands. 1982. Liver haem as a target of drug toxicity. In *Advances in Pharmacology and Therapeutics* II (ed. H. Yoshida, Y. Hagihara, S. Ebashi) vol. 5, p. 131. Pergamon Press, Oxford.

Diaz Gomez, M.I., P.F. Swann, and P.N. Magee. 1977. The absorption and metabolism in rats of small oral doses of dimethylnitrosamine. *Biochem. J.* **164**:497.

Doll, R. and R. Peto. 1981. The causes of cancer. *J. Natl. Cancer Inst.* **66**:1191.

Eisenbrand, G., B. Spiegelhalder, and R. Preussman. 1981. Analysis of human biological specimens for nitrosamine contents. *Ban. Rep.* **7**:275.

Fine, D.H., R. Ross, D.P. Rounbehler, A. Silvergleid, and L. Song. 1977. Formation *in vivo* of volatile N-nitrosamines in man after ingestion of cooked bacon and spinach. *Nature* **265**:753.

Gabridge, M.G. and M.G. Legator. 1969. A host-mediated microbial assay for the detection of mutagenic compounds. *Proc. Soc. Exp. Biol. Med.* (N.Y.) **130**:831.

Garro, A.J., H.K. Seitz, and C.S. Lieber. 1981. Enhancement of dimethylnitrosamine metabolism and activation to a mutagen following chronic ethanol consumption. *Cancer Res.* **41**:120.

Gibel, von W. 1967. Experimentelle Untersuchungen zur Synkarcinogenese beim Oesophaguskarzinom. *Arch. Geschwulstforsch.* **30**:181.

Goth, R. and M.F. Rajewsky. 1974. Persistence of O^6-ethylguanine in rat brain DNA. *Proc. Natl. Acad. Sci. U.S.A.* **71**:639.

Griciute, L., M. Casteganaro, J.C. Bereziat. 1981. Influence of ethyl alcohol on carcinogenesis with N-nitrosodimethylamine. *Cancer Lett.* **13**:345.

Grilli, S. and P. Prodi. 1975. Identification of dimethylnitrosamine metabolites *in vitro. Gann* **66**:473.

Heath, D.F. 1962. The decomposition and toxicity of dialkylnitrosamines in rats. *Biochem. J.* **85**:72.

Hecht, S.S., D. Lin, and C.B. Chen. 1981. Comprehensive analysis of urinary metabolites of N-nitrosonornicotine. *Carcinogenesis* **2**:833.

Hodgson, R.M., M. Wiessler, and P. Kleihues. 1980. Preferential methylation of target organ DNA by the oesophageal carcinogen N-nitrosomethylbenzylamine. *Carcinogenesis* **1**:861.

Jensen, D.E., P.D. Lotlikar, and P.N. Magee. 1981. The *in vitro* methylation of DNA by microsomally-activated dimethylnitrosamine and its correlation with formaldehyde production. *Carcinogenesis* 2:349.

Keefer, L., W. Lijinsky, and H. Garcia. 1973. Deuterium isotope effect on the carcinogenicity of dimethylnitrosamine in rat liver. *J. Natl. Cancer Inst.* 51:299.

Klement, U. and A. Schmidpeter. 1968. Structure of dimethylnitrosamine copper (II) chloride. *Angew Chem. Int. Ed. Engl.* 7:470.

Kroeger-Koepke, M.B. and C.J. Michejda. 1979. Evidence for several demethylase enzymes in the oxidation of dimethylnitrosamine and phenylmethylnitrosamine by rat liver fractions. *Cancer Res.* 39:1587.

Kroeger-Koepke, M.B., S.R. Koepke, G.A. McClusky, P.N. Magee, and C.J. Michejda. 1981. α-Hydroxylation pathway in the *in vitro* metabolism of carcinogenic nitrosamines: N-nitrosodimethylamine and N-nitroso-N-methylaniline. *Proc. Natl. Acad. Sci. U.S.A.* 78:6489.

Kurechi, T., K. Kikugawa, and T. Kato. 1980. Effect of alcohol on nitrosamine formation. *Food Cosmet. Toxicol.* 18:591.

Lai, D.Y. and J.C. Arcos. 1980. Dialkylnitrosamine bioactivation and carcinogenesis. *Life Sci.* 27:2149.

Lawley, P.D. 1980. DNA as a target of alkylating carcinogens. *Br. Med. Bull.* 36:19.

Leung, K.H. and M.C. Archer. 1981. Urinary metabolites of N-nitrosodipropylamine, N-nitroso-2-hydroxypropylpropylamine and N-nitroso-2-oxopropylpropylamine in the rat. *Carcinogenesis* 2:859.

Li, M., P. Li, and B. Li. 1980. Recent progress in research on oesophageal cancer in China. *Adv. Cancer Res.* 33:173.

Lijinsky, W. and M.D. Reuber. 1980. Carcinogenicity in rats of nitrosomethylethylamines labelled with deuterium in several positions. *Cancer Res.* 40:19.

Lijinsky, W. and H.W. Taylor. 1975. Increased carcinogenicity of 2,6-dimethylnitrosomorpholine compared with nitrosomorpholine in rats. *Cancer Res.* 35:2123.

_____. 1977. Carcinogenicity of nitrosoazetidine and tetradeuteronitrosoazetidine in Sprague Dawley rats. *Z. Krebsforsch.* 89:215.

Lijinsky, W., H.W. Taylor, and L.K. Keefer. 1976. Reduction of rat liver carcinogenicity of nitrosomorpholine by alpha deuterium substitution. *J. Natl. Cancer Inst.* 57:1311.

Maling, H.N., B. Stripp, J. Sipes, B. Highman, W. Saul, and M.A. Williams. 1975. Enhanced hepatotoxicity of carbon tetrachloride, thioacetamide and dimethylnitrosamine by pretreatment of rats with ethanol and some comparisons with potentiation by isopropanol. *Toxicol. Appl. Pharmacol.* 33:291.

Melikian, A.A., E.J. LaVoie, D. Hoffmann, and E.L. Wynder. 1981. Volatile nitrosamines: analysis in breast fluid and blood of non-lactating women. *Food Cosmet. Toxicol.* 19:757.

Michejda, C.J., M.B. Kroeger-Koepke, S.R. Koepke, and R.J. Kupper. 1979. Oxidative activation of nitrosamines: model compounds. In *N-nitrosamines* (ed. J-P. Anselme) *ACS Symp. Ser.* 101:77.

Mochizuki, M., T. Anjo, and M. Okada. 1980. Isolation and characterization of

N-alkyl-N-(hydroxymethyl)nitrosamines from N-alkyl-N-(hydroperoxymethyl) nitrosamines by dehydrogenation. *Tetrahedron Lett.* 21:3693.

Montesano, R. and P.N. Magee. 1970. Metabolism of dimethylnitrosamine by human liver slices *in vitro*. *Nature* 228:173.

Moss, R.A. 1974. Some chemistry of alkanediazotates. *Accs. Chem. Res.* 7:421.

Müller, E., H. Haiss, and W. Rundel. 1960. Uber das Kalium-methyldiazotat, ein stabilisiertes Diazomethan und das Monomethylnitrosamin. *Chem. Ber.* 93:1541.

Neutze, J.M., F. Wyler, and A.M. Rudolf. 1968. Use of radioactive microspheres to assess distribution of cardiac output in rabbits. *Am. J. Physiol.* 215: 486.

Okada, M., E. Suzuki, J. Aoki, M. Iiyoshi, and Y. Hashimoto. 1975. Metabolism and carcinogenicity of N-butyl-N-(4-hydroxybutyl)-nitrosamine and related compounds with special reference to induction of urinary bladder tumours. *Gann. Monogr. Cancer Res.* 17:161.

Pegg, A.E. 1977. Formation and metabolism of alkylated purines: possible role in carcinogenesis by N-nitroso compounds and alkylating agents. *Adv. Cancer Res.* 25:195.

Pegg, A.E. and W. Perry. 1981. Alkylation of nucleic acids and metabolism of small doses of dimethylnitrosamine in the rat. *Cancer Res.* 41:3128.

Peto, R., R. Doll, J.D. Buckley, and M.B. Sporn. 1981. Can dietary β-carotene materially reduce human cancer rates? *Nature* 290:201.

Phillips, J.C., B.G. Lake, S.D. Gangolli, P. Grasso, and A.G. Lloyd. 1977. Effects of pyrazole and 3-amino-1,2,4-triazole on the metabolism and toxicity of dimethylnitrosamine in the rat. *J. Natl. Cancer Inst.* 58:629.

Rao, M.S., D.G. Scarpelli, and W. Lijinsky. 1980. N-nitroso-2,6-dimethylmorpholine induced haemangiosarcomas in the livers of random bred guinea pigs. *J. Natl. Cancer Inst.* 64:529.

Reznik, G., U. Mohr, and W. Lijinsky. 1978. Carcinogenic effects of N-nitroso-2,6-dimethylmorpholine in Syrian golden hamsters. *J. Natl. Cancer Inst.* 60:371.

Rosenberg, L., D. Slone, S. Shapiro, D.W. Kaufman, S.P. Helmrich, O.S. Miettinen, P.D. Stolley, M. Levy, N.B. Rosenheim, D. Schottenfeld, and R.L. Engle. 1982. Breast cancer and alcoholic beverage consumption. *Lancet* 1:267.

Schmähl, D. 1976. Investigations on oesophageal carcinogenicity by methylphenylnitrosamine and ethyl alcohol in rats. *Cancer Lett.* 1:215.

Schmähl, D., F.W. Kruger, M. Habs, and B. Diehl. 1976. Influence of disulphiram on the organotropy of the carcinogenic effects of dimethylnitrosamine and diethylnitrosamine in rats. *Z. Krebsforsch.* 85:271.

Schmähl, D., C. Thomas, W. Sattler, and G.F. Scheld. 1965. Experimentelle Untersuchungen zur Syncarcinogenese. *Z. Krebsforsch.* 66:526.

Schwarz, M., K.E. Appel, D. Schrenk, and W. Kunz. 1980. Effect of ethanol on microsomal metabolism of dimethylnitrosamine. *J. Cancer Res. Clin. Oncol.* 97:233.

Singer, B. 1979. N-nitroso alkylating agents: formation and persistence of alkyl derivatives in mammalian nucleic acids as contributing factors in carcinogenesis. *J. Natl. Cancer Inst.* 62:1329.

Swann, P.F. and A.E.M. Mclean. 1971. The effect of a protein-free high-carbohydrate diet on the metabolism of dimethylnitrosamine in the rat. *Biochem. J.* **124**:283.

Swann, P.F., D.G. Kaufman, P.N. Magee, and R. Mace. 1980. Induction of kidney tumours by a single dose of dimethylnitrosamine: Dose response and influence of diet and benzo(a)pyrene treatment. *Br. J. Cancer* **41**: 285.

Suzuki, E., M. Mochizuki, and M. Okada. 1981. Metabolic fate of N-methyl-N-dodecylnitrosamine in the rat in relation to its carcinogenicity in the urinary bladder. *Gann* **72**:713.

Tipping, E. and B. Ketterer. 1981. The influence of soluble binding proteins on lipophile transport and metabolism in hepatocytes. *Biochem. J.* **195**:441.

Thomson, C., D. Provan, and S. Clark. 1977. Quantum mechanical investigations of unstable intermediates relevant to the mechanism of chemical carcinogenesis by N-nitrosamines. *Int. J. Quantum Chem. Symp.* **4**:205.

Tuyns, A.J. 1979. Epidemiology of alcohol and cancer. *Cancer Res.* **39**:2840.

Umbenhauer, D.R. and A.E. Pegg. 1981. Alkylation of intracellular and extracellular DNA by dimethylnitrosamine following activation by isolated rat hepatocytes. *Cancer Res.* **41**:3471.

Yang, C.S. 1980. Research on oesophageal cancer in China: A review. *Cancer Res.* **40**:2633.

Yamamoto, M., T. Yamada, and A. Tanimura. 1980. Volatile nitrosamines in human blood before and after ingestion of a meal containing high concentrations of nitrate and secondary amines. *Food Cosmet. Toxicol.* **18**:297.

Nitrogen Formation During In Vivo and In Vitro Metabolism of *N*-Nitrosamines

CHRISTOPHER J. MICHEJDA, MARILYN B. KROEGER-KOEPKE,
STEVEN R. KOEPKE
Chemical Carcinogenesis Program
National Cancer Institute
Frederick Cancer Research Facility
Frederick, Maryland 21701

PETER N. MAGEE, CECILIA CHU
Fels Research Institute
Temple School of Medicine
Philadelphia, Pennsylvania 19140

The metabolism of *N*-nitrosamines is a complicated process which undoubtedly involves several pathways, most of which result in the harmless excretion of the xenobiotics. Some pathways, however, result in the formation of highly electrophilic intermediates, which interact with a host of nucleophilic substances in a cell. Again, most of these electrophile-nucleophile interactions cause no permanent damage. A small fraction, however, results in the initiation of a complex series of events which eventually lead to tumor formation. The most widely accepted hypothesis for the metabolic activation of nitrosamines to the reactive, electrophilic agents is the α-hydroxylation hypothesis (Fig. 1). The only enzyme-mediated step in this reaction sequence is the formation of the α-hydroxylated nitrosamine; the subsequent steps involve a nonenzymatic cascade of reactions which lead to the formation of the reactive diazonium ion. This substance then reacts randomly with a variety of nucleophiles, including water. An obligatory result of the formation of the diazonium ion, particularly if R is an alkyl group, is the formation of molecular nitrogen. Thus, the measurement of the amount of molecular nitrogen formed during metabolism should provide a measurement of the contribution of the α-hydroxylation pathway to the metabolism of nitrosamines, provided that the extent of total metabolism can be determined. This concept was applied to the in vitro and in vivo metabolism of two nitrosamines, *N*-nitrosodimethylamine (NDMA) and *N*-nitroso-*N*-methylaniline (NMA). In the case of NDMA, α-hydroxylation gives rise to the methyldiazonium ion, while in the case of NMA, the far less reactive benzenediazonium ion is formed.

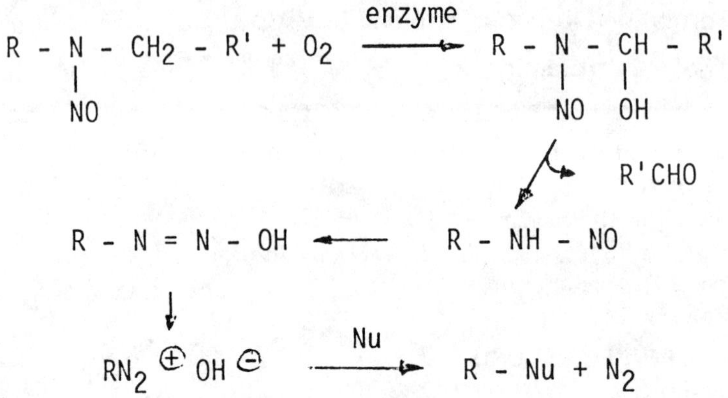

$$
\begin{array}{c}
R - \underset{\underset{\displaystyle NO}{|}}{N} - CH_2 - R' + O_2 \xrightarrow{\text{enzyme}} R - \underset{\underset{\displaystyle NO}{|}}{N} - \underset{\underset{\displaystyle OH}{|}}{CH} - R'
\end{array}
$$

$$
\xrightarrow{\hspace{1cm}} R'CHO
$$

$$
R - N = N - OH \longleftarrow R - NH - NO
$$

$$
\downarrow
$$

$$
RN_2 \overset{\oplus}{} OH \overset{\ominus}{} \xrightarrow{\hspace{0.3cm}Nu\hspace{0.3cm}} R - Nu + N_2
$$

Figure 1
α-Hydroxylation pathway of nitrosamine metabolism, (Nu) nucleophile.

METHODS

Preparation of Labeled Nitrosamines

Dimethyl$[^{15}N_2]$nitrosamine, 99% labeled in both nitrogens, was prepared from dimethyl$[^{15}N]$amine hydrochloride (Stohler) and sodium$[^{15}N]$nitrite in 80% yield. The final product was purified by column chromatography. $[^{13}C_2]$Dimethylnitrosamine was prepared in an analogous manner from 99% enriched $[^{13}C_2]$dimethylamine hydrochloride (Prochem). The preparation of N-$[^{15}N_2]$-nitroso-N-methylaniline was achieved by formylation of $[^{15}N]$aniline (Stohler) with ethyl formate followed by reduction of the formanilide with LiAlH$_4$, and nitrosation of the N-methylaniline with sodium $[^{15}N]$ nitrite. The product, formed in 88% yield, was purified by chromatography on silica gel and crystallization from pentane at -80°C. Mass spectrometry (MS) indicated 99% enrichment in both nitrogens. N-$[^{15}N_2]$-Nitroso-N-methylurea (NMU) was prepared from methyl$[^{15}N]$amine by an adaptation of the procedure of Murray and Williams (1958).

In Vitro Experiments: Preparation of S9 Fraction

The post-mitochondrial supernatant (S9 fraction) from rat livers was prepared by conventional methods (Kroeger-Koepke and Michejda, 1979). Ten-week-old, uninduced, male Fischer 344 rats were used in this study. The S9 fractions from 10-20 rats were pooled and stored at -80°C in 15 ml portions until used.

Determination of Formaldehyde Formation and Nitrosamine Loss

The detailed procedures have been described (Kroeger-Koepke et al. 1981). The initial concentrations of the nitrosamines in the incubation mixtures were 5.0 mM. Each mixture also contained 15 ml of the S9 fraction which corresponded to 5 g of wet liver. Incubations were carried out for 1 hour. The formaldehyde determinations were carried out by the colorimetric method of Nash (1953). The determination of nitrosamine loss was carried out by high pressure liquid chromatography (HPLC). Aliquots (1 ml) of the incubation mixture were taken at time 0 and at 60 min. To this was added a known amount of internal standard, diethylnitrosamine (NDEA) (0.5 ml of 1.00 mg/ml solution), and the proteins were precipitated with $ZnSO_4$ and $Ba(OH)_2$. After centrifugation (8000 $\times$ g for 10 min at 0°C), the supernatant was filtered through an ultrafilter, which excluded materials with molecular weight > 1000. The filtrates were immediately analyzed on HPLC, using a Bondapack phenyl 10 μm column (Alltech Associates), on a Laboratory Data Control Constametric pumping system. Detection was carried out using an LDC UVII detector at 254 nm and the data were processed through a Hewlett Packard 3354 computer, interfaced to the instrument. Chromatograms were developed using non-linear gradients, described in the original paper. The amount of nitrosamine loss was calculated with reference to the internal standard. The ratio of the areas at times 0 and 60 min of NDEA was defined as the normalization factor. This factor was multipled by the areas of NDMA (or NMA) at times 0 and 60 min. This procedure normalized the injection. The amount of nitrosamine loss was then simply given by: $([NA]_0 - [NA]_{60})/[NA]_0$.

In Vivo Experiments

The procedure was similar to that used by Magee (see Magee 1980). A female Sprague-Dawley rat (110-140g) was treated by IP injection with 0.26 mmoles/kg of a given nitroso compound. It was immediately placed in a respiration chamber whose top was a collapsible polyvinylidine chloride bag. The air was pumped out of the chamber to the volume of 100 ml and then refilled with a mixture of 50% oxygen and 50% sulfur hexafluoride. This procedure was repeated several times. A known amount of internal standard, neon, was then allowed to diffuse into the chamber. After 6 hours, the rat was killed by injecting 1 ml of chloroform into the chamber. The gases were then allowed to expand into a vacuum line, which caused the complete collapse of the plastic bag. The gases were passed through traps containing sodium dithionite in an alkaline solution to remove oxygen and carbon dioxide, and then through a liquid nitrogen cooled trap to remove the condensible gases. The residual gases were collected into a calibrated gas bulb by means of a Toepler pump. The contents of the gas bulb were analyzed by MS.

MS Analysis of Molecular Nitrogen

The details of the procedures were described earlier (Kroeger-Koepke et al. 1981). In the in vitro reactions, incubations were carried out in precisely calibrated 100 ml gas bulbs, using double the amounts of materials used in the other assays. Analyses were carried out with $[^{13}C_2]$NDMA, $[^{15}N_2]$NDMA, $[^{15}N_2]$-NMA and $[^{15}N_2]$NMU as substrates. Bulbs containing all the reactants were chilled to $0°C$ and outgassed on a specially constructed vacuum line. The atmosphere in the bulbs was replaced, by backfilling, with oxygen containing 1% (wt/wt) of neon (Matheson, primary standard, analyzed). After incubation at $37°C$ for 1 hour, the sample bulb was reattached to the vacuum line and the head gases were transferred to a 50 ml bulb with a Toepler pump. The sample gases were then expanded into a 1 liter gas probe of a VG Micromass ZAB-2F mass spectrometer. The relative ratios of Ne and $^{15}N_2$ were then determined. The mass spectrometer was calibrated with primary standard gas mixtures, containing Ne and $^{15}N_2$ in oxygen (Scott Specialty Gases). This allowed the determination of correction factors for mass discriminations and ionization efficiencies. Control experiments were carried out to measure the recovery of the nitrogen produced and of the internal standard introduced.

The gas measurements in the in vivo experiments were carried out in the same manner as above. In order to determine recovery efficiencies, primary gas standard mixtures were carried through the entire experimental procedure. It was determined that $^{15}N_2$ was lost preferentially. This loss was shown to be relatively constant and independent of the concentration of $^{15}N_2$, in the range used in the study. This allowed the calculation of a recovery factor. Control experiments were repeated nine times. The formation of $^{15}N_2$ (χ) was calculated from the equation, $\chi = M(V_2/V_1)/0.871 R$, where M is moles of Ne standard, V_2 is volts for m/z 30, and V_1 the volts for m/z 20. The response factor R was determined from the equation, $R = (S_2/S_1)C^{-1}$, where S_2 and S_1 are volts for the primary standards for m/z 30 and 20, respectively, and C in the concentration factor used to adjust the N_2/Ne ratio to 1% N_2 and 1% Ne. This factor was calculated from the known ratios of $^{15}N_2$ and Ne in the primary standards.

RESULTS

Determination of the Extent of In Vitro Metabolism of NDMA and NMA

The data in Table 1 compare the extent of nitrosamine metabolism as measured by formaldehyde formation and by direct measurement of nitrosamine loss. Formaldehyde formation was measured by the standard Nash (1953) assay.

Nitrosamine loss was determined by HPLC using a reversed-phase column. Semicarbazide is frequently used in assays which involve the measurement of formaldehyde to prevent the loss of that substance. We found, however, that semicarbazide itself gave rise to some formaldehyde (16% of the total formalde-

Table 1

Comparison of Extent of Nitrosamine Metabolism by Two Different Methods

Substrate	H_2CO Detected (μmol/g liver/hr)	Nitrosamine consumed (μmol/g liver/hr)
NDMA	0.169 ± 0.050 (6)	0.732 ± 0.184 (5)
NMA	0.039 ± 0.010 (4)	1.570 ± 0.173 (5)

Results are expressed as the mean ± SD (number of observations).

hyde) as well as molecular nitrogen, at the rate of 2.5 μmol/g liver/hr. Consequently, this trapping agent was not included in our incubation mixtures.

Determination of Molecular Nitrogen in the In Vitro Experiment

These measurements were carried out by MS, using neon as an internal standard. Although neon was ionized less efficiently than $^{15}N_2$, the ratio of nitrogen to neon, as obtained by MS readings, was directly proportional to the relative concentrations. Control experiments, where the entire experimental protocol minus the nitrosamines was conducted with primary standard gas mixtures, indicated that the ratio of $^{15}N_2$ to Ne was unchanged and that the recovery of the gases was greater than 90%. The experimental values for $^{15}N_2$ formation are indicated in Table 2. The data show that 33% of the theoretical nitrogen was formed during the S9 metabolism of NDMA. The figure for NMA was only 19%. The evolution of $^{15}N_2$ from labeled NMU was used as a positive control, yielding 96% of the theoretical amount. The metabolism of unlabeled NDMA gave the expected low value of $^{15}N_2$; this experiment served as a negative control. The unlikely possibility that formaldehyde was being oxidized to CO_2 was checked by the analysis of the total gases formed during the metabolism of

Table 2

Quantitation of $^{15}N_2$ in the In Vitro Metabolism of Labeled Nitrosamines

Substrate	$^{15}N_2$ Produced (μmol/g liver/hr)[a]	% of theory[b]
[$^{15}N_2$] NDMA	0.240 ± 0.031 (4)	33.1
[$^{15}N_2$] NMA	0.296 ± 0.074 (3)	18.8
[$^{15}N_2$] NMU	0.912 ± 0.010 (2)[c]	96.0
[$^{14}N_2$] NDMA	0.014 ± 0.001 (2)	—

[a]Mean value ± standard deviation (number of determinations)
[b]Molecular nitrogen formed as compared to total metabolism
[c]One sample of NMU was decomposed in pH 7.4 phosphate buffer with no S9, the other was decomposed in the presence of S9.

$[^{13}C_2]$ NDMA. The ratio of the masses for $^{14}CO_2$ and $^{13}C_2$ (m/z 44 and 45, respectively) was precisely the same as that obtained from unlabeled NDMA. The total gases from the ^{15}N-labeled substrate were also checked for the presence of ^{15}N-labeled nitrogen oxides and isotopically mixed nitrogen (^{15}N-^{14}N). None were detected above natural background levels.

Nitrogen Determination from the In Vivo Experiments

Each rat was kept in the respiration chamber in an atmosphere of 50% O_2 and 50% SF_6, containing a known amount of neon for 6 hours. It was assumed that all of the substrates were fully metabolized during that time. The rats were killed by injection of chloroform into the chamber. The gases were then pumped through a series of traps to remove all the condensibles and the residual gases were collected in a calibrated gas bulb and measured in precisely the same manner as had been done for the in vitro experiments. Table 3 shows the values obtained for ^{15}N-labeled NDMA, NMA, and NMU. These data indicate that up to about 80% of NDMA is metabolized by the α-hydroxylation pathway, but only about 50% of NMA released its nitrogen. The positive control, NMU, led to about 90% molecular nitrogen release. This was somewhat less than the in vitro experiment.

Table 3
$^{15}N_2$ Analysis of in vivo Metabolism of Labeled Nitrosamines

Substrate	moles substrate injected ($\times 10^5$)	yield $^{15}N_2$ (moles $\times 10^5$)	% of injected dose	
NDMA	3.83	2.73	71.23	
	4.14	3.08	73.83	
	3.04	1.81	59.77	67.1 ± 11.1
	4.03	3.18	78.97	
	4.03	2.08	51.78	
NMA	3.69	2.53	68.57	
	3.75	1.76	46.85	52.4 ± 10.9
	4.02	1.95	48.67	
	3.48	1.58	45.43	
NMU	3.81	3.29	86.33	
	4.04	3.71	91.90	
	3.44	2.90	86.89	88.0 ± 2.6
	4.11	2.52	61.20	
	4.07	3.33	87.01	

DISCUSSION

Nitrogen Evolution During Metabolism

There is a substantial body of indirect evidence that α-hydroxylation is an important pathway in determining the formation of carcinogenic metabolites of many nitrosamines. The carcinogenicity of NDMA is substantially reduced by deuteration (Keefer et al. 1973). In a similar manner, N-nitrosomorpholine is significantly more carcinogenic than its deuterated analog, 3,3,5,5-tetradeutero-N-nitrosomorpholine (Lijinsky et al. 1976). The α-hydroxylation pathway has been demonstrated to be important in the in vitro metabolism of cyclic nitrosamines. Thus, N-nitrosopyrrolidine is α-hydroxylated by rat liver homogenates (Hecht et al. 1978; Hecker et al. 1979), and by human liver enzymes (Hecht et al. 1979). Similarly, α-hydroxylation has been shown to occur in the metabolism of N-nitrosopiperidine (Leung et al. 1978), N-nitrosopiperazine (Krüger et al. 1976) and N-nitrosonornicotine (Chen et al. 1978), as well as other cyclic nitrosamines. This evidence for the α-hydroxylation of the cyclic nitrosamines was deduced from the analysis of the stable products of the resulting diazonium ions; no α-hydroxylated nitrosamine has ever been detected as a metabolite. Recently, however, the first synthetic examples of α-hydroxynitrosamines have been reported (Mochizuki et al. 1980). Predictably, these substances are unstable in aqueous solutions, particularly at pH > 5.

Some years ago, Magee (1980) showed that doubly $[^{15}N]$-labeled NDMA injected into a rat contained in a respiration chamber, was metabolized in such a way that up to 90% of the label was exhaled as doubly-labeled molecular nitrogen. The pathway of metabolism indicated by Fig. 1 shows that for each equivalent of α-hydroxylation there ought to be an equivalent of molecular nitrogen. Cottrell et al. (1977) also studied the metabolism of $[^{15}N_2]$-NDMA by the S10 fraction of uninduced and phenobarbital-induced Sprague-Dawley rat livers. These workers followed the metabolism by measuring formaldehyde formation and the formation of nitrogen was measured mass spectroscopically. They concluded that only 5% of the metabolism proceeded by α-hydroxylation. On the other hand, Milstein and Guttenplan (1979), using unlabeled NDMA and both mouse and rat microsomes, found nearly quantitative nitrogen evolution, based on formaldehyde formation. In contrast to these results, our data (Kroeger-Koepke et al. 1981) indicated that about 33% of NDMA was metabolized by the α-hydroxylation pathway, when uninduced Fischer 344 rat S9 was used as the metabolizing medium. The yield of molecular nitrogen from NDMA under these conditions was even lower (19%), a reason for this is suggested below. The apparent discrepancy of our value for NDMA metabolism with those obtained by other workers must be taken in context of the differences between the experimental protocols. Cottrell and coworkers (1977) used Sprague-Dawley rat livers and there were significant differences in their experimental protocol, as compared to ours. Milstein and Guttenplan (1979) used microsomes from unspecified strains of rats and unlabeled NDMA, the latter made the measurements particularly difficult. Our data appear to reflect the true in vitro metabolic picture accurately. It is significant that the bulk (60-70%) of NDMA must be metabolized in vitro by pathways other than α-hydroxylation. These could include denitrosation (Appel et al. 1980), as well as reductive pathways (Grilli and Prodi 1975). Our experimental protocol, however, was not designed to determine the nature of these reactions.

The apparently low amount of α-hydroxylation of NMA, as determined by the nitrogen evolution technique, may not mirror the true extent of that reaction. NMA, on demethylation, gives the rather stable benzenediazonium ion. In contrast to the alkyldiazonium ions, the aromatic analogues do not lose their nitrogen very readily. Reactions, such as azo coupling reactions with activated aromatics, are well known. Indeed, the benzenediazonium ion is known to couple with purines (see below). In the case of NMA, we were able to determine that no ring hydroxylation occurs in vitro, and we know that rat liver enzymes actually demethylate NMA more rapidly than they do NDMA (Kroeger-Koepke and Michejda 1979). Consequently, we made an effort to trace the fate of the benzenediazonium ion indirectly. Metabolism of [ring-^{14}C]NMA was carried out with the S9 mix in presence of phenol. After 1 hour, the reaction was stopped (6% metabolism) and treated with unlabeled p-hydroxyazobenzene. The reisolated (HPLC) p-hydroxyazobenzene contained 70% of the theoretical radioactivity, based on 6% of total metabolism. This result suggests that the metabolically-formed benzenediazonium ion was stable enough to be trapped by coupling with phenol. In absence of phenol, it was probably trapped by other aromatic substances present in the mix. Thus, the nitrogen evolution technique is not adequate to measure the true extent of α-hydroxylation in the case of NMA.

Formaldehyde formation is not a reliable way of measuring the extent of N-demethylation in the presence of S9 since formaldehyde is apparently oxidized to formate by oxidases present in the mix. In absence of mitochondria, the formate is not oxidized to carbon dioxide, as is also evident from our data on the metabolism of [$^{13}C_2$]NDMA. The usual practice of adding semicarbazide to suppress formaldehyde loss was inappropriate in our experiment because semicarbazide was an active substrate for the oxidase enzymes, producing a little formaldehyde and a substantial amount of nitrogen.

The in vivo data indicate that α-hydroxylation is the principal pathway for NDMA metabolism in the intact organism. While it does not appear to be as high as the 90% found earlier by Magee, Holsman and Halliday (Magee 1980), it is likely to be the path which produces the majority of reactive metabolites. It is tempting to speculate that the reason for the at least two-fold increase in the extent of α-hydroxylation in vivo, as compared to in vitro, is due to the fact that the in vitro experiments were carried out with liver homogenates, while the in vivo metabolism was due to all the organs of the entire animal. This argument, however, cannot be supported, for at least two reasons. The first is that the in vivo experiments were conducted with Sprague-Dawley rats, while the homogenates were prepared from Fischer 344 rats. Thus, the inter-strain variations may account for some of the difference. More importantly, sub-cellular fractions are not an ideal mirror of the situation in the intact organ or the intact cell. Cellular architecture must play an important role in the determination of partition between various metabolic channels. This was, in fact, found to be the case in the metabolite profile of 7,12-dimethylbenz[a]anthracene (Bigger et al. 1980).

The amount of nitrogen release from NMA in the intact animal was again about two-fold higher than that observed with liver homogenates. NMA is an esophageal carcinogen (Druckrey et al. 1967). It is, however, metabolized significantly in the liver. This raises the yet unanswered question as to whether a reactive metabolite, formed in the liver, can be transported to distal sites, where its reactions with particularly sensitive cells may lead to tumor initiation. The present data do not provide a direct answer to this important question but they do indicate that a potentially reactive metabolite is formed in the liver, however no information is available on whether it gets out of the liver.

The Nature of Reactive Metabolites from Nitrosamines

It has been assumed widely that metabolism of nitrosamines leads to electrophilic, alkylating intermediates which interact with DNA and other cellular nucleophiles. In the case of dialkylnitrosamines, alkylation of DNA has been established for NDMA (Swann and Magee 1968), NDEA (Ross et al. 1971) and dipropylnitrosamine (Park et al. 1980). The originally proposed alkylating intermediate was the diazoalkane (Schoental 1960), formed by C-deprotonation of one of the unstable intermediates indicated in Fig. 1. However, the work of Lijinsky and his coworkers on NDMA (Lijinsky et al. 1968) and NDEA (Ross et al. 1971) has shown that the intact methyl group and ethyl group were transfered to the RNA and DNA, isolated from the livers of rats treated in vivo with the deuterated nitrosamines. These data supported the notion that an alkyldiazonium ion was the alkylating species. Theoretical support for this came from the work of Andreozzi et al. (1980), who, on the basis of semiempirical MINDO 3 calculations, concluded that the dissociation of the diazohydroxide to the diazonium ion was more favorable energetically than the dissociation to the diazoalkane. Unfortunately, these types of calculations only considered unimolecular dissociations in absence of solvent, hence, they are not particularly useful in describing the real-life situation. Another theoretical calculation on the methyldiazonium ion (Demontis et al. 1981) indicated the profound importance of solvation on that ion's stability. The experimental results of Lijinsky et al. 1968 however, provide a firm basis for the notion that the reactive intermediate in the case of NDMA and NDEA was the diazonium ion. However, the energy differences between the pathways leading to the diazonium ion and the

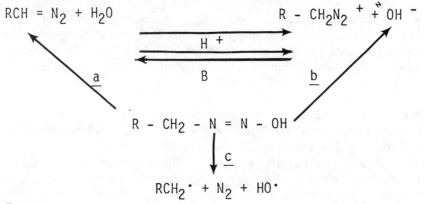

Figure 2
Modes of decomposition of alkyldiazohydroxides

diazoalkane are not large (for a discussion of this problem see: McGarrity [1978] and Hegarty [1978]). Consider the scheme shown in Figure 2. It is generally assumed that the initial product of dealkylation of dialkylnitrosamines is the diazohydroxide (as shown in Fig. 1). The present data strongly support the notion that alkylation of nucleic acids proceeds through the alkyldiazonium ion. This would suggest that the diazohydroxide dissociates via path b, (Fig. 2). Lijinsky's data also suggest reaction through path b, rather than path a, followed by protonation of the diazoalkane. However, one must note that path a, leading to the diazoalkane, would be subject to a significant isotope effect when the hydrogens are substituted by deuterium. This isotope effect would not exist for path b, except for a much smaller secondary isotope effect. Thus, the presence of deuterium in the substrate may have predetermined the path of the reaction. At the present time there is no compelling evidence to support the diazoalkane intermediate in the metabolism of simple dialkylnitrosamines. However, the alkyldiazonium ion is not a stable entity and therefore must be formed close to its ultimate reaction site. An elegant study by McGarrity and Smyth (1980) established that the half-life of the methyldiazonium ion in a tetrahydrofuran-water mixture was about 0.4 seconds. Thus, the attractiveness of a diazoalkane intermediate, which can then be protonated to the diazonium ion, stems from the fact that it is a relatively stable species which can be transported intact in a neutral environment. Diazomethane is protonated very rapidly; the second order rate constant for the reaction is 4×10^8 M^{-1} sec^{-1} (McGarrity and Smyth 1980). At neutral or slightly alkaline pHs, however, diazomethane has a relatively long life.

The decomposition of the alkyldiazohydroxide by path a or path b is dictated by a number of factors. Generally, factors which stabilize carbonium ions will tend to favor decomposition by path b, that is to the diazonium ion (or carbonium ion directly). Thus, methyldiazohydroxide may either decompose by one path or the other, but isopropyldiazohydroxide would tend to decompose to the isopropyl cation. By the same token, factors which destabilize the carbonium ion also tend to stabilize the diazoalkane (path a). One fascinating case of such a situation would be the diazohydroxide formed from the demethylation of methyl(2-oxopropyl)nitrosamine. This diazohydroxide would be expected to decompose via path a.

$$CH_3 - \overset{\overset{O}{\|}}{C} - CH_2 - N(NO)CH_3 \rightarrow CH_3 - \overset{\overset{O}{\|}}{C} - CH_2 - N = N - OH \rightarrow CH_3 - \overset{\overset{O}{\|}}{C} - CH = N_2$$

Finally, Figure 2 also indicates a third path of decomposition, namely one that involves the formation of free radical intermediates (path c). This is considered to be unlikely in most cases, because such reactions generally involve appreciable activation energies. It might be pointed out, however, that factors which tend to stabilize carbonium ion intermediates also stabilize the corresponding radicals. Moreover, homolytic dissociation may be aided sometimes by electron transfer processes.

Several reactive intermediates also can be envisioned from nitrosamines such as NMA, which give rise to aryldiazonium ions. The scheme shown in Figure 3 indicates some of the possibilities. This is by no means an exhaustive listing of possible reactions of aryldiazonium ions. These reactions are those that might occur in a biological system (for a complete discussion see Patai [1978]). While space limitations do not permit a complete discussion of these reactions, it would be worth pointing out that all of them are possible, even probable, reactions of metabolically formed aryldiazonium ions. Path e, which involves the coupling of the diazonium ion with an appropriate nucleophile provides for

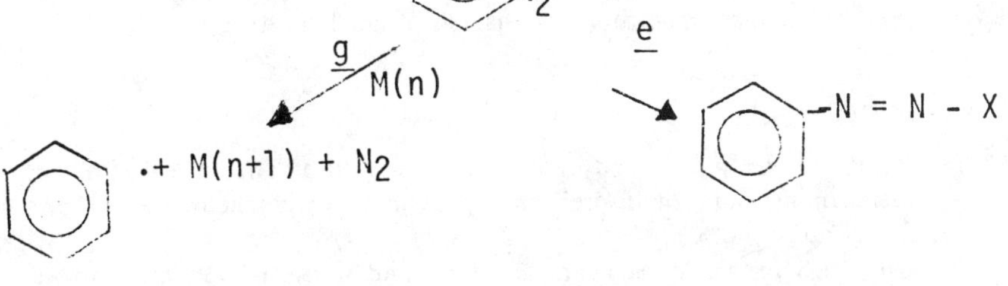

Figure 4
Some reactions of aryldiazonium ions with nucleophiles and low-valent metal ions

a covalent product which may prevent nitrogen release. Alternatively, path *e* may provide a route for the formation of a metastable, covalent product, which could be transported. For example, the reaction of aryldiazonium ions with thiophenolates is well known (Price and Tsanawski 1963). Such an adduct with a thiol group of a serum albumin could provide a transportable form of the diazonium ion. It is also possible that various substances, capable of undergoing electron transfer reactions, could generate the highly reactive aryl radicals (path *f*). A special, particularly attractive, electron transfer reaction of diazonium ions, is analogous to the well known Gomberg-Bachmann reaction (path *g*). The reactivity of diazonium ions with nucleic acid bases is not well understood, but some reactions of adenine, adenosine and adenylic acid (Chin et al. 1981) and guanine, guanosine, and guanylic acid (Hung and Stock 1982) have been examined recently.

SUMMARY

The purpose of the foregoing discussion was to reemphasize that even if we know something about the gross metabolism of nitrosamines, we know very little about the nature and the fate of the various possible reactive intermediates formed by that metabolism. Subtle structural differences may give entirely different reactivity patterns. Some of the reactive metabolites may be quasi-stable. These could then be transported away from the site of the initial metabolism, only to wreak havoc at distant sites.

Finally, it has to be pointed out that α-hydroxylation may not be a unique mode of nitrosamine activation. It is well known that hydroxylation of nitrosamines is not a particularly selective reaction. We have shown, for example, that β-hydroxylation, followed by sulfate conjugation, leads to electrophilic intermediates (Michejda et al. 1981).

ACKNOWLEDGMENTS

This work was supported in part by Contract No. NO1-CO-75380 and also by Grant No. CA-23451 with the National Cancer Institute, NIH, Bethesda, Maryland 20205. We are very grateful to Dr. Gary A. McClusky for his effort in the development of the mass spectrometric analysis of labeled nitrogen.

REFERENCES

Andreozzi, P., G. Klopman, and A.J. Hopfinger. 1980. Theoretical study of *N*-nitrosamines and their presumed proximate carcinogens. *Cancer Biochem. Biophys.* **4**:209.

Appel, K.E., D. Schrenk, M. Schwarz, B. Mahr, and W. Kunz. 1980. Denitrosation of *N*-nitrosomorpholine by liver microsomes: Possible role of cytochrome P450, *Cancer Lett.* **9**:13.

Bigger, C.A.H., J.E. Tomaszewski, A. Dipple, and R.S. Lake. 1980. Limitations of metabolic activation systems used with *in vitro* test for carcinogens. *Science* **209**:503.

Chen, C.B., G.D. McCoy, S.S. Hecht, D. Hoffmann, and E.L. Wynder. 1978. High pressure liquid chromatographic assay for α-hydroxylation of *N*-nitrosopyrrolidine by isolated rat liver microsomes. *Cancer Res.* **38**:3812.

Chin, A., M-H. Hung, and L.M. Stock. 1981. Reactions of benzenediazonium ions with adenine and its derivatives. *J. Org. Chem.* **46**:2203.

Cottrell, R.C., B.G. Lake, J.C. Phillips, and S.D. Gangolli. 1977. The hepatic metabolism of ^{15}N-labelled dimethylnitrosamine in the rat. *Biochem. Pharmacol.* **26**:809.

Demontis, P., R. Ercoli, A. Gamba, G.P. Suffritti, and M. Simonetta. 1981. A theoretical investigation of the energy and structure of ion-molecule pairs in polar solvents. Part 2. Methanediazonium cation in water. *J. Chem. Soc., Perkin Trans. II* 488.

Druckrey, H., R. Preussmann, S. Ivankovic, and D. Schmahl. 1967. Organotrope carcinogene wirkungen bei 65 verschiedenen *n*-nitrosoverbindungen an d-bd-ratten. *Z. Krebsforsch.* **69**:103.

Grilli, S. and G. Prodi. 1975. Identification of dimethylnitrosamine metabolites *in vitro. Gann.* **66**:473.

Hecht, S.S., L.B. Chen, and D. Hoffmann. 1978. Evidence for metabolic α-hydroxylation of *N*-nitrosopyrrolidine. *Cancer Res.* **38**:215.

Hecht, S.S., C.B. Chen, G.C. McCoy, and D. Hoffmann. 1979. α-Hydroxylation of *N*-nitrosopyrrolidine and *N'*-nitrosonornicotine by human liver microsomes. *Cancer Lett.* **8**:35.

Hecker, L.I., J.G. Farrelly, J.H. Smith, J.E. Saavedra, and P.A. Lyon. 1979. Metabolism of the liver carcinogen *N*-nitrosopyrrolidine by rat liver microsomes. *Cancer Res.* **39**:2679.

Hegarty, A.F. 1978. Kinetics and mechanisms of reactions involving diazonium and diazo groups, in *The Chemistry of Diazonium and Diazo Groups*, Part 2 (S. Patai, ed.) p. 511. John Wiley and Sons, New York.

Hung, M.-H. and L.M. Stock. 1982. Reactions of benzenediazonium ions with guanine and its derivatives. *J. Org. Chem.* **47**:448.

Keefer, L.K., W. Lijinsky, and H. Garcia. 1973. Deuterium isotope effect on the carcinogenicity of dimethylnitrosamine in rat liver. *J. Natl. Cancer Inst.* **51**:299.

Kroeger-Koepke, M.B. and C.J. Michejda. 1979. Evidence for several demethylase enzymes in the oxidation of dimethylnitrosamine and phenylmethylnitrosamine by rat liver fractions. *Cancer Res.* **39**:1587.

Kroeger-Koepke, M.B., S.R. Koepke, G.A. McClusky, P.N. Magee, and C.J. Michejda. 1981. α-Hydroxylation pathway in the *in vitro* metabolism of carcinogenic nitrosamines: *N*-nitrosodimethylamine and *N*-nitroso-*N*-methylaniline. *Proc. Natl. Acad. Sci. U.S.A.* **78**:6487.

Krüger, F.W., B. Bertram, and G. Eisenbrand. 1976. Metabolism of nitrosamines *in vivo*. V. Investigation on $^{14}CO_2$ exhalation, liver RNA labelling and isolation of two metabolites from urine after administraton of [2,5-^{14}C-]-dinitrosopiperazine to rats. *Z. Krebsforsch.* **85**:125.

Leung, K.H., K.K. Park, and M.C. Archer. 1978. α-Hydroxylation of the metabolism of N-nitrosopiperidine by rat liver microsomes: Formation of 5-hydroxypentanal. *Res. Commun. Chem. Pathol. Pharmacol.* **19**:201.

Lijinsky, W., J. Loo, and A.E. Ross. 1968. Mechanism of alkylation of nucleic acids by nitrosodimethylamine. *Nature* **218**:1174.

Lijinsky, W., H.W. Taylor, and L.K. Keefer. 1976. Reduction of rat liver carcinogenicity of 4-nitrosomorpholine by α-deuterium substitution. *J. Natl. Cancer Inst.* **57**:1311.

Magee, P.N. 1980. Metabolism of nitrosamines: An overview. In *Microsomes, Drug Oxidations and Chemical Carcinogenesis*, Vol. 2, p. 1081. Academic Press, New York.

McGarrity, J.F. 1978. Basicity, acidity and hydrogen bonding, in *The Chemistry of Diazonium and Diazo Groups*, Part 1 (S. Patai, ed.) p. 179. John Wiley and Sons, New York.

McGarrity, J.F. and T. Smyth. 1980. Hydrolysis of diazomethane—kinetics and mechanism. *J. Am. Chem. Soc.* **102**:7303.

Michejda, C.J., M.B. Kroeger-Koepke, S.R. Koepke, and D.H. Sieh. 1981. Activation of nitrosamines to biological alkylating agents, in *N-Nitroso Compounds*. ACS Symposium Series (eds. R.A. Scanlan and S.R. Tannenbaum), No. 174, p. 3. American Chemical Society, Washington.

Milstein, S. and J.B. Guttenplan. 1979. Near quantitative production of molecular nitrogen from metabolism of dimethylnitrosamine. *Biochem. Biophys. Res. Commun.* **87**:337.

Mochizuki, M., T. Anjo, and M. Okada. 1980. Isolation and characterization of N-alkyl-(N-hydroxymethyl)nitrosamines from N-alkyl-N-(hydroperoxymethyl)-nitrosamines by deoxygenation. *Tetrahedron Lett.* 3693:

Murray, A. and D.L. Williams. 1958. *Organic Syntheses with Isotopes, Part I*, p. 583. Interscience, New York.

Nash, T. 1953. The colorometric estimation of formaldehyde by means of the Hantzsch Reaction. *Biochem. J.* **55**:416.

Park, K.K., MC. Archer, and J.S. Wishnok. 1980. Alkylation of nucleic acids by N-nitrosodi-n-propylamine: Evidence that carbonium ions are not significantly involved. *Chem. Biol. Interact.* **29**:139.

Patai, S. (Ed.). 1978. *Chemistry of Diazonium and Diazo Groups*, Parts 1 and 2, Chapters 6, 8, 12, 13, 14, John Wiley and Sons, New York.

Price, C.C. and S. Tsanawski. 1963. Polycondensation of mercaptobenzenediazonium salts. *J. Org. Chem.* **28**:1867.

Ross, A.E., L. Keefer, and W. Lijinsky. 1971. Alkylation of nucleic acids of rat liver and lung by deuterated N-nitrosodiethylamine *in vivo*. *J. Natl. Cancer Inst.* **47**:789.

Schoental, R. 1960. Carcinogenic action of diazomethane and of N-nitroso-N-methylurethane. *Nature* (Lond.) **188**:420.

Swann, P.F. and P.N. Magee. 1968. Nitrosamine-induced carcinogenesis: The alkylation of nucleic acids of the rat by N-methyl-N-nitrosourea, dimethylnitrosamine, dimethylsulphate and methylmethanesulfonate. *Biochem. J.* **110**:39.

COMMENTS

PREUSSMANN: Could your data on nitrogen formation be confounded by the reaction of nitrite to form nitrogen? Nitrite might be formed in vivo by enzymatic deamination. So your conclusion that the amount of nitrogen evolution as an indicator of the α-hydroxylation pathway, may be somewhat compromised.

MICHEJDA: Well, if nitrite were formed by denitrosation I think one would then expect to get mixed nitrogen and we don't. In fact, we looked for it, but did not get mixed nitrogen.

YANG: I have some data on that. I think the nitrite formation is also derived from α-oxidation. It is parallel to cytochrome P450-dependent reaction. With NDMA it accounts for about 2-3%. With this compound, methylphenylnitrosamine it is about 5%.

MICHEJDA: It may be a difference in protocols, because we would have seen that. In this experiment, the MS analysis is done very precisely. This would demand the formation of mixed nitrogen, N^{15}-N^{14}. Isotopically mixed nitrogen would be formed because nitrite only has one nitrogen, and another nitrogen, which would be unlabeled, would have to be found.

YANG: In my case you get a methylamine and nitrite. I think that is the pathway. You break the nitrogen bond.

MICHEJDA: Perhaps you are correct. If Dr. Yang is forming methylamine from the nitrosamine, then my theory is incorrect. I cannot tell if the methylamine and the nitrite would find each other. Dr. Preussmann may have found something very important. This experiment is a kind of a unidimensional experiment since we are only looking at the nitrogen evolution. It is hard to discuss other possible pathways in metabolism. For example, with NMA we know that other things occur, but we only get a small amount of nitrogen. So one would be led to a rather false conclusion, that α-hydroxylation is relatively unimportant here. Only 20% of this nitrosamine releases its nitrogen, but in fact I think that most of it is metabolized by demethylation, except that most of the nitrogen is not lost.

ARCHER: In some of the work I am going to describe we have looked at least at the in vitro metabolism of nitrosomethylbenzylamine, and we find no evidence for denitrosation. We looked quite hard for the methylbenzylamine and didn't find it. I think we would have found it had it been there.

YANG: How about nitrite?

ARCHER: We didn't look for nitrite.

LIJINSKY: Chris, this probably isn't a fair question, but do you have any reflections from your work on why NMA is an esophageal carcinogen?

MICHEJDA: We are very interested in that particular problem. If I knew why NMA was an esophageal carcinogen, I would know a great deal about how chemicals cause cancer. Unfortunately, I don't know yet.

NMA is an esophageal carcinogen, not a liver carcinogen, yet it is metabolized very rapidly in the liver.

TANNENBAUM: Well, so is methylbenznitrosamine.

MICHEJDA: It seems to me that the active metabolite from NMA might actually be formed in the liver and then transported out. In fact, we are at present doing an experiment to try to demonstrate this.

LIJINSKY: The difference between methylbenzyl and methylphenyl is that methylphenyl cannot form a methylating agent. That is why I asked my original question.

TANNENBAUM: One of the really interesting things that comes out of your work, which hasn't been discussed at all, is the big difference between the in vitro and the in vivo results. For example, if you really believe those numbers, then you have to place a lot of doubt upon whether or not the experiments that are being done in vitro are really telling us what we want to know.

MICHEJDA: Absolutely. I think that is a very important conclusion to draw. I was hoping that I would have our data on hepatocytes available for this meeting, but we haven't completed the experiment yet. That would tell us whether the intact cell will reproduce the in vivo situation a little bit better.

CONNEY: I am also very struck by the difference between the in vitro and the in vivo experiments. You have much less nitrogen formation in the in vitro experiments as compared to the in vivo experiments. Also in the in vivo experiments you can't account for everything by nitrogen formation when you compare it with NMU. I assume that the control animal is a normal animal.

MICHEJDA: Yes.

CONNEY: Did you try to modulate metabolism by any modulators (either inducers or inhibitors) to see if you would alter the amount of nitrogen formation?

MICHEJDA: No we have not done this. These were uninduced animals. You are absolutely correct, it needs to be done. This is definitely, as Steve points out, one of the crucial questions that one needs to ask. But it is not unusual. I hasten to add that in the polycyclic aromatic hydrocarbon field, the pattern of metabolites that one gets with subcellular fractions is quite different from what you get in the intact cell.

CONNEY: There are explanations for that, though, as certainly an explanation must exist for the nitrosamines. One has to try to figure out explanations for these differences.

MICHEJDA: That is right. They are simply not available yet.

PEGG: In your in vitro experiments, you have a very major analytical problem, because an extremely small amount of your nitrosamine is being metabolized. That therefore leads me to be somewhat skeptical that you could actually measure the difference between 100% and 97% with the precision which would enable you to make the calculation. It would be much nicer if you could repeat that under conditions where most of the nitrosamine went away.

MICHEJDA: Unfortunately, unless you can get me an S9 mix that is exceedingly active, I don't think that can be done. Those of you who have worked with these subcellular fractions know that the degree of metabolism that one gets out of that is not very large. You are looking at small differences between two rather large numbers.

I am fairly confident of these results. There is some scatter, and there is a sizeable error, but I think that the numbers are real.

On the Mode of Action of *N*-Nitrosomethylbenzylamine, an Esophageal Carcinogen in the Rat

MICHAEL C. ARCHER AND GEORGE E. LABUC
Department of Medical Biophysics
University of Toronto
Ontario Cancer Institute
500 Sherbourne Street
Toronto M4X 1K9, Canada

A primary target for many carcinogenic nitrosamines, particularly unsymmetrical dialkylnitrosamines, is the rat esophagus (Druckrey et al. 1967; Magee and Barnes 1967). These nitrosamines induce high incidences of basal cell and squamous cell tumors, independent of the route of administration of the carcinogen. There is some evidence that nitrosamines may be causative factors of human esophageal cancer in certain parts of the world, particularly China (Yang 1980). Few other chemicals apart from nitrosamines and nitrosamides have been reported to induce esophageal tumors in experimental animals (Pozharisski 1973; Ito 1981). Little is known, however, about the mechanism of this remarkable sensitivity of the rat esophagus to nitrosamines.

In order to study the mode of action of nitrosamines as esophageal carcinogens, we chose initially to compare the metabolism of nitrosomethylbenzylamine (NMBzA) and nitrosodimethylamine (NDMA) in both target and nontarget tissues. NMBzA is a potent esophageal carcinogen in the rat that produces no liver tumors (Druckrey et al. 1967), while NDMA is a potent hepatocarcinogen that produces no esophageal tumors (Druckrey et al. 1967; Magee and Barnes 1967). Metabolic activation of NMBzA is expected to yield formaldehyde and a benzylating agent from hydroxylation at the methyl carbon, or benzaldehyde and a methylating agent from hydroxylation at the benzylic position (Lai and Arcos 1980). Activation of NDMA, of course, is well known to yield formaldehyde and a methylating agent.

Since our metabolic studies showed that rat liver microsomes extensively metabolize NMBzA to yield both methylating and benzylating agents, we decided to investigate the ability of this nitrosamine to initiate neoplasia in the liver. More detailed accounts of these studies will appear elsewhere (Labuc and Archer 1982a,b).

METHODS

Male Sprague-Dawley rats, 21-23 days old, were maintained on Teklad 6% fat rat-mouse diet ad lib for 5-10 days prior to sacrifice by a blow to the head.

Esophageal mucosa was prepared from the excised organ by physically shearing the outer muscle and submucosa layers away from the mucosa. Histological examination showed that the resulting mucosa was intact and free from contamination by muscle or submucosa. Mucosae from 7-10 rats were slit longitudinally, cut into small pieces, combined, and homogenized in 9 volumes of buffer (1.15% KCl, 50 mM Tris-HCl, pH 7.4) with 30 passes of a motor-driven Duall all-glass homogenizer. After removal of the 9000 g pellet, the supernatant was centrifuged at 100,000 g for 60 min. The resulting microsomal pellet was resuspended in buffer to a final concentration of 5 mg protein/ml. A yield of about 4.5 mg microsomal protein/g mucosa was obtained. Liver microsomes were prepared by standard procedures.

Incubation mixtures contained 5 mM substrate (NMBzA; [methyl-C^{14}]-NMBzA, 0.33 mCi/mmole; [methylene-C^{14}]-NMBzA, 0.33 mCi/mmol; or [methyl-C^{14}]-NDMA, 0.33 mCi/mmole), 20 mM semicarbazide, 2 mM NADP$^+$, 10 mM glucose-6-phosphate (G-6-P), 2 units/ml G-6-P dehydrogenase, 10 mM MgCl$_2$, 50 mM Tris (pH 7.40), and 0.1 ml of microsomal suspension about 0.5 mg protein), in a final volume of 0.6 ml. Samples were incubated at 37° under air with shaking for 20 minutes (NMBzA) or 40 minutes (NDMA). Reaction rates were linear with respect to both incubation time and protein concentration. Samples were deproteinized by addition of 0.3 ml of 20% ZnSO$_4$ and 0.3 ml saturated Ba(OH)$_2$ solution and the supernatants were stored at -20° overnight prior to analysis to minimize nonenzymatic formation of benzaldehyde. Benzaldehyde semicarbazone, benzyl alcohol, and benzoic acid were analyzed by liquid chromatography on a C18-μBondapak column eluted with 15% methanol/3% acetic acid, pH 4.2, at a flow rate of 2 ml/min. Detection was at 260 nm. The identities of benzyl alcohol and benzaldehyde semicarbazone were confirmed by gas chromatography-mass spectrometry (GC/MS). Free benzaldehyde was liberated from the semicarbazone by treatment with HNO$_2$ (Goldschmidt and Veer 1946). C^{14}-formaldehyde formed from [methyl-C^{14}]-NMBzA or -NDMA was analyzed as the dimedone derivative (Paik and Kim 1974). Controls were mixtures incubated at 37° in the absence of tissue or complete mixtures incubated at 0°. Cytochrome P450 was determined spectrophotometrically using dithionite as reducing agent (Jakobsson and Cinti 1973).

In order to compare the tumor initiating activities of NDMA and NMBzA, two assays were used. First, in a modification of the assay of Tsuda et al. (1980), rats maintained on a Bio-Serv semisynthetic high protein diet were given a single i.p. dose of solvent (25% dimethylsulfoxide in 0.9%-NaCl, 0.2 ml/80 g body weight), NDMA (33.5 μmol/kg or 115 μmol/kg), NMBzA (33.5 μmol/kg or nitrosomethylamylamine (NMAmA) (115 μmol/kg) 18 hours after partial hepatectomy (ph). After 3 weeks, groups of 4 rats per cage were given the diet suplemented with 0.04% acetoaminofluorene (AAF) by a modified pair-feeding regimen. Each group of rats received identical quantities of diet. The amount corresponded to the lowest amount consumed by any group the previous day (invariably the NMBzA-treated rats). After 1 week on the AAF diet, each rat was given a single intragastric dose of CCl_4 in corn oil (1:1; 4.0 ml/kg). Two weeks later, the rats were returned to the basal diet ad libitum for 1 week then sacrificed. Three slices from each liver (1.5-3 cm^2) were fixed in acetone at 4°, then processed for γ-glutamyltranspeptidase (GGT) staining (Rutenburg et al. 1969; Ogawa et al. 1980).

The second assay was a modification of the method of Pitot et al. (1978). Rats, maintained on Teklad diet, were given a single i.p. dose of solvent as before, NDMA, nitrosodiethylamine (NDEA), or NMBzA (all at 33.5 µmol/kg) 18 hours after ph or sham hepatectomy (sh). After 4 weeks, the drinking water was supplemented with sodium phenobarbital. The concentration of phenobarbital was maintained throughout at 0.05% for control, NDMA- and NDEA-treated rats but was continually adjusted between 0.05% and 0.075% for NMBzA-treated groups such that the intake was the same for all rats. The experiment was terminated 26 weeks after beginning the phenobarbital treatment, and liver slices were processed for GGT staining as before. Treated groups were compared with control groups in the assays by the Behrens-Fisher test (Snedecor and Cochran 1967), since population variances were significantly different.

RESULTS AND DISCUSSION

NMBzA was metabolized to benzaldehyde and formaldehyde by microsomes from either liver or esophageal mucosa (Table 1). Benzyl alcohol was formed with liver microsomes but not with esophageal microsomes. We showed, however, that a large portion of the benzyl alcohol produced with liver microsomes came from the reduction of benzaldehyde (0.73 nmol/min/mg protein at a benzaldehyde concentration of 16.7 µM). Inclusion of 20 mM semicarbazide in the incubation mixtures minimized benzaldehyde reduction without altering nitrosamine metabolism. Mucosal microsomes lacked benzaldehyde reductase activity. There was no oxidation of benzaldehyde to benzoic acid in either preparation. Formaldehyde was stable with both tissues. Radioactivity profiles

Table 1
NMBzA and NDMA Metabolism by Microsomes from Rat Liver and Esophageal Mucosa

Substrate	Metabolite	Hepatic microsomes (nmol/min/mg protein)	Mucosal microsomes (nmol/min/mg protein)
NMBzA	Benzaldehyde	0.978 ± 0.108[a] (4)[b]	0.549 ± 0.055 (18)
	Benzyl alcohol	2.0 ± 0.3 (4)	≤ 0.1
	Formaldehyde	0.289 ± 0.087 (4)	0.005 ± 0.001 (6)
NDMA	Formaldehyde	0.871 ± 0.102 (4)	≤ 0.03

(Reprinted with permission from Labuc and Archer 1982a)
[a] Mean ± S.E.M.
[b] Number of replicate assays.

of the chromatograms revealed the absence of metabolites of $[C^{14}$-methyl]- or $[C^{14}$-methylene]-NMBzA other than those described above, in either hepatic or mucosal incubations. NDMA was extensively metabolized to formaldehyde by hepatic microsomes as expected, but microsomes prepared from esophageal mucosa lacked detectable NDMA demethylase activity (Table 1).

The relative rates of metabolism of NMBzA and NDMA by microsomes from liver and esophageal mucosa are shown in Figure 1 (the rate of formation of benzaldehyde has been corrected for the benzaldehyde that is lost by reduction to benzyl alcohol). It is clear that rat esophageal mucosa contains an enzyme which can metabolize the esophageal carcinogen NMBzA at a high rate, but the hepatocarcinogen NDMA is a poor substrate for this enzyme. It is also clear that whereas hepatic microsomes oxidize NMBzA at the benzylic carbon 10 times faster than the methyl carbon, this differential was 100-fold in the case of mucosal metabolism. A high rate of metabolism of NMBzA to benzaldehyde and absence of metabolism to formaldehyde has been reported by Schweinsberg and Kouros (1979) for microsomes prepared from whole rat esophagus. These workers did not detect hepatic metabolism of NMBzA to formaldehyde. It should be noted, however, that Schweinsberg and Kouros measured formaldehyde by the Nash colorimetric method which is much less sensitive than the dimedone assay; they did not use an aldehyde trapping agent, nor did they measure formation of benzyl alcohol.

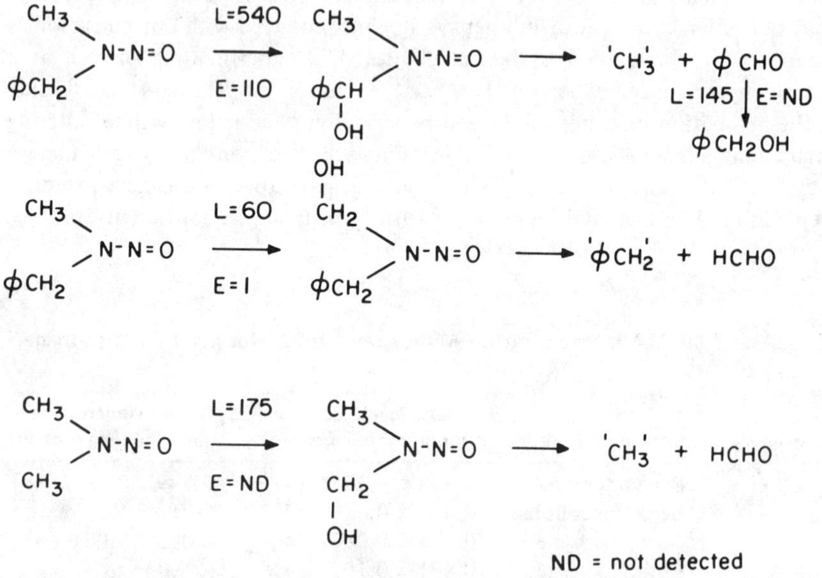

Figure 1
Relative rates of metabolism of NMBzA and NDMA by microsomes from liver (L) and esophageal mucosa (E).

From our results we would predict that since esophageal mucosa metabolizes NMBzA to benzaldehyde at approximately 100 times the rate of metabolism to formaldehyde, formation of a methylating intermediate would occur similarly at a 100-fold faster rate than formation of a benzylating intermediate. This prediction is born out by studies by Hodgson et al. (1980) in which they showed that esophageal DNA was methylated following a single i.v. dose of NMBzA whereas benzylation of DNA was undetectable.

We have examined the characteristics of the metabolizing system of the mucosa in some detail (Labuc and Archer 1982a). Briefly, esophageal metabolism of NMBzA was exclusively located in the mucosa, preferentially in the microsomal faction, was NADPH-dependent, and was inhibited by CO and SKF5-25-A. Thus the metabolism of NMBzA within the esophageal mucosa appears to involve a typical cytochrome P450 pathway. Using the method of Jakobsson and Cinti (1973) in which microsomes are preincubated with succinate to remove mitochondrial interference, reduced CO-difference spectroscopy revealed a typical cytochrome P450 spectrum with a λmax at 450 nm. We estimated that the level of cytochrome P450 was about 15% of that detected in hepatic microsomes. Hepatic metabolism of NMBzA was inducible by phenobarbital pretreatment, whereas mucosal metabolism was not altered by either phenobarbital or 3-methylcholanthrene pretreatment.

Our results show that the difference in carcinogenic activity of NMBzA and NDMA in rat esophagus may be related to the capacity of this tissue to activate NMBzA at a high rate, and its inability to activate NDMA. Our results also suggest, however, that the difference in carcinogenic activities of NMBzA and NDMA in the liver is not related to differences in the metabolic activation of the two nitrosamines in this tissue. This conclusion is corroborated by studies that have shown that both nitrosamines methylate DNA to similar extents in liver slices, and produce the same spectrum of methylated adducts (Pegg 1977; Fong et al. 1979; Hodgson et al. 1980). Other studies have shown that the tissue specificity of NDMA and NMBzA is not caused by preferential uptake into their respective target organs (Magee 1956; Johansson and Tjälve 1978; Iizuka et al. 1978; Kraft and Tannenbaum 1980; Hodgson et al. 1980). Since the liver is a major tissue for uptake of NMBzA and since the nitrosamine is rapidly metabolized and methylates DNA in the liver, we decided to determine whether NMBzA can initiate neoplasia in the liver using the established assays of Pitot et al. (1978) and Tsuda et al. (1980).

We considered that it was essential to administer NMBzA at the same molar dose that would produce a positive response in the initiation assays by the control hepatocarcinogen, NDMA. Although a dose of 5 mg (33.5 μmol)/kg administered 18 hours post-ph killed about half of the rats within 3-4 days, this level of lethality was considered to be acceptable for the purposes of the initiation assays. A lower dose would have been more desirable, but it was precluded by the uncertainty of obtaining a positive result with NDMA even at 33.5 μmol/kg. In view of the necessity to use low doses, we included NDEA as a second

Table 2
Initiation Assay—AAF/CCl₄ Selection

Treatment (μmol/kg)		Number of GGT positive (foci/cm² liver)
Control		0.7 ± 0.3^a
NDMA	(33.5)	14.6 ± 4.1^b
NDMA	(115)	44.3 ± 14.2^b
NMBzA	(33.5)	1.0 ± 0.4
NMAmA	(115)	2.1 ± 0.5

[a] Mean ± S.E.M.
[b] Significantly different from control, $p < 0.05$.

positive control in the initiation assay using phenobarbital selection (Pitot et al. 1978), and NMAmA as an additional test compound in the assay using AAF/CCl₄ selection (Tsuda et al. 1980). NMAmA, like NMBzA, induces esophageal but not hepatic tumors in the rat (Druckrey et al. 1967), but is less toxic than NMBzA, and was administered at a higher dose (15 mg (115 μmol)/kg) that resulted in no deaths from acute toxicity.

For the AAF/CCl₄ selection assay, two modifications of the original protocol of Tsuda et al. (1980) were made. First, in order to increase the recovery of NMBzA-treated rats, the interval between nitrosamine administration and commencement of AAF-feeding was lengthened from 2 weeks to 3 weeks. Alteration of the interval between initiation and selection has been shown to have no effect on the number of preneoplastic foci detected (Solt et al. 1980). Second, in order to ensure that all rats consumed an equal quantity of AAF each day, they were given a diet containing 0.04% AAF using a modified pair-feeding regimen. The rats consumed an average of 7 g/rat/day, which is similar to the quantity of AAF consumed by normal rats given free access to diet containing 0.02% AAF.

The results of this assay are shown in Table 2. It is clear that NDMA increased the number of GGT positive foci above background at both dose levels. Neither NMBzA nor NMAmA, however, significantly increased the number of foci.

For the phenobarbital selection assay of Pitot et al. (1978), the concentration of phenobarbital in the drinking water was continually adjusted so that on average, all rats ingested the same amounts of phenobarbital throughout the entire period. Although most NMBzA rats gained weight at a lower rate than the other groups, the liver/body weight ratios at time of sacrifice were virtually identical in all groups.

The results of this assay are shown in Table 3. Again it is clear that the hepatocarcinogens NDMA and NDEA increased the number of GGT positive foci in the livers by 3- to 5-fold. Although the number of foci in the NDMA and NDEA treated animals in the ph group was greater than the sh group, NDMA

Table 3
Initiation Assay—Phenobarbital Selection

Treatment[a]		Number of GGT positive foci/cm^2 liver
Partial hepatectomy	Control	1.1 ± 0.3[b]
	NDMA	4.0 ± 0.8[c]
	NDEA	3.8 ± 0.5[c]
	NMBzA	0.6 ± 0.1
Sham hepatectomy	Control	0.4 ± 0.1
	NDMA	1.2 ± 0.2[c]
	NDEA	2.2 ± 0.4[c]
	NMBzA	0.8 ± 0.2

[a]All compounds administered at 33.5 μmol/kg.
[b]Mean $\pm$ S.E.M.
[c]Significantly different from control, $p < 0.05$

and NDEA did increase the number of foci in the sh group compared to the control for that group. This positive result was anticipated since the rats used in this experiment were young (28-30 days) and hepatocyte division would therefore be occurring to some extent. As before, NMBzA did not significantly increase the number of foci above background in either the sh or the ph groups.

One reason why NMBzA gave a negative result in these assays while NDMA gave a positive result could have been that metabolism of the two nitrosamines was altered differentially in regenerating liver so that metabolism of NDMA proceeded at a significantly faster rate than that of NMBzA. When microsomes isolated from rats 18 hours following ph were used to compare metabolism of NMBzA and NDMA, however, their capacity to metabolize both nitrosamines was somewhat lower than microsomes from intact liver, but the decrease in activity was similar for both compounds (Labuc and Archer 1982b). Another reason for the negative result with NMBzA could have been that NMBzA was a more potent inhibitor than NDMA of the first wave of DNA synthesis following ph. However we have shown that neither NDMA nor NMBzA inhibit DNA synthesis in vivo in the regenerating liver (Labuc and Archer 1982b).

Our results indicate that in contrast to NDMA and NDEA, NMBzA, and NMAmA lack tumor initiating activity in rat liver. In view of previous work on the distribution, metabolism, and methylating ability of NMBzA, this result was unexpected. There are, however, a number of possible explanations for the inability of NMBzA to initiate neoplasia in the liver. NDMA and NMBzA produce the same spectrum of methylated bases in DNA, but there may be quantitative differences in the relative abundance of the various adducts. Such a result has been suggested in experiments with liver slices (Fong et al. 1979). There may also be differences in the relative distribution of methylated adducts or differences in their repair. Differences in abundance or distribution of DNA adducts would not be unreasonable to expect if, for example, the α-hydroxy-nitrosamine interacts with DNA prior to release of a methylating moiety as has been suggested (Park et al. 1980). Presence of a benzyl group would be expected to confer stricter steric requirements on such an interaction compared to a methyl group. Finally, NMBzA and NDMA may attack different cell populations within the liver, a suggestion that has been made to explain hepatic repair activity following pretreatment of rats with nitrosomethylurea and NDMA (Margison 1981).

CONCLUSIONS

Rat esophageal mucosa contains an enzyme which activates the esophageal carcinogen NMBzA at a high rate. NMBzA was also extensively activated by hepatic microsomes. The hepatocarcinogen NDMA, on the other hand, was extensively activated by hepatic microsomes, but not by esophageal microsomes. The esophageal enzyme may play a role in determining which compounds induce tumors in that organ. In contrast to the hapatocarcinogens NDMA and NDEA, the esophageal carcinogens NMBzA and NMAmA at equimolar doses lack tumor initiating activity in rat liver. Others have shown that NDMA and NMBzA methylate DNA to similar extents in liver slices (Fong et al. 1979) and produce the same spectrum of methylated adducts (Pegg et al. 1977; Fong et al. 1979; Hodgson et al. 1980). We may conclude therefore that while carcinogen activation and DNA modification per se may be necessary, they are not sufficient for initiation of neoplasia. Care must be exercised in the interpretation of data on the activity of nitrosamines in human tissues in terms of their potential for cancer induction.

ACKNOWLEDGMENTS

The authors thank Kwan Leung and Louis Marai for performing the gas chromatography-mass spectrometry, V. Eng for assistance with the surgical operations and Dr. E. Farber and G. Lee for helpful discussions. This work was supported by the Ontario Cancer Treatment and Research Foundation and Grant Number MT-7025 from the Medical Research Council of Canada.

REFERENCES

Druckrey, H., R. Preussmann, S. Ivankovic, and D. Schmähl. 1967. Organotrope carcinogene Wirkungen bei 65 verschiedenen N-Nitroso-Verbindungen an BD-Ratten. *Z. Krebsforsch.* **69**:103.

Fong, L.Y., H.J. Lin, and C.L. Lee. 1979. Methylation of DNA in target and nontarget organs of the rat with methylbenzylnitrosamine and dimethylnitrosamine. *Int. J. Cancer* **23**:679.

Goldschmidt, S.T. and W.L. Veer. 1946. A simple method for the fission of semicarbazone. *Recl. Trav. Chim. Pays-Bas* **65**:796.

Hodgson, R.M., M. Wiessler, and P. Kleihues. 1980. Preferential methylation of target organ DNA by the oesophageal carcinogen N-nitroso-methylbenzylamine. *Carcinogenesis* 1:861.

Iizuka, T., S. Ichimura, and T. Kawachi. 1978. Autoradiography and organ distribution of N-methyl-N-nitrosobenzylamine in rats. *Gann* 69:487.

Jakobsson, S.V. and D.L. Cinti. 1973. Studies on the cytochrome P-450-containing mono-oxygenase system in human kidney cortex microsomes. *J. Pharmacol. Exp. Ther.* 185:226.

Johansson, E.B. and H. Tjälve. 1978. The distribution of [^{14}C] dimethylnitrosamine in mice. Autoradiographic studies in mice with inhibited and noninhibited dimethylnitrosamine metabolism and a comparison with the distribution of [^{14}C] formaldehyde. *Toxicol. Appl. Pharmacol.* 45:565.

Kraft, P.L. and S.R. Tannenbaum. 1980. Distribution of N-nitrosomethylbenzylamine evaluated by whole-body radioautography and densitometry. *Cancer Res.* 40:1921.

Labuc, G.E. and M.C. Archer. 1982a. Esophageal and hepatic metabolism of N-nitrosomethylbenzylamine and N-nitrosomethylamine in the rat. *Cancer Res.* (in press).

———. 1982b. Comparative tumor initiating activities of N-nitrosomethylbenzylamine and N-nitrosodimethylamine in rat liver. *Carcinogenesis* 3:519.

Lai, D.Y. and J.C. Arcos. 1980. Dialkylnitrosamine bioactivation and carcinogenesis. *Life Sci.* 27:2149.

Magee, P.N. 1956. Toxic liver injury. The metabolism of dimethylnitrosamine. *Biochem. J.* 64:676.

Magee, P.N. and J.M. Barnes. 1967. Carcinogenic nitroso compounds. *Adv. Cancer Res.* 10:163.

Margison, G.P. 1981. Effect of pretreatment of rats with N-methyl-N-nitrosourea on the repair of O^6-methylguanine in liver DNA. *Carcinogenesis* 2:431.

Ogawa, K., D.B. Solt, and E. Farber. 1980. Phenotypic diversity as an early property of putative preneoplastic hepatocyte populations in liver carcinogenesis. *Cancer Res.* 40:725.

Paik, W.K. and S. Kim. 1974. ε-alkyllysinase. New assay method, purification, and biological significance. *Arch. Biochem. Biophys.* 165:369.

Park, K.K., M.C. Archer, and J.S. Wishnok. 1980. Alkylation of nucleic acids by N-nitrosodi-n-propylamine: Evidence that carbonium ions are not significantly involved. *Chem. Biol. Interact.* 29:139.

Pegg, A.E. 1977. Formation and metabolism of alkylated nucleosides: possible role in carcinogenesis by nitroso compounds and alkylating agents. *Adv. Cancer Res.* 25:195.

Pitot, H.C., L. Barsness, T. Goldsworthy, and T. Kitagawa. 1978. Biochemical characterisation of stages of hepatocarcinogenesis after a single dose of diethylnitrosamine. *Nature* 271:456.

Pozharisski, K.M. 1973. Tumours of the oesophagus. In *Pathology of Tumours in Laboratory Animals.* Vol. 1. *Tumours of the Rat,* Part 1. (ed. V.S. Turusov), publication no. 5, p. 87. International Agency for Research on Cancer, Lyon, France.

Rutenburg, A.M., H. Kim, J.W. Fischbein, J.S. Hanker, H.L. Wasserkrug, and A.M. Seligman. 1969. Histochemical and ultrastructural demonstration of γ-glutamyl transpeptidase activity. *J. Histochem. Cytochem.* **17**:517.

Schweinsberg, F. and M. Kouros. 1979. Reactions of N-methyl-N-nitrosobenzyl-amine and related substrates with enzyme-containing cell fractions isolated from various organs of rats and mice. *Cancer Lett.* **7**:115.

Snedecor, G.W. and W.G. Cochran. 1967. *Statistical Methods,* 6th ed., p. 115. Iowa State University Press, Ames, Iowa.

Solt, D.B., E. Cayama, D.S. Sarma, and E. Farber. 1980. Persistence of resistant putative preneoplastic hepatocytes induced by N-nitrosodiethylamine or N-methyl-N-nitrosourea. *Cancer Res.* **40**:1112.

Tsuda, H., G. Lee, and E. Farber. 1980. Induction of resistant hepatocytes as a new principle for a possible short-term *in vivo* test for carcinogens. *Cancer Res.* **40**:1157.

Yang, C.S. 1980. Research on esophageal cancer in China: A review. *Cancer Res.* **40**:2633.

COMMENTS

LIJINSKY: Mike, could I ask you the same question I asked Chris? Could you reflect on the fact that nitrosomethylaniline is an esophageal carcinogen in the rat, based on your results, when it cannot be oxidized to a methylating agent?

ARCHER: We chose not to use that compound as a model, because presumably metabolism can only take place at the methyl group. Until we know how it is handled by the esophagus, I wouldn't care to speculate. I assume that the esophagus would metabolize the compound very readily at the methyl carbon atom.

PREUSSMANN: Why doesn't it metabolize NDMA?

ARCHER: I don't know.

LIJINSKY: That is why I asked for reflection and not information.

CONNEY: If I am correct, the amount of DNA binding in esophagus and in liver is about the same with NMBzA, comparing liver and esophagus.

ARCHER: Hodgson et al. (1980) have shown that in the rat, DNA methylation is higher in the esophagus than in the liver, but in the mouse (Kleihues 1981), the liver, a nontarget organ, is more extensively methylated than the target organs—lung and forestomach.

CONNEY: What about RNA and protein, has that been done?

ARCHER: I don't believe it has been done.

TANNENBAUM: With regard to that specific point, we used whole-body autoradiography at a series of times following NMBzA treatment. Most of what is bound would be bound to RNA and protein, not DNA. The esophagus after 24 hours still contains almost all the ratioactivity that it contained at 4 hours, but the liver is substantially cleared within 24 hours, and certainly after 48 hours. The implication is that there is an extensive amount of repair in the liver, whereas there isn't in the esophagus. But I don't remember whether Kleihues (Kleihues et al. 1981) or Louise Fong's data (Fong et al. 1979) support that or not, when they looked specifically at DNA. Do you remember whether they looked at repair?

ARCHER: No, I don't think repair has been looked at. I think Kleihues measures his alkylation levels after 4 hours, at one time point.

PEGG: But I don't think that autoradiography experiment can be interpreted unless you know what you are measuring. You not only have adducts, you have metabolic incorporation—label gets into normal amino acids, it gets into normal purine bases. Your labeling is made up of a mixture of alkylated materials.

TANNENBAUM: I agree you can't interpret it in terms of types of molecules that are being either alkylated or synthesized, but what I am saying is that the label is gone in the liver after a day or so, and it is not in the esophagus. Whatever it was in the liver, it is gone.

PEGG: Well, that doesn't have to be repair. It can be a turnover of those constituents which were labeled.

TANNENBAUM: That is why I asked whether or not anyone had specifically looked at DNA. I don't think we can interpret our results as repair.

ARCHER: It would also be interesting to know whether there is a difference in DNA methylation and repair in the liver by NMBzA and NDMA.

MICHEJDA: May I offer a comment, a comment without any explanation? Nitrosomethylaniline does not appear to be bound, is not mutagenic at all, does not give sister chromatid exchange in three cell types, but yet gives tumors of the esophagus.

HECHT: Mike, do your results suggest a role for formaldehyde in hepatocarcinogenesis by NDMA?

ARCHER: O, I don't think so. I wouldn't go that far.

HECHT: Isn't that one of the major differences between these two compounds—one gives formaldehyde, the other doesn't?

ARCHER: Yes it is, but it is certainly premature to use that to explain differences in carcinogenic activity, although it has to remain a possibility.

WEISBURGER: Wouldn't a direct way be to look at what is bound to DNA in esophagus and/or liver?

ARCHER: Yes. We intend to follow up our experiments by measuring DNA methylation under the conditions we carried out these initiation assays. I think that is important.

WEISBURGER: It would seem to me that would give you the definitive answer.

ARCHER: Well, it may or may not be definitive. It seems to me if the differences between NDMA and NMBzA are small, the interpretation will be difficult.

MIRVISH: I just want to point out—it doesn't answer your question—NMBzA is very lipophilic. We pointed out, (Mirvish et al. 1976) and so have others, that the more lipophilic nitrosamines tend to cause esophageal cancer, other things being equal. This doesn't explain your results, but somehow it is part of the picture.

   I wonder if the dose of NMBzA that you used was so small that it didn't cause any liver changes. There is no reason, really, to choose equimolar doses of NMBzA and NDMA. If you could have used ten times more, you might have seen changes.

ARCHER: We couldn't have used ten times more, because we would kill the animals from acute toxic effects of NMBzA.

MIRVISH: How would you have killed the animals?

ARCHER: They die of esophageal necrosis.

PEGG: So you don't know if you would have been able to get liver tumors under those circumstances.

GOLDFARB: I would like to raise a technical point about the assessment of the foci. When you take a section through liver, you have to keep in mind that it is very important to know the size of the foci. If you have several large ones, you will see them more frequently in random sections through the liver. So I think it is improper to quantitate the number of foci in transsections. It can't be done since we don't know how big they are.

ARCHER: Well, we do know how big they are. They are all roughly 10-30 cells in diameter. And there are large areas of diffuse staining, which we don't count as foci. I think we are counting areas which are all pretty much the same size.

GOLDFARB: You determine that they are a certain size on the basis of serial section reconstruction? How do you know that they are this size?

ARCHER: You can count the cells in any particular focus, and we have looked at many sections.

GOLDFARB: You are saying that they are exactly equivalent, that the sizes of the foci are the same with the different agents. You really don't know that. You also have to prove that they are spherical.

ARCHER: We don't know that they are spheres. All I can say is that we have looked at the size distribution. The foci that we are counting are all approximately the same size. We have done multiple sections.

LIJINSKY: Did you look at the metabolism of NDEA in your esophageal preparation? NDEA is an esophageal carcinogen.

ARCHER: Our studies are now being extended to other compounds. We haven't yet done NDEA, but we have done NMAmA. This compound is interesting because, of course, it is not aromatic. It is a dialkylnitrosamine. Very preliminary results do suggest that there is a high degree of selectivity towards metabolism on the amyl as opposed to the methyl group.

LIJINSKY: But what I was thinking of is that, because NDMA seems not to be metabolized at all, it would be interesting to see if NDEA is or is not.

ARCHER: Yes, it will be interesting to compare NDMA and NDEA. These experiments are underway in our lab. I do not at the moment understand your result in which you were able to measure metabolism of nitrosopyrrolidine (a liver carcinogen) in the esophagus, but not 2,6-dimethyldinitrosopiperazine (an esophageal carcinogen).

LIJINSKY: I don't understand it either. It is one of those odd results that is there.

MICHEJDA: Mike, how many rats did you use for these preparations? I think Scanlon used something like 50 or 60 rats to prepare esophageal microsomes.

ARCHER: Oh, it takes a lot of rats. We combined esophageal mucosa from, typically, 10 to 15 animals, to give just a few data points.

MIRVISH: Did you try a control like, for example, the forestomach or the trachea?

ARCHER: No.

MIRVISH: The forestomach looks like the esophagus, but it doesn't behave like it.

References

Fong, L.Y.Y., H.J. Lin, and C.L.H. Lee. 1979. Methylation of DNA in target and non-target organs of the rat with methylbenzylnitrosamine and dimethyl-nitrosamine. *Int. J. Cancer* **23**:679.

Hodgson, R.M., M. Wiessler, and P. Kleihues. 1980. Preferential methylation of target organ DNA by the esophageal carcinogen N-nitrosomethylbenzyl-amine. *Carcinogenesis* **1**:861.

Kleihues, P., C. Veit, M. Wiessler, and R.M. Hodgson. 1981. DNA methylation by N-nitrosomethylbenzylamine in target and non-target tissues of NMRI mice. *Carcinogenesis* **2**:897.

Mirvish, S.S., P. Issenberg, and H.C. Sornson. 1976. Air-water and ether-water distribution of N-nitroso compounds: Implications for laboratory safety, analytical methodology, and carcinogenicity for rat esophagus, nose and liver. *J. Natl. Cancer Inst.* **56**:1125.

Recent Studies on the Metabolic Activation
of Cyclic Nitrosamines

STEPHEN S. HECHT, ANDRE CASTONGUAY, FUNG-LUNG CHUNG, AND DIETRICH HOFFMANN
Naylor Dana Institute for Disease Prevention
American Health Foundation
Valhalla, New York 10595

GARY D. STONER
Department of Pathology
Medical College of Ohio
Toledo, Ohio 43614

Cyclic nitrosamines are important because of their environmental occurrence and their organospecific carcinogenicity. (International Agency for Research on Cancer 1978). Environmentally prevalent cyclic nitrosamines include N-nitroso-pyrrolidine (NPYR), N-nitrosomorpholine (NMOR), N'-nitrosonornicotine (NNN), N'-nitrosoanabasine (NAB), and N'-nitrosoanatabine (NAT). The latter three are tobacco specific nitrosamines to which human exposure is particularly high as discussed by D. Hoffmann (this volume). The organospecific properties of cyclic nitrosamines provide a good lead for understanding mechanisms of chemical carcinogenesis. For example, under comparable conditions NPYR (see Fig. 1) induces exclusively liver tumors in F-344 rats whereas N-nitrosopiperidine (NPIP) gives primarily esophageal tumors. NNN, a 3-pyridyl derivative of NPYR, causes esophageal tumors rather than liver tumors and NAB, the corresponding derivative of NPIP, is practically inactive (Boyland et al. 1964; Hoffmann et al. 1975; Lijinsky and Reuber 1981). Since cyclic nitrosamines require metabolic activation, it is necessary to delineate their metabolic pathways and DNA binding properties in order to provide a foundation for understanding their carcinogenic activities. Extensive studies in the past several years have shown that, in general, cyclic nitrosamines are metabolized by ring hydroxylation to give the types of intermediates and products illustrated in Figure 2 and that α-hydroxylation is a likely activation step (Hecht et al. 1981b). However, little is known about the properties of the DNA adducts formed from cyclic nitrosamines.

If α-hydroxylation is important in cyclic nitrosamine activation, then it is essential to understand target tissue metabolism since the electrophilic intermediates that are formed may have short lifetimes. We have investigated the metabolism of NNN in cultured tissues from experimental animals and humans,

This study is dedicated to the founder of the American Health Foundation, Dr. Ernst L. Wynder, on the occasion of the tenth anniversary of the Naylor Dana Institute for Disease Prevention.

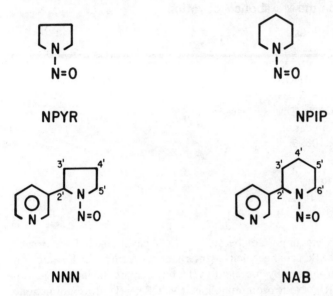

Figure 1
Structures of NPYR, NPIP, NNN, and NAB. Under comparable conditions in F-344 rats, NPYR induces liver tumors, NPIP and NNN induce tumors of the esophagus, and NAB is inactive.

and have also done experiments on the reaction of α-acetoxyNPYR and related compounds with deoxyguanosine (dG). These studies are described in this report.

MATERIALS AND METHODS

Metabolism in tissue culture

The metabolism of [2'-^{14}C] NNN in short-term organ cultures of F-344 rat and Syrian golden hamster esophagus, and in liver slices from F-344 rats, was carried out according to the procedure developed by B. Reiss and G. M. Williams (Hecht et al. 1982a). Similar procedures were employed to study the metabolism of [2'-^{14}C] NAB (Hecht and Young 1982b). The metabolism of [2'-^{14}C] NNN in short-term cultures of A/J mouse peripheral lung was carried out as described in Castonguay et al. 1982.

For the studies with human tissues, grossly normal tissues were taken from patients at autopsy within 2-6 hours of the time of death. Tissues were immersed in ice-cold L-15 medium immediately after removal from the patient. They were then cut into 0.5 cm × 0.5 cm pieces and cultured for 24 hours in supplemented

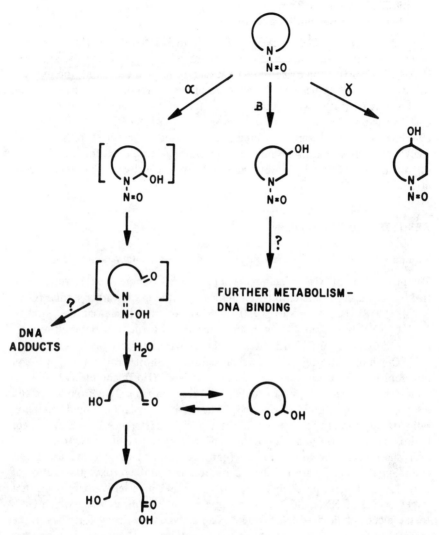

Figure 2
Generalized scheme for the metabolism of cyclic nitrosamines.

PFMR-4 medium. At the end of this time, the medium was removed and re-placed with medium containing $[2'\text{-}^{14}C]$ NNN. After a 24-hour-incubation period, the medium was analyzed by high pressure liquid chromatography (HPLC). HPLC conditions for all the metabolic studies were as described in Hecht et al. 1981a.

Reactions of α-acetoxyNPYR and
4-(carbethoxynitrosamino)butanal with dG

Typically, α-acetoxyNPYR (2g) was allowed to react with dG (2.5g) at 37°C in pH 7.0 phosphate buffer in the presence of 2700 units hog liver esterase (EC 3.1.1.1). After the α-acetoxyNPYR had all reacted (4 hours), the mixture was extracted with ether and the aqueous phase was lypophilized. The resulting residue was extracted with ethanol/methanol:1/1 and analyzed by HPLC on a C_{18} reverse-phase column with elution by 20-50% $MeOH/H_2O$ in 50 minutes. UV-absorbing peaks were collected, concentrated at reduced pressure, and analyzed spectroscopically. Similar conditions were employed for the reactions of 4-(carbethoxynitrosamino)butanal and crotonaldehyde (2-butenal) with dG.

RESULTS AND DISCUSSION

Metabolism of NNN in Cultured Tissues from Experimental Animals

The metabolism of NNN is summarized in Figure 3. All metabolites were identi-fied by their spectral and chromatographic properties in our earlier studies (Chen et al. 1978; Hecht et al. 1980, 1981a). In the tissue culture studies, $[2'-^{14}C]$ NNN was incubated with the appropriate tissue, the metabolites were separated by HPLC and identified by coelution with reference markers.

Our initial investigations were carried out in short-term cultures of F-344 rat esophagus since this is a target organ of NNN (Hoffmann et al. 1975). As indicated in Table 1, the major metabolites resulted from 2'-hydroxylation and 5'-hydroxylation (α-hydroxylation). The 2'-hydroxylation/5'-hydroxylation ratio of 3.0 for rat esophagus indicates a clear preference in this tissue for hydroxylation of the more sterically hindered 2'-carbon of NNN. In contrast, liver slices from the same animals (data not shown) or cultured esophagus from Syrian golden hamsters had 2'-hydroxylation/5'-hydroxylation ratios of only 1.4 or 0.3, respectively. Since rat liver and hamster esophagus are not target organs of NNN, these results suggest that 2'-hydroxylation which leads to the electrophilic diazohydroxide 8 is an activation pathway for NNN in the rat esophagus. However, the studies with cultured A/J mouse lung, another target tissue of NNN (Hecht et al. 1978a; Castonguay et al. 1982), indicate that the 2'-hydroxylation/5'-hydroxylation ratio (0.6) alone is not sufficient as an indicator of target tissue specificity. Nevertheless, the results do clearly demonstrate that NNN is extensively metabolized by α-hydroxylation in target tissues and that there is a high degree of tissue dependent regiospecificity that may influence susceptibility to tumor development. Analogous results have been obtained with N-nitroso-N-methylbenzylamine (NMBzA) (Schweinsberg and Kouros 1979; Hodgson et al. 1980; Kleihues et al. 1981).

The regiospecificity of the rat esophagus in the metabolism of cyclic nitrosamines was further demonstrated by the results of comparative studies

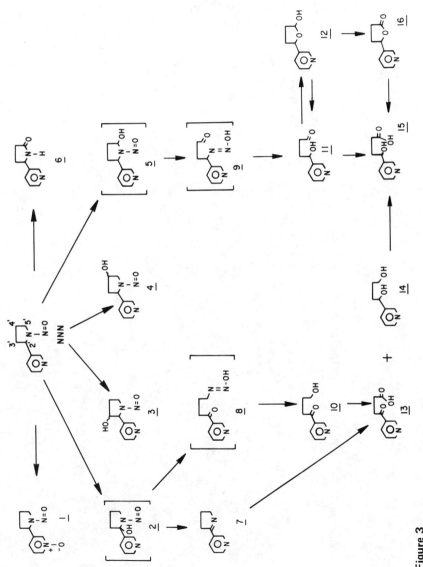

Figure 3
Metabolism of NNN in the F-344 rat.

Table 1
Metabolism of [2'-^{14}C] NNN in Cultured Human and Animal Tissues

Species and Tissue	Number of Determinations	Metabolites (% of initial concentration of NNN in the medium)[a,b,c]				
		N-oxidation	2'-hydroxylation			5'-hydroxylation
		NNN-1-N-oxide 1	Keto Alcohol 10	Keto Acid 13	Diol 14	Hydroxy Acid 15
F-344 rat esophagus	3	0.87 ± 0.02	8 ± 1	10 ± 1	2.4 ± 0.4	6.8 ± 1.1
Syrian golden hamster esophagus	2	3.6 ± 0.1	1.4 ± 0.1	2.2 ± 0.1	1.8 ± 0.1	21.0 ± 1.3
Human esophagus	6	0.3 ± 0.3	N.D.	N.D.	N.D.	0.1 ± 0.07
A/J Mouse lung	4	3.2 ± 0.3	1.3 ± 0.5	13 ± 2	6.5 ± 1.0	36 ± 4
Human lung	6	0.6 ± 0.3	N.D.	N.D.	N.D.	0.2 ± 0.3
Human bronchus	6	0.2 ± 0.3	N.D.	N.D.	N.D.	0.1 ± 0.06

[a] Numbers refer to Fig. 3
[b] N.D. = Not detected.
[c] Explants were cultured for 24 hrs.

on NNN and NAB. In contrast to NNN, the major metabolite of $[2'-^{14}C]$ NAB in 48-hour cultures of rat esophagus was 5-hydroxy-5-(3-pyridyl)pentanoic acid, resulting from 6'-hydroxylation. This result provides further support for the hypothesis that 2'-hydroxylation is the major activation pathway for NNN in the esophagus since it is a much more potent esophageal carcinogen than is NAB.

Metabolism of NNN in Cultured Tissues from Humans

The results for esophagus, bronchus, and peripheral lung are summarized in Table 1. In all cases, the principal metabolites detected were hydroxy acid *15*, from 5'-hydroxylation, and NNN-1-N-oxide (*1*), from N-oxidation. A wide interindividual variation in metabolism was observed, as reported in other studies of carcinogen metabolism by cultured human tissues (Autrup et al. 1979; Autrup and Stoner 1982). In comparing the results from human and experimental animal tissues, we observed both quantitative and qualitative differences in metabolism. The conversion of NNN to metabolites (up to 0.8%) was considerably lower in human tissues compared to those from experimental animals (30-60%). The distribution of metabolites was also quite different. For example, in the human esophagus, N-oxidation was observed to a greater extent than was 5'-hydroxylation, and 2'-hydroxylation was not detected. In contrast, 2'-hydroxylation was the major metabolic pathway in rat esophagus and 5'-hydroxylation was the predominant mode of metabolism in hamster esophagus. Since human tissues can metabolically carry out the α-hydroxylation of NNN, they can be considered as potential target tissues. However, the observed differences in regiospecificity between the human and animal tissues in NNN metabolism suggests that NNN may have different target organs in man and experimental animals. The distribution of metabolites in the human samples is also likely to be affected by exposure to exogenous enzyme inducers.

Reactions of α-acetoxyNPYR, 4(carbethoxynitrosamino)-butanal, and Crotonaldehyde with dG

The structures of the DNA adducts resulting from metabolism of cyclic nitrosamines are not known. As an approach to this problem we have studied the reactions of α-acetoxyNPYR (*1*, see Fig. 6, page 113) and 4-(carbethoxynitrosamino)butanal (*3*) with dG in the presence of esterase. Compounds *1* and *3* are mutagenic toward *Salmonella typhimurium* without activation and are model compounds for the intermediates *2* and *4* that are formed by α-hydroxylation of NPYR (Hecht et al. 1978b).

Under our conditions, the intermediates formed in the hydrolyses of *1* and *3* reacted mainly with H_2O to give products such as *12*. However, approximately 0.5-2% reaction with dG was observed and from both *1* and *3* the same two major dG adducts (peaks 4 and 5 of Fig. 4) were formed. We did not detect

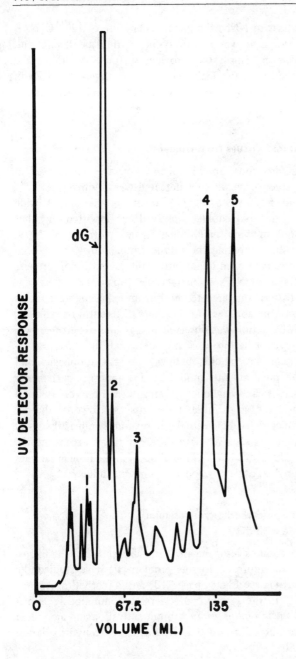

Figure 4
Chromatogram obtained by HPLC analysis of the products formed in the reaction
with 4-(carbethoxynitrosamino)butanal.

Table 2
Ultraviolet and Mass Spectral Properties of Peaks 4 and 5[a]

UV^b pH 1:	max 284 nm (sh), 262 nm
pH 7:	max 280 nm (sh), 258 nm
pH 13:	max 278 nm (sh), 261 nm

MS (Chemical desorption ionization): m/e 338 (M+H), 222[b]

MS (High resolution): peak 4, m/e 625.2966 (M$^+$) $\Big\}$ $C_{14}H_{17}N_5O_5$.4TMS

peak 5, m/e 625.2979 (M$^+$)

[a]Peaks 4 and 5 of Fig. 4.
[b]Peaks 4 and 5 had identical spectra.

any other major products containing the dG moiety. The ultraviolet (UV), mass, and nuclear magnetic resonance (NMR) spectra of peaks 4 and 5 were similar if not identical. UV and mass spectral data are summarized in Table 2. The UV data indicate substitution at the 1 or N^2 positions of dG. The mass spectral data are consistent with the addition of a single oxobutyl residue (e.g. 7 in Fig. 6, page 113) to dG. In agreement with the high resolution mass spectral data, silylation of either peak 4 or 5 followed by combined gas chromatography/ mass spectrometry (GC/MS) gave a product with m/e 625 corresponding to the formation of a tetratrimethylsilyl derivative.

The NMR spectrum of peak 4 and its assigned structure are illustrated in Figure 5. Important features include the presence of a methyl doublet at δ 1.21 which collapsed to a singlet upon irradiation of the C_6 methine proton at δ 3.70. The axial and equatorial protons at C_7 were assigned to the doublet of doublets at δ 1.41 and the doublet at δ 2.00, respectively. Analysis of the coupling constants indicated that the C_8–OH and C_6–CH$_3$ were axial and equatorial, respectively. The C_8–OH, N_5–H, 3′–OH, and 5′–OH resonances disappeared upon treatment with D_2O. The NMR spectrum of peak 5 was essentially identical to that shown in Figure 5.

The spectral data are consistent with the diastereomeric structures 9 and 10 of Figure 6 for peaks 4 or 5. Hydrolysis of peak 4 proceeded smoothly in 0.1N HCl (37°C, 16 hours) to give a single product with UV, MS, and NMR spectral properties entirely consistent with the corresponding tricyclic guanine derivative. Hydrolysis of peak 5 gave a product which was identical to that obtained from peak 4 except that its circular dichroism spectrum was of opposite polarity. Thus, the hydrolysis products of peaks 4 and 5 are enantiomeric tricyclic guanine derivatives. Treatment of the tricyclic guanine derivatives with aqueous NaOH in the presence of $NaBH_4$ resulted in the formation of a single major product which was identified by its UV, IR, and NMR spectrum as N^2-[2(4-hydroxybutyl)]guanine. These results are in agreement with the assigned structures.

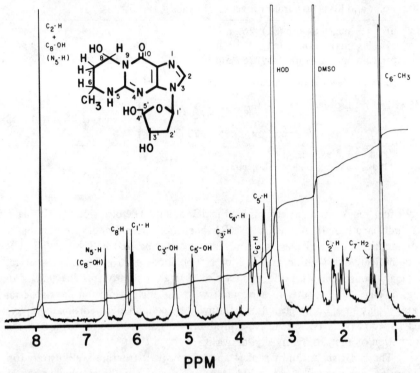

Figure 5
NMR spectrum of peak 4 of Fig. 4.

To obtain further structural evidence, we examined the reaction of dG with crotonaldehyde (2-butenal, *8*). Depending on conditions, yields as high as 30-40% of compounds *9* and *10* were obtained. In this reaction, as well as those described above, the R,R and S,S isomers were formed to the apparent exclusion of the R,S and S,R isomers. This stereoselectivity requires further investigation.

Simple alkylating agents such as methyl-, ethyl- and butylnitrosourea, methyl- and ethylmethanesulfonate, dimethyl and diethylsulfate, methyl- and ethyl iodide, propylene oxide, and α-hydroxydimethylnitrosamine tend to react preferentially at the 7 position of guanosine. Depending on reaction conditions, varying amounts of products resulting from reaction at the 1 or 3 positions, or at N^2 or O^6 may also be formed but their yields seldom exceed those of the 7-alkyl derivatives (Lawley and Brookes 1963; Shapiro 1968; Lawley and Jarman 1972; Singer 1972; Singer 1979; Moschel et al. 1979; Ortleib and Kleihues 1980; Mochizuki et al. 1981). In contrast, the major products observed in the present study resulted from reaction at the 1 and N^2 positions of dG. We did not detect O^6 or 7-adducts of dG although they could have been

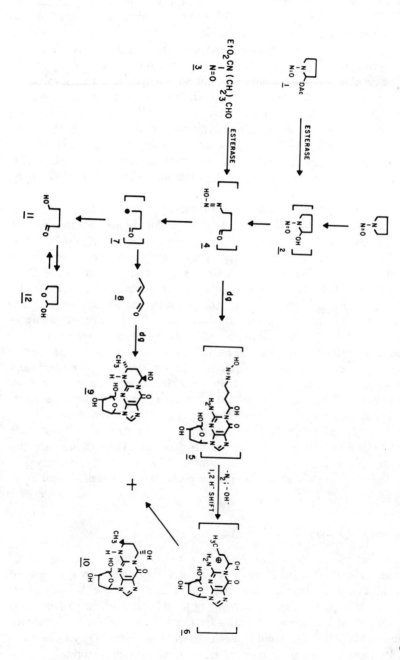

Figure 6

Formation of dG adducts from α-acetoxyNPYR (*1*), 4-(carbethoxynitrosamino)butanal (*3*) and crotonaldehyde (*8*). Structures *9* and *10* are peaks 4 or 5 of Fig. 4.

formed in trace amounts. It is not clear at present whether the tricyclic adducts *9* and *10* were formed from the 4-oxobutyl diazohydroxide *4*, from the 4-oxobutylcarbonium ion *7*, or from crotonaldehyde (*8*) which is a minor product of the solvolyses of *1* and *3*. It is apparent, however, that the aldehyde group of these electrophiles is involved in directing the reaction toward the 1 and N^2 positions of dG. Since electrophiles bearing an aldehyde group are involved in the metabolism of all cyclic nitrosamines studied so far, these results suggest that the products of DNA alkylation and possibly the mechanism of action of cyclic nitrosamines may differ significantly from those of the acyclic nitrosamines. Recently, evidence for the presence of a fluorescent adduct in the liver DNA of rats treated with NPYR has been reported (Hunt and Shank 1982). Whether or not that adduct is identical to the one characterized in this study requires further investigation.

The relatively facile reaction of crotonaldehyde with dG to give *9* and *10* suggests a possible role in carcinogenesis. Crotonaldehyde has been shown to be mutagenic toward *S. typhimurium* without activation (Lutz et al. 1982). A bioassay of crotonaldehyde for carcinogenicity is currently in progress. The reaction of other α, β unsaturated aldehydes and related compounds with dG and DNA requires further study. It is possible that such reactions may be involved in the toxic or carcinogenic properties of such compounds as acrolein and acrylonitrile.

Unsaturated tricyclic guanine derivatives with the same ring structure as observed in the present study have been prepared previously by reaction of substituted malondialdehydes with guanine (Moschel and Leonard 1976). We are not aware of any examples of tricyclic guanine derivatives in which the additional six-membered ring is fully saturated. The corresponding five-membered derivatives (1-N^2-ethano- or 1-N^2-ethenoguanines) are well characterized (Shapiro and Hachmann 1966; Shapiro et al. 1969; Sattsangi et al. 1977; Czarnik and Leonard 1980). They are formed from reaction of compounds such as glyoxal and chloroacetaldehyde with guanosine. These adducts and the related ones formed from adenine and cytosine derivatives could be involved in the biological properties of compounds such as chloroacetaldehyde and vinyl chloride (Hathway 1981).

ACKNOWLEDGMENTS

These studies were supported by National Cancer Institute Grants CA-21393, CA-23901, and CA-30133. Chemical desorption ionization mass spectra were obtained at the Rockefeller University Mass Spectrometric Biotechnology Resource. NMR spectra were obtained using the 7T spectrometer at the Rockefeller University purchased in part with funds from the National Science Foundation (PCM-7912083) and from the Camille and Henry Dreyfus Foundation. NMR and circular dichroism spectra were also obtained through the cooperation of the Columbia University Chemistry Department. We thank Dr. James McCloskey, Department of Medicinal Chemistry, College of Pharmacy, University of Utah, for high resolution mass spectra.

REFERENCES

Autrup, H., A.M. Jeffrey, and C.C. Harris. 1979. Metabolism of benzo[a]-pyrene in cultured human bronchus, trachea, colon, and esophagus. In *Polynuclear aromatic hydrocarbons: Chemistry and biological effects* (ed. A. Bjorseth and A.J. Dennis), p. 89. Battelle Press, Columbus, Ohio.

Autrup, H. and G.D. Stoner. 1982. Metabolisn of N-nitrosamines by cultured human and rat esophagus. *Cancer Res.* 42:1307.

Boyland, E., F.J.C. Roe, J.W. Gorrod, and B.C.V. Mitchley. 1964. The carcinogenicity of nitrosoanabasine, a possible constituent of tobacco smoke. *Br. J. Cancer* 18:265.

Castonguay, A., D. Lin, G.D. Stoner, P. Radok, K. Furuya, S.S. Hecht, H.A.J. Schut, and J.E. Klaunig. 1982. Comparative carcinogenicity in A/J mice and metabolism by cultured mouse peripheral lung of N'-nitrosonornicotine, 4-(methylnitrosamino)-1-(3-pyridyl)-1-butanone and their analogues. *Cancer Res.* (in press).

Chen, C.B., S.S. Hecht, and D. Hoffmann. 1978. Metabolic α-hydroxylation of the tobacco specific carcinogen N'-nitrosonornicotine. *Cancer Res.* 38:3639.

Czarnik, A.W. and N.J. Leonard. 1980. Unequivocal assignment of the skeletal structure of the guanine-glyoxal adduct. *J. Org. Chem.* 45:3514.

Hathway, D.E. 1981. Mechanisms of vinyl chloride carcinogenicity/mutagenicity. *Br. J. Cancer* 44:597.

Hecht, S.S. and R. Young. 1982. Regiospecificity in the metabolism of the homologous cyclic nitrosamines, N'-nitrosonornicotine and N'-nitrosoanabasine. *Carcinogenesis* (in press).

Hecht, S.S., C.B. Chen, and D. Hoffmann. 1978b. Evidence for metabolic α-hydroxylation of N-nitrosopyrrolidine. *Cancer Res.* 38:215.

_____. 1980. Metabolic β-hydroxylation and N-oxidation of N'-nitrosonornicotine. *J. Med. Chem.* 23:1175.

Hecht, S.S., D. Lin, and C.B. Chen. 1981a. Comprehensive analysis of urinary metabolites of N'-nitrosonornicotine. *Carcinogenesis* 2:833.

Hecht, S.S., G.D. McCoy, C.B. Chen, and D. Hoffmann. 1981b. The metabolism of cyclic nitrosamines. In *N-Nitroso Compounds* (eds. R.A. Scanlan and S.R. Tannenbaum) *ACS Symp. Ser.* 174:49.

Hecht, S.S., B. Reiss, D. Lin, and G.M. Williams. 1982. Metabolism of N'-nitrosonornicotine by cultured rat esophagus. *Carcinogenesis* (in press).

Hecht, S.S., C.B. Chen, N. Hirota, R.M. Ornaf, T.C. Tso, and D. Hoffmann. 1978a. Tobacco specific nitrosamines: formation by nitrosation of nicotine during curing of tobacco and carcinogenicity in strain A mice. *J. Natl. Cancer Inst.* 60:819.

Hodgson, R.M., M. Wiessler, and P. Kleihues. 1980. Preferential methylation of target organ DNA by the oesophageal carcinogen N-nitrosomethyl-benzylamine in rats. *Carcinogenesis* 1:861.

Hoffmann, D., R. Raineri, S.S. Hecht, R.R. Maronpot, and E.L. Wynder. 1975. A study of tobacco carcinogenesis. XIV. Effects of N'-nitrosonornicotine and N'-nitrosoanabasine in rats. *J. Natl. Cancer Inst.* 55:977.

Hunt, E.J. and R.C. Shank. 1982. Evidence for DNA adducts in rat liver after administration of N-nitrosopyrrolidine. *Biochem. Biophys. Res. Commun.* 104:1343.

International Agency for Research on Cancer. 1978. Some N-Nitroso Compounds. *IARC (Monogr. Eval. Carcinog. Risk Chem. Hum.)* 17:263.

Kleihues, P., C. Veit, M. Wiessler, and R.M. Hodgson. 1981. DNA methylation by N-nitrosomethylbenzylamine in target and non-target tissues of NMRI mice. *Carcinogenesis* 2:897.

Lawley, P.D. and P. Brookes. 1963. Further studies on the alkylation of nucleic acids and their constituent nucleotides. *Biochem. J.* 89:127.

Lawley, P.D. and M. Jarman. 1972. Alkylation by propylene oxide of deoxyribonucleic acid, adenine, guanosine and deoxyguanylic acid. *Biochem. J.* 126:893.

Lijinsky, W. and M.D. Reuber. 1981. Carcinogenic effect of nitrosopyrrolidine, nitrosopiperidine and nitrosohexamethylenemine in Fischer rats. *Cancer Lett.* 12:99.

Lutz, D., E. Eder, T. Neudecker, and D. Henschler. 1982. Structure-mutagenicity relationship in α,β-unsaturated carbonylic compounds and their corresponding allylic alcohols. *Mutat. Res.* 93:305.

Mochizuki, M., T. Anjo, K. Takeda, E. Suzuki, N. Sekiguchi, G.F. Huang, and M. Okada. 1981. Chemistry and mutagenicity of α-hydroxynitrosamines. *IARC Sci. Publ.* 41:(in press).

Moschel, R.C. and N.J. Leonard. 1976. Fluorescent modification of guanine. Reaction with substituted malondialdehydes. *J. Org. Chem.* 41:294.

Moschel, R.C., W.R. Hudgins, and A. Dipple. 1979. Selectivity in nucleoside alkylation and aralkylation in relation to chemical carcinogenesis. *J. Org. Chem.* 44:3324.

Ortleib, H. and P. Kleihues. 1980. Reaction of N-n-butyl-N-nitrosourea with DNA *in vitro. Carcinogenesis* 1:849.

Sattsangi, P., N.J. Leonard, and C.R. Frihart. 1977. 1,N^2-Ethenoguanine and N^2,3-ethenoguanine. Synthesis and comparison of the electronic spectral properties of these linear and angular triheterocycles related to the Y bases. *J. Org. Chem.* 42:3292.

Schweinsberg, F. and M. Kouros. 1979. Reaction of N-methyl-N-nitrosobenzylamine and related substances with enzyme containing cell fractions isolated from various organs of rats and mice. *Cancer Lett.* 1:115.

Singer, B. 1972. Reaction of guanosine with ethylating agents. *Biochemistry* 11:3939.

_____. 1979. N-Nitroso alkylating agents: Formation and persistence of alkyl derivatives in mammalian nucleic acids as contributing factors in carcinogenesis. *J. Natl. Cancer Inst.* 62:1329.

Shapiro, R. 1968. Chemistry of guanine and its biologically significant derivatives. *Progr. Nucleic Acid Res. Mol. Biol.* 8:73.

Shapiro, R. and J. Hachmann. 1966. The reaction of guanine derivatives with 1,2-dicarbonyl compounds. *Biochemistry* 5:2799.

Shapiro, R., B.I. Cohen, S.J. Shiuey, and H. Maurer. 1969. On the reaction of guanine with glyoxal, pyruvaldehyde, and kethoxal, and the structure of the acylguanines. A new synthesis of N^2-alkylguanines. *Biochemistry* 8:238.

COMMENTS

MICHEJDA: Reznick-Schuller showed in the hamster lung that of approximately 40 epithelial cell types, only two cell types are responsible for all lung tumors (Reznick-Schuller and Reznick 1980).

HECHT: Our studies were done with A/J mice and human lungs.

HARRIS: Well, I don't know if N-nitrosamines cause lung cancer in humans.

MICHEJDA: Assuming that this is true, you may simply not see the right kinds of metabolites because they're caused by those particular types of cells.

HECHT: That's entirely possible. In fact, the levels of DNA alkylation in these studies are very low. Cyclic nitrosamines such as NNN apparently alkylate but the levels of alkylation are very low.

TANNENBAUM: Since you ran this reaction in dilute solution, maybe it's not surprising to find this cyclization. But suppose it happened on DNA? Then the possibility of a cross-link might be equally probable. Have you looked for cross-links—particularly since the initial reaction here probably is taking place at N^2—is N^1 accessible in DNA?

HECHT: We're doing the DNA studies now. We don't know what will happen in DNA, whether we'll see it or not. I assume we will. You're quite right; however, we don't really know if the initial reaction is at N^1 or N^2.

SIMENHOFF: Do you know whether the tissues from those autopsy studies were from smokers or nonsmokers?

CASTONGUAY: Among the six cases reported in the present study, only one was a smoker. The levels of N-oxidation and $5'$-hydroxylation of NNN by tissues of this smoker were no different from the other cases.

MIRVISH: How long does the cultured esophagus maintain its ability to metabolize the nitrosamine?

HECHT: We have only done organ cultures up to 48 hours.

MICHEJDA: Are these adducts exclusively deoxyguanosine adducts?

HECHT: We have only looked at dG so far.

MICHEJDA: Have you tried DNA?

HECHT: The study of DNA alkylation is in progress.

ANDERSON: Is the metabolism influenced qualitatively or quantitatively by inducers, such as might also be found in cigarette smoke?

HECHT: That's a very good point. We haven't done any inducer studies in esophagus, but we have done them in liver. The various inducers induce the 2′-and 5′-hydroxylations differently. For example, methylcholanthrene induces mainly 2′; phenobarbital induces mainly 5′. So it's quite possible that in the human studies we may be seeing an induction phenomenon.

YANG: The question has been raised whether nitrosamines are metabolized by the cytochrome P-450 dependent monooxygenase system. Although several lines of evidence indicate that nitrosamines are metabolized by P-450, there are suggestions that nitrosodimethylamine demethylase (NDMAd) activity is due to other enzyme systems. Part of the controversy

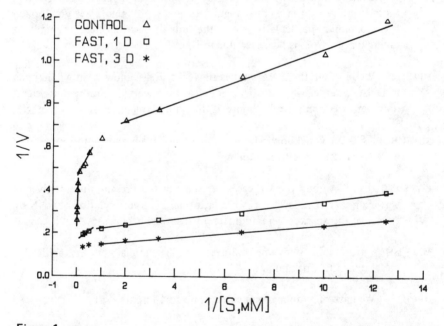

Figure 1
Gel electrophoresis of microsomal proteins. The samples in different wells are: *A*, purified cytochrome P-450 (induced by phenobarbital, M_r 52,000); *B*, control microsomes; *C*, *D*, and *E*, microsomes from rats which had been fasted for 1, 2, and 3 days, respectively; *F*, microsomes from acetone treated rats. Each well contained 10 μg protein. Well G contained 7 protein standards. Wells H to M contained 5.3 g protein in each well. *H*, control; *I*, fast (1 day); *J*, fast plus actinomycin D; *K*, fast plus $CoCl_2$; *L*, fast plus cycloheximide; *M*, fast plus ethionine. Well N contained purified P-450 (M_r 52,000).

is derived from the fact that microsomal NDMAd activity is affected differently by classical P-450 inducers such as phenobarbital (Pb) and 3-methylcholanthrene (3-MC) in comparison to many well established mono-oxygenase activities. The existence of multiple K_m values for NDMAd also complicates the issue. The problem, however, may be resolved if we consider the multiplicity of P-450 in microsomes. That is, the different P-450 isozymes have different affinities and catalytic activities for nitrosamines, and the major forms of P-450 induced in rat liver by Pb and 3-MC have low affinities for nitrosamines. This working hypothesis has been quite useful in our laboratory. Many investigators have studied the kinetics of NDMAd and observed K_m values of 0.3-0.5 mM and 30-50 mM. As shown in Figure 1, we observed similar K_m values (0.38 and 38.6 mM) for

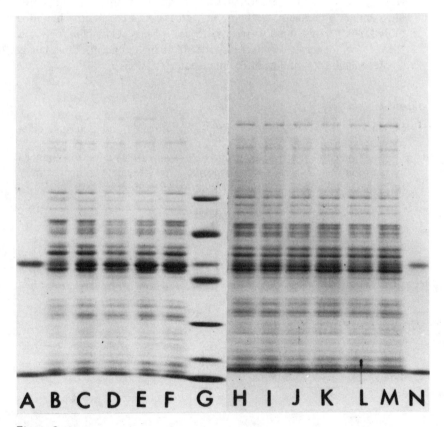

Figure 2
Double reciprocal plots of the NDMAd reaction. Activity was assayed in the presence of microsomes from control (△); 1-day fasted (□); and, 3-day fasted (*) rats at concentrations corresponding to 0.47, 0.44, and 0.47 my protein/ml, respectively.

NDMAd. In addition, we found a K_m of 0.07 mM which has not been reported previously for rat liver microsomes. This low K_m form of NDMAd was induced by fasting. The V_{max} was increased from 1.59 to 4.84 and 7.07 nmol/min/mg, respectively, after 1 and 3 days of fasting. The induction is correlated with the appearance of a 50,000 dalton protein and the induction was inhibited by $CoCl_2$ as well as inhibitors of RNA and protein synthesis (Fig. 2). This and other results suggest that the enhanced NDMAd activity is due to the induction of a P-450 isozyme which has high affinity for NDMA. Similar high affinity isozymes were also induced by pyrazole, acetone, isoproponol, and other factors (Tu et al. 1981; Yang, unpubl. results). These treatments also enhanced the metabolism of several other nitrosamines tested. The high affinity NDMAd may play an important role in carcinogenesis because animal cells are rarely exposed to high concentrations of nitrosamines. Elucidation of the properties of this enzyme system may help us understand certain aspects of carcinogenesis, for example, concerning the alteration of organ specificity of nitrosamines by ethanol. We know that ethanol is a competitive inhibitor of NDMAd (Yang, unpubl. results); thus, it is a weak inhibitor when NDMA (or other nitrosamines) is present at high concentrations but is a potent inhibitor with low nitrosamine concentrations.

References

Reznick-Schuller, H. and G. Reznick. 1980. Experimental pulmonary carcinogenesis. *Int. Rev. Exp. Pathol.* **20**:211.

Tu, Y.Y., J. Sonnenberg, K.F. Lewis, and C.S. Yang. 1981. Pyranzole-induced cytochrome P-450 in rat liver microsomes: An isozyme with high-affinity for dimethylnitrosamines. *Biochem. Biophys. Res. Commun.* **103**:905.

Metabolism of N-Nitrosamines and Repair of DNA Damage in Cultured Human Tissues and Cells

CURTIS C. HARRIS, ROLAND C. GRAFSTROM,
JOHN F. LECHNER AND HERMAN AUTRUP
Laboratory of Human Carcinogenesis
National Cancer Institute
National Institutes of Health
Bethesda, Maryland 20205

The possible role of N-nitrosamines in the etiology of human cancer can be assessed by several approaches: epidemiology, animal models, clinical investigations, and model systems using human tissues and cells. We are currently focusing our attention on the latter approach.

Impressive progress in the culture of human epithelial tissues and cells has been made during the last decade (Harris et al. 1980). Methods have been developed to culture normal tissues and cells from the major sites of human cancer. Chemically defined media have been devised for explant culture of human bronchus, colon, esophagus, and pancreatic duct and for culture of human bronchial epithelial cells (Lechner et al. 1982) and skin keratinocytes (Maciag et al. 1981).

The extrapolation of data from studies of N-nitrosamine carcinogenesis between experimental animals and humans is a pressing problem. Abundant evidence of N-nitrosamine carcinogenesis from both in vitro and in vivo studies using experimental animals has accumulated (Magee et al. 1976). Although N-nitrosamines are widespread pollutants, the carcinogenicity of these chemicals in humans has been difficult to prove by epidemiological studies. In vitro studies comparing pathobiological responses of N-nitrosamines in humans and experimental animals offers an approach to solve this problem at least at the cellular and tissue level of biological organization.

MATERIAL AND METHODS

Human tissues were collected at the time of surgery and immediate autopsy and transported to the laboratory in L-15 medium at $4°C$. Prior to the addition of the radiolabeled N-nitrosamine (generally for 24 hours) explants were maintained in culture for 7 days as previously described (Harris et al. 1978; Harris et al. 1979; Autrup et al. 1980) to minimize the effects acquired by the donor from diet, exogenous agents, etc. Methods for the culture of human cells have also been published (Lechner et al. 1981; 1982).

Nucleic acids were isolated from cells and the mucosal layers of explants by treatment with proteinase K and then by phenol extraction. Following sequential exposure to RNAse and proteinase K, DNA was purified by CsCl gradient centrifugation (Harris et al. 1976). The binding values were determined by radioactivity associated with purified DNA.

Metabolites with an oxo-group were detected as derivatives of 2,4-dinitrophenylhydrazine and the hydrazines were separated either by thin layer chromatography or high pressure liquid chromatography (HPLC) (Autrup and Stoner 1982). $[C^{14}]CO_2$ was isolated by a published method (Harris et al. 1977).

Cytotoxicity for formaldehyde and X-rays were determined by plating either 500 bronchial fibroblasts or 5000 epithelial cells/60 mm tissue culture dish; colony forming efficiency (CFE) and growth rate measured as previously described (Lechner et al. 1981).

Measurement of DNA single strand breaks (SSB) and DNA-protein cross-links by alkaline elution methodology has been described in detail (Kohn et al. 1981; Fornace 1982).

The levels of methylated DNA purines after exposure to alkylating agents were analyzed by hydrolyzing DNA in 0.1N HCl at 70° for 30 minutes followed by subsequent separation by HPLC using a Magnum 9 Partisil SCX column and 0.4 M ammonium formate (pH 4.3, 1.2 ml/min). Optical markers for O^6-methylguanine and N7-methylguanine were included.

RESULTS AND DISCUSSION

Metabolism of N-Nitrosamines

Following enzymatic hydroxylation and chemical heterolysis, N-nitrosodimethylamine (NDMA) yields equal molar quantities of carbonium ions and aldehydes (Fig. 1). Both of these metabolites can react with nucleophilic sites in cellular macromolecules; carbonium ions by alkylation and aldehydes via formation of unstable alkyl-ol derivatives preferably with amine groups $(R-HN-CHOH-R_1)$. The monomethylol derivatives of formaldehyde can form intermediary labile products that, by secondary reaction, can yield stable methylene bridges between macromolecules. The amounts of carbonium ion and aldehyde bound to macromolecules are dependent on many physicochemical factors (Auerbach et al. 1977; Hemminki 1981), and for aldehydes, such as formaldehyde, the rate of degradation by cellular enzymes (Fig. 2). In addition to measuring association of radioactivity of carbonium ions and aldehydes to cellular macromolecules, metabolites of N-nitrosamines can be measured by formation of (1) N_2 by using $[N^{15}]$ labeled N-nitrosamines, (2) aldehydes detected as 2,4-dinitrophenylhydrazone derivatives, and (3) CO_2 by using $[C^{14}]$-labeled N-nitrosamines.

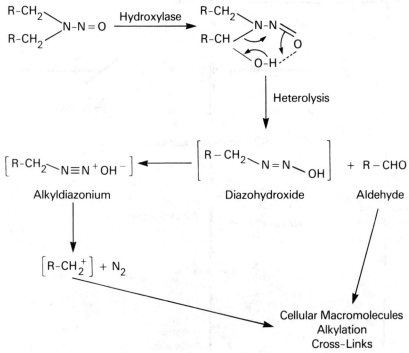

Figure 1
Metabolic activation of N-nitrosamines.

Both acyclic and cyclic *N*-nitrosamines can be activated to metabolites that are associated with DNA in cultured human epithelial tissues and cells (Table 1; Harris et al. 1982). Human bronchus can activate all of the *N*-nitrosamines tested to date. Radioactivity associated with DNA was observed in human colon incubated with *N*-nitrosopyrrolidine (NPYR) but not with *N*-nitrosopiperidine. Neither of these cyclic *N*-nitrosamines was activated to metabolites associated with DNA in cultured human esophagus although radioactivity associated with proteins was observed. In contrast, cultured rat esophagus can readily activate cyclic *N*-nitrosamines to metabolites associated with DNA including the potent organotrophic carcinogen in the rat, N-nitrosomethylbenzylamine (Table 2; Autrup and Stoner 1982). Experimental studies using NDMA have also demonstrated alkylation of guanine in DNA to form N7-methylguanine and O^6-methylguanine in explants of human colon, bronchus, bladder, and esophagus (Harris et al. 1977, 1979; Autrup et al. 1978a,b; 1981). Alkylated DNA bases have also been detected in a liver sample from an individual presumably poisoned with NDMA. Additional investigations

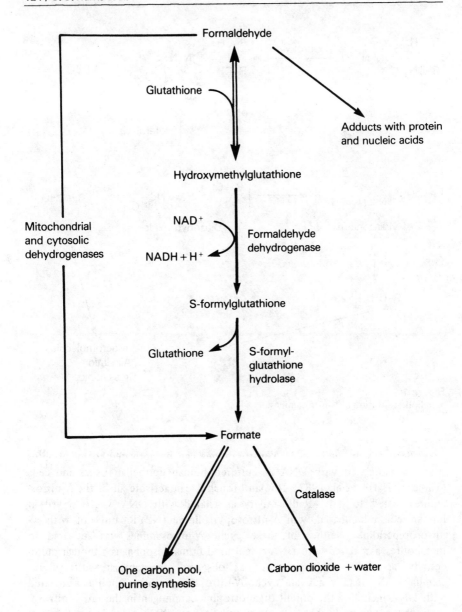

Figure 2
Metabolism of formaldehyde.

Table 1
N-Nitrosamines Activated to Form Metabolites Associated with DNA by Cultured Human Tissues and Cells

N-Nitrosamine	Bronchus	Colon	Esophagus	Pancreatic Duct	Bladder
NDMA	+[a]	+	+	+	+
NDEA	+	+	+		
NPYR	+	+	−[b]		+
NPIP	+	−	−		
Dinitrosopiperazine	+	+			
NMBzA		−			

[a](+) positive
[b]no radioactivity associated with DNA
[c](no symbol) not tested.

are needed to identify the alkylation products of the other N-nitrosamines with DNA in human tissues.

The amount of N-nitrosamine metabolite(s) associated with DNA varies among individuals (Table 3) and in a single person, among different tissues (Table 4). Interindividual differences are in the range of 50- to 150-fold for several classes of chemical carcinogens including N-nitrosamines (Harris et al. 1982).

Oxidation of N-nitrosamines at both α- and β-positions gives rise to formation of aldehydes and CO_2. These products have been detected even in cases where no radioactivity was associated with DNA. A positive correlation between the amount of CO_2 formed and radioactivity associated with DNA was found in human colon (6 cases) but not in the other organs (Autrup et al. 1978b). In intact tissues, oxidation occurs at most carbon atoms. In case of NPYR, oxidation was detected at both α- and β-positions, whereas in subcellular fraction of human liver, only α-oxidative products could be detected (Autrup et al. 1978b). α-Oxidation was also the predominant metabolic pathway in human bladder cells, but evidence for β-oxidation was shown by formation of NPYR-3-al (Nebelin et al. 1981).

DNA Damage and Repair

DNA repair has been extensively studied in human fibroblasts, lymphoid cells, and neoplastic cells (Setlow 1978; Hanawalt et al. 1982; Cleaver et al. 1982). However, little information is available concerning DNA repair in normal human epithelial cells (Taichman and Setlow 1979; Hanawalt et al. 1981; Fornace et al. 1981). Using the methodology to culture human bronchial epithelial and fibroblastic cells developed in our laboratory (Lechner et al. 1981; 1982), we have initiated a series of studies to investigate DNA damage and repair caused

Table 2
Metabolism of *N*-Nitrosamines by Cultured Human and Rat Esophagus. Radioactivity Bound to DNA

N-Nitrosamine	Rat		Human	
	dpm per mg DNA	pmoles per 10 mg DNA	dpm per mg DNA	pmoles per 10 mg DNA
NDMA	3,380 ± 735 (3)[a]	380[b]	<10-11,000[c] (3370;[b] 10[a])	335[b]
NEMA				
[¹⁴C]-Methyl	4,040 ± 670 (4)		<100 (3)	
[¹⁴C]-Ethyl	680 ± 120 (3)		<100 (3)	
Nitrosoethylamine	1,270 ± 99 (4)	390	<100-4,540 (990; 5)	384
NMBzA				
[¹⁴C]-Methyl	19,300 ± 3,480 (4)	20,940	<100-200 (74; 3)	240
[¹⁴C]-Benzyl	300 ± 430 (4)		n.d. (3)	
NPYR	2,720 ± 270 (3)	770	n.d. (3)	

[a] number of individual experiments
[b] mean value
[c] range of values

Table 3

Activation of N-Nitrosodimethylamine (NDMA) and NPYR to Metabolites Associated with DNA in Cultured Human Tissues

Tissue	NDMA (100 μM)	NPYR (100 μM)
Bronchus	906[a] (15)[b]	73 (4)
Esophagus	503 (8)	<20 (4)
Colon	215 (24)	38 (6)
Pancreatic duct	161 (2)	N.T.[c]

[a]Mean value expressed as pmoles/10 mg DNA
[b]Number of cases studied
[c](N.T.) not tested

Table 4

Interindividual Differences in DNA Binding Values of Chemical Carcinogens in Cultured Human Epithelial Tissues

Tissue	Benzo[a]pyrene (1.5 μM)	Aflatoxin B_1 (1.5 μM)	NDMA (100 μM)
Bronchus	75	120	60
Esophagus	99	70	90
Colon	130	150	145
Bladder	68	90	N.T.
Endometrium	70	N.T.[a]	N.T.

[a](N.T.) not tested.

by chemical and physical carcinogens as examined by alkaline elution methodology, Benzoylated Naphthoylated DEAE (BND) cellulose chromatography, unscheduled DNA synthesis (UDS) and HPLC analysis of the formation and removal of carcinogen-DNA adducts. Human bronchial epithelial cells can repair SSB in DNA damaged by X-radiation, UV-radiation, polynuclear aromatic hydrocarbons or N-nitrosamides (Fornace et al. unpubl. results; Grafstrom et al. 1982).

Physical Agents

SSBs in DNA are readily caused by either ionizing radiation or during excision repair of UV-induced DNA damage. The number of SSB and the rate of their removal is nearly equal in both normal epithelial and fibroblastic cells (Fornace et al. 1982). As shown in Table 5, asbestos fibers did not cause either DNA-protein crosslinks or a detectible increase in SSB even in the presence of the combination of arabinofuranosyl cytosine (ara-C) and hydroxyurea (Snyder et al. 1981), which inhibit the polymerase step during excision repair and, thus, enhance the sensitivity of the assay by allowing SSB to accumulate.

Table 5
Effects of Asbestos Fibers or Formaldehyde in Bronchial Cells

Cell	Agent	R	SSB/10^{10}d	R,Ara-C	Net Ara-C SSB/10^{10}d	Fraction of DNA Protein Cross-links Remaining
E	–	.90	–	.50	–	–
F	–	.99	–	.70	–	–
E	Amosite	.90	0	.51	0	–
F	Amosite	.98	< 1	.77	0	–
E	Crocodolite	.83	< 1	.48	< 1	–
F	Crocodolite	.94	< 1	.78	0	–
E	Formaldehyde	.87	< 1	.09	11.0	.23
F	Formaldehyde	.99	0	.11	11.8	.25

Epithelial (E) or fibroblastic (F) cells were exposed to amosite or crocodolite asbestos (100 μg/4 mls) in 60 mm tissue culture plates for 14.5 hr and analyzed for DNA SSB by alkaline elution. R indicates the relative retention of the cells treated with the indicated agent alone. 10 μM Ara-C and 2 mM Hydroxyurea (HU) were added to some of the samples for the final 4.5 hr of exposure to asbestos; "R,Ara-C" indicates the relative retention obtained with this regimen. Net Ara-C SSB represents the SSB frequency induced by the agent with Ara-C minus that obtained with Ara-C alone in each cell type. Cells were treated with 0.8 mM formaldehyde in serum-free medium for 1 hr and incubated in medium with serum for an additional 3.5 hr. "Fraction of crosslinks remaining" represents the crosslink level determined after exposure to formaldehyde for 1 hr and 3 hr of incubation in fresh medium divided by that obtained immediately after formaldehyde exposure.

Chemical Agents

Both procarcinogens, e.g., 7,12-dimethylbenz[a]anthracene (DMBA), and direct acting carcinogens, such as benzo[a]pyrene-diol-epoxide (BPDE) and N-methyl-N'-nitro-N-nitrosoguanidine (MNNG), cause DNA damage in bronchial cells (Fornace et al. 1982). When compared to DMBA, BPDE produced more SSB in DNA. MNNG also caused SSB that were nearly completely repaired by 15 hours. Metabolism of NDMA yields formaldehyde in quantities equivalent to production of methylcarbonium ions as seen in Figure 1. In addition to binding to cellular macromolecules, formaldehyde reacts with glutathione, a reaction that reduces NAD^+, and is enzymatically oxidized to formate and eventually CO_2 as shown in Figure 2. Therefore, the intracellular fate of formaldehyde is dependent on availability and quantity of macromolecular binding targets, concentrations of glutathione and NAD^+, and activities of degrading enzymes.

When human cells are exposed to formaldehyde, a number of pathobiological effects are seen. Formaldehyde at concentrations up to 300 μM is only slightly toxic to human bronchial fibroblasts (Table 6). Inhibition of CFE is only slightly larger at 300 μM as compared to 100 μM formaldehyde, although the growth rate is significantly decreased at the higher concentration. A con-

Table 6
CFE and Clonal Growth Rate of Human Bronchial Fibroblasts after Exposure to
Formaldehyde (HCHO) and X-Rays

Treatment	CFE[a]	PD/D[b]
Control	100	0.85 ± 0.02
100 μM HCHO 1 hr	76	0.84 ± 0.02
300 μM HCHO 1 hr	69	0.73 ± 0.02^c
X-ray, 200 R	55	0.79 ± 0.03
X-ray, 400 R	21	0.67 ± 0.03^c
X-ray, 200 R + 100 μM HCHO 1 hr	17	0.60 ± 0.04^d
X-ray, 200 R + 300 μM HCHO 1 hr	5	0.53 ± 0.04^d
X-ray, 400 R + 100 μM HCHO 1 hr	7	0.53 ± 0.04^d
X-ray, 400 R + 300 μM HCHO 1 hr	2	0.51 ± 0.03^d

[a]Mean CFE was expressed as percent of control and determined from colonies containing at least 16 cells after 8-day post-treatment culture of 500 cells/dish.
[b]Clonal growth rate was expressed as population doublings per day (PD/D ± SEM) and estimated as the mean number of cells/clone in 18 randomly selected colonies (2 replicate dishes) for each treatment.
[c]$p < 0.05$, compared to control.
[d]$p < 0.05$, compared to X-ray or HCHO.

centration of 1 mM is required to decrease CFE to less than 10% of control (data not shown). Interestingly, when cells were pre-exposed to ionizing radiation (200R or 400R), formaldehyde markedly increased the toxicity of radiation which resulted in both decreased CFE and growth rate. The effect of the combined exposure to X-ray and formaldehyde was significantly higher than the combined effect of each agent alone. Similar effects of these agents were also obtained in bronchial epithelial cells (data not shown). Since formaldehyde has been used as an agent for chemical modification of DNA (Feldman 1975) and gives rise to DNA damage in bacteria (Nishioka 1973), yeast (Magana-Schwenke and Bernard 1978), and mouse tumor cells (Ross and Shipley 1980), its effect in bronchial cells was investigated. DNA-protein crosslinks are caused by formaldehyde in human bronchial cells (Table 5). These crosslinks are rapidly removed at a rate similar to that found in rodent cells (Fornace et al. unpubl.). DNA-protein crosslinks are also caused by the pulmonary carcinogen, chromate, in human bronchial epithelial cells (Fornace et al. 1981) and in skin fibroblasts by *trans*diamminedichloroplatinate (Fornace and Little 1980; Fornace 1982), UV-radiation (Braun and Merrick 1975), formaldehyde (Fornace 1982), and polyfunctional alkylating drugs (Kohn et al. 1981). Although these chemical and physical agents are carcinogenic, the role of DNA-protein crosslinks, if any, in their oncogenic effects is unknown. DNA-protein crosslinks caused by formaldehyde are considered to be less cytotoxic lesions than are DNA-DNA crosslinks (Bedford and Fox 1981) which were not detected in bronchial cells (Grafstrom et al. 1982). Repair of DNA damage by formaldehyde results in the formation of DNA SSB. When human bronchial cells are exposed to formaldehyde and the DNA polymerase combination of ara-C and hydroxyurea, substantial DNA SSB accumulated. Studies using excision-deficient cells from patients with xeroderma pigmentosum indicate that these SSB are generated during DNA excision repair (Fornace 1982).

The effect of formaldehyde on the repair of X-ray-induced DNA SSB was investigated. Human bronchial cells were exposed to 800R of X-rays and then incubated with or without the presence of 100 μM formaldehyde and the repair of DNA SSB measured (Fig. 3). The presence of formaldehyde significantly inhibited the repair of the X-ray-induced SSB correlating with the potentiation of cytotoxicity by the combinations of these agents. Effects of formaldehyde on other DNA repair pathways is also being investigated. For example, preliminary experiments indicate that the removal of O^6-methylguanine in human bronchial cells is inhibited by formaldehyde (data not shown). One can also speculate that during the demethylation reaction putative O^6-methyl transferase may be inactivated by the generation of formaldehyde.

Formaldehyde has been shown to have many pathobiological effects in addition to those described above. In *Drosophilia*, mutations and enhancement of X-ray-induced mutation are caused by formaldehyde (Auerbach et al. 1977). One report suggests that formaldehyde acts as an initiating agent in the in vitro malignant transformation of mouse 10T½ cells (Ragen and Boreiko 1981). Nasal cavity carcinomas have been produced in rats by chronic inhalation of formaldehyde in parts per million levels (Swenberg et al. 1980). Although the carcinogenic effects, if any, of formaldehyde have not been demonstrated in humans, its toxicity as an irritant to the skin, mucous membranes, and respiratory tract is well known. Formaldehyde is also an important industrial product—annual U.S. production of 6 billion pounds in 1979—and is found in the gaseous phase of tobacco smoke so that tobacco smokers may inhale approximately 0.38 mg formaldehyde by smoking one pack of cigarettes (Yodaiken 1981).

SUMMARY

N-nitrosamines can be metabolized by cultured human epithelial tissues and cells. Quantitative differences in metabolism and alkylation of DNA are found among humans and among various organs within an individual. Whether or not these differences are sufficient to influence an individual's cancer risk and organ site is as yet unknown.

While the alkylating metabolites of *N*-nitrosamines and their cytotoxic, mutagenic, and carcinogenic effects have been extensively studied, the possible contribution of other metabolites, especially aldehydes, has not received much attention. Results from studies using experimental animals and our results showing multiple effects (DNA-protein crosslinks, DNA SSB, inhibition of DNA repair and cytotoxicity) of formaldehyde in cultured human bronchial cells suggest that the major metabolites of *N*-nitrosamines, i.e., carbonium ions and

FRACTION OF INTERNAL STANDARD DNA RETAINED ON FILTER

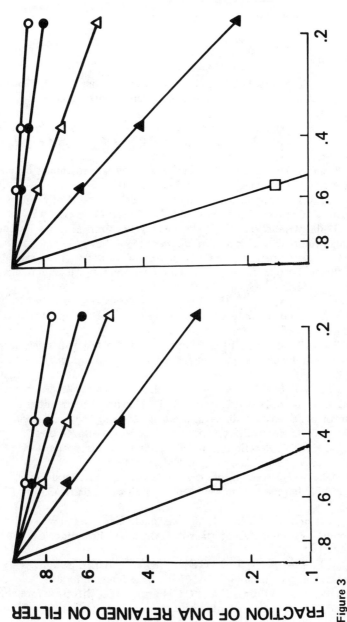

Figure 3

Effect of formaldehyde on the repair of X-ray-induced DNA SSB in human bronchial epithelial cells and fibroblasts. Epithelial cells (left); fibroblasts (right) (○———○) control; (●———●) 100 μM formaldehyde, 1 hr; (□———□) 800 R, no repair incubation; (△———△) 800 R and subsequently incubated for 1 hr in fresh medium at 37°; (▲———▲) 800 R and subsequently incubated for 1 hr in medium with 100 μM formaldehyde.

aldehydes, may act in concert in producing the toxic, mutagenic, and carcinogenic effects of N-nitrosamines.

ACKNOWLEDGMENT

We appreciate the secretarial assistance of Mrs. Norma Paige.

REFERENCES

Auerbach, C., M. Moutschen-Dahmen, and J. Moutschen. 1977. Genetic and cytogenetical effects of formaldehyde and related compounds. *Mutat. Res.* 39:317.

Autrup, H. 1980. Explant culture of human colon. In *Normal human tissue and cell culture, Methods in Cell Biology* 21B (eds. C.C. Harris et al.), p. 358. Academic Press, New York.

Autrup, H. and G.D. Stoner. 1982. Metabolism of N-nitrosamines by cultured rat and human esophagus. *Cancer Res.* 42:1307.

Autrup, H., C.C. Harris, and B.F. Trump. 1978a. Metabolism of N-nitrosamines by cultured human tissues. *Proc. XII Int. Cancer Congress* 1:12.

_____. 1978b. Metabolism of acyclic and cyclic N-nitrosamines by cultured human colon. *Proc. Soc. Exp. Biol. Med.* 159:111.

Autrup, H., R.C. Grafstrom, B. Christensen, and J. Kieler. 1981. Metabolism of chemical carcinogens by cultured human and rat bladder epithelial cells. *Carcinogenesis* 2:763.

Bedford, P. and B.W. Fox. 1981. The role of formaldehyde in methylene di-methanesulphonate-induced DNA cross-links and its relevance to cytotoxicity. *Chem.-Biol. Interact.* 38:119.

Braun, A. and B. Merrick. 1975. Properties of the ultraviolet-light-mediated binding of bovine serum albumin to DNA. *Photochem. Photobiol.* 21:243.

Cleaver, J.E., W.J. Bodell, D.C. Gruenert, L.N. Knapp, W.K. Kaufmann, S.D. Park, and B. Zelle. 1982. Repair and replication abnormalities in various human hypersensitive diseases. In *Mechanisms of chemical carcinogenesis* (eds. C.C. Harris and P. Cerutti). A.L. Liss, New York. (In press).

Feldman, M.Y. 1975. Reactions of nucleic acids and nucleoproteins with formaldehyde. *Progr. Nucleic Acid Res. Mol. Biol.* 13:1.

Fornace, A.J. 1982. Detection of DNA single-strand breaks produced during the repair of damage by DNA-protein cross-linking agents. *Cancer Res.* 42:145.

Fornace, A.J. and J.B. Little. 1980. Malignant transformation by the DNA-protein crosslinking agent trans-Pt(II)diamminedichloride. *Carcinogenesis* 1:989.

Fornace, A.J., D.S. Seres, J.F. Lechner, and C.C. Harris. 1981. DNA-protein crosslinking by chromium salts. *Chem.-Biol. Interact.* 36:345.

Grafstrom, R.C., A.J. Fornace, and C.C. Harris. 1982. Effect of formaldehyde on DNA damage and repair in human bronchial, epithelial and fibroblastic cells. *Proc. Am. Soc. Cancer Res.* 23:68.

Hanawalt, P.C., P.K. Cooper, A.K. Ganesan, R.S. Lloyd, C.A. Smith, and M.E. Zolan. 1982. Repair responses to DNA damage: Enzymatic pathways in *E. coli* and human cells. In *Mechanisms of Chemical Carcinogenesis* (eds. C.C. Harris and P. Cerutti), A.L. Liss, New York (In press).

Harris, C.C., B.F. Trump, and G.D. Stoner. (eds.) 1980. Culture of normal human tissues in cells. *Meth. Cell Biol.* 21A, 21B.

Harris, C.C., H. Autrup, G. Stoner, and B.F. Trump. 1978. Carcinogenesis studies in human respiratory epithelium: An experimental model system. In *Pathogenesis and Therapy of Lung Cancer* (ed. C.C. Harris), p. 559. Marcel Dekker, New York.

Harris, C.C., B.F. Trump, R.C. Grafstrom, and H. Autrup. 1982. Differences in metabolism of chemical carcinogens in cultured human epithelial tissues and cells. In *Mechanisms of Chemical Carcinogenesis* (ed. C.C. Harris and P. Cerutti). A.L. Liss, New York. (In press).

Harris, C.C., H. Autrup, G. Stoner, E. McDowell, B. Trump, and P. Schafer. 1977. Metabolism of acyclic and cyclic N-nitrosamines in cultured human bronchi. *J. Natl. Cancer Inst.* 59:1401.

Harris, C.C., H. Autrup, G.D. Stoner, B.F. Trump, E. Hillman, P.W. Schafer, and A.M. Jeffrey. 1979. Metabolism of benzo[a]pyrene, N-nitrosodimethylamine, and N-nitrosopyrrolidine and identification of the major carcinogen-DNA adducts in cultured human esophagus. *Cancer Res.* 39: 4401.

Harris, C.C., A. Frank, C. Van Haaften, D. Kaufman, R. Connor, F. Jackson, L. Barret, E. McDowell, and B. Trump. 1976. Binding of [^{3}H]Benzo(*a*)-pyrene to DNA in cultured human bronchus. *Cancer Res.* 36:1011.

Hemminki, K. 1981. Reactions of formaldehyde with guanosine. *Toxicol. Lett.* 9:161.

Kohn, K.W., R.A.G. Ewig, L.C. Erikson, and L.A. Zwelling. 1981. Measurement of strand breaks and crosslinks of alkaline elution. In *DNA Repair, A Laboratory Manual of Research Procedures* (eds. E.C. Friedberg and P.C. Hanawalt), p. 379. Marcel Dekker, New York.

Lechner, J.F., A. Haugen, I.A. McClendon, and E.W. Pettis. 1982. Clonal growth of normal adult human bronchial epithelial cells in a serum-free medium. *In Vitro* (in press.)

Lechner, J.F., A. Haugen, H. Autrup, I. McClendon, B.F. Trump, and C.C. Harris. 1981. Clonal growth of epithelial cells from normal adult human bronchus. *Cancer Res.* 41:2294.

Maciag, T., R.E. Nemore, R. Weinstein, and B.A. Gilchrest. 1981. An endocrine approach to the control of epidermal growth: Serum-free cultivation of human keratinocytes. *Science* 211:1452.

Magana-Schwenke, N. and E. Bernard. 1978. Biochemical analysis of damage induced in yeast by formaldehyde. II. Induction of crosslinks between DNA and protein. *Mutat. Res.* 51:11.

Magee, P.N., R. Montesano, and R. Preussmann. 1976. N-nitroso compounds and related compounds. In *Chemical Carcinogens* (ed. C. Searle), Monograph 173, p. 491. American Chemical Society, Washington, D.C.

Nebelin, E., H. Autrup, B. Christensen, and G. Blomkvist. 1982. Detection of metabolites of N-nitrosopyrrolidine and N-nitrosomethylamine in cultures of human bladder epithelial cells of normal origin. *IARC Sci. Publ.* 41 (In press)

Nishioka, H. 1973. Lethal and mutagenic action of formaldehyde in HCr$^+$ and HCr$^-$ strains of *Escherichia coli. Mutat. Res.* **17**:261.

Ragen, D.L. and G.J. Boreiko. 1981. Initiation of C3H/10T1/2 cell transformation by formaldehyde. *Cancer Lett.* **13**:325.

Ross, W.E. and N. Shipley. 1980. Relationship between DNA damage and survival in formaldehyde treated mouse cells. *Mutat. Res.* **79**:277.

Setlow, R.B. 1978. Repair deficient human disorders and cancer. *Nature* **271**: 713.

Swenberg, J.A., W.D. Kerns, R.I. Mitchell, E.J. Caralla, and K.L. Pavkov. 1980. Induction of squamous cell carcinomas of the rat nasal cavity by inhalation exposure to formaldehyde vapor. *Cancer Res.* **40**:3398.

Snyder, R.D., W.L. Carrier, and J.D. Regan. 1981. Application of arabinofuranosyl cytosine in the kinetic analysis and quantitation of DNA repair in human cells after ultraviolet irradiation. *Biophys. J.* **35**:339.

Taichman, L.B. and R.B. Setlow. 1979. Repair of ultraviolet light damage to the DNA of cultured human epidermal keratinocytes and fibroblasts. *J. Invest. Dermatol.* **73**:217.

Yodaiken, R.E. 1981. The uncertain consequences of formaldehyde toxicity. *J. Am. Med. Assoc.* **246**:1677.

COMMENTS

PEGG: Wouldn't you expect there to be a striking difference between the actions of MMU and NDMA, since one of them is generating the aldehyde and the other one isn't?

HARRIS: It may relate to the organ specificity, more so than just using a direct-acting agent. So the organ specificity might be, in part, related to the aldehyde formation and their subsequent metabolism.

TANNENBAUM: There is one other very significant difference, though, with nitrosourea, it also generates cyanates.

MONTESANO: Cyanates are not mutagenic.

TANNENBAUM: No, but they interact very rapidly with sulfhydryl compounds, which could have a role in the whole process. It's not just a simple comparison.

CHALLIS: They could also act as a cross-linking agent, like formaldehyde since they have very structurally similar features.

MILO: Curt, do you know whether nuclear protein might be involved in the cross-linking?

HARRIS: We're very interested in that. There are several different possibilities. A whole series of DNA-associated proteins could be cross-linked by formaldehyde. Of course, the repair enzymes could be directly inactivated. In addition, cross-links between the enzymes and DNA could be formed.

MILO: Do you think they are structural proteins?

HARRIS: I think we need further investigation.

PETO: You showed that NDMA actually alkylates, or at least binds to, the esophogeal DNA in the rat quite effectively. And yet, it's just not carcinogenic to the esophagus of the rat. We have just completed an experiment in which 1800 rats were treated over a very long lifespan with quite high doses of NDMA, and not a single one of those 1800 rats got an esophageal hyperplasia or benign esophageal tumor. And yet, the degree of alkylation of the DNA is really on the same order of magnitude; it differed only by a factor of 2 from the amount of alkylation that was produced by NDEA, which in the other half of the same experiment produced something like 1200 esophageal tumors. It really seemed as though the alkylation of DNA wasn't a sufficient explanation for the carcinogenicity of these nitrosamines. I mean, there has to be some other qualitatively different process involved. There has been almost an overemphasis on their effect of alkylating DNA, because the repair systems are so neat and they're interesting to work on. That makes them attractive, but there just has to be some qualitatively different process involved. Have you any idea what is likely to be involved? Has anyone any comment on that? Presumably, it's related to the cytoxicity.

HARRIS: Well, yes carcinogenesis is more than alkylation.

PETO: Certainly, carcinogenesis by nitrosamines appears to be a lot more than alkylation. There must be something else very, very specific.

SWANN: Can we just get one thing clear? The data you presented was actually alkylation, not just bound counts?

HARRIS: The only thing we can say for sure is that it is alkylation for NDMA, NEMA, and NMBzA, and NPYR and NIP were just bound counts.

ARCHER: Do you know whether they were covalently-bound counts?

HARRIS: They go through cesium chloride gradients and are not removed by extensive extraction with organic solvents.

ARCHER: Have you ever hydrolyzed to see if . . .

HARRIS: No, we haven't done that with NDEA or NPYR; only with NDMA, NEMA, and NMBzA.

HARTMAN: It has already been mentioned that perhaps only one cell type is important. In an esophageal cell preparation, if a large percentage of your cells are differentiated and contain DNA, they are likely not to make DNA any more. Perhaps, it will repair very well when that DNA is alkylated. Then the kind of numbers found will tell nothing about what happens to stem cells.

HARRIS: I agree.

PETO: Why the difference between NDMA and NDEA? When they're binding to a similar extent, why the gross qualitative difference in their effects on the esophagus in the rat?

PEGG: As Dr. Swann tried to point out, the total counts, which is what is being measured, is not entirely indicative of the amount of alkylation of the particular specific site.

MAGEE: I was going to say, in reply or to make a comment on Richard Peto's remark, that I think it would be important, if these comparisons are made, to remember that the cultured cell doesn't necessarily reflect the precise situation that occurs in the intact animal. We haven't really got, for obvious reasons, those comparative measurements between human beings and the various animals. I think when we get down to making quantitative comparisons they could be a bit misleading.

HARRIS: That is one of the reasons that we focused mostly on using cultured tissues instead of cultured cells, because we wanted to get as close as we could to the intact human.

SWANN: I think there is one thing which is really rather important, and that is that, of course, part of the experiment of Lee, et al. (1964) which was measurement, after NDMA administration, of the amount of alkylation in the esophageal nucleic acids—there wasn't any.

MAGEE: No, very low effect. But the sensitivity was much lower in those days, remember.

WEISBURGER: I have two questions: (1) On the question of carcinogenicity of formaldehyde—although many people in pathology have been exposed to sizable levels, there hasn't been a striking effect of formaldehyde exposure in humans. I am, however, intrigued with your comment, that perhaps aldehydes, and formaldehydes specifically, might affect the repair systems. The question is whether in your studies in your organ cultures you might have a carcinogen and formaldehyde, and see if you get more binding, or whatever you call it.

HARRIS: Well, two comments. One is that, unfortunately, epidemiology is a very insensitive approach for identifying specific carcinogens in the environment.

The second is as we are very interested in doing co-carcinogenesis experiments with bronchial epithelial cells using carcinogens plus different aldehydes.

MIRVISH: You stated that the human esophagus didn't metabolize the nitrosamines much, in commenting on Peter Magee's question. Just what do you mean by human esophagus? Are they taken freshly from autopsy, or are they cultured?

HARRIS: These are from trauma patients who are kidney donors from which we have obtained the tissues for the purposes of this research.

MIRVISH: Do you do the experiment as soon as they die, or keep them for a week?

HARRIS: No, because we culture the tissue for varying periods of time, usually one week, to minimize the effects of exogenous agents that the host might have been exposed to.

MIRVISH: How do you know they don't lose the activity while you culture them?

HARRIS: Because they have substantial activity, even at 1 day v. 7 days.

MIRVISH: It doesn't drop off?

HARRIS: We haven't looked further than 7 days.

MONTESANO: You mentioned the effects of formaldehyde in DNA synthesis and protein synthesis. I think you suggested that formaldehyde may inhibit DNA repair, which also was raised in relation to TPA some years ago. That data shows that this was completely aspecific, because TPA was affecting many cellular functions.

HARRIS: At 100 μm formaldehyde, the CFE of both bronchial epithelial cells and fibroblast was over 80%. We looked at growth rate, too, and the growth rate of the cells was not much different than without formaldehyde.

MONTESANO: But you mentioned here that there seemed to be an effect on DNA synthesis.

HARRIS: We are doing those experiments now, not only DNA, but also on protein and RNA.

ARCHER: I have a question which may be too complicated. One thing that bothers me with these kind of studies is a similar reservation as Sid Mirvish has, and that is how do you know that these cells, after they are being maintained 1 week in culture, are anything like normal? What are your criteria for normalcy?

HARRIS: That is less of a problem when you work with intact tissues than when you work in the cell system in which you are selecting out cells in monolayer culture.

What do we mean by "normal?" When we compare the explants and the tissue from the intact individual by electron microscopy and a number of other morphological methods, they are quite similar. We can't do many of the experiments on humans that perhaps would be suggested from your question.

ARCHER: You don't have any functional criteria, just morphological?

HARRIS: They make keratins and have a normal complement of keratins that are found in the bronchial epithelium. The cultured tissues incorporate amino acids, uridine, etc. But, again, we don't have the intact human comparison because most of us don't like to take tritiated thymidine and uridine.

PEGG: But you have done rat tissue comparison and you can also do the whole animal experiments in the rats. Can you do that and show that that works?

HARRIS: Yes, that could be done.

ARCHER: Why don't you do these studies with freshly isolated human tissue? Why culture it at all?

HARRIS: For a very simple reason: Freshly-isolated tissue is not fresh, because there has been a period of ischemia in that tissue, which we have characterized. Even in the immediate autopsy patients, it takes anywhere from 1-3 hours before that tissue is actually into the laboratory, under the best of circumstances. You do electron microscopy, look at the mitochondria, and they show all the signs of ischemic injury. You put them in culture for 3 hours, those signs of ischemic injury reverse themselves. Fresh tissue is not as good, in my opinion, as tissue that has been cultured.

TANNENBAUM: I just wonder whether Bill Hartman's statement about the stem cells isn't really the critical one. Perhaps the critical criterion shouldn't be whether or not you could show that those stem cells really are slowing or undergoing division.

HARRIS: Using tritiated thymidine, the basal cells will incorporate thymidine, as shown by autoradiography.

Metabolism of Dimethylnitrosamine and Repair of O^6-Methylguanine in DNA by Human Liver

RUGGERO MONTESANO AND HENRIETTE BRÉSIL
International Agency for Research on Cancer
Lyon Cedex 02, France

ANTHONY E. PEGG
Department of Physiology and Specialized Cancer Research Center
The Milton S. Hershey Medical Center
The Pennsylvania State University
Hershey, Pennsylvania 17033

The carcinogenicity of a variety of nitrosamines has been shown in a variety of animal species and tissues (Druckrey et al. 1967; Magee et al. 1976; Bogovski and Bogovski 1981) and there is now substantial evidence that this adverse biological effect is dependent upon the capacity of the target organ or cell to metabolize these carcinogens into reactive and mutagenic metabolites which react with various cellular macromolecules (see Swann, this volume).

The liver is the main target organ for dimethylnitrosamine (NDMA) in various animal species for tumor induction after chronic administration (Magee et al. 1976). In all instances it has been shown that metabolic activation is a necessary condition for such biological effects (Pegg 1980).

Among the different sites of base alkylation in the DNA, there is growing evidence that alkylation of the oxygen of guanine in DNA (in particular O^6-alkylguanine) is critical for the carcinogenic effect of these types of alkylating agents (Goth and Rajewsky 1974; Pegg 1977; Montesano 1981). The probability that an organ develops tumors appears to be associated with the accumulation of O^6-alkylguanine in its DNA. This has been attributed to the lower efficiency (in comparison to main target organs) of the enzyme system(s) involved in the removal of such damage from DNA. The persistence of this promutagenic base in DNA presumably increases the probability that a miscoding event will take place during DNA synthesis and result in a permanent heritable change in the base sequence (mutation) (Loveless 1969; Lawley 1976). Other mechanisms have also been proposed by Karran and Marinus (1982).

A series of experiments are summarized here examining the capacity of human liver to metabolize DMN and to repair from DNA the biologically important lesion, O^6-methylguanine. More detail of these experiments are reported elsewhere (Montesano and Magee 1970, 1974; Montesano et al. 1973; Pegg et al. 1982).

Metabolism of NDMA

The metabolism of NDMA has been determined in vitro using liver slices from rats, Syrian golden hamsters, trout, newts, monkeys, and man. Briefly, the tissue slices were incubated at 37°C for 90 minutes, using O_2 as gas phase in 2.0 ml of Krebs-Ringer phosphate buffer, containing 20 μM of glucose in a conventional Warburg apparatus. ^{14}C-NDMA (70 μg - 0.1 μCi) in 0.2 ml of buffer was added from the side arms. The labeled [14]CO_2 produced was trapped in 10% NaOH, converted to Ba_2[14]CO_3 and the radioactivity was measured. Total nucleic acids were extracted from the pooled slices according to the procedure of Schneider (1945). The nucleic acid, after hydrolysis in 1N HCl for 1 hour at 100°C, were chromatographed on a Dowex-50 W (H^+ form) column with an exponential 1N to 4N HCl gradient in order to separate the purine bases. The amount of 7-methylguanine formed was calculated according to Swann and Magee (1968). The respiration rates were also monitored to assess the viability of the various tissues examined. The metabolism of NDMA is expressed as the production of radioactive [14]CO_2 (percentage of the ^{14}C added as ^{14}C-NDMA) that is produced in 90 minutes by 160 mg of tissue and the percentage of 7-methylguanine formed in total nucleic acids. The present knowledge on the metabolism of DMN (see Pegg 1980) indicates that these are reliable parameters of the metabolism of this carcinogen.

The results are summarized in Table 1, which shows that the two parameters measured (production of [14]CO_2 and formation of 7-methylguanine) are proportional to each other. Metabolism of NDMA was observed in the liver of all species tested, all of which are known to be susceptible to the carcinogenic activity of NDMA. The liver of Syrian golden hamster showed the highest rate of metabolism followed by the rat liver. The human liver slices showed a metabolism capacity to activate NDMA similar to that detected in rat liver slices. Much lower activities were observed in the tissues from other species. These in vitro results parallel the result obtained in vivo, since the ratio of liver nucleic acid methylation in hamster, to that of rat liver, closely corresponds to the ratio of methylation determined in vivo in these two species (Margison et al. 1976). The ratio between the rates at which rat liver and kidney slices metabolize NDMA in vitro (see Table 1) also reflects the ratio observed in NDMA methylation studies in vivo in the same species (Swann and Magee 1968). More recently, alkylation in the O^6-position of guanine has been detected in the liver DNA of human beings exposed to NDMA (Herron and Shank 1980; Shank, this volume) and postmitochondrial fractions of human liver have been shown to metabolize nitrosamines into mutagenic metabolites (Sabadie et al. 1980).

In summary, these data indicate that human liver is able to metabolize NDMA and therefore there is no reason to suppose that man should be resistant to the toxic and other adverse biological effects of NDMA.

Table 1

In Vitro Metabolism of NDMA in Tissue Slices From Various Species Including Human Beings

Species	Tissues	$^{14}CO_2$ Production (% of ^{14}C added as ^{14}C-NDMA)	7-methylguanine (mol/100 mol of guanine)
Newt *(Triturus Helveticus)*	liver	0.31	N.D.[a]
Trout *(Rainbow)*	liver	0.16	0.0004
Hamster *(Syrian golden)*	liver	8.6	0.29
Rat *(Wistar)*	liver	5.2	0.19
	kidney	0.5	0.01
Monkey *(Macacus cynomolgus)*	liver	0.56	0.018
	kidney	0.16	0.0001
Man	liver	3.0	0.13

Data from Montesano and Magee (1970); Montesano et al. (1973); Montesano and Magee (1974).

[a]N.D. = not determined.

Repair of O^6-methylguanine

Methylating agents, such as NDMA, are known to alkylate DNA at various sites (Lawley 1976; Pegg 1977; Singer 1979) and each of these DNA adducts is repaired by a specific repair process (see Lindahl 1979; Pegg and Bennett 1982). Most of these repair reactions involve various glycosylases, but O^6-methylguanine is removed by a methyltransferase, that transfers the methyl group from the O^6-position of guanine to a receptor protein containing cysteine residues. This new process of DNA repair was originally characterized in *Escherichia coli* (Olsson and Lindahl 1980) and is also present in rodent liver cells (Bogden et al. 1981; Pegg and Perry 1981).

In our in vitro assay using methylated DNA as a substrate, we have examined the capacity of human liver fractions to catalyze the repair of O^6-methylguanine and compared this to the activity found in rat liver. A total of 10 samples of human livers (6 males and 4 females of different ages) were tested. These samples were obtained shortly after circulatory arrest from kidney transplant donors with total cerebral infraction (von Bahr et al. 1980). The assay is described in detail elsewhere (Pegg et al. 1982). Briefly, [^{3}H-methyl]-methylated calf thymus DNA (containing 1.2 pmol of O^6-methylguanine) was

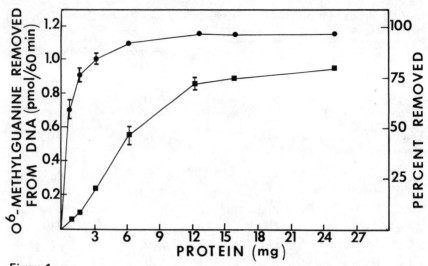

Figure 1
The results ± S.E.M. of the amount of O^6-methylguanine removed in a 60 min incubation
with the protein indicated are shown. The DMA substrate contained 1.20 pmol of O^6-
methylguanine. The right-hand ordinate indicates the percentage of the total removed.
(■━━━━━■) rat livers; (●━━━━━●) human liver.

incubated at 37° with different amounts of liver extracts in 66 mM Tris-HCl
(pH, 8.3) in the presence of 1.3 mM dithiothreitol, and 0.3 mM Edetic Acid
(EDTA). At the end of incubation the reaction was stopped with cold $HC10_4$,
the DNA hydrolyzed in 0.1 N HCl at 70°C for 30 minutes and chromatographed
on a Sephadex G-10 column. The results are presented (Fig. 1) as the amount of
O^6-methylguanine removed in 60 minutes and the data obtained with human
liver compared to that observed with rat liver fractions. It can be seen that the
human liver samples were considerably more active.

With human liver fractions less than 1 mg of protein was needed to remove more than 50% of the total O^6-methylguanine from the DNA substrate,
while with rat liver, more than 6 mg of protein was required to remove the same
amount of O^6-methylguanine. When the comparison is made based on measurements in which less than 60% of the substrate was removed [conditions which
give results proportional to the protein added (Pegg et al. 1981)], the human
liver fractions were about 10 times more active. A higher capacity to remove
O^6-methylguanine from DNA in vivo was also observed in cultured human
fibroblasts (Medcalf et al. 1981) and in human peripheral blood lymphocytes
(Harris et al. 1981) as compared to rodent cells but in these experiments the
repair process was not characterized using subcellular extracts.

Separate experiments (Pegg et al. 1982) have also shown that the
mechanism of repair of O^6-methylguanine results [as in bacteria (Olsson and

Lindahl 1980) and in rodent cells (Bogden et al. 1981; Pegg and Perry 1981)], in the stoichiometric transfer of the methyl group from the O^6-position of guanine in DNA to an acceptor protein. This process forms S-methylcysteine in the protein and restores guanine in the DNA (Pegg et al. 1982).

CONCLUSIONS

The results presented here show that human liver is able to metabolize NDMA efficiently into reactive metabolites which bind to DNA. These findings are consistent with the toxic effect observed in the liver of subjects exposed to NDMA (Freund 1937; see Kimbrough and Flieg, this volume). Human liver was able to repair a biologically important adduct formed in DNA (O^6-methylguanine) and was substantially more active than rat liver in carrying out this repair. The accumulation of such data among various animal species including man may provide a more scientific basis in the future for the qualitative and quantitative extrapolation of carcinogenicity animal data to man.

REFERENCES

von Bahr, C., C.-G. Groth, H. Jansson, G. Lundgren, M. Lind, and H. Glaumann. 1980. Drug metabolism in human liver *in vitro*: establishment of a human liver bank. *Clin. Pharmacol. Ther.* **27**:711.

Bogden, J.M., A. Eastman, and E. Bresnick. 1981. A system in mouse liver for the repair of O^6-methylguanine lesions in methylated DNA. *Nucl. Acid Res.* **81**:3089.

Bogovski, P. and S. Bogovski. 1981. Animal species in which N-nitroso-compounds induce cancer. *Int. J. Cancer* **27**:471.

Druckrey, H., R. Preussmann, S. Ivankovic, and D. Schmähl. 1967. Organotrope carcinogene Wirkungen bei 65 vershiedenen N-nitroso Verbindungen an BD-ratten. *Z. Krebsforsch.* **69**:103.

Freund, H.A. 1937. Clinical manifestations and studies in parenchymatous hepatitis. *Ann. Intern. Med.* **10**:1144.

Goth, R. and M.F. Rajewsky. 1974. Persistence of O^6-ethylguanine in rat brain DNA: correlation with nervous system-specific carcinogenesis by ethyl nitrosourea. *Proc. Natl. Acad. Sci. U.S.A.* **71**:639.

Harris, G., P.D. Lawley, and I. Olsen. 1981. Mode of action of methylating carcinogens: comparative studies of murine and human cells. *Carcinogenesis* **5**:403.

Herron, D.C. and R.C. Shank. 1980. Methylated purines in human liver DNA after probable dimethylnitrosamine poisoning. *Cancer Res.* **40**:3116.

Karran, P. and M.G. Marinus. 1982. Mismatch correction at O^6-methylguanine residues in *E. coli* DNA. *Nature* **296**:868.

Lawley, P.D. 1976. Carcinogenesis by alkylating agents. In: Chemical Carcinogenesis (ed. C.E. Searle), ACS Monograph Series **173**:No. 4, p. 83.

Lindahl, T. 1979. DNA glycosylases, endonucleases for apurinic/apyrimidinic sites and base excision-repair. *Prog. Nucleic Acid Res. Mol. Biol.* **22**:135.

Loveless, A. 1969. Possible relevance of O^6-alkylation of deoxyguanosine to the mutagenicity and carcinogenicity of nitrosamines and nitrosamides. *Nature* 223:206.

Magee, P.N., R. Montesano, and R. Preussmann. 1976. N-nitroso compounds and related carcinogens. *ACS Monogr.* 173(11):491.

Margison, G.P., J.M. Margison, and R. Montesano. 1976. Methylated purines in the deoxyribonucleic acid of various Syrian gold hamster tissues after administration of a hepatocarcinogenic dose of dimethylnitrosamine. *Biochem. J.* 157:627.

Medcalf, A.S.C. and P.D. Lawley. 1981. Time course of O^6-methylguanine removal from DNA of MNU-treated human fibroblasts. *Nature* 289:796.

Montesano, R. 1981. Alkylation of DNA and tissue specificities in nitrosamine carcinogenesis. *J. Supramol. Struct. Cell. Biochem.* 17:259.

Montesano, R. and P.N. Magee. 1970. Metabolism of dimethylnitrosamine by human liver slices *in vitro*. *Nature* 228:173.

––––––. 1974. Comparative metabolism *in vitro* of nitrosamines in various animal species including man. *IARC Sci. Publ.* 10:39.

Montesano, R., A.J. Ingram, and P.N. Magee. 1973. Metabolism of dimethyl-nitrosamine by amphibians and fish *in vitro*. *Experientia* 29:599.

Olsson, M. and T. Lindahl. 1980. Repair of alkylated DNA in Escherichia coli: methyl group transfer from O^6-methylguanine to a protein cysteine residue. *J. Biol. Chem.* 255:10569.

Pegg, A.E. 1977. Formation and metabolism of alkylated nucleosides: possible role in carcinogenesis by nitroso compounds and alkylating agents. *Adv. Cancer Res.* 25:195.

––––––. 1980. Metabolism of N-nitrosodimethylamine. *IARC Sci. Publ.* 27:3.

Pegg, A.E. and W. Perry. 1981. Stimulation of transfer of methyl groups from O^6-methylguanine in DNA to protein by rat liver extracts in response to hepatoxins. *Carcinogenesis* 2:1195.

Pegg, A.E. and R.A. Bennett. 1982. Mammalian DNA repair enzymes. In: *Enzymes of Nucleic Acid Synthesis and Processing*: CRC Series on Biochemistry and Molecular Biology of the Cell Nucleus, CRC Press, Inc. Boca Raton, Florida. (In press).

Pegg, A.E., W. Perry, and R.A. Bennett. 1981. Effect of partial hepatectomy on removal of O^6-methylguanine from alkylated DNA by rat liver extracts. *Biochem. J.* 197:195.

Pegg, A.E., M. Roberfroid, C. von Bahr, R.S. Foote, S. Mitra, H. Brésil, A. Likhachev, and R. Montesano. 1982. Removal from DNA on O^6-methyl-guanine by human liver fractions. *Proc. Natl. Acad. Sci. U.S.A.* (in press).

Sabadie, N., C. Malaveille, A.-M. Camus, and H. Bartsch. 1980. Comparison of the hydroxylation of benzo(a)pyrene with the metabolism of vinyl chloride, N-nitrosomorpholine and N-nitroso-N′-methylpiperazine to mutagens by human and rat liver microsomal fractions. *Cancer Res.* 40: 119.

Schneider, W.C. 1945. Phosphorus compounds in animal tissues. I. Extraction and estimation of desoxypentose nucleic acid and of pentose nucleic acid. *J. Biol. Chem.* 161:293.

Singer, B. 1979. N-nitroso alkylating agents: formation and persistence of alkyl derivatives in mammalian nucleic acids as contributing factors in carcinogenesis. *J. Natl. Cancer Inst.* 62:1329.

Swann, P.F. and P.N. Magee. 1968. Nitrosamine-induced carcinogenesis. The alkylation of nucleic acids of the rat by N-methyl-N-nitrosourea, dimethyl-nitrosamine, dimethylsulphate and methylmethane sulphonate. *Biochem. J.* **110**:39.

COMMENTS

YANG: Have you looked at tissue distribution? Does liver have the highest activity?

MONTESANO: In all the species tested, the liver shows the highest capacity to repair by O^6-methylguanine. In the case of the hamster, however, the rate of removing O^6-methylguanine is not as good as the rat liver. (Montesano et al. 1980).

TANNENBAUM: I think Ron Shank just published a paper on hydrazine which showed that this causes O^6-methylguanine formation. Is there some physiological significance to these enzymes?

MONTESANO: Ron Shank's group found O^6-methylguanine was produced after administration of substances that are not methylating agents. Production of O^6-methylguanine may therefore arise though other mechanisms than direct alkylation (Barrows and Shank 1981).

TANNENBAUM: Is this repair enzyme a toxic response to the cell? Perhaps it has physiological functions other than just what we are discussing.

MONTESANO: The repair process is the same. You can induce alkylation with various types of agents in the O^6-position, but the mechanism of removal of O^6 doesn't look as though it is dependent on the agents which you use for the alkylation.

WEISBURGER: If I understand you correctly, your findings are the reverse of Ron Shank's, that is, to remove methyl from a key alkylation site. How would you rate this transfer process in relation to the efficient repair for the methyl and ethyl groups in liver, compared to the nucleases which strip out in a whole segment of codon that may affect this?

Is this transfer or dealkylation a more efficient way of, quote, "repairing," liver specifically, than the more classic endonucleases that operate differently?

MONTESANO: In adapted *E. coli*, the removal of O^6-methylguanine is very rapid, with a half-life of less than 1 second (Cairns 1980). The maximum number of O^6-methylguanine molecules required to saturate this rapid repair system has been calculated to be about 3000 molecules per bacterium. Protein synthesis is required to build up a pool of molecules responsible for this repair process, that is one of the most efficient forms of DNA repair reported (Cairns 1980).

WEISBURGER: Just as a follow-up on your review of the bacterial systems: would it seem that the bacterial systems are more efficient than the mammalian systems, because they have many cell duplications in the 90 minutes of preexposure, so that a new generation of cells coming in actually has more of the enzyme and you almost get a mutational effect? In other words, if you remove the alkylating agent and continue collecting cells do you maintain this high level, or does it drop down again?

MONTESANO: Following this rapid removal in adapted bacteria it has been shown that protein synthesis is required to build up a pool of proteins which is responsible for the removal of the O^6.

PEGG: How do you know the mammalian system isn't already partly induced?

WEISBURGER: That's what one wonders about, of course.

MONTESANO: One may assume that during evolution the "adaptive" response became constitutive in mammalian cells.

PEGG: But it may have been induced, because of the exposure to nitrosamines or some other alkylating agent or to Dr. Shank's physiological mechanism.

MAGEE: I think, in this connection, that Dr. Louis Barrows (Barrows and Magee 1982) has recently found that S-adenosylmethionine (SAM) will methylate DNA on O^6 without an enzyme in vitro. We believe this to be correct, because Dr. Lindahl has a paper (Rydberg and Lindahl 1982) proving the same thing.

MICHEJDA: On the other hand, SAM is not mutagenic, though.

HARTMAN: Michael Benders and Richard Setlow's (unpubl. results) reported at the Environmental Mutagenesis Society meeting that they measured this activity in lymphocytes and several other blood cells, and the activity is different for different cell types.

PEGG: I was really very surprised to learn that with that many human samples the activities were all so similar.

HARRIS: There is always a level of variation between different human samples. I believe that Setlow found over a 40-fold variation in the activity of this enzyme in lymphocytes.

WEISBURGER: Many years ago at the NIH when we were working on the metabolism of acetylaminofluorene (AAF) in five clinical center patients, we found them to be almost the same as concerned 7-hydroxylation. They were quite markedly different as regards the key N-oxidation activities. I guess even the same sample would have different activities depending on which enzyme you are looking at.

HARTMAN: Between the ages of 20 and 60, there didn't seem to be any difference in the activities measured with lymphocytes in Setlow's experiments. They were laboratory personnel examined. Also, males and females showed no difference.

MONTESANO: In our human samples, the ages go from 19-65.

HARTMAN: I did notice only four people were in their sixties. But that is not an adequate sample size.

MIRVISH: Does this enzyme put the methyl group onto cysteine of itself, or is there another protein, or does the enzyme then get used up very quickly?

PEGG: With the bacterial enzyme, it's fairly clear that it puts the methyl group onto itself, and is used only once since the acceptor cannot be regenerated.

   With the mammalian systems, it is not really so clear, but the regeneration of the acceptor protein is slow if it occurs at all.

   I would like to mention some experiments we have done in collaboration with James Swenberg (unpubl. results) on the removal of O^6-methylguanine from DNA in rat liver cells. Such removal is increased about threefold by chronic exposure to carcinogens including NDMA or 1,2-dimethylhydrazine when you consider the liver as a whole. We have now assayed the enzyme activity in isolated hepatocytes and in nonparenchymal cells from the liver. The activity in the hepatocytes which make up the bulk of the liver mass is induced threefold, peaking at 8 days in agreement with the total liver activity. But the activity in the nonparenchymal cells is much lower than in the hepatocytes and is not induced at all. In considering DNA repair it is important to know how active this is in the cell populations which actually are targets for carcinogens.

PETO: What sort of nonparenchymal cells were they?

PEGG: These were a mixed population of nonparenchymal cells, which included several different cell types not including the bile duct cells.

MIRVISH: How did you separate them?

PEGG: They were separated using an elutriation technique. Dr. Swenberg has, as I'm sure you know, published in *Nature* studies for the persistence of O^6-alkylguanine in vivo under these conditions, and the enzyme data goes along with that (Lewis and Swenberg 1980).

KIMBROUGH: Has anybody looked at embryonic tissues?

MONTESANO: Dr. M. Rajewsky (Goth and Rajewsky 1974) has done a quite comprehensive study on the removal of O^6 to see if O^6-ethylguanine is removed from the brain tissue in rat embryos. In the last days of pregnancy they are able to remove O^6-ethylguanine from liver DNA but in the brain tissue they were not.

PEGG: We actually isolated the enzyme from very young rats immediately afrer birth, and at that time the amount of extractable enzyme was rather low. But, of course, the number of actual hepatocytes in the liver is also rather low, and it seemed to fit rather well with the number of hepatocytes.

CONNEY: Does the enzyme level go up in partial hepatectomy, where you stimulate liver growth?

PEGG: Yes, it goes up sixfold. That's the biggest induction we have found in mammalian cells.

CONNEY: Does anything happen with those compounds with phenobarbital administration or compounds that stimulate liver growth?

PEGG: A 3-4-day treatment with phenobarbital did not induce the activity but we did not try for longer times.

References

Barrows, L.R. and P.N. Magee. 1982. Nonenzymatic methylation of DNA by S-adenosylmethionine *in vitro. Carcinogenesis* 3:349.

Barrows, L.R. and R.C. Shank. 1981. Aberrant methylation of liver DNA in rats during hepatotoxicity. *Toxicol. Appl. Pharmacol.* 60:334.

Cairns, J. 1980. Bacteria as proper subjects for cancer research. *Proc. R. Soc. Lond. B Biol. Sci.* 208:121.

Goth, R. and M.F. Rajewsky. 1974. Persistence of O^6-ethylguanine in rat brain. DNA: Correlation with nervous system-specific carcinogenesis by ethyl nitrosourea. *Proc. Natl. Acad. Sci. U.S.A.* 71:639.

Lewis, J.G. and J.A. Swenberg. 1980. Differential repair of O^6-methylguanine in DNA of rat hepatocytes and nonparenchymal cells. *Nature* **288**:185.

Montesano, R., A.E. Pegg, and G.P. Margison. 1980. Alkylation of DNA and carcinogenicity of N-nitroso-compounds. *J. Toxicol. Environ. Health* **6**:1001.

Rydberg, B. and T. Lindahl. 1982. Nonenzymatic methylation of DNA by the intracellular methyl group donor S-adenosyl-L-methionine is a potential mutagenic reaction. *EMBO J.* **1**:211.

Methylation of Human Liver DNA After Probable
Dimethylnitrosamine Poisoning

RONALD C. SHANK AND DEBORAH C. HERRON*
Department of Community and Environmental Medicine
University of California Southern Occupational Health Center
University of California
Irvine, California 92717

Development of a rapid, highly sensitive, and inexpensive technique to quanti-tatively measure the concentration of small amounts of alkylated bases in DNA was required for recent investigations on the methylation of liver DNA by S-adenosylmethionine in response to administration of the inorganic hepatotoxin and carcinogen, hydrazine (Barrows and Shank 1978, 1980; Becker et al. 1981) and for studies on the dose-dependent pharmacokinetics of the formation and removal of methylguanines following administration of 1,2-dimethylhydrazine (Herron and Shank 1981). In those studies, the use of radioactive precursors was either not useful in quantifying DNA methylation (the case of hydrazine in which the specific activity of the metabolic pool of the methylating agent varied greatly with time) or not economically feasible (the case of 1,2-dimethyl-hydrazine which involved analysis of over a thousand DNA samples). Friedman and coworkers (1963) and Loveless (1969) called attention to the intense fluorescence of 7-methylguanine (7-MeGua) and O^6-methyldeoxyguanosine in UV light, and Taylor and Cooney (1976) described the slow, liquid chromato-graphic separation and quantitation of methylated derivatives of nucleic acids using a fluorescence detector rather than radiolabeled tracers. On the basis of these observations, Herron and Shank (1979) developed a highly sensitive high-pressure liquid chromatographic (HPLC) technique for the optical detection of alkylated purines in DNA hydrolysates that was complete in 15 minutes. At that time that method permitted the quantitative analysis of as little as 7 ng 7-MeGua and 150 pg of O^6-methylguanine (O^6-MeGua) in 500 μg DNA; for levels of DNA methylation resulting from exposures to toxic doses of methylating carcinogens only 50 μg of DNA were required for quantitative analysis.

*Present address: Atlantic Richfield Company, Los Angeles, California.

A fluorescence detector with a 150-watt xenon lamp was used because of its especially high sensitivity to materials which fluoresce at excitation wavelengths between 275 and 300 nm. A fluorescence spectrophotometer using a deuterium lamp was unable to detect the levels of methylated guanines normally encountered in fractionated hydrolysates of DNA derived from animals treated with high doses of methylnitrosourea, 1,2-dimethylhydrazine, or even dimethylnitrosamine (NDMA); the lower sensitivity of the deuterium lamp detector was due, presumably, to the lower photon output of such lamps at the longer UV wavelengths.

In the chromatographic separation of DNA guanine bases chosen for this study, baseline resolution between adenine and 7-MeGua could not be achieved. In this instance monitoring base elution with a fluorescence spectrophotometer has an added benefit: 7-MeGua fluoresces strongly, but adenine does not; this difference decreases the size of the large adenine chromatographic peak and increases the size of the small 7-MeGua peak and gives a much greater apparent resolution between the two materials.

This analytical procedure has been extremely useful in the quantitative determination of not only 7-MeGua and O^6-MeGua but also 7-ethylguanine, O^6-ethylguanine, 3-methyladenine, 1-methyladenine, 7-methyladenine, and 1-methylguanine (1-MeGua) as well, all without the need for radiolabeled material (Herron and Shank 1979; R.A. Becker and R.C. Shank unpubl. results). A quantitative study (Herron and Shank 1979) comparing the formation of 7-MeGua and O^6-MeGua in liver, kidney, and colon DNA of rats treated with equal doses of either $1,2$-^{14}C dimethylhydrazine or unlabeled dimethylhydrazine demonstrated that the radioactivity and fluorescence detection techniques gave nearly identical results (radioactivity: 2450 μ mol 7-MeGua and 254 μ mol O^6-MeGua/mol guanine; fluorescence: 2510 μ mol 7-MeGua and 214 μ mol O^6-MeGua/mol guanine).

Having developed this method, our laboratory was asked in August 1979 to examine specimens of human tissues to determine whether any of the tissues had come from persons exposed to methylating agents, and, in particular, whether any of the tissues contained methylated DNA that would be consistent with NDMA poisoning.

METHODS

Eight frozen samples of liver and kidney (2-8 g/sample) from human subjects were received from the Center for Disease Control, Atlanta, Georgia, and DNA was isolated by the phenolic extraction method of Kirby (1957) and purified by the method of Swann and Magee (1968). After purification the DNA was dissolved in water and one-ninth volume 1 M HCl was added (final mixture: 5 mg DNA/ml 0.1 M HCl). The DNA was depurinated at 70° for 30 min. The

DNA hydrolysate was filtered through a 0.65 μm pore size Millipore filter and fractionated on a Partisil-10 strong cation-exchange column (4.5 mm ID, 25 cm long; Whatman, Inc., Clifton, New Jersey) using a mobile phase of 0.06 M ammonium phosphate (pH 2.0) at a flow of 2.0 ml/min (Herron and Shank 1979). Elution of pyrimidine oligonucleotides and free purine bases was monitored using a Farrand fluorescence spectrophotometer LCF-100 with an excitation wavelength of 286 nm and interference emission filter of 366 nm. The amounts of guanine, 7-MeGua and O^6-MeGua in each hydrolysate were quantitated by measuring the area of the respective chromatographic peaks using electronic integration and calibration with authentic standards of guanine and 7-MeGua (Sigma Chemical Company, St. Louis, Missouri) and O^6-MeGua (prepared according to Balsiger and Montgomery 1960). At the time of analysis it was known that the tissues were derived from victims of Reye's syndrome, methyl bromide poisoning and a suspected NDMA poisoning, one of the cases described at this meeting by Dr. Renate Kimbrough (this volume); however, the source of any one tissue at that time was not known to us.

RESULTS

Only one DNA sample contained detectable amounts of 7-MeGua (1363 μmol/ mol guanine) and O^6-MeGua (273 μmol/mol guanine). The code number on the tissue specimen from which the DNA was obtained was communicated to Dr. Renate Kimbrough of the Center for Disease Control in Atlanta, and a request was made for a second specimen from the same tissue to confirm the analytical results. Another frozen liver specimen was received from the Center for Disease Control, and frozen specimens of liver, kidney, and heart were received from the Poison Laboratory in Denver, Colorado. DNA was isolated from these specimens and again only one, a liver DNA sample, contained methylated purines. That sample of DNA contained 1373 μmol 7-MeGua/mol guanine and 317 μmol O^6-MeGua/mol guanine and was subsequently identified by Dr. Kimbrough as a liver specimen taken from a 24-year old male victim of probable NDMA poisoning, as was the earlier liver specimen from which DNA containing methylated purines was obtained. The DNA samples prepared from the remaining tissues were derived from victims of methyl bromide poisoning and Reye's syndrome cases; analyses of 500 μg of DNA from those tissues failed to detect methylguanines. Figure 1 compares the elution profiles of fractionated DNA hydrolysates (100 μg DNA) prepared from a methyl bromide poisoning and the suspected NDMA poisoning. The O^6-MeGua elution peak appears greater than that for 7-MeGua because the relative fluorescence of O^6-MeGua is 18:1 at a 286-nm excitation. Analyses on the two liver specimens from the NDMA poisoning were in close agreement, with only a 0.7% variation between 7-MeGua values and 7.5% variation between O^6-MeGua values.

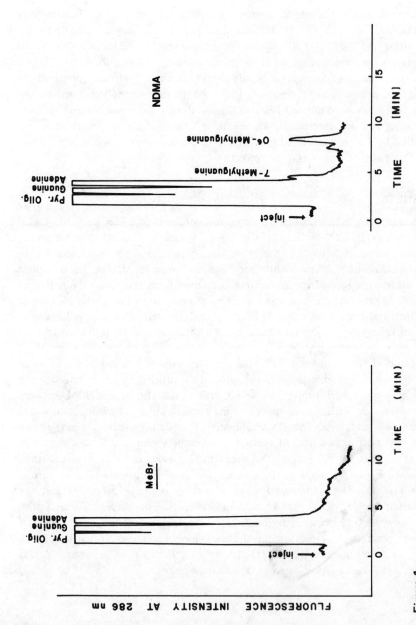

Figure 1
Elution profiles of liver DNA hydrolysate from victims of methyl bromide (MeBr) and NDMA poisonings; pyrimidine oligonucleotides (Pyr. Olig.). (Redrawn from the original chromatogram and reprinted, with permission, from Herron and Shank 1980.)

DISCUSSION

An attempt was made to determine whether these levels of DNA methylation were consistent with exposure to a dose of NDMA likely to be lethal to a 24-year old man, based on what is known about experimental NDMA poisoning in animals. If it is assumed that 7-MeGua in the DNA of the victim's liver had a half-life of approximately 48 hours, which is consistent with several reports in the literature for rodent liver DNA (Pegg and Nicoll 1976), then the level of 1300 μmol 7-MeGua/mol guanine 5 days after apparent exposure to NDMA would imply a maximum level of approximately 6000-7000 μmol 7-MeGua/mol guanine on the day of intoxication. According to Craddock (1969) and Pegg (1977), such alkylation levels can result from a dose of approximately 20 mg NDMA/kg body wt to the rat. Montesano and Magee (1970) suggested that the human may metabolize NDMA at a rate somewhat slower than the rat and therefore the actual amount of NDMA to which the poisoning victim may have been exposed could be greater than 20 mg/kg body wt. The published oral LD_{50} for NDMA in the rat is 27-41 mg/kg body wt (Heath and Magee 1962), hence, the methylation levels observed in the victim's liver DNA are consistent with the young man in this study receiving a lethal dose of NDMA.

If the assumption that the maximum level of 7-MeGua in the victim's liver DNA was 6000-7000 μmol/mol guanine, and if one assumes the ratio of O^6-MeGua to 7-MeGua at lethal doses of NDMA is approximately 0.10, as shown in the rat by Pegg (1977), then the estimated maximum level of O^6-MeGua in the human liver DNA would have been approximately 600-700 μmol/mol. The measured level of O^6-MeGua in DNA of the deceased's liver was approximately 300 μmol/mol or about half as much as there may have been 5 days before, a few hours after NDMA exposure; that is, in 5 days it appears that only half of the O^6-MeGua was removed from the DNA. This, then, might suggest that O^6-MeGua was removed from the human liver DNA at a slow rate, similar to that seen in the hamster and unlike that seen in the rat (Stumpf et al. 1979).

Nine years before these analyses were done, Dr. Ruggero Montesano and Professor Peter N. Magee reported the formation of 7-MeGua in DNA of human liver slices incubated with NDMA (Montesano and Magee 1970), and Dr. Montesano has reported further on those scientific studies at this conference (Montesano et al., this volume). The findings regarding the probable NDMA poisoning, reported by Herron and Shank (1980), appear to confirm the results of Montesano and Magee (1970), that human liver is capable of metabolically activating NDMA to an alkylating agent which methylates DNA at at least two sites, one of which is a base-pairing site. Such aberrant methylation of target organ DNA is considered a promutagenic event (Loveless 1967; Lawley 1976). If indeed the somatic mutation hypothesis for chemical induction of cancer is valid, that is, DNA damage is causally related to the initiation of cancer, then NDMA, because it can be metabolically activated to a DNA methylating agent in man, would be expected to have potential as a human carcinogen.

REFERENCES

Balsiger, R.W. and J.A. Montgomery. 1960. Synthesis of potential anticancer agents. XXV. Preparation of 6-alkoxy-2-aminopurines. *J Org. Chem.* **25**: 1573.

Barrows, L.R. and R.C. Shank. 1978. Chemical modification of DNA in rats treated with hydrazine. *Toxicol. Appl. Pharmacol.* **45**:324.

_____. 1980. DNA methylation in hydrazine-treated animals. *Proc. Am. Assoc. Cancer Res.* **21**:110.

Becker, R.A., L.R. Barrows, and R.C. Shank. 1981. Methylation of liver DNA guanine in hydrazine hepatotoxicity: dose-response and kinetic characteristics of 7-methylguanine and O^6-methylguanine formation and persistence in rats. *Carcinogenesis* **2**:1181.

Craddock, V.M. 1969. Stability of deoxyribonucleic acid methylated in the intact animal by administration of dimethylnitrosamine. Rate of breakdown *in vivo* and *in vitro* at different dosages. *Biochem. J.* **111**:497.

Friedman, O.M., G.N. Malapatra, and R. Stevenson. 1963. Methylation of deoxyribonucleosides by diazomethane. *Biochim. Biophys. Acta* **68**:144.

Heath, D.F. and P.N. Magee. 1962. Toxic properties of dialkylnitrosamines and some related compounds. *Br. J. Ind. Med.* **19**:276.

Herron, D.C. and R.C. Shank. 1979. Quantitative high-pressure liquid chromatographic analysis of methylated purines in DNA of rats treated with chemical carcinogens. *Anal. Biochem.* **100**:58.

_____. 1980. Methylated purines in human liver DNA after probable dimethylnitrosamine poisoning. *Cancer Res.* **40**:3116.

_____. 1981. *In vivo* kinetics of O^6-methylguanine and 7-methylguanine formation and persistence in DNA of rats treated with symmetrical dimethylhydrazine. *Cancer Res.* **41**:3967.

Kirby, K.S. 1957. New method for the isolation of deoxyribonucleic acids: evidence on the nature of bonds between deoxyribonucleic acid and protein. *Biochem. J.* **66**:495.

Lawley, P.D. 1976. Carcinogenesis by alkylating agents. *ACS Monogr.* **173**:83.

Loveless, A. 1969. Possible relevance of O-6 alkylation of deoxyguanosine to the mutagenicity and carcinogenicity of nitrosamines and nitrosamides. *Nature* **223**:206.

Montesano, R. and P.N. Magee. 1970. Metabolism of dimethylnitrosamine by human liver slices *in vitro*. *Nature* **228**:173.

Pegg, A. 1977. Alkylation of rat liver DNA by dimethylnitrosamine: effect of dosage on O^6-methylguanine levels. *J. Natl. Cancer Inst.* **58**:681.

Pegg, A. and J.W. Nicoll. 1976. Nitrosamine carcinogenesis: the importance of the persistence in DNA of alkylated bases in the organotropism of tumour induction. *IARC Sci. Publ.* **12**:571.

Stumpf, R., G.P. Margison, R. Montesano, and A.E. Pegg. 1979. Formation and loss of alkylated purines from DNA of hamster liver after administration of dimethylnitrosamine. *Cancer Res.* **39**:50.

Swann, P.F. and P.N. Magee. 1968. Nitrosamine-induced carcinogenesis. The alkylation of nucleic acids of the rat by N-methyl-N-nitrosourea, dimethyl-nitrosamine, dimethylsulphate, and methyl methanesulphonate. *Biochem. J.* **110**:39.

Taylor, B. and D. Cooney. 1976. Liquid chromatographic separation and quantitation of methylated derivatives of nucleic acids. *Fed. Proc.* **35**:523.

COMMENTS

PEGG: Were there any other tissues available which were looked at and found negative? It would be very interesting to know whether other tissues were alkylated.

KIMBROUGH: I had no frozen tissues from the child at all. That was one reason we only had one case. The child died a day earlier, and I was not really involved. After the child died, they found that the next victim would also die, they then called me and asked me what to collect. That's how we got the frozen tissues.

I have to admit we did have brain and a few other tissues on this one patient. I may have something in my freezer, and I have to look.

PEGG: That would actually be quite interesting, because, as Dr. Shank knows— and Dr. Swann has worked on this too—there are even more sensitive methods which are available using specific antibodies to O^6-MeGua, for example. So it would theoretically be possible to really use quite small amounts of tissue to get a measurement. It would certainly be very interesting to see whether there was alkylation.

PETO: I don't think that you can infer that the repair processes for O^6-MeGua are less effective in humans than in rats, because if you give such a massive dose the rat repair system goes very slowly, as well. It seems that there is an enzyme which is consumed and involved in the repair. At low doses, if anything, the human repair system seems to be better than the rat's.

SHANK: What is the half-life of O^6-MeGua using an LD-50?

PETO: There is none. The concept of a half-life is simply not an appropriate one for those kind of kinetics.

PEGG: While that is true, you don't know—and, in fact, nobody here knows— that there is only one process for repairing O^6-MeGua. It certainly looks as though there is more than one in the rat and one of them is a slower process, which would then have a half-life.

SHANK: If we give an LD-50 of an alkylating carcinogen and measure the amount of O^6-MeGua several hours later, we see much less than 50%. Oftentimes, we don't see anything in the rat liver after 5 or 6 days have elapsed; the O^6-MeGua in DNA is gone. I realize that I should not refer to these as half-life and repair, but I was surprised at the level of O^6-MeGua: 7-MeGua. In this case there is something wrong in this relationship.

CASTONGUAY: I assume you used only one column. Is it possible to have a better separation of adenine and 7-Me-Gua by using two columns?

SHANK: No. What happens is the O^6-MeGua peak spreads. Whatman has now produced a much better column, and we get baseline resolution between adenine and 7-MeGua. The data I presented were obtained in 1979. Now the columns are much better.

MAGEE: Perhaps I heard you wrong, but didn't you say that you tried to get DNA from the kidney of one of those victims and it was too degraded to get it?

SHANK: Yes, that's correct.

MAGEE: I was wondering if it might be possible, if that happened again, to do a cruder method of extracting the DNA with trichloroacetic acid.

LIJINSKY: Again? What do you mean "again?"

MAGEE: Well, because Dr. Kimbrough said that she had more tissues and perhaps would be able to get an answer in terms of 7-MeGua by a much cruder method.

PEGG: But, you mustn't forget that the 7-MeGua is present normally in RNA, of course.

MAGEE: Ah, yes, that's a problem.

ELDER: Just as a point of information, do you know, in taking a sample of a liver, if your result is typical of the whole liver, or could this be a regional phenomenon in certain bits of liver?

SHANK: That's a very good question. I don't know. I grind up whole rat livers and whole mouse livers. But, in the case of the human liver, we had just a few grams. The specimen may have been atypical. I have no idea.

KIMBROUGH: The pathology was quite uniform throughout the entire liver, so I would assume that a few grams might be more or less representative, but that is only an assumption.

SHANK: We received two entirely separate specimens over a couple of weeks and got similar alkylation levels in both specimens; unless they were adjacent segments, the close agreement in analytical results would tend to dampen the argument of nonuniformity.

ELDER: Sometimes carcinogenesis appears to be focal in a particular area of an organ, at least in the stomach.

PEGG: Yes, it may be. This particular case is not very well—well, it's a very big dose, so it's less relevant. But it is certainly an extremely important question.

MILO: Again, we have heard that there appears to be difference in the repair and persistence of damage.

What appears to be happening is that the type of insult that we are dealing to the cell, whether it's an acute toxic situation such as this, or a chronic toxic situation, or a carcinogenic insult, might be very relevant in this, as far as the types of repair processes. If the nucleus and the DNA or the repair process is going to be perturbed, why can't the physiological interaction of those proteins with the removal of the persistence damage also be perturbed? Would you or Dr. Harris care to comment on this?

SHANK: I'm not sure I've got your point. Certainly, if this was NDMA at a lethal dose, the processes which govern the rate of removal of something like O^6-MeGua from the target DNA are going to be quite different compared to lower doses. Several people have shown this experimentally.

I shouldn't have said the word "repair." We have no idea of what kind of repair mechanisms may have been working in this patient.

SESSION III:

ANALYTICAL METHODS FOR NITROSAMINES IN BIOLOGICAL MEDIA

Analytical Methods for Nitrosamines—An Overview

DAVID H. FINE
New England Institute for Life Sciences
125 Second Avenue
Waltham, Massachusetts 02254

For a proper understanding of N-nitroso compounds in the environment, it is important to understand where they come from. They are formed from their precursors, the amino substances (amines, ureas, amides, etc.) and the nitrosating agents (nitrite, nitrogen oxides, organic nitro, and nitroso compounds) under a wide range of conditions (hydrophilic or lipophilic) and pH (acid, neutral, alkaline). From secondary amines and nitrite, for example, nitrosamines can only form under acidic conditions (pH 3-5). If nitrogen oxides are involved (either directly or as a reaction product from an organic nitro or nitroso compound), then the reaction proceeds rapidly under neutral or alkaline conditions. The formation of N-nitroso compounds can also be increased, decreased, or completely blocked by the presence of enhancing or inhibiting compounds (thiocyanate, iodide, polyphenols). The effect of these catalysts and inhibitors is strongly pH-dependent, and some compounds, such as sulphamic acid, have been shown to inhibit reaction at one pH and catalyze it at another. Most importantly, it must be realized that wherever N-nitroso compounds are found, their precursors are also present, often in as much as one thousand- to one-million-fold excess. It is not surprising, therefore, that the literature on the presence of N-nitroso compounds in the environment is confused and often contradictory.

Because N-nitroso compounds are found in a sea of precursors, it is difficult to be sure that the perturbation introduced into the system by the very act of sampling, concentrating and analyzing, has not altered the system. Although it is relatively easy for the analyst to generate data, it is difficult to ensure that the data are a true reflection of the original sample, and not an artifact. In order to properly understand the validity of the analytical data, it therefore becomes necessary to study not only the N-nitroso compounds, but also the amino compounds, the nitrosating agents, the catalysts and inhibitors, and the sample conditions.

The analyst divides N-nitroso compounds into two broad categories: the volatiles and the nonvolatiles. The volatile nitroso compounds are those which are amenable to separation by gas chromatography (GC). Dimethylnitrosamine, diethylnitrosamine, nitrosomorpholine (NMOR), N-nitrosodiethanolamine (NDELA) all fall into this class. Analytical methodologies for this class of compounds is well advanced and includes the major part of the technical literature. The nonvolatile nitroso compounds are those which are not sufficiently volatile to survive a GC column without decomposition. Compounds in this class include the large molecular weight nitrosamines, as well as the nitroso ureas, carbamates, amino acids, amides, etc. Specific analytical methods for only a few of these, such as nitroso carbaryl (Krull et al. 1980), nitrosonornicotine (Hoffmann et al. 1979) and nitrosoproline (Ohshima and Bartsch 1981) have been developed. For the vast majority of compounds in this class, analytical procedures are not currently available.

VOLATILE NITROSAMINES

Artifacts

The TEA Analyzer and the high-resolution mass spectrometer, when used as detectors for GC have become the instruments of choice for volatile N-nitroso compounds (IARC 1978, 1980, 1982). With the widespread availability of this equipment over the last few years, the literature is swollen with data on the environmental occurrence of nitrosamines. It has become routine to analyze for nitrosamines at the part per billion (ppb) level (1 μg/kg) and be entirely confident of the identity and quantitation. Unfortunately, the increase in data has also led to an increase in the number of papers with questionable data. The culprit is usually not misidentification, but rather the introduction of artifacts due to a lack of understanding of the true nature of the matrix being analyzed. It is instructive to examine the following examples:

1. Deionized water has been shown by several workers to contain volatile nitrosamines at the ppb level (Kimoto et al. 1980). A field trip searching for airborne industrial nitrosamines was ruined when deionized water was used to dilute the potassium hydroxide impingers (Cohen and Bachman 1978).
2. Sunlight and heat—Labile compounds such as the pesticide derivatives, N-nitrosocarbaryl and N-nitrosoatrazine, decompose under fluorescent light. Special handling precautions are required including the avoidance of temperatures above 30°C (Fine 1980).
3. Solvents often contain traces of volatile nitrosamines. Eisenbrand et al. (1978) reported NMOR in samples of highly purified methylene chloride and chloroform; whereas less pure grades of the same solvent were nitrosamine-free. Bottle to bottle variations were found by Tannenbaum (1981a). The only effective approach to overcome this difficulty is to run parallel control samples on a daily basis, and especially if solvents from different bottles were used.

4. Rubber products all contain nitrosamines (Fajen et al. 1982; Spiegelhalder and Preussmann 1982). Rubber tubing, rubber septum syringe pistons, rubber gaskets, etc., are all sources of laboratory contamination. Care should be taken to avoid all rubber products when carrying out analyses for nitrosamines.

5. Amines, especially secondary alkyl amines, often contain significant nitrosamine impurities (Eisenbrand et al. 1978). The problem is difficult to avoid, with the U.S. Environmental Protection Agency setting the allowable nitrosamine impurity in amine and amine salt herbicides at mg/L (EPA 1980). It is essential to check all amines which may come in contact with the sample so as to quantitate the nitrosamine contamination.

6. Cross-contamination occurs readily with the volatile nitrosamines. The storage of high level nitrosamine standards and trace level samples in the same refrigerator will virtually guarantee cross-contamination. On defrosting a refrigerator where samples containing nitrosamines had been stored, it is common to be able to detect nitrosamines in the thawing accumulated ice. Another common source of cross-contamination in the laboratory arises from the use of volatile amines. We have found, for example, that the use of morpholine in a neighboring laboratory contaminated the analytical laboratory with NMOR. E.A. Walker (pers. comm.), in Lyon, experienced a similar problem, where amine usage in one laboratory led to contamination in the analytical laboratory.

7. GC injector port. Fan and Fine (1978) demonstrated a positive artifact occurring inside the heated injector port of a GC. Concentrated samples of the dimethylamine salt of 2,4,6 trichlorobenzoic acid were being analyzed by GC/TEA. Dilution of the sample, or extraction with a solvent, gave results which were much lower than that observed when the sample was injected directly, without clean-up. The problem was traced to a nitrosating agent in the sample, which nitrosated the amine salt inside the hot port.

8. Exposure to ambient nitrogen oxides in the laboratory were shown by Eisenbrand et al. (1978) to cause the N-nitrosodimethylamine (NDMA) content of aminopyrine tablets to increase from approximately 100 μg/kg to 5000 μg/kg. Nitrosation is rapid in the presence of nitrogen oxides, even in organic solvents, or at alkaline pH.

9. Kuderna Danish evaporator. The final step in most analyses of volatile nitrosamines is to distill off excess methylene chloride in a Kuderna Danish evaporator. Fajen et al. (1979) used dilute potassium hydroxide impingers to sample air from a chemical factory, where diphenylnitrosamine was being manufactured. The impingers were extracted with methylene chloride, and then concentrated on a Kuderna Danish evaporator. The final concentrate was shown to contain diphenylnitrosamine, morpholine and NMOR. A check for artifacts showed that some of the

measured NMOR was being formed in the Kuderna Danish evaporator by diphenylnitrosamine transnitrosation of morpholine.

10. Solid absorbents, such as activated charcoal and Tenax GC, were shown by Rounbehler et al. (1980) to readily form nitrosamines in the presence of the precursor amine and ambient levels of nitrogen oxides. Use of these absorbents for airborne nitrosamine measurements should be avoided, since it is not possible to distinguish the artifactually formed nitrosamine from what was present in the ambient air. A special absorbent package, with built-in artifact inhibitors, has been developed to overcome these difficulties (Rounbehler et al. 1980).

11. Alkali. Part of the nitrosamine mythology of the early 1970s was to "freeze" nitrosamine forming reactions by the addition of alkali, since it was argued that the rate of nitrosation was infinitely slow at high pH. The finding of NDELA at levels as high as 3% in aqueous cutting fluids (pH 12), stopped this erroneous belief. While alkali does stop nitrosation by nitrite, it actually accelerates nitrosation by oxides of nitrogen. The oxides of nitrogen could be derived from the decomposition of organic nitro or nitroso compounds.

12. Fragmentation by alkali of β-hydroxynitrosamines (those having a hydroxyl, aldehyde, keto or carboxyl function at the second carbon atom from the nitrosyl function) was shown by Loeppky and Christiansen (1978) to eliminate aldehyde, giving the corresponding smaller molecular weight nitrosamine. Thus, nitrosodiethanolamine could, for example, give NDMA, by this mechanism. This reaction is another strong reason to avoid the use of alkali in the isolation and analysis of nitrosamines from complex matrices.

13. Solid-phase sodium nitrite in nonaqueous solutions was shown by Angelis et al. (1978) to be capable of nitrosating amines. A 0.024M solution of pyrrolidine in methylene chloride, for example, was nitrosated to N-nitrosopyrrolidine in 10% yield if solid sodium nitrite was present. A similar effect was observed for chloroform, tetrahydrofuran, and bromochloromethane.

14. Freezing. Fan and Tannenbaum (1973) showed that the rate of nitrosation of dilute amines in aqueous nitrite solutions was increased by chilling to below 0°C and then thawing. The reason for the increase was due to the increase in effective concentration of the unfrozen solution brought about by the freezing.

15. Bacterial conversion of nitrate to nitrite has been shown to occur in a wide variety of matrices, including human saliva (Ishiwata et al. 1975a,b,c). Bacterial contamination of a sample high in nitrate can therefore lead to conversion of nitrate to nitrite, resulting in nitrosamine formation.

16. Biological fluids are the most difficult matrices of all to analyze, especially for the nitrosamines which are metabolized rapidly. Early experiments

on the presence of volatile nitrosamines in blood (Lakritz et al. 1979; Kowalski et al. 1980; Yamamoto et al. 1980), in urine (Hicks et al. 1977; El Merzabani et al. 1979; Kakizoe et al. 1979) and in feces (Wang et al. 1978) were not able to be repeated when appropriate analytical control protocols were instituted (Archer et al. 1981; Eisenbrand et al. 1981; Tannenbaum 1981b).

It is obvious from the above discussion that there can be no foolproof cookbook approach that can be used to analyze for volatile nitrosamines. Each matrix needs to be evaluated carefully with respect to amino compounds, nitrosating agents, and conditions. Because of these problems, it is prudent to assume that any new report of the presence of volatile nitrosamines (especially at the sub ppb level in biological fluids) is due to an artifact, unless all of the following control protocols have been carried out:

• Nitrosation inhibitors, such as α-tocopherol (fat soluble) and ascorbic acid (water soluble) have been added in excess of the amount required for complete inhibition.

• A readily nitrosatable amine, such as 2,6 dimethylmorpholine, has been added to the sample. The presence of the N-nitroso derivative of the marker amine in the final extract can be used to estimate the extent to which artifacts have formed.

• Glassware, solvents, and other testing equipment has been checked, at least daily, for contamination. Zero controls (everything but the sample of interest) must be carried out at least daily.

• The minimum number of analytical steps have been used. If possible, it is advisable to analyze at least one sample without any clean-up whatsoever, by introducing the crude sample directly onto a GC/TEA (Fan et al. 1977).

CONFIRMATION

An important part of the experimental protocol for the first finding of a new nitrosamine contamination is independent confirmation of the identity of the compound itself. If GC/TEA or GC/mass spectrometry (GC/MS) is used, alternative confirmatory procedures are generally only necessary during personnel training, setting up, and the first reports of new contaminated matrices.

Aesthetically, the most defensible approach is to carry out the confirmatory analysis using an entirely different experimental apparatus or technique. Thus, if GC/TEA is used for analysis, GC/high resolution MS is often used for confirmation, and vice versa (Krull et al. 1979). Attention must be taken to use MS critically, since it can lead to false identifications if not used with care (Groenen et al. 1982; Gough et al. 1977).

Three TEA techniques have been described for confirming the identity of compounds found by GC/TEA. The first is parallel GC/TEA and HPLC/TEA (Fine 1980), which relies on the fact that in GC, compounds elute as a function of their relative vapor pressure and solubility in the liquid phase, whereas in HPLC, compounds elute according to either their size, polarity, solubility in the liquid phase, and (or) ionic properties. Because of these differences, elution order is quite different in GC and HPLC. Positive identification is made if the compound of interest elutes at the correct retention time, and if quantitation of the peak is identical by both GC and HPLC. A second TEA approach is to use the GC/TEA in its nitrogen mode (Rounbehler and Fine 1982), which gives a response for both the N atoms of the N-nitrosamine functionality. Again, the approach requires quantitation of the peak according to the number of nitrogen atoms in the molecule. The third TEA approach, was developed by Sen et al. (1982), who oxidized the nitrosamine to the nitramine, and then rechromatographed the nitramine derivative by GC/TEA. Confirmation is obtained by observing the disappearance of the nitrosamine peak and the appearance of the nitramine peak. As above, the confirmation is strengthened by obtaining quantitative conversion.

Other techniques which have been used, with mixed success, include denitrosation by either UV-light or a mixture of hydrobromic and acetic acids.

NONVOLATILE N-NITROSO COMPOUNDS

Specific analytical procedures for nonvolatile nitroso compounds, such as the N-nitroso ureas, amides, and carbamates have only recently been developed. For example, a colorimetric method for urea can be used to determine nitrosoureas and nitrosocyanamides (Mirvish et al. 1979), and Saul et al. (1982) have recently reported a method for detecting nitrosamides. The method involved the release of nitrite, which was detected with the Griess reagent using HPLC-UV (ultraviolet). There are also some broad screening techniques that can be used for some nonvolatile N-nitroso compounds (Fan et al. 1978; Fine 1980). For example, screening techniques have been used successfully to identify a variety of nonvolatile nitrosamines in pesticide products (Wolf et al. 1980; Zweig and Garner 1982). Final detection has generally been made by HPLC-UV or HPLC-TEA techniques. In tobacco and tobacco smoke, the presence of tobacco-specific nonvolatile nitrosamines has been detected by HPLC-TEA and other HPLC procedures (Hecht et al. 1978; Hoffmann et al. 1979).

Procedures have been developed to analyze foodstuffs for such compounds as the nitrosamino acids. N-nitrosoproline and other nitrosamino acids have been determined on GC/TEA following esterification with diazomethane (Ohshima and Bartsch 1981; Sen et al. 1982). Nitroso-3-hydroxypyrrolidine, which was found in cured meat products (Janowski et al. 1978), was determined by trifluoroacetylation, followed by GC/TEA and GC-high-resolution MS. Sen et al. (1977a) have also described a mass spectrometric method to detect this compound in cooked bacon. More recently, Roussin's red methyl ester $[(NO)_2 Fe(CH_3 S)]_2$ was isolated and identified by GC/MS from the ether extracts of Chinese vegetables (Lu et al. 1981). The total N-nitroso compound content of food samples has been assayed by Walters et al. (1978), who used a chemical denitrosation procedure, followed by the detection of the nitrosyl radical by its chemiluminescence reaction with ozone. Bavin et al. (1982) have further refined the Walters approach by adjusting to pH 4, destroying nitrite with hydrazine sulphate, and then injecting the sample into refluxing ethyl acetate containing hydrobromic acid and acetic acid, releasing the nitrosyl radical. Their technique allows for the rapid processing of many samples.

REFERENCES

Angelis, R.M., L.K. Keefer, P.P. Roller, and S.J. Uhm. 1978. Chemical models for possible nitrosamine artifact formation in environmental analysis. *IARC Sci. Publ.* **19**:109.

Archer, M. 1981. Hazards of nitrate, nitrite, and N-nitroso Compounds. In *Nutritional Toxicology* (ed. J. Hathcock). Academic Press, New York (In press).

Bavin, P.M.G., D.W. Darkin, and N.J. Viney. 1982. Total nitroso compounds in gastric juice. *IARC Sci. Publ.* **41**:(In press).

Cohen, J.B., and J.D. Bachman. 1978. Measurement of environmental nitrosamines. *IARC Sci. Publ.* **19**:357.

Eisenbrand, G., B. Spiegelhalder, and R. Preussmann. 1981. Analysis of human biological specimens for nitrosamine contents. *Ban. Rep.* **7**:275.

Eisenbrand, G. B. Spiegelhalder, C. Janowski, J. Kann, and R. Preussmann. 1978. Volatile and non-volatile N-nitroso compounds in foods and other environmental media. *IARC Sci. Publ.* **19**:311.

El-Merzabani, M.M., A.A. El-Aasser, and N.I. Zakhary. 1979. A study on the aetiological factors of bilharzial bladder cancer in Egypt–1. Nitrosamines and their precursors in urine. *Eur. J. Cancer* **15**:287.

Fajen, J.M., D.P. Rounbehler, and D.H. Fine. 1982. Summary report on N-nitroso compounds in the factory environment. *IARC Sci. Publ.* **41**: (In press).

Fajen, J.M., G.A. Carson, D.P. Rounbehler, T.Y. Fan, R. Vita, E.U. Goff, M.H. Wolf, G.S. Edwards, D.H. Fine, V. Reinhold, and K. Biemann. 1979. N-nitrosamines in the rubber and tire industry. *Science* **205**:1262.

Fan, T.Y. and D.H. Fine. 1978. Formation of N-nitrosodimethylamine in the injection port of a gas chromatograph: An artifact in nitrosamine analysis. *J. Agric. Food Chem.* **26**:1471.

Fan, T.Y. and S.R. Tannenbaum. 1973. Factors influencing the rate of formation of Nitrosomorpholine from morpholine and nitrite. II. Rate enhancement in frozen solution. *J. Agric. Food Chem.* **21**:967.

Fan, T.Y., I.S. Krull, R.D. Ross, M.H. Wolf, and D.H. Fine. 1978. Comprehensive analytical procedures for the determination of volatile and non-volatile, polar and nonpolar N-nitroso compounds. *IARC Sci. Pub.* **19**:3.

Fan, T.Y., J. Morrison, D.P. Rounbehler, R. Ross, D.H. Fine, W. Miles, and N.P. Sen. 1977. N-nitrosodiethanolamine in synthetic cutting fluids: A part per hundred impurity. *Science* **196**:70.

Fine, D.H. 1980. N-nitroso compounds in the environment. In *Advances in Environmental Science and Technology* (eds. J. Pitts and R. Metcalf), Vol. 10, p. 40. John Wiley & Sons, Inc., New York.

Gough, T.A., K.S. Webb, M.A. Pringuer, and B.J. Wood. 1977. A comparison of various mass spectrometric and a chemiluminescent method for the estimation of volatile nitrosamines. *J. Agric. Food Chem.* **25**:663.

Groenen, P.J., J.B. Luten, J.H. Dhont, M.W. de Cock-Bethbeder, A.A. Prins, and J.W. Vreeken. 1982. Formation of volatile N-nitrosamines from food products, especially fish, under simulated gastric conditions. *IARC Sci. Publ.* **41**:(In press).

Hecht, S.S., C.B. Chen, N. Hirota, R.M. Ornaf, T.C.Tso, and D. Hoffmann. 1978. Tobacco-specific nitrosamines: formation from nicotine *in vitro* and during tobacco curing and carcinogenicity in strain A mice. *J. Natl. Cancer Inst.* **60**:819.

Hicks, R.M., C.L. Walters, I. Elsebai, A.-B. El Aasser, M. El-Merzabani, and T.A. Gough. 1977. Demonstration of nitrosamines in human urine: Preliminary observations on a possible etiology for bladder cancer in association with chronic urinary tract infections. *Proc. R. Soc. Med.* **70**:413.

Hoffmann, D., J.D. Adams, K.D. Brunnemann, and S.S. Hecht. 1979. Assessment of tobacco-specific N-nitrosamines in tobacco products. *Cancer Res.* **39**:2505.

International Agency for Research on Cancer. 1978. Environmental Aspects of N-nitroso Compounds. *IARC Sci. Publ.* **19**:566.

———. 1980. N-nitroso Compounds: Analysis, Formation, and Occurrence. *IARC Sci. Publ.* **31**:841.

———. 1982. N-nitroso compounds: Occurrence and Biological Effects. *IARC Sci. Publ.* **41**:(In press).

Ishiwata, H., A. Tanimura, and M. Ishidate. 1975c. Studies on *in vivo* formation of nitroso compounds (III). Nitrite and nitrate concentrations in human saliva collected from salivary ducts. *J. Food Hyg. Soc. Jpn.* **16**:89.

Ishiwata, H., P. Boriboon, M. Harada, A Tanimura, and M. Ishidate. 1975a. Studies on *in vivo* formation of nitroso compounds (IV): Changes of nitrite and nitrate concentration in incubated human saliva. *J. Food Hyg. Soc. Jpn.* **16**:93.

Ishiwata, H., P. Boriboon, Y. Nakamura, M. Harada, A. Tanimura, and M. Ishidate. 1975b. Studies on *in vivo* formation of nitroso compounds (II). Changes of nitrite and nitrate concentrations in human saliva after ingestion of vegetables or sodium nitrate. *J. Food Hyg. Soc. Jpn.* **16**:19.

Janowski, C., G. Eisenbrand, and R. Preussmann. 1978. Occurrence and determination of N-nitroso-3-hydroxypyrrolidine in cured meat products. *J. Chromatogr.* **150**:216.

Kakizoe, T., T. Wang, W.S. Eng, R. Furrer, P. Dion, and W.R. Bruce. 1979. Volatile N-nitrosamines in the urine of normal donors and of bladder cancer patients. *Cancer Res.* **39**:829.

Kimoto, W.I., C.J. Dooley, J. Carre, and W. Fiddler. 1980. Roles of strong ion exchange resins in nitrosamine formation in water. *Water Res.* **14**:869.

Kowalski, B., C.T. Miller, and N.P. Sen. 1980. Studies on the *in vivo* formation of nitrosamines in rats and humans after ingestion of various meals. *IARC Sci. Publ.* **31**:609.

Krull, I.S., E.U. Goff, G.G. Hoffman, and D.H. Fine. 1979. Confirmatory methods for the thermal energy determination of N-nitroso compounds at trace levels. *Anal. Chem.* **51**:1706.

Krull, I.S., K. Mills, G. Hoffman, and D.H. Fine. 1980. The analysis of N-nitrosocarbaryl in whole mice. *J. Anal. Toxicol.* **4**:260.

Lakritz, L., M.L. Simenhoff, S.R. Dunn, and W. Fiddler. 1979. N-nitroso-dimethylamine in human blood. *Food Cosmet. Toxicol.* **18**:77.

Loeppky, R.N. and R. Christiansen. 1978. The fragmentation reaction of beta-hydroxynitrosamines: possible environmental and biochemical significance for nitrosamine carcinogenicity. *IARC Sci. Publ.* **19**:117.

Lu, S.-H., A.-M. Camus, L. Tomatis, and H. Bartsch. 1981. Mutagenicity of extracts of pickled vegetables collected in Linhsien County, a high-incidence area for esophageal cancer in Northern China. *J. Natl. Cancer Inst.* **66**:33.

Mirvish, S.S., J. Sams, and S. Arnold. 1979. Spectrophotometric method for determining ureas applied to nitrosoureas, nitroso cyanamides and a cyanamide. *Fresenius Z. Anal. Chem.* **298**:408.

Ohshima, H. and H. Bartsch. 1981. Quantitative estimation of endogenous nitrosation in man by monitoring N-nitrosoproline excreted in the urine. *Cancer Res.* **41**:3658.

Rounbehler, D.P. and D.H. Fine. 1982. Specific detection of amines and other nitrogen containing compounds with a modified TEA Analyzer. *IARC Sci. Publ.* **41**:(In press).

Rounbehler, D.P., J. Reisch, J. Coombs, and D.H. Fine. 1978. Nitrosamine air sampling sorbents compared for quantitative collection and artifact formation. *Anal. Chem.* **52**:273.

Rounbehler, D.P., J. Reisch, and D.H. Fine. 1980. Nitrosamine air sampling using a new artifact resistant solid sorbent. In *Symposium on Sampling and Analysis of Toxic Organics in the Atmosphere,* ASTM STP 271, p. 80. American Society for Testing and Materials, Philadelphia.

Saul, R.L., W.R. Bruce, and M.C. Archer. 1982. An analytical method for simple N-nitrosamides. *IARC Sci. Publ.* **41**:(In press).

Sen, N.P., D.E. Coffin, S. Seaman, B. Donaldson, and W. Miles. 1977. Extraction, clean-up and estimation as methyl ether of 3-hydroxyl-1-nitroso-pyrrolidine, a non-volatile nitrosamine in cooked bacon at mass fractions of μg/kg. In *Proceedings of the Second International Symposium on Nitrite in Meat Products,* (eds. B.J. Tinbergen and B. Krol), p. 179. Centre for Agricultural Publishing and Documentation, Wageningen, The Netherlands.

Sen, N.P., S. Seaman, and L. Teissier. 1982. A rapid and sensitive method for the determination of nonvolatile N-nitroso compounds in foods and some recent data on the levels of volatile N-nitrosamines in dried foods and multi-based beverages. *IARC Sci. Publ.* **41** (In press).

Spiegelhalder, B., and R. Preussmann. 1982. Nitrosamines and rubber. *IARC Sci. Publ.* **41**:(In press).

Tannenbaum, S.R. 1981b. Endogenous Formation of N-Nitroso Compounds. *Ban. Rep.* 7:269.

U.S. Environmental Protection Agency. 1980. Pesticides Contaminated with N-nitroso Compounds: Proposed Policy. *Fed. Regist.* 45(124):42854.

Walters, C.L., M.J. Downes, M.W. Edwards, and P.L.R. Smith. 1978. Determination of a nonvolatile N-nitrosamine on a food matrix. *Analyst* 103:1127.

Wang, T., T. Kakizoe, P. Dion, R. Furrer, A.J. Varghese, and W.R. Bruce. 1978. Volatile nitrosamines in normal human faeces. *Nature* 276:280.

Wolf, M.H., W.C. Yu, and D.H. Fine. 1980. Analysis of N-nitroso compounds in pesticide formulations. In *Analytical Methods for Pesticides and Plant Growth Regulators, Updated General Techniques and Additional Pesticides* (eds. G. Zweig and J. Sherma), Vol. 11, p. 363. Academic Press, New York.

Yamamoto, M., T. Yamada, A. Tanimura. 1980. Volatile nitrosamines in human blood before and after ingestion of a meal containing high concentrations of nitrate and secondary amines. *Food Cosmet. Toxicol.* 18:297.

Zweig, G. and W. Garner. 1982. Policy and regulatory aspects of N-nitroso contaminants in pesticide products. In *N-nitroso Compounds* (eds. R.A. Scanlan and S.R. Tannenbaum), ACS Symp. Ser. (In press).

Electrochemical Detection of N-Nitrosamines with High Performance Liquid Chromatography

GEORGE W. HARRINGTON, SAROJ K. VOHRA, AND JEAN FU WANG
Department of Chemistry
Temple University
Philadelphia, Pennsylvania 19122

Electrochemical detection for high performance liquid chromatography (HPLC-EC) is a relatively new development in the field of chromatography. It has grown rapidly in recent years and has found applications in a wide variety of areas (Hanekamp et al. 1982). Electroanalytical methods, especially differential pulse polarography, have been shown, as noted in a recent review (Vohra 1982), to be sensitive, accurate, and versatile when applied to N-nitrosamines. When used in the differential pulse mode one particular Electrochemical (EC) detector, the dropping mercury electrode (DME), is particularly suitable for N-nitrosamines (Vohra et al. 1980, 1981). This article summarizes these applications.

EXPERIMENTAL

The EC detector consisted of an EG&G PARC (Princeton, N.J.) Model 310 polarographic detector. Potentials were applied with a PARC Model 174A polarographic analyzer. All potentials are reported with respect to a silver-silver chloride reference electrode. The HPLC was equipped with a U6K injector valve and a Waters Associates (Milford, MA.) model 6000 reciprocating pump. A Waters Associates reversed-phase, μBondapak-C_{18} column was used. A Perkin-Elmer Series Two HPLC equipped with a Whatman Partisil PXS 10/25 ODS C-18 column was also used. The flow rate was 2.0 ml/min. Mobile phases were degassed with helium. All analyses were carried out in an oxygen-free atmosphere. Reagents for the various mobile phases were all glass distilled. The pH was controlled by Britton-Robinson buffers. The various N-nitrosamines were synthesized by the usual means (Vogel 1957). N-nitrosodiethanolamine (NDELA) was prepared by the method of Preussmann (1962).

RESULTS

This study was conducted in three parts. The first part was a general evaluation of the EC detector for various nitrosamines by class. The second was an application of the method for the determination of NDELA in cosmetic products and the third was a comparison of Gas Chromatography-Thermal Energy Analyzer (GC/TEA) to HPLC-EC for the determination of *N*-nitroso-pyrrolidine (NPYR) in fried bacon.

Nitrosamines can be characterized into four classes (Fan et al. 1978) based on various physical properties such as volatility, ionic character, and polarity. The four classes are as follows: (1) volatile nitroso compounds such as dialkylnitrosamines, (2) low polarity, nonvolatile nitroso compounds such as diphenylnitrosamine and methylphenylnitrosamine, (3) high polarity nonionic, nonvolatile nitroso compounds, such as NDELA, and (4) high polarity, ionic, nonvolatile nitroso compounds such as nitrosoamino acids.

Different mobile phases were used for each class as follows: Class I: Methanol-water-glacial acetic acid (50:47:3 by vol); Class II: Methanol-water-glacial acetic acid (41:56:3 by vol); Class III: Water-glacial acetic acid (98:2 v/v); Class IV: Water-glacial acetic acid (95:5 v/v).

The EC conditions found suitable for each class were as follows: drop size, large; modulation amplitude, 50-100 mv; drop time, 0.5-1.0 sec.; mode, differ-

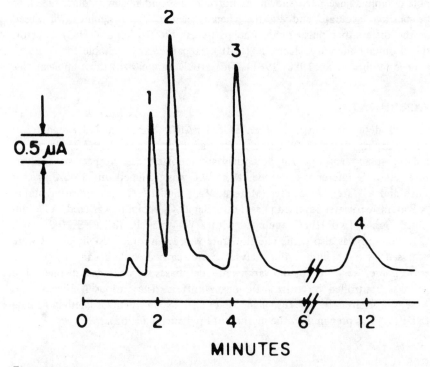

Figure 1

Chromatogram for Class I *N*-nitrosamines. 1: Dimethylnitrosamine (NDMA) (37 ng), 2: *N*-nitrosodiethylamine (34 ng), 3: *N*-nitrosodipropylamine (27 ng), 4: *N*-nitrosodibutylamine (27 ng). Reprinted, with permission, from Vohra and Harrington (1980).

ential pulse or sampled DC. The electrode potentials for each class were, -0.77v for Class I, -0.740v for Class II, -0.820v for Class III, and -0.77v for Class IV.

The appropriate drop size, drop time, modulation amplitude, and flow rate were found by using *N*-nitrosodipropylamine as a model compound. It was found that drop size large, gave as expected, greatest sensitivity. Drop times over 1.0 sec resulted in loss of information. This was due to the instrument sampling mode of operation in which the current is measured only near the end of the life of the drop. If long drop times are used, the species eluting from the column may pass the DME before current is sampled and hence go undetected.

The results of the evaluation study can best be seen by reference to Figures 1, 2, and 3 which show typical chromatograms for different classes of

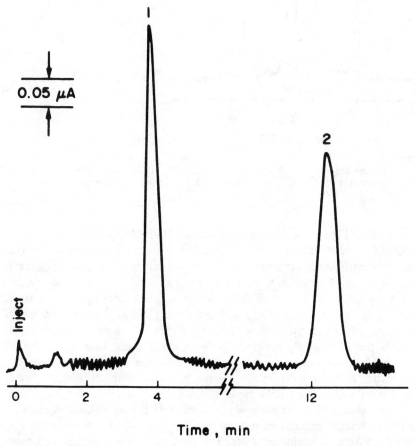

Figure 2
Chromatogram for Class II *N*-nitrosamines. 1: *N*-Nitroso-*N*-Methylaniline (90 ng), 2: *N*-nitrosodiphenylamine (150 ng). Reprinted, with permission, from Vohra and Harrington (1981).

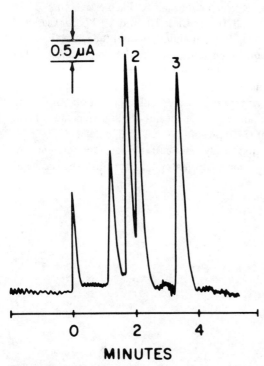

Figure 3
Chromatogram for Class IV *N*-nitrosamines. 1: *N*-nitroso-4-hydroxyproline (43.5 ng), 2: *N*-nitrososarcosine (45.4 ng), 3: NPRO (36.1 ng). Reprinted, with permission, from Vohra and Harrington (1980).

nitrosamines. Figure 4 shows a plot of amount injected v. peak height, using the sampled DC mode. It will be noted that in this mode, in which only one current measurement is made per drop, the detection limit is about 20 ng. Figure 5, however, shows a similar plot for the differential pulse mode. In this mode, current is sampled twice on each drop, before and after pulsing, and the signal recorded is the difference (Parry and Osteryoung 1965). This method results in better signal:noise ratio, hence better sensitivity. It can be seen from Figure 5 that in the differential pulse mode the detection limit is < 1 ng.

Figure 6 shows plots of amount injected v. peak height for representative compounds from each of the four classes. In each case the conditions were as stated and the differential pulse mode was used.

The second phase of the study involved determining NDELA in cosmetic products. Sample preparation utilized the fact that NDELA is not soluble in chloroform, but is soluble in water. The extraction procedure has been previously described (Vohra et al. 1981). Results are shown in Table 1. Samples 1, 2, 4, and 5 were hand and face creams, and sample 3 was a shampoo. This

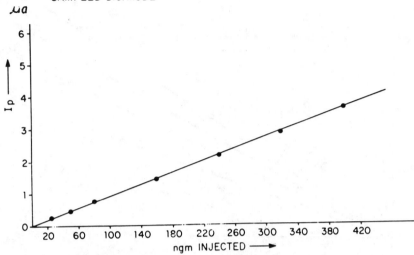

Figure 4
Amount injected v. peak height, *N*-nitrosodipropylamine. Sampled DC mode. Reprinted, with permission, from Vohra and Harrington (1980).

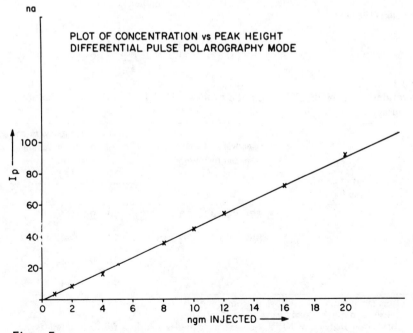

Figure 5
Amount injected v. peak height, *N*-nitrosodipropylamine. Differential pulse mode. Reprinted, with permission, from Vohra and Harrington (1980).

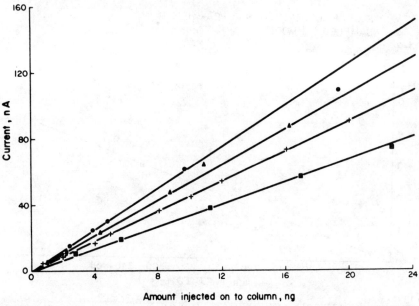

Figure 6

Chromatopolarography of 4 *N*-nitrosamines. (+) *N*-nitrosodipropylamine; (●) NDELA; (▲) NPRO; (■) *N*-nitroso-*N*-methylaniline. Reprinted, with permission, from Vohra and Harrington (1981).

Table 1

Determination of NDELA in cosmetic products by HPLC and differential pulse polarography

Prepared concentration of NDELA in sample (ppm)	Recovery of NDELA[a] in sample number [%]					Corrected recovery of NDELA[b] in sample number [%]				
	1	2	3	4	5	1	2	3	4	5
0·5	87	89	41	70	83	94	95	44	76	89
1·0	88	89	40	74	85	94	95	44	80	90
1·5	91	88	44	80	89	96	94	48	85	94
2·0	90	90	42	82	90	95	94	44	87	95

Data reprinted, with permission, from Vohra and Harrington (1981).
[a]Mean of duplicate analyses.
[b]Based on analyses of NDELA-containing aqueous solutions for each determination in place of the cosmetic product.

Table 2
NPYR in Fried Bacon

Sample Number	GC/TEA (ppb)	HPLC-EC (ppb)
1[a]	8.56	10.0
2[a]	9.60	10.6
3[a]	4.88	5.56
4[b]	10.00	10.72
5[b]	7.69	5.88
6[b]	11.6	9.55

sample size = 25.0g
[a] nitrite-free bacon, spiked at 10, 10, and 5 ppb, respectively
[b] USDA samples containing natural levels of NPYR

latter sample consistently yielded low recoveries. These variations of recoveries in the determination of NDELA in cosmetic products have been reported by others (Fan et al. 1977).

The third part of this study consisted of determining NPYR in fried bacon by GC/TEA and HPLC-EC. Bacon samples were prepared by the method of Fazio et al. (1972). At the last step in this procedure, the sample is contained in methylene chloride for injection into the GC. Water-immiscible solvents cannot be used with the HPLC-EC, hence the sample was transferred to mobile phase prior to injection. This was accomplished by adding mobile phase and evaporating the methylene chloride with a stream of nitrogen. Two types of samples were run. One was nitrite-free bacon spiked with NPYR at the desired level, and the second was nitrite-processed bacon known to contain NPYR. Sample results are shown in Table 2. It will be noticed that at these low levels, the comparison between the GC/TEA method and the HPLC-EC is quite good. The error for the individual values reported is approximately ± 1.5 ppb.

Thus it can be seen that HPLC-EC holds considerable promise as an alternate method of analysis for *N*-nitrosamines in a variety of matrices. The technique can determine volatile and nonvolatile nitroso compounds, and requires relatively simple, inexpensive instrumentation that can also serve other analytical purposes in the analytical laboratory.

ACKNOWLEDGMENTS

This work was supported in part by Grant No. CA 18618, awarded by the National Cancer Institute, DHEW, and by the U.S. Department of Agriculture, Broad Form Cooperative Agreement No. 58-32U4-9-47. The authors would also like to express their appreciation to the staff of the Food Safety Laboratory, U.S.D.A., Eastern Regional Center for the GC/TEA analyses.

REFERENCES

A High Resolution Mass Spectrometry Assay for
N-Nitrosodimethylamine in Human Plasma

WILLIAM A. GARLAND, HALYNA HOLOWASCHENKO,
WOLFGANG KUENZIG, EDWARD P. NORKUS, AND ALLAN H. CONNEY
Department of Biochemistry and Drug Metabolism
Hoffmann-La Roche Inc.
Nutley, New Jersey 07110

The report of N-nitrosodimethylamine (NDMA) in the blood of one individual (Fine et al. 1977) has been confirmed by three additional studies. Lakritz et al. (1980), using distillation of blood and analysis of the methylene dichloride extract of the distillate by gas chromatography/thermal energy analysis (GC/TEA), found a mean NDMA concentration of 600 pg/ml in blood samples from 38 normal volunteers. Yamamoto et al. (1980) found the same mean blood concentration of NDMA in blood samples from 8 normal volunteers. These workers examined the methylene dichloride extract of a steam distillate of blood by GC/TEA. Webb et al. (1979) analyzed the methylene dichloride extract of a vacuum distillate of blood from 14 normal volunteers by gas chromatography/high resolution mass spectrometry (GC-[HR]MS) and found a mean NDMA concentration of about 300 pg/ml.

In this article, we report a sensitive and highly specific GC-[HR]MS assay for NDMA in human plasma. We also report the analyses of plasma samples taken 1 hour before and 1 hour after lunch from 64 normal volunteers. Our assay differs from that of Webb et al. (1979) in that it (1) uses mild chemical ionization instead of electron ionization, (2) uses a stable isotope analog of NDMA ($[^{15}N_2]$-NDMA) as an internal standard, (3) does not use a distillation "clean-up" step, and (4) includes procedures to prevent and detect the measurement of artifactual concentrations of NDMA.

METHODS

Precautions

To avoid artifacts, all solvents (including water) and the borate buffer solution are irradiated just prior to use for at least 15 minutes under a 200-watt high pressure quartz mercury vapor lamp (Hanovia 654A, Conrad-Hanovia, Newark, NJ). All scintillation vials, Pasteur pipets, centrifuge tubes, and culture tubes are thoroughly rinsed by sonication just prior to use first with irradiated methanol and then with irradiated methylene dichloride.

Sample Collection

Two 10-ml blood samples are obtained from each volunteer using two Becton-Dickinson No. 6527 Vacutainers (heparinized) and a single Luer adaptor and hub and a single Yale No. 5191 needle. The blood samples in the Vacutainers are stored on ice for between 0.25 and 2.0 hours and are then centrifuged for 30 minutes at 1200 x g at 2°C. The resulting 9-ml pooled plasma sample from each individual is immediately transferred using a Pasteur pipet into a glass scintillation vial containing 1 ml of a "morpholine-azide solution" consisting of 50 μl of a 5 μg/ml aqueous solution of morpholine, 100 μl of a 2.0M aqueous solution of sodium azide and 850 μl of water. Post-collection nitrosation of plasma dimethylamine is detected by monitoring the amount of nitrosomorpholine generated from the morpholine during the analysis of the sample (S.R. Tannenbaum, pers. comm.). Sodium azide is used to inhibit post-collection nitrosation reactions (Eisenbrand et al. 1981).

Sample Analysis

A 5-ml aliquot of the fortified plasma sample described above is transferred with a Pasteur pipet into a 10-ml culture tube (Pyrex 9825 with Teflon lined screw cap) which was previously spiked with 20 μl of a 45 pg/μl aqueous solution of $[^{15}N_2]$-NDMA. The $[^{15}N_2]$-NDMA was synthesized from 99% $[^{15}N]$-dimethylamine (Merck and Co., Inc. [Isotopes Division], St. Louis, MO) using a published method (Vogel 1956). The tube is vortexed and allowed to stand for 5 minutes. One ml of 1.0 molar pH 10 borate buffer and 7 ml of methylene dichloride are added, and the tube is shaken (60 strokes/min) for 30 minutes on a reciprocating shaker (Eberbach Inc.). The tube is centrifuged for 15 minutes at 1200 x g, the aqueous layer is aspirated off, and 5 ml of the organic layer is transferred using a Pasteur pipet into a 5-ml centrifuge tube (Pyrex 8061). The volume of the methylene dichloride is reduced to approximately 100 μl by gentle evaporation of the solution under a stream of argon (prepurified by bubbling the gas through a trap containing concentrated sulfuric acid).

Two to 5 μl of this methylene dichloride solution are injected onto a 2 mm x 1.9 m glass gas chromatography column packed with 10% SP 1000 on acid washed 100/120 mesh Chromosorb W (Supelco, Inc.). The oven and injector temperatures of the gas chromatograph (Carlo Erba) are 128° and 148°C, respectively. Hydrogen (1.6 kg/cm^2) is the carrier gas. The retention times of NDMA and $[^{15}N_2]$-NDMA under these conditions are both 90 seconds. The effluent from the gas chromatography column is directed 45 seconds after injection (divert valve) via an all-glass jet separator into the chemical ionization ion source of a Kratos MS-50 high resolution mass spectrometer set to monitor at a mass resolution of m/Δm = 10,000 (10% valley definition) the ions at m/z 75.0558 (MH$^+$) of NDMA) and m/z 77.0499 (MH$^+$ of [^{15}N$_2$]-NDMA). The separator oven and ion source are both operated at 150°C. Sufficient isobutane is introduced via the chemical ionization direct insertion probe to give an ion source pressure of approximately 20 pascals. A small amount of isobutanol (MH$^+$ = 75.0810) is added to the ion source via the perfluorokerosine inlet to aid in tuning and to check the mass scale calibration.

Calculations

The m/z 75 to m/z 77 ion ratio (y) in an experimental sample ("unknown") is calculated and converted to an uncorrected concentration of NDMA (x) using the formula x = $\frac{y-b}{m}$, where m (slope) and b (intercept) are constants generated from the least squares linear regression analysis of the ion ratio (ordinate) versus concentration (abscissa) data from the analysis in duplicate of 5-ml water samples each fortified with 900 pg of [^{15}N$_2$]-NDMA and either 0, 100, 200, 400, 800, or 1600 pg of NDMA (Tables 1 and 2). The working solution used to prepare the calibration samples is prepared from a 1-liter aqueous solution containing 1.00 ml of authentic NDMA purchased from the Aldrich Chemical Co. (1.01 mg/ml).

A corrected concentration of NDMA is calculated as described below. We first subtract from the uncorrected concentration: (1) the mean apparent NDMA concentration from the duplicate analysis of a 5-ml water sample drawn up through a randomly picked needle into a randomly picked Vacutainer and shaken for 15 minutes with the water continually in contact with the stopper, and (2) one-half of the mean NDMA concentration from the duplicate analysis of a solution consisting of 1 ml of the "morpholine-azide solution" and 4 ml of water. We then multiply the resulting value by 1.11 to correct for the initial

Table 1

Parameters from the Least Squares Analysis of the Four Sets of Calibration Curve Samples Used to Generate the Data in Table 3

Curve	Slope[a] ± SD[a] (RSD)[b]	Intercept ± SD	Correlation Coefficient
1	42.0 ± 0.8 (1.9%)	0.012 ± 0.012	.998
2	38.9 ± 0.5 (1.3%)	0.014 ± 0.008	.999
3	39.2 ± 0.7 (1.8%)	0.007 ± 0.010	.999
4	40.2 ± 0.6 (1.5%)	0.012 ± 0.009	.999

[a]Multiplied by 10^4
[b]Relative standard deviation

Table 2

Inter-assay Precision from the Four Calibration Curves Used to Generate the Data in Table 3

NDMA added (pg/ml)	m/z 75 ÷ m/z 77 [mean ± SD (RSD)[a]]	NDMA found (pg/ml) [mean ± SD (RSD)[a]]	(found-added) × 100 added
0	0.013 ± 0.003 (24%)	0.26 ± 0.19 (73%)	—
20	0.092 ± 0.009 (10%)	20 ± 2 (10%)	0%
40	0.16 ± 0.010 (6.3%)	37 ± 2 (5.4%)	−7.5%
80	0.32 ± 0.014 (4.4%)	76 ± 3 (3.9%)	−5.0%
160	0.67 ± 0.026 (3.8%)	164 ± 7 (4.2%)	+2.5%
320	1.31 ± 0.073 (5.5%)	324 ± 12 (3.8%)	+1.3%

[a]Relative standard deviation

dilution of the 9-ml plasma sample with the 1 ml of "morpholine-azide solution."

RESULTS AND DISCUSSION

Typical selected ion current profiles at m/z 75 and m/z 77 from the analysis of 5-ml water samples fortified with 180 pg/ml of $[^{15}N_2]$-NDMA and either 0 or 20 pg/ml of NDMA are shown in Figures 1 and 2, respectively. In viewing these profiles, the reader should note that for display purposes the profile for m/z 75 has been multiplied by a factor of 3 relative to the profile for m/z 77. It can be seen (Fig. 2) that the analysis of the sample containing 20 pg/ml of NDMA gives a peak for NDMA which is more than ten times both the background "noise" and the NDMA response from the analysis of the 0 pg/ml sample. The peaks in the selected ion current profiles which are generated from the irradiated methylene dichloride are starred.

The selected ion current profiles from the analysis of plasma samples from normal volunteers are shown in Figures 3 and 4. The profiles in Figure 3 are typical of most of the plasma samples analyzed. In this plasma sample the concentration of NDMA is below the limit of quantitation of the assay. The profiles in Figure 4 are from the analysis of a plasma sample from the rare normal volunteer who had a quantifiable concentration of NDMA. In this plasma sample the uncorrected concentration of NDMA is 90 pg/ml and the corrected concentration is 86 pg/ml.

A number of experiments were performed with fresh blood samples that were fortified with NDMA to give a concentration of 100 pg/ml above the small NDMA concentration normally present. These experiments showed that:

1. No NDMA is either lost or gained when the blood samples are shaken for 30 minutes in Vacutainers with the blood in constant contact with the stoppers.

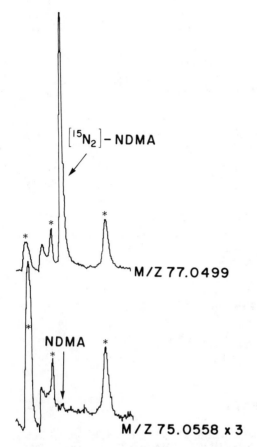

Figure 1
Selected ion current profiles from the analysis of a 5 ml water sample fortified with 0 pg/ml of NDMA (m/z 75) and 180 pg/ml of $[^{15}N_2]$-NDMA (m/z 77). The response for m/z 75 has been multiplied by three for display. The starred peaks come from the irradiated methylene dichloride.

2. Assuming a hematocrit of 0.46 (Diem and Lentner 1970), the plasma-red blood cell partition coefficient for NDMA is approximately 1.6. Thus, 100 pg/ml of NDMA in a blood sample when centrifuged gives an observed NDMA concentration of 121 pg/ml in the plasma and a calculated 76 pg/ml in the red blood cells (for the formula used in the calculation see, Sheiner et al. 1981).

3. The Vacutainer stoppers have no effect on the plasma/red blood cell partition coefficient for NDMA.

4. NDMA is stable in blood for at least 2 hours when the sample is stored in a Vacutainer placed in ice.

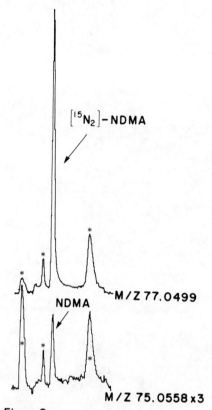

Figure 2
Selected ion current profiles from the analysis of a 5 ml water sample fortified with 20 pg/ml of NDMA (m/z 75) and 180 pg/ml of $[^{15}N_2]$-NDMA (m/z 77). The response for m/z 75 has been multiplied by three for display. The starred peaks come from the irradiated methylene dichloride.

5. The addition of morpholine and azide to plasma samples causes no significant change in NDMA concentration, even if the fortified plasma samples are stored for 3 days at 2°C.

Data from the four calibration curves used in the analysis of the plasma samples from 64 normal volunteers are given in Table 1. The intra-assay precision, from a consideration of the relative standard deviation of the slopes of the four calibration curves, is better than 2%. In addition, the actual values for the slope and intercept are seen to change very little during the 4-week period in which the measurements were made. For all four curves the correlation coefficients for the least squares fit of the ion ratio versus concentration data are greater than 0.997.

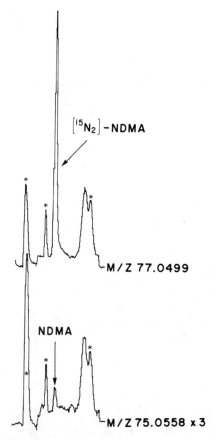

Figure 3
Selected ion current profiles from the analysis of 5 ml of plasma from a normal volunteer. The sample has been fortified with 180 pg/ml of [$^{15}N_2$]-NDMA (m/z 77). The response for NDMA (m/z 75) has been multiplied by three for display. The starred peaks come from irradiated methylene dichloride. This sample contains a nonquantifiable amount of NDMA.

Inter-assay precision from the four calibration curves is shown in Table 2. Excluding the value for 0 pg/ml added, the mean precision (± SD) for all concentrations of NDMA is 5.5 ± 2.6% and the mean percent difference (± SD) between the amount of NDMA found and the amount of NDMA added is 3.3 ± 3.0%.

The limit of quantitation of the assay is calculated using the concepts set forth in the guidelines of the American Chemical Society for data acquisition and data quality evaluation in environmental chemistry (ACS Committee on Environmental Improvement and Subcommittee on Environmental Analytical Chemistry 1980). These guidelines set the limit of quantitation of an assay as

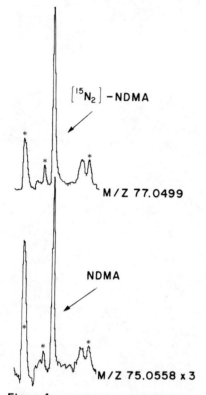

Figure 4
Selected ion current profiles from the analysis of 5 ml of plasma from a normal volunteer. The sample has been fortified with 180 pg/ml of [$^{15}N_2$]-NDMA (m/z 77). The response for NDMA (m/z 75) has been multiplied by three for display. The starred peaks come from irradiated methylene dichloride. This sample contains 86 pg/ml of NDMA.

any signal, i.e., concentration, which exceeds the sum of the signal from the analysis of an analyte-free matrix plus the signal equivalent to ten times the standard deviation of the response from the analysis of the analyte-free matrix. The limit of quantitation for NDMA in the plasma samples from the 64 normal volunteers is calculated as follows. The mean (± SD) response for NDMA from the analysis of the Vacutainer and needle and one-half the mean ± SD response for NDMA from the "morpholine-azide solution" are 1.7 ± 2.5 pg/ml (n = 6) and 1.9 ± 0.3 pg/ml (n = 6), respectively. Dividing the intercept of the calibration curve by the slope of the calibration curve gives a value for NDMA in the water blank samples. Using the data in Table 1, the mean value (± SD) for such a calculation for all 4 curves is 2.8 ± 0.8 pg/ml. Summing this value and the value for apparent NDMA from the Vacutainer and needle and the "morpholine-azide solution" gives a value of 6.4 pg/ml. Ten times the SD for the most uncertain concentration, i.e., the apparent NDMA from the Vacutainers and needles, gives an apparent NDMA concentration of 25 pg/ml. Summing this value and the 6.4 pg/ml value gives the assay a limit of quantitation of 31 pg/ml.

The concentrations of NDMA in plasma samples obtained from 64 normal volunteers 1 hour before lunch and 1 hour after lunch are given in Table 3. Most of the samples had nonmeasurable concentrations of NDMA and the mean concentration of NDMA in the few samples which had measurable amounts of NDMA were considerably less than the mean concentrations reported in the literature.

Because the results of our assay for NDMA in human plasma did not agree with the data reported in the literature, we analyzed five additional human plasma samples for NDMA by both our GC-[HR]MS method and by vacuum distillation–GC/TEA. The mean concentration (± S.D.) of apparent NDMA in the 5 plasma samples was 448 ± 185 pg/ml when the samples were analyzed by the GC/TEA procedure. We found < 31 pg/ml of NDMA when the same plasma samples were assayed by our GC-[HR]MS method.

CONCLUSION

A GC-[HR]MS method which utilizes chemical ionization and stable isotope dilution has been developed for the measurement of NDMA in human plasma. The limit of quantitation of the method was 31 pg NDMA/ml plasma. The assay has been used to analyze plasma samples from 64 normal volunteers. The concentrations of NDMA in the plasma samples were considerably less than those reported previously in the literature.

Table 3
NDMA in Plasma Samples from 64 Normal Volunteers

Plasma Sample	Number of Subjects	NDMA in Plasma (pg/ml)
1 Hour before lunch	59	< 31
	5	$89 \pm 66^{a,b}$
1 Hour after lunch	60	< 31
	4	$59 \pm 24^{a,b}$

[a]Mean ± SD
[b]Only two of the normal volunteers had quantifiable concentrations of NDMA both before and after lunch. The plasma samples from these subjects were reanalyzed 30 days after the original analyses. The new concentrations were within 5% of old values. In addition, the NDMA peak vanished upon irradiation with UV light for 15 minutes.

ACKNOWLEDGMENT

Mr. F. De Grazia of the Department of Pharmacokinetics and Biopharmaceutics helped with a number of experiments during assay development. Ms. S. Boyle of the Product Development Department made the GC/TEA measurements. Ms. D. Matuszewski of the Immunology Department drew most of the blood samples from the normal volunteers.

REFERENCES

ACS Committee on Environmental Improvement and Subcommittee on Environmental Analytical Chemistry. 1980. Guidelines for data acquisition and data quality evaluation in environmental chemistry. *Anal. Chem.* 52:2242.

Diem, K. and C. Lentner, eds. 1970. *Documenta Geigy*, p. 617. J.R. Geigy S.A., Basle, Switzerland.

Eisenbrand, G., B. Spiegelhalder, and R. Preussmann. 1981. Analysis of human biological specimens for nitrosamine content. *Ban. Rep.* 7:275.

Fine, D.H., R. Ross, D.P. Rounbehler, A. Silvergleid, and L. Song. 1977. Formation in vivo of volatile N-nitrosamines in man after ingestion of cooked bacon and spinach. *Nature* 265:753.

Lakritz, L., M.L. Simenhoff, S.R. Dunn, and W. Fiddler. 1980. N-Nitrosodimethylamine in human blood. *Food Cosmet. Toxicol.* 18:77.

Sheiner, L.B., L.Z. Benet, and L.A. Pagliaro. 1981. Pharmacokinetic data: a standard approach to compiling clinical pharmacokinetic data. *J. Pharmacokinet. Biopharm.* 9:59.

Vogel, A.I. 1956. *A Textbook of Practical Organic Chemistry*, 3rd edition, p. 426. Longman, London.

Webb, K.S., T.A. Gough, A. Carrick, and D. Hazelby. 1979. Mass spectrometric and chemiluminescent detection of picogram amounts of N-nitrosodimethylamine. *Anal. Chem.* 51:989.

Yamamoto, M., T. Yamada, and A. Tanimura. 1980. Volatile nitrosamines in human blood before and after ingestion of a meal containing high concentrations of nitrate and secondary amines. *Food Cosmet. Toxicol.* 18:297.

COMMENTS

FINE: I would like to make two comments: In my next presentation I point out that most published work on nitrosamines in the blood did not include the critical experiment of adding a precursor amine. In fact, the old data is suspect because they didn't have the amine additive and, therefore we don't know if there was an artifact or not. Recent data from Eisenbrand et al. (1979) showed that they have not been able to reproduce any background blood levels in agreement with your findings. In the comparison of TEA and MS analyses, the data of Webb et al. (1979) showed a very good correlation. Do you have any possible explanation for this?

GARLAND: No I don't.

TANNENBAUM: Did the TEA peaks disappear on irradiation?

GARLAND: We haven't tried that yet, but when I set up the TEA procedure, I looked at the chromatograms and the peaks looked like they were from NDMA.

BRUNNEMANN: One would assume from your talk that there is no difference between the NDMA levels before and after lunch.

GARLAND: I don't think we have enough data to establish that.

BRUNNEMANN: You had five individuals before lunch with rather high NDMA levels. Did you have data on who were smokers and who were nonsmokers?

GARLAND: We carefully recorded whether the individuals were smokers or nonsmokers, and what they had eaten for lunch, and we found no correlations of these data and the individuals' NDMA plasma levels.

ARCHER: Was the lunch controlled?

GARLAND: The particular lunch was served at the Roche cafeteria.

MIRVISH: Was any beer ingested?

CONNEY: No.

FINE: I don't understand the mean levels you give for the few individuals who had measurable levels. When you say 59 ± 24 pg/ml, that will take these measurements near your limit of quantitation.

GARLAND: No. These are just the mean concentrations from the five samples that had measurable levels. The five had values of, for instance, 30, 40, 60 and so on.

FINE: If you've got a lot of error range, aren't you getting below the level that you can quantitate?

GARLAND: No. The wide SD just happens to reflect the range of the values.

FINE: All right.

BRUNNEMANN: You say the vacuum distillation was not the factor that gave elevated values. Do you have other explanation?

GARLAND: It is possible that there is an interfering peak in the TEA chromatograms.

MIRVISH: You used azide to scavenge for nitrite. Does azide work at neutral pH?

GARLAND: I don't know.

MIRVISH: What's the point of adding it if it doesn't work? The advantage of ascorbic acid is that at least it does work around pH 4.

CHALLIS: I can answer that question. It's the best one to use in neutral and alkaline conditions, but it's not anywhere near as efficient as it is under acidic conditions.

GARLAND: There are very few options.

ARCHER: It doesn't matter anyway, because it's just scavenging. You're reacting with azide instead of reacting with amine. Amines don't nitrosate well in neutral pH.

CHALLIS: They do at neutral and alkaline pH. That's the problem.

ARCHER: Well, okay. It depends on what the nitrosating agent is.

PETO: Your method is actually somewhat better than you presented it to be: To take a mean $\pm$ 10 SD as the limit of detectability seems completely inappropriate and doesn't seem to give your method credit for its probable quality.

For example, you could perfectly well have values at 10 pg/ml or 15 pg/ml being meaningfully detected and discriminated between. If, for example, you find that plotting duplicate analyses of the same sample one against the other gives a reasonable correlation between the duplicate measurements, but that the difference between different samples are consistent at 10, or 5, or 15 pg/ml level, then this is the measure of the limit of detectability, not your criteria. I think your method must surely be giving meaningful results well below 31 pg/ml and you shouldn't use that as a cutoff but should look at the actual value below that. I am sure you would find that there is a lot of information at a much lower level.

GARLAND: That's possible, but I am very comfortable with the 31 pg/ml cutoff. In addition, we have reanalyzed samples with low concentrations, and found considerable imprecision; 6 pg/ml becomes 12, and 12 becomes 15, and 15 becomes 3.

PETO: Well, that suggests then that something like 10 pg/ml is perhaps the cutoff of what is meaningful.

GARLAND: I think that the concept expressed in the ACS (1980) article does a good job of differentiating between what is detectable and what is quantifiable. I think we are using a good criteria for quantitation.

TANNENBAUM: Does the blank value ± SD correspond to a certain signal-to-noise ratio?

GARLAND: No.

FINE: When you did your GC/TEA analyses, did you go to as elaborate lengths in terms of artifacts as you did on the mass spectrometer?

GARLAND: Yes, we did the best we could. I feel confident about that.

MICHEJDA: Why should the TEA method have such consistently high values? You offer no explanation for it. Is it just an artifact of some kind? It's not an instrumental artifact. Four different methods give more or less the same values.

BRUNNEMANN: At the time no internal nitrosation monitor was used so you don't really know if the original papers are the true values.

GARLAND: When I go back to my lab, I will start doing additional studies, looking for co-eluting peaks at m/z 75 in the plasma extracts.

FINE: I understand that they analyzed blood samples at Heidelberg by GC/ TEA and got zero values, not values of 500 pg/ml. So I don't quite understand the discrepancy between your MS results and the TEA results.

PREUSSMANN: Nor do I.

ARCHER: Does your calibration curve go that far down for the TEA? Have you actually injected known samples?

GARLAND: Yes, we did. We actually brought spiked water samples through the method. But the lowest concentration we analyzed was 100 pg/ml.

ARCHER: Is that what it measures?

GARLAND: Yes.

CHALLIS: Did you have morpholine in the samples analyzed by GC/TEA? Did you see NMOR?

GARLAND: We haven't gone back and analyzed for NMOR.

CHALLIS: That would answer the problem about formation of NDMA on the column. It is possible that the NMOR in the extract rearranged when injected on the column?

GARLAND: Well, you've got to remember that the TEA procedure and the MS procedures use the same GC-column, so that is a common feature.

References

Eisenbrand, G., B. Spiegelhalder, and R. Preussmann. 1981. Analysis of human biological specimens for nitrosamine content. *Ban Rep.* 7:275.
Webb, K.S., T.A. Gough, A. Carrick, and D. Hazelby. 1979. Mass spectrometric and chemiluminescent detection of picogram amounts of N-nitrosodimethylamine. *Anal. Chem.* 51:989.

SESSION IV:

EXPOSURE OF HUMAN BEINGS TO NITROSAMINES

Nitrosamines in the General Environment and Food

DAVID H. FINE
New England Institute for Life Sciences
125 Second Avenue
Waltham, Massachusetts 02254

The highest known concentrations of exogenous nitrosamines occur in the workplace, especially in the rubber and leather-tanning industries.

OCCUPATIONAL SETTINGS

Rubber Industry

The rubber industry uses nitrosodiphenylamine (NDPhA) as a vulcanization retarder. It is labile, can participate in transnitrosation reactions, and may contribute to the formation of other carcinogenic N-nitroso compounds.

Fajen et al. (1979) measured levels of nitrosamines in three rubber factories. NDPhA was found at the 0.2 to 47 $\mu g/m^3$ level in the air of a factory where the compound was being manufactured. In addition to the presence of NDPhA in chemical manufacturing areas, curing and extrusion sections of the rubber factories were found to contain nitrosomorpholine (NMOR) in concentrations ranging from 0.5-27 $\mu g/m^3$. (The NMOR presumably arises from the use of bismorpholinecarbamylsulfenamide, which is used as an accelerator). Nitrosodimethylamine (NDMA) was detected at lower levels (0.05-0.5 $\mu g/m^3$) as an air pollutant in several of the factories.

More recently, McGlothlin et al. (1981) conducted an in-depth study of nitrosamine levels in a rubber factory. Initial measurements indicated that one area air sample contained NMOR at 250 $\mu g/m^3$. Within 7 months, airborne nitrosamine levels were reduced dramatically (McGlothlin et al. 1981) to only 14 $\mu g/m^3$.

Preussmann et al. (1980) measured nitrosamine levels in 19 rubber factories in the Federal Republic of Germany. Initial concentrations of NDMA and NMOR ranged from 1 to 20 $\mu g/m^3$. In one working area (tire-tube curing), an extremely high concentration of NDMA (140 $\mu g/m^3$) was detected. More recently, Spiegelhalder and Preussmann (1982) reported a concentration of 1060 $\mu g/m^3$ NDMA and 4,700 $\mu g/m^3$ NMOR during injection moulding and curing of conveyor belts.

Leather Tanning

An investigation of airborne nitrosamine levels in a typical leather tannery was undertaken because of Acheson's (1976) report of a possible increase in nasal cancer incidence among leather workers. In their initial study, Rounbehler et al. (1979) reported that NDMA was detected as an airborne pollutant at all sites in the tannery on three separate visits. The highest level, 47 $\mu g/m^3$, was found in the retanning, coloring, and fatliquoring areas. Eight leather-tanning facilities have been surveyed in the United States (Fajen et al. 1982). Four of the eight plants were found to have airborne concentrations of NDMA greater than 0.5 $\mu g/m^3$.

Amine Factories

Bretschneider and Matz (1973, 1976) reported levels of NDMA in the air of between 1 and 43 $\mu g/m^3$ on the site of a plant manufacturing dimethylamine (DMA). Fine et al. (1976c) reported NDMA concentrations ranging from 0.01-1 $\mu g/m^3$ in the ambient air outside a factory in Belle, West Virginia in which DMA was manufactured and used. Atmospheric concentrations of NDMA in the neighboring towns of Belle and Charleston ranged from 0.001-0.04 $\mu g/m^3$. Apparently, most of the NDMA detected had been produced in the chemical plant and not by the reaction of DMA with oxides of nitrogen in the atmosphere (Fine et al. 1977b).

Rocket Fuel Factory

Fine et al. (1976a,b) reported that NDMA was present as an air pollutant in Baltimore, Maryland. The prime source was subsequently found to be a chemical plant that used NDMA in the manufacture of a rocket fuel—unsymmetrical-dimethylhydrazine (UDMH). Typical NDMA levels ranged from 6-36 $\mu g/m^3$ at the factory site. Approximately 1 $\mu g/m^3$ was measured in the residential neighborhood adjacent to the factory, and approximately 0.1 $\mu g/m^3$ was found about 3.2 km away in downtown Baltimore (Fine et al. 1976a,c; 1977a,b,c).

Machine Shops

The finding of nitrosodiethanolamine (NDELA) in some industrial fluids at the 3% level (Fan et al. 1977b) triggered an effort to determine the extent of worker exposure to airborne NDELA. NDELA was not detected as an airborne pollutant in factories making the cutting fluids or in large and small machine shops using the fluids (Fine and Rounbehler 1982).

Despite the fact that NDELA is not sufficiently volatile to pose a problem as an air pollutant, significant exposure of workers can still occur by dermal contact, either through splashing or by handling metal parts that have been soaked in the fluids. Concern for these workers has increased as a result of recent reports that NDELA penetrates the skin of both rats (Lijinsky et al. 1981a) and humans (Edwards et al. 1979; Bronaugh et al. 1981) and that it is a more potent carcinogen than was previously surmised (Lijinsky et al. 1980b; Preussmann et al. 1982). NDELA is also present in cosmetics.

NONOCCUPATIONAL EXPOSURES

Tobacco Smoke

Human exposure to nitrosamines from tobacco smoke is greater than all other nonoccupational exposures combined. This is discussed by Dietrich Hoffmann (this volume).

Food

Extensive compilations of the volatile nitrosamine content of foodstuffs in various diets have been published by Scanlan (1975), Havery et al. (1978), the International Agency for Research on Cancer (1978), Kawabata et al. (1979), Preussmann et al. (1979), Schmähl (1980), and Gray (1982).

Meats

Over the past 9 years, the meat industry and various government and research laboratories have developed techniques to reduce volatile nitrosamines in cooked bacon. Although nitrosamines have not been eliminated, their concentrations have been reduced considerably (Sen et al. 1977). The nitrosamine content of cooked bacon is regulated in the U.S. with action level being 14 μg/kg.

In England, Gough et al. (1978) analyzed a variety of foodstuffs typical of the diet in that country. All 50 samples of fried bacon examined contained concentrations of N-nitrosopyrrolidine (NPYR) ranging from 1-20 μg/kg, and occasionally up to 200 μg/kg. In addition, all samples contained nitrosopiperidine (NPIP) (in concentrations up to 0.25 μg/kg) and NDMA (in concentrations as high as 5 μg/kg).

In recent surveys conducted in the United States to determine the nitrosamine content of cured meats other than bacon (Nitrite Safety Council 1980; Sen et al. 1979), the majority of the positive samples contained extremely low levels of nitrosamines—usually less than 1 μg/kg.

Dairy Products

Cheeses of the Gouda and Edam types as produced in certain European countries could contain nitrosamines because of the addition of nitrate to prevent the growth of clostridia (Gray et al. 1979). Gough et al. (1977) examined different varieties of cheese commonly available in England. Levels of NDMA were similar for all cheeses (1-5 μg/kg), except for one sample of Stilton, which contained 13 μg/kg. A similar range of concentrations was measured by Sen et al. (1978) in 31 samples of cheese imported into Canada.

Fish

Because of its relatively high amine content, fish has been regarded as a likely source of nitrosamines. However, fish products in the United States rarely contain nitrosamines in excess of 1 μg/kg.

The Japanese diet contains a relatively large amount of fish, some of which contains NDMA at levels of between 0.5 and 5.0 μg/kg. Dried squid is the exception, with NDMA levels being in the 15-84 μg/kg range (Kawabata et al. 1979). These investigations also showed that fish cooked in a gas oven contained much higher NDMA levels than fish cooked in an electric oven. Dried squid cooked in a gas oven had NDMA levels of between 24 and 310 μg/kg.

Alcoholic Beverages

Considerable attention has been focused over the past few years on the presence of nitrosamines in beer and other alcoholic beverages. Spiegelhalder et al. (1979) analyzed 158 samples of different types of beer in the Federal Republic of Germany and reported that 70% of them contained NDMA (mean concentration, 2.7 μg/kg). Goff and Fine (1979) reported NDMA levels ranging from 0.4-7.0 μg/kg in 18 brands of U.S. and imported beers. In addition, six of seven brands of Scotch whiskey, which is also made from malt, contained NDMA at levels between 0.3 and 2.3 μg/kg. Scanlan et al. (1980) reported NDMA in 23 of 25 beer samples, at levels ranging from 0-14 μg/kg and averaging 5.9 μg/kg.

Following the initial reports of nitrosamines in beer, changes in malting procedures were implemented. As a consequence, the NDMA levels in beer have dropped. They are now generally well below the level (5 μg/liter) at which the FDA would consider regulatory action (Food and Drug Administration 1980; Havery et al. 1981). A recent survey of domestic and imported beers conducted by the FDA following implementation of this "action level" showed that NDMA in 180 samples of domestic beer ranged from undetectable levels (0.2 or 0.4 μg/liter) to 13 μg/liter, averaging 1 μg/liter (Havery et al. 1981).

Cosmetics

Many cosmetics, soaps, and shampoos are contaminated with NDELA at levels ranging from less than 1 μg/kg to 48,000 μg/kg (Fan et al. 1977a). The source of the amine is triethanolamine, which is present in most cosmetic formulations.

The presence of nitrosamines in products containing lauramine oxide was analyzed by combined gas chromatography-thermal energy analyzer (GC/TEA) and high-pressure liquid chromatography-thermal energy analyzer (HPLC-TEA) (Hecht 1981). Of seven products analyzed, six gave positive responses on both HPLC-TEA and GC/TEA for nitrosododecylmethylamine (NDOMA). The concentrations of NDOMA in these products ranged from 0.02-0.60 μg/kg. Apparently, some NDOMA is also present in the lauramine oxide ingredient itself. These results show that NDOMA, a bladder carcinogen, is present in cosmetics formulated with lauramine oxide.

Analyses for nitrosobenzylmethylamine (NBMA) and nitrosomethylstearylamine (NMSA) in products containing stearalkonium chloride are currently in progress in Hecht's laboratories. Of eight samples screened by combined HPLC-TEA, three gave a positive response for NDMA and, .tentatively, NBMA. Further work is needed to confirm the presence of these nitrosamines in cosmetics. In addition, every cosmetic sample tested so far has given some positive TEA response, indicating the presence of other nitroso compounds, nitro compounds, or nitrite esters (Hecht 1981).

Pharmaceuticals

Many drugs contain chemically bound nitrogen and have sites for possible nitrosation. For example, cimetidine has received considerable attention recently, and its possible nitrosation products are being investigated (Jensen and Magee 1981). In addition, vasodilators derived from nitrate or nitrite esters can behave as potential nitrosating agents. Nitrosation may occur exogenously (within the drug itself) or it may occur endogenously in humans after ingestion of the drug.

Eisenbrand et al. (1979) analyzed 68 commercial formulations of the drug aminopyrine for the presence of preformed nitrosamines. Although this drug was available in the Federal Republic of Germany, none of the formulations have been licensed for sale in the United States. All formulations contained NDMA in amounts varying from 1-370 μg/kg.

Krull et al. (1979) reported that nitrosamine impurities were absent from 68 of 73 pharmaceutical products, consisting of both prescription and over-the-counter drugs available in the United States. The methods used by these investigators were designed to detect volatile and some nonvolatile N-nitroso compounds at levels as low as 1 μg/kg.

Pesticides

Fine et al. (1977b) reported that dinitroaniline herbicides, and formulations prepared as the amine salt, contained substantial nitrosamine impurities. For example, a formulation of the herbicide trifluralin was shown to contain 154 mg nitrosodipropylamine (NDPA)/liter (Ross et al. 1977). Two experimental field studies have demonstrated that the nitrosamine impurity in trifluralin is not detectable as an air pollutant on farms, even during application, presumably because the pesticide is generally applied by incorporation into the soil (Ross et al. 1978; West and Day 1979). Furthermore, NDPA was not detected in crops. Later EPA analyses of pesticides showed that concentrations of N-nitroso compounds ranged from 1.2-430 mg/liter. The chemical identity of the contaminants was usually predictable on the basis of the chemical structure and route of synthesis of the pesticide compound. For example, pendimethalin [N(1-ethylpropyl)-3,4-dimethyl-2,6-dinitrobenzenamine] yields nitrosopendimethalin, 2,4-D dimethylamine salt yields NDMA, and dinoseb triethanolamine salt yields NDELA.

Water

Nitrosamines have been observed in deionized water at concentrations ranging from 0.03-0.34 μg/kg (Kimoto et al. 1980). Volatile nitrosamines such as NDMA have also been identified in industrial wastewater in concentrations ranging from 0.2-5 μg/liter (Fine et al. 1977b; Cohen and Bachman 1978).

Air

Amines and oxides of nitrogen can react to form nitrosamines. This reaction is partially responsible for the nitrosamine contamination of workroom air in tanneries and rubber factories (see earlier discussion on occupational settings).

NMOR and NDMA have been found in the interior air of new 1979 model automobiles by Rounbehler et al. (1980). In the 38 automobiles tested, the concentrations ranged from 0.07-2.5 μg/m^3 for NMOR, from 0.04-0.39 μg/m^3 for NDEA.

NDMA pollution of indoor air from the burning of tobacco was investigated by Brunnemann and Hoffmann (1978). The appreciable amounts of NDMA detected in these environments were attributed largely to sidestream smoke.

REFERENCES

Acheson, E.D. 1976. Nasal cancer in the furniture and boot and shoe manufacturing industries. *Prev. Med.* **5**:295.

Bretschneider, K., and J. Matz. 1973. [In German; English summary.] [Nitrosamines (NA) in the atmospheric air and in the air at the places of employment.] *Arch. Geschwulstforsch.* **42**:36.

————. 1976. Occurrence and analysis of nitrosamines in air. In *Environmental N-nitroso Compounds: Analysis and Formation* (eds. E.A. Walker et al.), *IARC Sci. Publ.* **19**:395.

Bronaugh, R.L., E.R. Congdon, and R.J. Scheuplein. 1981. The effect of cosmetic vehicles on the penetration of N-nitrosodiethanolamine through excised human skin. *J. Invest. Dermatol.* **76**:94.

Brunnemann, K.D., and D. Hoffmann. 1978. Chemical studies on tobacco smoke. LIX. Analysis of volatile nitrosamines in tobacco smoke and polluted indoor environments. *IARC Sci. Publ.* **19**:343.

Cohen, J.B., and J.D. Bachman. 1978. Measurement of environmental nitrosamines. *IARC Sci. Publ.* **19**:357.

Edwards, G.S., M. Peng, D.H. Fine, B. Spiegelhalder, and J. Kann. 1979. Detection of N-nitrosodiethanolamine in human urine following application of a contaminated cosmetic. *Toxicol. Lett.* **4**:217.

Eisenbrand, G., B. Spiegelhalder, J. Kann, R. Klein, and R. Preussmann. 1979. Carcinogenic N-nitrosodimethylamine as a contamination in drugs containing 4-dimethylamino-2,3-dimethyl-1-phenyl-3-pyrazolin-5-one (amidopyrine, aminophenazone). *Arzneim. Forsch.* **29**:867.

Fajen, J.M., D.P. Rounbehler, and D.H. Fine. Summary report on N-nitroso compounds in the factory environment. *IARC Sci. Publ.* **41**:(In press).

Fan, T.Y., U. Goff, L. Song, D.H. Fine, G.P. Arsenault, and K. Biemann. 1977a. N-nitrosodiethanolamine in cosmetics, lotions and shampoos. *Food Cosmet. Toxicol.* **15**:423.

Fan, T.Y., J. Morrison, D.P. Rounbehler, R. Ross, D.H. Fine, W. Miles, and N.P. Sen. 1977b. N-nitrosodiethanolamine in synthetic cutting fluids: A part-per-hundred impurity. *Science* **196**:70.

Fine, D.H. and D.P. Rounbehler. 1982. N-nitroso compounds in the factory environment. NIOSH/Public Health Service, Cinncinnati, Ohio.

Fine, D.H., D.P. Rounbehler, N.M. Belcher, and S.S. Epstein. 1976a. N-nitroso compounds: Detection in ambient air. *Science* **192**:1328.

Fine, D.H., D.P. Rounbehler, T. Fan, and R. Ross. 1977a. Human exposure to N-nitroso compounds in the environment. *Cold Spring Harbor Conf. Cell Proliferation* **4**:293.

Fine, D.H., D.P. Rounbehler, E. Sawicki, K. Krost, and G.A. DeMarrais. 1976b. N-nitroso compounds in the ambient community air of Baltimore, Maryland. *Anal. Lett.* **9**:595.

Fine, D.H., J. Morrison, D.P. Rounbehler, A. Silvergleid, and L. Song. 1977b. N-nitrosamines in the air environment. In *Toxic Substances in the Air Environment.* Air Pollution Control Association, p. 168. Pittsburgh, Pennsylvania.

Fine, D.H., D.P. Rounbehler, A. Rounbehler, A. Silvergleid, E. Sawicki, K. Krost, and G.A. DeMarrais. 1977c. Determination of dimethylnitrosamine in air, water, and soil by thermal energy analysis: Measurements in Baltimore, Maryland. *Environ. Sci. Technol.* **11**:581.

Fine, D.H., D.P. Rounbehler, E.D. Pellizzari, J.E. Bunch, R.W. Berkeley, J. McCrae, J.T. Bursey, E. Sawicki, K. Krost, and G.A. DeMarrais. 1976c. N-nitrosodimethylamine in air. *Bull. Environ. Contam. Toxicol.* **15**:739.

Food and Drug Administration. 1980. Dimethylnitrosamine in malt beverages; Availability of guide. *Fed. Regist.* **45**(113):39341.

Goff, E.U., and D.H. Fine. 1979. Analysis of volatile N-nitrosamines in alcoholic beverages. *Food Cosmet. Toxicol.* **17**:569.

Gough, T.A., M.F. McPhail, K.S. Webb, B.J. Wood, and R.F. Coleman. 1977.

An examination of some foodstuffs for the presence of volatile nitrosamines. *J. Sci. Food Agric.* **28**:345.

Gough, T.A., K.S. Webb, and R.F. Coleman. 1978. Estimate of the volatile nitrosamine content in UK food. *Nature* **272**:161.

Gray, J.I. 1981. Formation of nitroso compounds in foods. *ACS Symp. Ser.* **174**:165.

Gray, J.I., D.M. Irvine, and Y. Kakuda. 1979. Nitrates and N-nitrosamines in cheese. *J. Food Prot.* **42**:263.

Havery, D.C., T. Fazio, and J.W. Howard. 1978. Trends in levels of N-nitrosopyrrolidine in fried bacon. *J. Assoc. Off. Anal. Chem.* **61**:1379.

Havery, D.C., J.H. Hotchkiss, and T. Fazio. 1981. Nitrosamines in malt and malt beverages. *J. Food Sci.* **46**:501.

Hecht, S.S. 1981. Investigation of new nitrosamine contaminants of cosmetics—Report on FDA contract studies. Paper presented at the SCC-FDA Scientific Seminar, Society of Cosmetic Chemists, Mid-Atlantic Chapter, April 15, 1981. Food and Drug Administration, Washington, D.C.

International Agency for Research on Cancer. 1978. Environmental Carcinogens: Selected Methods of Analysis, Vol. 1. *IARC Sci. Publ.* **18**:Vol. 1.

Jensen, D.E., and P.N. Magee. 1981. Methylation of DNA by nitrosocimetidine *in vitro. Cancer Res.* **41**:230.

Kawabata, T., H. Ohshima, J. Uibu, M. Nakamura, M. Matsui, and M. Hamano. 1979. Occurrence, formation, and precursors of N-nitroso compounds in Japanese diet. In *Naturally Occurring Carcinogens-Mutagens and Modulators of Carcinogenesis* (eds. E.C. Miller et al.), p. 195. Japan Scientific Society Press, Tokyo, Japan, and University Park Press, Baltimore, Maryland.

Kimoto, W.I., C.J. Dooley, J. Carre, and W. Fiddler. 1980. Role of strong ion exchange resins in nitrosamine formation in water. *Water Res.* **14**:869.

Krull, I.S., U. Goff, A. Silvergleid, and D.H. Fine. 1979. N-nitroso compound contaminants in prescription and nonprescription drugs. *Arzneim. Forsch.* **29**:870.

Lijinsky, W., A.M. Losikoff, and E.B. Sansone. 1981a. Mutagenicity of extracts of pickled vegetables collected in Linhsien County, a high-incidence area for esophageal cancer in Northern China. *J. Natl. Cancer Inst.* **66**:33.

———. 1981b. Penetration of rat skin by N-nitroso diethanolamine and N-nitroso morpholine. *J. Natl. Cancer Inst.* **66**:125.

McGlothlin, J.D., T.C. Wilcox, J.M. Fajen, and G.S. Edwards. 1981. A health hazard evaluation of nitrosamines in a tire manufacturing plant. *ACS Symp. Ser.* **149**:283.

Nitrite Safety Council. 1980. A survey of nitrosamines in sausages and dry-cured meat products. *Food Technol.* **34**(7):45-51, 53, 103.

Preussmann, R., G. Eisenbrand, and B. Spiegelhalder. 1979. Occurrence and formation of N-nitroso compounds in the environment and *in vivo.* In *Environmental Carcinogenesis* (eds. P. Emmelot and E. Kriek), p. 51. Elsevier/North Holland Biomedical Press, Amsterdam, The Netherlands.

Preussmann, R., B. Spiegelhalder, and G. Eisenbrand. 1980. Reduction of human exposure to environmental N-nitroso-carcinogens. Examples of possibilities for cancer prevention. In *Carcinogenesis: Fundamental*

Mechanisms and Environmental Effects. (eds. B. Pullman et al.), p. 273. D. Reidel Publishing Company, The Netherlands.

Preussmann, R., M. Habs, D. Schmähl, and G. Eisenbrand. 1982. Dose-response study on the carcinogenicity of N-nitrosodiethanolamine (NDELA) in male Sprague-Dawley rats. *IARC Sci. Publ.* **41** (In press).

Ross, R.D., J. Morrison, D.P. Rounbehler, S. Fan, and D.H. Fine. 1977. N-nitroso compound impurities in herbicide formulations. *J. Agric. Food Chem.* **25**:1416.

Ross, R., J. Morrison, and D.H. Fine. 1978. Assessment of dipropylnitrosamine levels in a tomato field following application of Treflan EC. *J. Agric. Food Chem.* **26**:455.

Rounbehler, D.P., J. Reisch, and D.H. Fine. 1980. Nitrosamines in new motor cars. *Food Cosmet. Toxicol.* **18**:147.

Rounbehler, D.P., I.S. Krull, E.U. Goff, K.M. Mills, J. Morrison, G.S. Edwards, D.H. Fine, J.M. Fajen, G.A. Carson and V. Rheinhold. 1979. Exposure to N-nitrosodimethylamine in a leather tannery. *Food Cosmet. Toxicol.* **17**:487.

Scanlan, R.A. 1975. N-nitrosamines in foods. *Crit. Rev. Food Technol.* **5**:357.

Scanlan, R.A., J.F. Barbour, J.H. Hotchkiss, and L.M. Libbey. 1980. N-nitrosodimethylamine in beer. *Food Cosmet. Toxicol.* **18**:27.

Schmähl, D. 1980. Risk assessment of N-nitroso compounds for human health. *Oncology* **37**:193.

Sen, N.P., S. Seaman, and W.F. Miles. 1979. Volatile nitrosamines in various cured meat products: Effect of cooking and recent trends. *J. Agric. Food Chem.* **27**:1354.

Sen, N.P., B. Donaldson, S. Seaman, B. Collins, and J.Y. Iyengar. 1977. Recent nitrosamine analyses in cooked bacon. *Can. Inst. Food Sci. Technol. J.* **10**:A13.

Sen, N.P., B.A. Donaldson, S. Seaman, J.R. Iyengar, and W.F. Miles. 1978. Recent studies in Canada on the analysis and occurrence of volatile and non-volatile N-nitroso compounds in food. *IARC Sci. Publ.* **19**:373.

Spiegelhalder, B., and R. Preussmann. 1982. Nitrosamines and rubber. *IARC Sci. Publ.* **41**:(In press).

Spiegelhalder, B., G. Eisenbrand, and R. Preussmann. 1979. Contamination of beer with trace quantities of N-nitrosodimethylamine. *Food Cosmet. Toxicol.* **17**:29.

West, S.D., and E.W. Day, Jr. 1979. Determination of volatile nitrosamines in crops and soils treated with dinitroaniline herbicides. *J. Agric. Food Chem.* **27**:1075.

COMMENTS

SEN: Some levels of certain nonvolatiles have been detected in food, for example nitrosoproline and nitrosohydroxyproline. Maybe the levels are so low you felt they weren't worth mentioning.

FINE: In fact, what I have focused on are the nitrosamine levels that can be analyzed, the knowledge of what we know today in terms of the volatiles.

PREUSSMANN: The action level for NDMA in beer in Germany is a voluntary 0.5 µg/l. This came easily in our country, and we have done a large survey of the changes in the production. The average concentration in beer now is below 0.2 µg/l. So this is really a dramatic reduction in the occurrence of NDMA in beer.

All the data which you are giving should always say "These are data from 1979." Nowadays, the total exposure is much lower than it used to be 3 years ago.

SEN: The same thing is true in Canada. The average level in that country is 0.3 ppb, both in imported and domestic beer.

KIMBROUGH: How well are nitrosamines absorbed through the skin?

FINE: The only one that I am aware that has been tested in humans is NDELA, in both excised human skin and through the skin of one of my colleagues applied some cosmetics on his skin. We picked up about 2 or 3% in the urine. It depends very much on the cosmetic base and what the constituents were.

KIMBROUGH: Actually, the amount absorbed through skin is not that great, is it?

PREUSSMANN: It can be.

FINE: It can be, in a cosmetic, but I think the constituents of the cosmetics determine how much goes through.

LIJINSKY: We did work on animals, and we found that both NDELA and NMOR were very readily absorbed, and particularly from certain media. From oily media, NDELA is readily absorbed, and from aqueous media, not so readily absorbed. The NMOR is absorbed readily from both. So those two compounds certainly are readily absorbed through rat skin.

FINE: I think one of the early poisonings in England was a floor spill of NDMA which was mopped up with paper towels and apparently a major intake was through the skin.

KIMBROUGH: I thought some of that was by inhalation.

FINE: Yes. Obviously.

PETO: Could you give us some details on German factories? What sort of numbers of workers have been exposed to these very high levels? What type of factories were they? How long is this exposure continued? What studies, if any, have been done? Would epidemiological studies be practical? The exposure is about 3 orders of magnitude above the national average. Perhaps, it represents the best estimate of what calibrates the carcinogenicity of nitrosamines to humans.

PREUSSMANN: The high levels that David [Fine] mentioned were not obtained by personal sampling, but just acquired by taking air samples at the production site. So, while the personal intake levels were higher than those measured here in America, they were not as high as the highest levels which could be measured in air.

I would agree that this is a very good chance for epidemiological studies.

PETO: What type of factories were these?

PREUSSMANN: Mainly tire and rubber factories. It is known that they have an increased incidence of cancer there, but the picture is a little bit compounded because other carcinogens were formerly used and still are in use. Nevertheless, I think there is a good chance, with these present estimates, on which to base a prospective epidemiological study. This is being done now in Germany, but the number of factories is probably not sufficient for a very good epidemiological study. If it could be combined with several other studies, I think that might be a good thing to do.

FINE: A study similar to the one in Germany is underway at NIOSH.

PETO: If your exposures are an order of magnitude lower, then it becomes much more difficult to pick up any trends.

PREUSSMANN: In Germany the levels are less than one order of magnitude higher. These are exceptional values taken directly at the source of the nitrosamine. Usually, this is diluted in the indoor atmosphere of the factory.

WEISBURGER: In certain occupations such as in the rubber industry there is an increased risk of diseases such as brain cancer. But one has to also state that the exposures 20 or 30 years ago weren't measured. There is no doubt one has to say they were higher.

N-Nitrosamines in Tobacco Carcinogenesis

DIETRICH HOFFMANN, KLAUS D. BRUNNEMANN, JOHN D. ADAMS,
ABRAHAM RIVENSON, AND STEPHEN S. HECHT
Naylor Dana Institute for Disease Prevention
American Health Foundation
Valhalla, New York 10595

The 1982 U.S. Surgeon General's Report on "The Health Consequences of Smoking" concluded that cigarette smoking is a major cause of cancer of the lung, larynx, oral cavity, and esophagus and is a contributing factor in the development of cancer of the pancreas, kidney, and urinary bladder (Public Health Service 1982). Smokers of cigars and pipes also face an increased risk for cancer of the lung, larynx, oral cavity, and esophagus (Public Health Service 1982). Two recent studies documented a correlation between long-term use of snuff and cancer of the oral cavity, particularly cancers of the cheek and gum (Axéll et al. 1978; Winn et al. 1981). Based on the observation that tobacco usage is also correlated with cancers at sites not directly exposed to tobacco products we initiated detailed studies with tobacco carcinogens which are organ-specific in the laboratory animal. Such groups of carcinogens include aromatic amines, nitro compounds, and N-nitrosamines (Public Health Service 1982).

The presence of volatile N-nitrosamines (VNA) in mainstream and sidestream smoke of cigarettes and in smoke-polluted environments has been established and repeatedly described in our previous reviews (Brunnemann and Hoffmann 1978; Hoffmann et al. 1980a; Rühl et al. 1980). More recently, in-depth analytical investigations on VNA, N-nitrosodiethanolamine (NDELA) and tobacco-specific N-nitrosamines (TSNA) were undertaken with snuff, since the use of this product has been correlated with oral cancer in man (Axéll et al. 1978; Winn et al. 1981).

N-NITROSOMORPHOLINE IN SNUFF TOBACCO

The analyses of snuff products led, among other findings, to the detection of N-nitrosomorpholine (NMOR) in 7 out of 10 commercial brands (Fig. 1; Brunnemann et al. 1982). In addition, morpholine (MOR) was found in several samples ranging from 2.0-4.0 ppm (Table 1). Levels of MOR and NMOR in the snuff did not appear to be correlated. It was therefore presumed, and later confirmed in model studies, that in addition to the concentration of MOR in

This study is dedicated to the founder of the American Health Foundation, Dr. Ernst L. Wynder, on the occasion of the tenth anniversary of the Naylor Dana Institute for Disease Prevention.

211

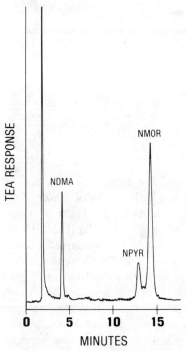

Figure 1
Gas chromatogram of volatile nitrosamines in snuff.

tobacco, the processing and aging of the snuff are important for NMOR formation (Hoffmann and Adams 1981). The presence of MOR in tobacco had thus far been reported only in one study (Singer and Lijinsky 1976). We considered that "casing solutions" used for snuff preparations could be one source for MOR (Warth 1956) but we were unable to evaluate such a possibility since we have no access to data for the commercial formulations of casings. However, further investigations revealed contamination of the snuff for all those samples that were packaged in containers made of waxed cardboard (Table 1).

A model study with MOR-^{14}C demonstrated that this amine indeed diffuses from the container waxes into the snuff, where it gives rise to NMOR (Brunnemann et al. 1982). It is unlikely that the hydrophilic NMOR would diffuse from the moist snuff into the wax-layer. This deduction and the well-known fact that MOR can be N-nitrosated in vivo (IARC 1978; Sander and Bürkle 1969), prompted us to investigate whether MOR and NMOR contamination occurred in other waxed containers. Table 2 lists our first analytical data on the presence of MOR and NMOR in various food containers and in the respective foods. NMOR formation as a procedural artifact was ruled out by completion of

Table 1

NMOR and MOR in Snuff and Snuff Containers (ppb)

Snuff brand		Snuff Tobacco		Snuff Container	
		NMOR	MOR	NMOR	MOR
USA	I	24	2,800	34	845
	II	690	1,500	10	170
	III	690	4,000	230	4,740
	IV	630	3,200	4	90
	V	31	2,200	3	140
Sweden	I	44	820	4	1,750
	II	(−)[a]	200	3	460
	III	(−)	780	13	4,830
	IV	10	940	23	4,290
	V	(−)	2,500	N.D.[b]	N.D.

Containers of USA I-III and Sweden I-IV were cardboard boxes with a metal lid, USA IV plastic containers with individual snuff portions in porous paper bags; USA V plastic container; Sweden V individual snuff portions in Al-bags. Based on dry weight in case of snuff; uncorrected for moisture in case of snuff container.
[a](−) Below detection limit (< 2 ppb).
[b]N.D. = not determined.

Table 2

NMOR and MOR in Food and Food Containers (ppb)

Sample	Food		Container	
	NMOR	MOR	NMOR	MOR
Butter	3.2	58	1.9	220
Cream cheese	0.9	77	n.d.	680
Yogurt	n.d.	38	n.d.	3,060
Cottage cheese	0.4	44	5.4	17,200
Frozen peas and carrots	n.d.	26	3.1	57
Cheese (semi-soft) FR	3.3	8.7	n.d.	26
Cheese (semi-soft) DK	3.1	9.7	1.6	25
Cheese (semi-soft) AU	0.7	4.9	1.2	22
Cheese (semi-soft) US	1.4	8.0	n.d.[a]	132
Gouda	1.6	35	n.d.	35

[a]n.d. = not detected (< 0.2 ppb)
[b]FR = France, DK = Denmark, AU = Austria, US = USA

the extractions and analytical steps with cis-2,6-dimethylmorpholine as a marker. With this technique, suggested earlier by Mirvish et al. (1981), even excessive (> 10 fold) addition of the marker yielded no more than 0.007% of N-nitroso-cis-2,6-dimethylmorpholine. At this time, we are not attaching any biological significance to the analytical findings regarding MOR and NMOR in food containers. If, on the other hand, measurable quantities of NMOR metabolites were found in the urine of individuals who had consumed products contaminated with the nitrosamine, one would need to assess this problem in terms of its possible biological consequences. Some of these aspects have been discussed during this conference (Hecht et al., this volume).

OTHER N-NITROSAMINES IN SNUFF TOBACCO

Recently, we reported the finding of nitrosamines in the saliva of snuff dippers and we discussed the formation of N-nitrosamines within the oral cavity during snuff dipping (Hoffmann and Adams 1981). Table 3 summarizes analytical data on VNA, NDELA, and TSNA which constitute the only known animal carcinogens in popular American and Swedish snuff brands (Brunnemann et al. 1982). A remarkable and significant reduction of the nitrosamines has occurred in recently introduced brands (Swedish brand V and American brand V). This trend is appreciable in view of the increasing popularity of snuff products which according to current estimates, involves 2 million consumers in the U.S. alone (Public Health Service 1982). Snuff use is increasingly substituted and even recommended by some physicians as a smokeless alternative to cigarettes (Hoffmann and Adams 1981). The reduction of nitrosamines in the newer snuff brands appears to be a consequence of changes in curing and fermentation processes as well as of packaging techniques that avoid aging of the snuff by exposure to air. Such trends should be encouraged and monitored by chemical and biochemical data and by bioassays.

TOBACCO-SPECIFIC N-NITROSAMINES

The inhibition of nitrosamine formation during tobacco processing should also lead to a reduction of the TSNA in cigarette smoke. As was reported in studies with ^{14}C-labeled TSNA as markers, about 40-50% of the N'-nitrosonornicotine (NNN) and between 26 and 37% of 4-(methylnitrosamino)-1-(3-pyridyl)-1-butanone (NNK) in the mainstream smoke originates by direct transfer from tobacco while the remainder of the NNN and NNK in the smoke is pyrosynthesized during smoking from nicotine and nornicotine (Figure 2; Adams et al. 1981; Hoffmann et al. 1980b). The overall yield of TSNA in the smoke is primarily determined by the nitrate content of cigarette tobacco. Thus, elevation of nitrate in U.S. cigarette tobacco blends from about 0.5% in 1960 to 1.2-1.5% in 1980, has contributed to increases in the formation of TSNA which are undesirable smoke constituents because of their carcinogenic potential.

Table 3
N-Nitrosamines in Snuff (ppb)

Snuff brand		Volatile N-nitrosamines[a,b]				Tobacco-specific N-nitrosamines[a,b]			
		NDMA	NPYR	NMOR	NDELA	NNN	NNK	NAT	NAB
USA	I	215	(−)[c]	24	760	2,200	600	1,700	100
	II	37	120	690	1,700	19,000	2,400	19,000	800
	III	100	360	690	3,300	33,000	4,600	40,000	1,900
	IV	92	110	630	290	20,000	8,300	9,100	500
	V	(−)	(−)	31	600	830	210	240	10
Sweden	I	22	(−)	44	240	5,700	1,700	900	140
	II	60	(−)	(−)	225	6,100	1,000	2,200	80
	III	14	210	(−)	390	5,300	1,400	2,400	70
	IV	30	50	10	310	4,000	610	1,400	80
	V	(−)	(−)	(−)	290	2,000	800	1,400	40

[a]Values are based on dry weight.
[b]Values for NDEA in snuff were below detection limit (< 2 ppb) except Sweden I, II, III and IV which had values of 6, 4, 12, and 5 ppb, respectively.
[c](−) Below detection limit (< 2 ppb).

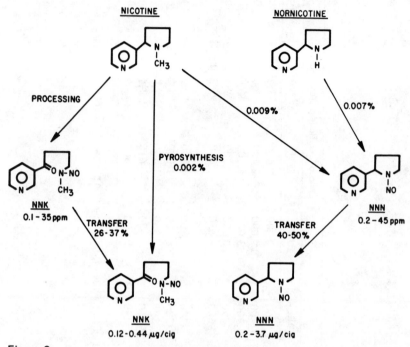

Figure 2
Formation of NNN and NNK in cigarette smoke.

We have explored whether selective reduction of TSNA in cigarette smoke is feasible. VNA can be selectively filtered from the smoke by use of cellulose acetate tips because of their hydrophilic nature and because they occur in the gas phase (Brunnemann et al. 1977). Reduction of TSNA by smoke filtration, on the other hand, is not selective due to the fact that, like nicotine and the other alkaloids, TSNA are an integral part of the smoke particulate phase. Preliminary studies had indicated that TSNA in the main stream smoke might be selectively reduced by substantial air dilution of the smoke. However, detailed studies did not confirm this finding and showed that smoke filtration and dilution achieve TSNA reduction merely to the same extent as reduction of nicotine (Table 4).

Another approach towards reduction of TSNA in cigarette smoke relates to tobacco ribs and stems. Today's cigarette blends contain about 15-20% of stems. However, ribs and stems of tobacco, and particularly those of Burley tobaccos, are rich in nitrate (< 5.5%; Jacin 1970). We calculated that up to 2/3 of the nitrate content of a U.S. cigarette blend can be attributed to the presence of ribs and stems. Thus, a reduction of nitrate in ribs and stems prior to their use in blending would be an effective means of lowering TSNA in the smoke. We are conducting several tests related to this concept.

Table 4
Reduction of Tar, Nicotine, and TSNA by Filtration

Filter Tip[a]	CO mg (% Reduction)	Tar mg (% Reduction)	Nicotine mg (% Reduction)	TSNA (µg) NNN	NNK	NAT	Total (% Reduction)
NF[b]	13.7 [+21]	24.8 [70]	2.29 [70]	122	79.7	137	339 [75]
F[c]	16.6	7.6	0.68	38.3	16.7	30.2	85.2
PF[d] (10%)	14.6 (12)	6.2 (18)	0.68 (0)	36.1	16.1	28.7	80.9 (5)
PF (25%)	11.8 (29)	6.0 (21)	0.66 (3)	37.0	15.2	31.7	83.9 (2)
PF (57%)	8.4 (49)	4.3 (44)	0.43 (37)	27.7	10.2	20.5	58.4 (32)
PF (76%)	2.9 (83)	1.1 (85)	0.19 (82)	15.9	4.8	8.7	29.4 (66)

[a] Dilution of smoke by air through filter perforation
[b] NF = nonfilter cigarette
[c] F = filter cigarette
[d] PF = filter cigarette with a perforated filter
[e] Numbers in square brackets = reduction or increase of smoke constituents by cellulose acetate filter tip
[f] Numbers in parentheses = reduction of smoke constituents in cigarettes with cellulose acetate filter tip by dilution of smoke with air

Table 5
Carcinogenic Activity of TSNA

Compounds	Species	Application	Principal Organ Affected
NNN	Mouse	i.p.	Lung (Adenoma, Adenocarcinoma), Salivary glands (?)
	Rat	s.c.	Nasal Cavity (Carcinoma)
		p.o. (water)	Esophagus (Papilloma, carcinoma)
	Hamster	s.c.	Pharynx (Papilloma), Nasal Cavity (Carcinoma)
NNK	Mouse	i.p.	Trachea (Papilloma), Nasal Cavity (Carcinoma)
	Rat	s.c.	Lung (Adenoma, Adenocarcinoma), Nasal Cavity (Carcinoma), Liver
	Hamster	s.c.	Lung (Adenoma, Carcinoma)
NAT	Rat	s.c.	Lung (Adenoma, Adenocarcinoma), Trachea (Papilloma), Nasal Cavity (Carcinoma)
	Rat	p.o. (water)	(not completed)
NAB	Hamster	s.c.	Esophagus (Papilloma, carcinoma), Pharynx (Papilloma), Inactive (?) (375 mg/hamster)

Table reprinted, with permission from Hoffmann et al. 1982

CARCINOGENICITY OF TSNA

Our major interest in the tobacco-specific nitrosamines is based on the facts that these compounds are the only known organic carcinogens in processed tobacco, that they occur in tobacco smoke in micrograms per cigarette and that they are carcinogenic in mice, rats, and hamsters (Table 5; Hoffmann et al. 1981; Public Health Service 1982).

The strongest carcinogen among the TSNA is NNK; in Syrian golden hamsters its potency appears to be about equal to that of NMOR.

One of the most intriguing aspects of the TSNA relates to their formation within the oral cavity during tobacco chewing (Hoffmann and Adams 1981). This observation points to the possibility of in vivo formation of TSNA in the lungs after smoke inhalation. Nicotine and the minor alkaloids would again be presumed to serve as precursors of the TSNA. We are investigating the possible in vivo formation of TSNA in inhalation studies with hamsters and by analysis of the urine of tobacco smokers and chewers for TSNA metabolites.

SUMMARY

Chemical analytical data have shown that snuff contains NMOR which was not previously found in either tobacco or smoke. One likely source of contamination is the wax-layer of the snuff packages from which MOR diffuses into the tobacco where it is *N*-nitrosated. Preliminary investigations indicate that MOR diffusion and *N*-nitrosation occurs also in foods which are packaged in waxed containers. However, analytical data on such food and food container samples are limited at this time and substantiation by identification of NMOR metabolites in the urine of consumers of such food products is needed before one would attach biological significance to these findings.

Several methods of reducing TSNA in tobacco and in cigarette smoke have been discussed. Such approaches are a major task in tobacco carcinogenesis because of the documented carcinogenic activity of all four identified TSNA and because of the possibility that inhaled or ingested nicotine and other alkaloids give rise to in vivo formation of these carcinogens.

ACKNOWLEDGMENTS

We thank Mrs. I. Hoffmann for her editorial assistance on this paper.

The studies discussed here are supported by American Cancer Society Research Grant BC-56 and by National Cancer Institute Grant 1PO1-CA-29580.

REFERENCES

Adams, J.D., A. Castonguay, S.J. Lee, N. Vinchkoski, and D. Hoffmann. 1981. Formation of 4-(methylnitrosamino)-1-(3-pyridyl)-1-butanone (NNK) during smoking. *35th Tobacco Chem. Res. Conf. Abstr.* p. 26.

Axéll, T., H. Moernstad, and B. Sundstroem. 1978. Snusning och munehale cancer—en retrospektiv studie. *Laekartidningen* 75:2224.

Brunnemann, K.D. and D. Hoffmann. 1978. Analysis of volatile nitrosamines in tobacco smoke and polluted indoor environment. *IARC Sci. Publ.* 9:343.

Brunnemann, K.D., J.C. Scott, and D. Hoffmann. 1982. N-Nitrosomorpholine and other volatile N-nitrosamines in snuff tobacco. *Carcinogenesis* 3: 693.

Brunnemann, K.D., L. Yu, and D. Hoffmann. 1977. Assessment of carcinogenic volatile N-nitrosamines in tobacco and in mainstream and sidestream smoke from cigarettes. *Cancer Res.* 37:3218.

Hoffmann, D. and J.D. Adams. 1981. A study of tobacco carcinogenesis XXIII. Carcinogenic tobacco-specific N-nitrosamines in snuff and in the saliva of snuff dippers. *Cancer Res.* 41:4341.

Hoffmann, D., J.D. Adams, K.D. Brunnemann, A. Rivenson, and S.S. Hecht. 1982. Tobacco-specific N-nitrosamines: Occurrence and bioassays. *IARC Sci. Publ.* 41(in press)

Hoffmann, D., C.H. Chen, and S.S. Hecht. 1980a. The role of volatile and non-volatile N-nitrosamines in tobacco carcinogenesis. *Ban. Rep.* 3:113.

Hoffmann, D., J.D. Adams, J.J. Piade, and S.S. Hecht. 1980b. Analysis of volatile and tobacco-specific nitrosamines in tobacco products. *IARC Sci. Publ.* 31:507.

Hoffmann, D., A. Castonguay, A. Rivenson, and S.S. Hecht. 1981. Comparative carcinogenicity and metabolism of 4-(methylnitrosamino)-1-(3-pyridyl)-1-butanone and N'-nitrosonornicotine in Syrian golden hamsters. *Cancer Res.* 41:2386.

International Agency for Research on Cancer. 1978. Some N-Nitroso Compounds. N-Nitrosomorpholine. *IARC Monogr.* 17:263.

Jacin, H. 1970. Quantitative determination of nitrate in tobacco using a specific ion electrode. *Tobacco Sci.* 4:28.

Mirvish, S.S., P. Issenberg, and J.P. Sams. 1981. N-Nitrosomorpholine synthesis in rodents exposed to nitrogen dioxide and morpholine. *Amer. Chem. Soc. Symp. Ser.* 174:181.

Public Health Service. 1982. Smoking and Health: A report of the Surgeon General. DHHS (PHS) Publication No. 82-50179. Government Printing Office, Washington, D.C.

Rühl, C., J.D. Adams, and D. Hoffmann. 1980. Chemical Studies on Tobacco Smoke LXVI. Comparative assessment of volatile and tobacco-specific N-nitrosamines in the smoke of cigarettes from the U.S.A., West Germany and France. *J. Anal. Toxicol.* 4:255.

Sander, J. and G. Bürkle. 1969. Induktion maligner Tumoren bei Ratten durch gleichzeitige Verfütterung von Nitrit and sekundären Aminen. *Z. Krebsforsch.* 74:54.

Singer, G.M. and W. Lijinsky. 1976. Naturally occurring nitrosatable amines. II. Secondary amines in tobacco and cigarette smoke condensate. *J. Agric. Food Chem.* 24:553.

Warth, A.H. 1956. *The chemistry and technology of waxes*, p. 856. Reinhold Publishing Corp., New York

Winn, D.M., W.J. Blot, C.M. Shy, L.W. Pickle, M.A. Toledo, and J.F. Fraumeni, Jr. 1981. Snuff dipping and oral cancer among women in the Southern United States. *N. Engl. J. Med.* 304:745.

COMMENTS

CONNEY: Dietrich, there are a number of compounds that block nitrosation. Have you considered adding some of those blocking agents to tobacco? Or would that have any practical application?

HOFFMANN: That has, of course, been considered. I heard that two companies made efforts to inhibit volatile nitrosamine formation by addition of ascorbic acid to tobacco. This approach, in my opinion, is a futile effort, although one may succeed to a degree. I am not sure that studies would need to be limited to ascorbic acid. In any case, one would have to take a careful look at the combustion products of ascorbic acid or any other inhibitor. Investigations on the addition of agents to tobacco are not at the top of the list of our priorities in respect to reducing toxic agents in the smoke. We rather believe in the selection of tobaccos that make up the blend for the cigarettes. In this manner, by modifying the precursors, we have a better chance of reducing nitrosamines in smoke. However, inhibitors are theoretically feasible alternatives and I believe—you have a patent on it, right? We tried inhibitors once without success. We would not put our cards primarily on inhibitors because their use may incur the chance that we increase benzo[*a*]pyrene, and other undesirable compounds in the smoke. Therefore, we prefer changing the precursors or eliminating them.

LIJINSKY: I think ascorbic acid doesn't inhibit gas-phase nitrosation.

HOFFMANN: There are two patents that I am aware of.

LIJINSKY: But that is not the substance of it.

HOFFMANN: We must remember that preventing the formation of nitrosamines, respectively their transfer into smoke, involves many more facets than the simple addition of a scavenger compound. Therefore, one should not exclusively focus on this approach.

CONNEY: I asked that question in a general sense, not specifically for ascorbic acid, since there are many compounds that block nitrosation.

HOFFMANN: There may well be compounds that are effective. We put our main emphasis on reducing the precursors for nitrosamine formation in tobacco and smoke.

WEISBURGER: Perhaps, as a compromise, one might wish to try your way and reduce the precursors; and Allan Conney's proposal, say BHA or Vitamin E, or some such inhibitor.

HOFFMANN: Obviously, we both try this, parallel though differently.

TANNENBAUM: It's not clear to me how much of the nitrosamines are actually present in the tobacco at the time of smoking, and how much is formed in the process of smoking.

HOFFMANN: Many variables affect the rates of nitrosamine formation and their transfer into main- and sidestream smoke. We have data on the range of nitrosamine formation in tobacco during fermentation. In the case of NNN, 50-60% is formed during smoking, the rest is derived from transfer from the tobacco into the smoke, as we learned from studying various tobacco types. We have added nicotine-2'-^{14}C to cigarette tobacco prior to smoking and, in this manner, determined that 50-60% of NNN is pyrosynthesized during cigarette smoking.

For NNK, we determined that 60-70% is pyrosynthesized. I would say a considerable portion of the tobacco-specific nitrosamines transfer from the tobacco into the mainstream smoke.

MAGEE: Just to confirm what you said, Dietrich, the filters do not retain the TSNA?

HOFFMANN: Cellulose acetate filters do retain TSNA nonselectively as they retain "tar". Perforated cellulose acetate filter tips are even more effective.

MAGEE: Still, a proportion still gets down into the pulmonary alveoli each time a drag is taken.

HOFFMANN: Yes, exactly. And it may well be that the endogenous formation of nitrosamines from nicotine is even more important. We have only begun to study in vivo reactions of this nature.

HARTMAN: I have heard that nitrate was intentionally added to keep the cigarette smoldering. Is that added to the paper?

HOFFMANN: No, the nitrate increases are largely due to the selection of tobacco. In order to facilitate burning, more nitrate-rich Burley tobacco is incorporated into blends for the U.S. cigarettes. The cigarettes manufactured in England continue to be mostly of Bright tobaccos which are low in nitrate ($\leq 0.1\%$). The U.S. blended cigarette is a mixture which used to be roughly 70% Bright, 30% Burley 20 years ago. Today, we have a greater proportion of Burley in American cigarettes. In addition, U.S. blended cigarettes as well as West German cigarettes incorporate stems from Burley, which are unusually high in nitrate—up to 5%.

MILO: I just want to ask whether the paper wrapping had anything to do with it, because the cellulose from there is taken through the stem.

HOFFMANN: The smoke yield of a cigarette is largely given by the filler—anywhere from 600-1100 mg of tobacco; roughly 50 mg of the cigarettes are paper. Mathematically, the impact of cellulose combustion products from the paper is minor. The wrapper porosity, however, has a major influence on the degree of combustion.

KIMBROUGH: I just have one comment. There are also very high levels of nitrosamines in the smoke of marijuana that have been determined by the National Institute of Drug Abuse (NIDA). I think in future studies, particularly epidemiology studies, we should take that into consideration.

HOFFMANN: I believe NIDA cited one of our studies which was done many years ago. Naturally, when you burn marijuana you do get volatile nitrosamines as well as a host of other toxins and carcinogens.

But, I guess when you smoke more than 2-3 marijuana cigarettes daily you will have other problems than lung cancer. I also think that you or I can't afford these cigarettes—at least not in N.Y. City, where they sell at $1.50-$2.00.

Relative to tobacco smoking—our concern needs to be with the cigarette smoker and his demonstrated risk for lung cancer. I doubt that many smokers would smoke marijuana to the extent they use tobacco. The concerns about marijuana, in my judgment, are other than those for respiratory cancer, because of the quantity and number of years it is being smoked.

In addition, we did not find a marijuana smoker who is not a cigarette smoker.

KIMBROUGH: That is true, but I wonder how much—when we did a survey on the use of marijuana, we found that there is a small subpopulation, within the United States at least, that may smoke as many as five joints a day. They have done this for many years and they have a lot of other health problems.

HOFFMANN: Perhaps I am oversimplyfying matters, so I apologize for that—but would we not have seen high rates of lung cancer in the near Orient, where marijuana has been smoked forever? We haven't seen that.

KIMBROUGH: Have you looked?

HOFFMANN: No, but we have statistics from WHO which are perhaps not as good as data from England or Denmark or Connecticut, but I think WHO would have noted a major incidence rate of respiratory cancer in the near Orient, if it existed.

BRUNNEMANN: Disregarding the inhaled amount of tobacco and marijuana cigarette smoke, the major nitrosamine present in tobacco smoke derives from alkaloids which are not present in marijuana cigarettes. That is a big difference.

The volatile nitrosamines are 10 times less than the tobacco-specific alkaloid-derived nitrosamines, so they are negligible in marijuana smoke.

HOFFMANN: Good point.

BRUNNEMANN: In addition to smoking much less of these cigarettes, hopefully, the nitrosamine concentration is also much lower.

KIMBROUGH: So you would feel that that would not be a problem?

BRUNNEMANN: I don't know whether that's a problem, but nitrosamines are much less concentrated in marijuana than in tobacco smoke.

PREUSSMANN: Dieter, perhaps I didn't listen, but where does the morpholine come from in the wax of the snuff containers? Is it an additive? We didn't find any NMOR in butter or milk products in our German survey.

HOFFMANN: It's in the wax. We believe it is a solvent effect.

BRUNNEMANN: It's a solvent of the wax manufacturer.

PREUSSMANN: Morpholine is used as a solvent?

BRUNNEMANN: Yes.

PREUSSMANN: I'm astonished.

CHALLIS: It is also used as an antioxidant in hot water systems.

SEN: Can I make a last comment about NMOR in butter and margarine. We found very low levels and we believe that they are originally found in the additives used in these products. We found very low levels and the incidence is also very low.

PETO: I just wanted to say, this idea that you can analyze the chemistry of tobacco smoke and marijuana and predict what their human effects are going to be is completely inappropriate. After 30 years of analysis, still one has no clear idea of what the carcinogenic components of tobacco smoke are. To say that you could, a priori, state whether marijuana would be more or less harmful could have some devastating effects. It could produce brain tumors. It has very strong effects on the central nervous system.

HOFFMANN: But, Richard [Peto], I spoke about snuff. I said if I were to study nitrosamines and their effects on man, I would do a retrospective epidemiological study, or case control on snuff users—a large population of snuff users in Scandinavia for example. I did not make that statement in reference to smoke. I know well enough from 20 years of research that tobacco smoke is such a complex mixture, I wouldn't dare single out any individual component. However, in addition to epidemiological data on oral cancer and snuff use, we finally know the chemistry.

PETO: But why would you dare say that marijuana is unlikely to be harmful in terms of carcinogenesis?

HOFFMANN: I said I would not put emphasis on marijuana in respect to respiratory carcinogenesis.

PETO: That's not a statement about marijuana.

HOFFMANN: I am glad we have some lively discussion. Since you are here, I expected that. (Laughter).

WEISBURGER: Druckrey and colleagues (1963) published a paper which I think some of us read with great relief, namely that when dimethylamine was given together with nitrite no cancers were found. It was a young man, Dr. Johannes Sander (Sander and Buerkle 1969) who a couple of years later came up with a bombshell, namely that when you used a less basic amine one could indeed get evidence of in vivo formation of nitrosamines, and get cancer. This opened then a big field, and many of you in the audience have contributed to the question of endogenous formation of nitrosamines.

References

Druckrey, H., D. Steinhoff, H. Beuthner, H. Schneider, and P. Klärner. 1963. Screening of nitrate for chronic toxicity in rats. *Arzneimittelforsch.* 13:320.
Sander, G. and G. Buerkle. 1969. Induktion maligner Tumoren bei Ratten durch gleichzeitige Verfütterung von Nitrit und sekundären Aminen. *Z. Krebs.-forsch.* 73:54.

In Vivo Formation of N-Nitroso Compounds: Formation from Nitrite and Nitrogen Dioxide, and Relation to Gastric Cancer

SIDNEY S. MIRVISH
Eppley Institute for Research in Cancer
and Allied Diseases
University of Nebraska Medical Center
Omaha, Nebraska 68105

I shall review the chemistry of N-nitroso compound formation from nitrite, the in vivo formation of N-nitroso compounds from nitrite, the possible in vivo nitrosation by nitrogen dioxide and evidence for the theory that gastric cancer (GC) is due to nitrosamides produced in the stomach.

CHEMISTRY OF N-NITROSO COMPOUND FORMATION FROM NITRITE

I refer the reader to an earlier review (Mirvish 1975). Nitrosation by nitrite is an acid-catalyzed reaction that, I believe, proceeds in vivo mainly in the stomach, where it is facilitated by the HCl. The nitrosation rate for secondary amines is proportional to nitrite concentration squared and that for N-alkylamides is proportional just to nitrite concentration. Amine nitrosation has a pH maximum of around 3, whereas amide nitrosation proceeds quicker as the pH drops below 3, without a pH maximum. If catalysts such as iodide, thiocyanate, or thiourea (Masui et al. 1982) are present, the kinetics change so that amine nitrosation is proportional only to nitrite concentration. The reaction rate under given conditions varies by factors of up to 3×10^5 for different amines or amides (Mirvish 1975). Among the amines, the nitrosation rate is intermediate for proline (the amino acid used by Ohshima and Bartsch [1981] to study in vivo nitrosation in man), rapid for morpholine and piperazine, and slow for dimethylamine and pyrrolidine. The nitrosation rate for amides is high for alkylureas, intermediate for N-alkylcarbamates, and least for simple N-alkylamides. Clearly, in vivo nitrosation of a reactive amine or amide is far more likely to be significant than that of an unreactive one. The significance obviously also depends on the extent of exposure to the amine or amide.

We found that ascorbic acid inhibited nitrosation of amines and amides by nitrite (Mirvish et al. 1972). Inhibition was efficient at pH 1-4, whereas urea and sulfamate inhibited well at pH 1 but poorly at pH 3-4. These compounds act by converting nitrite to NO or N_2. Ascorbate is effective at relatively high pH because the ascorbate anion, which predominates at about pH 4, reacts 240 times faster than ascorbic acid. α-Tocopherol (vitamin E), a fat soluble compound, can also inhibit nitrosation (reviewed by Mirvish 1981).

We suggested that ascorbate should be administered with readily nitrosated drugs, such as piperazine, to inhibit their in vivo nitrosation (Mirvish et al. 1972). Since Ohshima and Bartsch (1981) demonstrated that ascorbate inhibits the in vivo nitrosation of proline in man, this recommendation now has a firm experimental basis. In the meat industry, ascorbate or its isomer erythorbate is added to inhibit nitrosamine formation in fried bacon. We may further recommend that one should also eat fresh fruits and vegetables that contain vitamins C and E together with meals that might present a nitrosation hazard.

Phenols are common in many foods, including those prepared with wood smoke. Phenols such as catechol inhibit nitrosation because they react with nitrite to give benzoquinones and NO, or p-nitroso-phenols. Other polyhydric phenols, especially resorcinol, can catalyze nitrosation via a complex intermediate. As two successive reactions with nitrite are involved in the catalysis, this should not be important at low nitrite levels (reviewed by Mirvish 1981).

IN VIVO FORMATION OF N-NITROSO COMPOUNDS FROM NITRITE

This subject has been reviewed by Mirvish (1975). Several workers have gavaged amines, especially dimethylamine (DMA) and aminopyrine, and nitrite into rats or mice, and obtained acute liver damage attributed to intragastric formation of the derived nitrosamines. More significantly, in 1969, Sander and Bürkle showed that tumors were induced in rats by feeding nitrite together with certain amines and amides. In our studies, lung adenomas were induced in mice fed the readily nitrosated compounds morpholine, piperazine, N-methylaniline, methylurea (MU), and ethylurea (2-6 g/kg diet), given for 6 months together with sodium nitrite ($NaNO_2$) in drinking water (1 g/l). Tumors were not induced by feeding the slowly nitrosated dimethylamine with $NaNO_2$. When the mice received a constant piperazine level in diet, but varied $NaNO_2$ levels in drinking water, the lung adenoma yield was approximately proportional to nitrite concentration squared, in agreement with the kinetic data. Tumor incidence remained significant until $NaNO_2$ concentration fell below 250 mg/l water. When ascorbate was added to the diet containing an amine or amide, and $NaNO_2$ was again given in the water, we obtained up to a 90% inhibition of the tumors. To achieve this, sodium ascorbate concentration had to be 2.3% of the diet (Mirvish et al. 1975a).

We also treated rats continuously with morpholine (10 g/kg diet) and $NaNO_2$ (3 g/l water) with or without sodium ascorbate (23 g/kg diet) (Mirvish et al. 1976). Treatment with morpholine plus $NaNO_2$ induced liver tumors attributed to in vivo production of N-nitrosomorpholine (NMOR). The addition of ascorbate inhibited production of the liver tumors and increased their latency, indicating that in vivo NMOR production was about 50% inhibited. However, the group with ascorbate also developed forestomach papillomas and some forestomach carcinomas, which were absent in the morpholine plus nitrite group. The most likely explanation was that the ascorbate-treated rats did not die early from liver cancer and hence lived long enough to develop forestomach tumors, which showed a long latency and (like the liver tumors) were induced by the NMOR. A repetition of this experiment has confirmed this observation, with the exception that ascorbate given together with morpholine and nitrite probably induced the noncancerous lesions acanthosis and hyperkeratosis of the forestomach.

POSSIBLE IN VIVO NITROSATION BY NITROGEN DIOXIDE (NO_2)

When NO_2 gas was bubbled into aqueous solutions of amines at neutral pH, nitrosamines, and nitramines were produced (Challis and Kyrtopoulos 1976). In organic solvents such as dichloromethane (DCM), the reaction between nitrogen oxides and several amides to form nitrosamides was 90% complete within 5 seconds, as shown using a dried extract of nitrous acid that was actually a mixture of nitrogen oxides (Mirvish et al. 1978). This reaction was 30,000 times more rapid than that of nitrous acid with the same amides in aqueous solution. Nitrosation of N-butylacetamide by NO_2 in DCM solution was inhibited by α-tocopherol and butylated hydroxytoluene (BHT) (Mirvish 1981), presumably because these compounds reduce NO_2. These results suggested that inhaled NO_2 might form nitrosamines in vivo.

Accordingly, we gavaged rats with 1 g/kg morpholine and then exposed them to 12-21 ppm NO_2 for 30 minutes. The blood and stomach contents were analyzed for NMOR, after mixing the homogenized tissue with a "stopping solution" containing ascorbate and sulfamate and adjusted to pH 1, to prevent nitrosation during the workup. The stopping solution also contained cis-2,6-dimethylmorpholine and its conversion to 2,6-dimethylnitrosomorpholine (DMNM) indicated artifactual nitrosation. The mixture was extracted on a Celite column with DCM and the extract was analyzed by gas chromatography-thermal energy analysis (GC/TEA). We obtained more DMNM than NMOR and concluded that the NMOR was an artifact (Mirvish et al. 1981). In contrast, rats gavaged with both morpholine and $NaNO_2$ produced large amounts of NMOR.

About this time, Iqbal et al. (1980) reported that they had observed in vivo nitrosation of morpholine by inhaled NO_2. They gavaged mice with morpholine, immediately exposed them to 50 ppm NO_2 for 4 hours, killed the mice by immersion in liquid N_2, homogenized them in 35% aqueous methanol, and analyzed DCM extracts by GC/TEA. They did not use any means to prevent artifactual nitrosation. We repeated this procedure and obtained 140 ng/g tissue of NMOR, similar to Iqbal's results. The discrepancy between these results and our earlier ones suggested that the NMOR was artifactual and this was confirmed in further experiments. We concluded that a nitrosating agent (NSA) was formed in vivo from NO_2 and produced NMOR when the homogenate was worked up.

Since our last report (Mirvish et al. 1981), we have improved our technique. We expose mice to 50 ppm NO_2 for 4 hours (without gavage of an amine), kill the mice by immersion in liquid N_2, homogenize in 0.9% aqueous NaCl (100 ml/5 g tissue) and extract the homogenate with ether. The ether extract (200 ml/5 g tissue) is incubated with 25 mg morpholine in ether, concentrated in a Kuderna-Danish apparatus and then in an N_2 stream to 1.5 ml, kept for 1 day, and analyzed by GC/TEA. We obtained 1200 $\mu g/g$ tissue of NMOR, 12 times more than before. This corresponds to 10.3 $\mu mol/g$ tissue of NSA, if 1 mole NSA forms 1 mole NMOR.

The NSA was nonvolatile and stable when stored at $-15°C$. Similar nitrosamine yields were obtained when morpholine, 1,6-dimethylmorpholine, pyrrolidine, or a mixture of all 3 amines were reacted with an NSA-solution in ether, suggesting that our method for determining NSA was fairly quantitative.

Mice were exposed to 50 ppm NO_2 for 4 hours, killed, and dissected into various tissues. Each tissue was separately homogenized and worked up, as for the whole mouse. The total skin contained 65% of the NSA, with 60 nmol/g tissue of NSA, and the hair had the highest NSA concentration (300 nmol/g). The carcass and individual organs had 1-8 nmol/g (7.8 nmol/g for the stomach and 1.0-1.8 nmol/g for the blood, liver, and lungs). These results suggested that the principal exposure route for NO_2 was the skin and not inhalation. High NSA-concentrations in the skin occurred when the bodies but not when the heads of mice were exposed to NO_2. Under both conditions, the carcass and combined internal organs contained similar NSA-concentrations to those observed previously. This suggested that NSA reached these tissues by both inhalation and skin exposure. It is known that nitrosamines produced in the skin would be absorbed into the body.

In conclusion, by using an improved method for measuring NSA, we showed that 80% of the NSA occurs in the skin (including the hair) and that this is derived from direct exposure of the skin to NO_2. We have not yet demonstrated that the NSA can produce N-nitroso compounds in vivo, but expect that this will be achieved.

EVIDENCE FOR THE THEORY THAT GC IS DUE TO NITROSAMIDES PRODUCED IN THE STOMACH

General Points

The hypothesis that nitrosamides are concerned in GC-induction in man was introduced because these compounds have induced glandular stomach cancer in rodents and are direct-acting carcinogens that could act in the stomach, if they were formed there (reviewed by Mirvish 1977). This theory is supported by the correlation observed between GC and nitrate exposure in different countries (National Academy of Sciences 1981; Fine et al. 1982). Subjects from areas of high GC incidence showed elevated nitrate and nitrite levels in their saliva and gastric juice and (for nitrate) urine (Cuello et al. 1976; Tannenbaum et al. 1979). Furthermore, GC incidence shows a negative correlation with consumption of fresh fruits and vegetables that contain ascorbic acid. This has been observed in a number of countries (Haenszel and Correa 1975) and is attributed to inhibition by ascorbate of intragastric nitrosation, though other factors could also be involved.

Once nitrite enters the acidic stomach, it is converted to nitrous acid (HNO_2, pK_a 3.4) and becomes unstable. Hence gastric nitrite levels are lower than one would otherwise expect. For example, we studied nitrite disappearance from the stomach of rats given a "meal" containing $NaNO_2$ (Mirvish et al. 1975b). In the glandular stomach, which had a pH down to 2.0, nitrite concentration dropped 3 times due to emptying followed by dilution with drinking water or gastric juice, and 3 times due to other factors, presumably chemical decomposition and direct absorption through the stomach wall.

Stages for GC Development

Let us assume that GC develops in two stages. In stage 1, the normal gastric mucosa is altered to give chronic atrophic gastritis and intestinal metaplasia (considered together here). In stage 2, these precursor lesions are converted into GC. The question that arises is: At which stage are nitrosamides most likely to act? Following the model of Moolgavkar and Knudsen (1981) for cancer in various organs, stage 1 is induced by a genotoxic chemical and leads to the production of initiated cells, whereas stage 2 involves selective growth of these cells and is induced by promoting agents. The model implies that the genotoxic nitrosamides would act at stage 1 or stages 1 and 2 (since most initiators are also complete carcinogens), but not at stage 2 alone.

From studies by Haenszel (1961) on migrants from Japan to the United States, the important events in GC induction occur during the first two decades of life, since GC incidence in people migrating after this age resembles that of the country of origin. Atrophic gastritis is not uncommon below age 20 in high-incidence populations (Correa et al. 1976), suggesting that stage 1 is critical. This fits in with the kinetic data (Mirvish 1975) showing that nitrosamide production is acid-catalyzed, whereas the lesions produced by stage 1 are associated with achlorhydria.

A high GC incidence is correlated with the consumption of high-starch low-protein diets (Modan et al. 1974). (The reverse is not true; i.e., all populations on a high-starch diet do not have a high GC incidence.) This association may be due to a more acidic stomach associated with this diet, which would favor nitrosamide production and hence, perhaps, stage 1. The basis for this view is a study in which we fed rats MU and $NaNO_2$ in a meal and measured

232 / S. S. Mirvish

methylnitrosourea (MNU) formation in the stomach (Mirvish et al. 1980a). With a 5%-protein semisynthetic diet, we obtained a 4 times higher average MNU concentration in the stomach than with a 40% protein diet. The stomachs of the low-protein rats had a pH about 1 unit less than those of the high-protein rats. We think the low-protein diet favored MNU formation simply because this diet was a poorer buffer and hence produced a lower gastric pH, which favors MU nitrosation (Mirvish 1975).

The main factor favoring the view that stage 2 is where nitrosamides act is that the precancerous lesions produced by stage 1 lead to achlorhydria, which allows bacteria to multiply in the stomach. These reduce nitrate to nitrite, which may favor nitrosamide production despite the elevated pH. This view was propounded by Tannenbaum and Moran (1980). They pointed out that pH may be high in part of the stomach where nitrite is synthesized, and low in another part where nitrosamides might be formed, or that temporal changes in pH would achieve the same end. Of course, both views may be correct and nitrosamides may act on both stages, or more than 2 stages may be involved.

Foods Associated with GC

Table 1 shows foods that have been associated with GC. If the nitrosamide theory is correct, these foods may contain amides that react with nitrite to produce nitrosamides. The most general association is that with dried, smoked or salted fish; however, the associations with salted meat and salted vegetable products are also rather firm.

Nitrosamides that might be produced in vivo have been sought for by treating the foods with excess nitrite and testing the product for direct-acting

Table 1
Foods that Have Been Associated with GC

Food	Countries or areas	References
Dried, salted or smoked fish	Japan Europe	Sato et al. 1959 Sato et al. 1961
Salted or pickled meat	Europe Colombia	Sato et al. 1961 Haenszel et al. 1976
Salted pickled vegetables	Japan	Hirayama 1967
Fried foods (bacon)	United States and Holland	Haenszel and Correa 1975
Fava beans	Colombia	Haenszel et al. 1976
Corn cooked with lime	Colombia	Haenszel et al. 1976
Alcohol and coffee	Hawaii	Haenszel et al. 1972

mutagens. Weisburger et al. (1980) found an unidentified, direct-acting mutagen in a nitrosated Japanese fish product that produced glandular stomach cancer in 5 of 12 rats fed the nitrosated fish. A mutagen was detected in nitrosated fava beans but has not been identified (Piacek-Llancs et al. 1982).

We treated food extracts with 100 g $NaNO_2$/250 g food and then with strong acid to denitrosate any nitrosoureas formed, and isolated and identified the resultant ureas. Both a dried Japanese fish product and fried bacon yielded 25 mg/kg MU (Mirvish et al. 1980b). Nitrosation of the fish product without de-nitrosation yielded MNU. The MU did not arise from MU already present in the fish since alkylureas do not occur in foods, or from methylguanidine, which can yield MNU on nitrosation (Mirvish 1975). In fact, the MU was shown to originate mainly from creatinine (CRN) (Mirvish et al. 1982). The fish product and bacon were analyzed for CRN and creatine. CRN constituted 0.41% of the dried fish and 0.32% of the fried bacon by weight. Vertebrate muscle contains creatine and its phosphate, but very little of the dehydrated cyclic product CRN. This compound is the excretion form of creatine found in the urine and is also produced when foods are subjected to dehydrating conditions, such as when fish is dried or bacon is fried (Mirvish et al. 1982).

Using 100 g $NaNO_2$/700 ml water, nitrosation-denitrosation of pure CRN gave a 2.7% yield of MU, whereas creatine produced only an 0.15% yield of total ureas. CRN-5-oxime and 1-methylhydantoin-5-oxime are known products of CRN nitrosation (Archer et al. 1971). Methylhydantoin oxime was probably the immediate MU precursor, since nitrosation-denitrosation under similarly mild conditions gave MU yields of < 0.05% for CRN and CRN oxime, and 7% for methylhydantoin oxime. It seems that conversion to MU involves the following reactions with nitrite: CRN → CRN-oxime → methylhydantoin oxime → MU. Since MU readily produces MNU, the high CRN level in dried fish and fried bacon might produce MNU in the human stomach and this might induce GC. However, the large nitrite concentrations needed for the conversion militate against this hypothesis.

ACKNOWLEDGMENTS

Recent research was supported by NIH grant PO1-CA25100 from the National Cancer Institute. I thank Dr. P. Issenberg for advice and Mr. J.P. Sams for technical assistance in the NO_2 study.

REFERENCES

Archer, M.C., S.D. Clark, J.S. Thilly, and S.R. Tannenbaum. 1971. Environmental nitroso compounds: Reaction of nitrite with creatine and creatinine. *Science* 174:1341.

Challis, B.C. and S.A. Kyrtopoulos. 1976. Nitrosation under alkaline conditions. *J. Chem. Soc. Chem. Commun.* 877.

Correa, P., C. Cuello, E. Duque, L.C. Burbano, F.T. Garcia, O. Bolanos, C. Brown, and W. Haenszel. 1976. Gastric cancer in Colombia. III. Natural history of precursor lesions. *J. Natl. Cancer Inst.* **57**:1027.

Cuello, C., P. Correa, W. Haenszel, G. Gordillo, C. Brown, M. Archer, and S. Tannenbaum. 1976. Gastric cancer in Colombia. I. Cancer risk and suspect environmental agents. *J. Natl. Cancer Inst.* **57**:1015.

Fine, D.H., B.C. Challis, P. Hartman, and J. Van Ryzin. 1982. Human exposure assessment of nitrosamines from endogenous and exogenous sources: Model calculations and risk assessment. *IARC Sci. Publ.* **41**: (In press).

Haenszel, W. 1961. Cancer mortality among the foreign-born in the United States. *J. Natl. Cancer Inst.* **26**:37.

Haenszel, W. and P. Correa. 1975. Developments in the epidemiology of stomach cancer over the past decade. *Cancer Res.* **35**:3452.

Haenszel, W., P. Correa, C. Cuello, N. Guzman, L.C. Burbano, H. Lores, and J. Munoz. 1976. Gastric cancer in Colombia. II. Case-control epidemiologic study of precursor lesions. *J. Natl. Cancer Inst.* **57**:1021.

Hirayama, T. 1967. The epidemiology of cancer of the stomach in Japan with special reference to the role of diet. *UICC Monograph* **10**:37.

Iqbal, Z.M., K. Dahl, and S.S. Epstein. 1980. Role of nitrogen dioxide in the biosynthesis of nitrosamines in mice. *Science* **207**:1475.

Masui, M., H. Fugisawa, and H. Ohmori. 1982. N-Nitrosodimethylamine formation catalyzed by alkylthioureas—a kinetic study. *Chem. Pharm. Bull. (Tokyo)* **30**:593.

Mirvish, S.S. 1975. Formation of *N*-nitroso compounds: Chemistry, kinetics, and *in vivo* occurrence. *Toxicol. Appl. Pharmacol.* **31**:325.

_____. 1977. N-Nitroso compounds: Their chemical and *in vivo* formation and possible importance as environmental carcinogens. *J. Toxicol. Environ. Health* **2**:1267.

_____. 1981. Inhibition of the formation of carcinogenic *N*-nitroso compounds by ascorbic acid and other compounds. In *Cancer 1980: Achievements, Challenges, Prospects for the 1980's* (eds. J.H. Burchenal and H.F. Oettgen), p. 557. Grune and Stratten Inc., New York.

Mirvish, S.S., L. Wallcave, M. Eagen, and P. Shubik. 1972. Ascorbate-nitrite reaction: Possible means of blocking the formation of carcinogenic *N*-nitroso compounds. *Science* **177**:65.

Mirvish, S.S., P. Issenberg, and J.P. Sams. 1981. A study of N-nitrosomorpholine synthesis in rodents exposed to nitrogen dioxide and morpholine. *ACS Symp. Ser.* **174**:181.

Mirvish, S.S., A. Cardesa, L. Wallcave, and P. Shubik. 1975a. Induction of mouse lung adenomas by amines and ureas plus nitrite and by N-nitroso compounds: Effect of ascorbate, gallate, thiocyanate and caffeine. *J. Natl. Cancer Inst.* **55**:633.

Mirvish, S.S., K. Patil, P. Ghadirian, and V.R.C. Kommineni. 1975b. Disappearance of nitrite from the rat stomach: Contribution of emptying and other factors. *J. Natl. Cancer Inst.* **54**:869.

Mirvish, S.S., A.F. Pelfrene, H. Garcia, and P. Shubik. 1976. Effect of sodium ascorbate on tumor induction in rats treated with morpholine and sodium nitrite, and with nitrosomorpholine. *Cancer Lett.* **2**:101.

Mirvish, S.S., K. Karlowski, J.P. Sams, and S.D. Arnold. 1978. Studies related to nitrosamide formation: Nitrosation in solvent:water and solvent systems, nitrosomethylurea formation in the rat stomach, and analysis of a fish product for ureas. *IARC Sci. Publ.* **19**:161.

Mirvish, S.S., K. Karlowski, D.F. Birt, and J.P. Sams. 1980a. Dietary and other factors affecting nitrosomethylurea (MNU) formation in the rat stomach. *IARC Sci. Publ.* **31**:271.

Mirvish, S.S., D.A. Cairnes, N.H. Hermes, and C.R. Raha. 1982. Creatinine: A food component that is nitrosated-denitrosated to yield methylurea. *J. Agric. Food Chem.* (in press).

Mirvish, S.S., K. Karlowski, D.A. Cairnes, J.P. Sams, R. Abraham, and J. Nielsen. 1980b. Identification of alkylureas after nitrosation-denitrosation of a bonito fish product, crab, lobster and bacon. *J. Agric. Food Chem.* **28**: 1175.

Modan, B., F. Lubin, V. Barell, R.A. Greenberg, M. Modan, and S. Graham. 1974. The role of starches in the etiology of gastric cancer. *Cancer* **34**: 2087.

Moolgavkar, S.S. and A.G. Knudson. 1981. Mutation and cancer: a model for human carcinogenesis. *J. Natl. Cancer Inst.* **66**:1037.

National Academy of Sciences. 1981. *The Health Effects of Nitrate, Nitrite, and N-Nitroso Compounds,* Part 1. National Academy of Sciences, Washington, D.C.

Ohshima, H. and H. Bartsch. 1981. Quantitative estimation of endogenous nitrosation in humans by monitoring N-nitrosoproline excreted in the urine. *Cancer Res.* **41**:3658.

Piacek-Llancs, B.G., D.E.G. Shuker, and S.R. Tannenbaum. 1982. N-Nitrosamides of natural origin. *IARC Sci. Publ.* **41**:(In press).

Sander, J. and G. Bürkle. 1969. Induktion maligner tumoren bei Ratten durch gleichzeitige Verfutterung von Nitrit und sekondären Aminen. *Z. Krebsforsch.* **73**:54.

Sato, T., T. Fukuyama, T. Suzuki, J. Takayanagi, T. Murakami, N. Shiotsuki, R. Tanaka, and R. Tsuji. 1959. Studies of the causation of gastric cancer. 2. The relation between gastric cancer mortality rate and salted food intake in several places in Japan. *Bull. Inst. Public Health (Tokyo)* **8**: 187.

Sato, T., T. Fukuyama, T. Suzuki, J. Takayanagi, and Y. Sakai. 1961. Studies on the causation of gastric cancer. Intake of highly brined foods in several places with high mortality rate in Europe. *Bull. Inst. Public Health (Tokyo)* **10**:9.

Tannenbaum, S.R. and D. Moran. 1980. Epidemiological studies of nitrate, nitrite and gastric cancer. *Safety Evaluation of Nitrosatable Drugs and Chemicals* (eds. G.G. Gibson and C. Ioannides), p. 234. Taylor and Francis, Ltd., London.

Tannenbaum, S., D. Moran, W. Rand, C. Cuello, and P. Correa. 1979. Gastric cancer in Colombia. IV. Nitrite and other ions in gastric contents of residents from a high-risk region. *J. Natl. Cancer Inst.* **62**:9.

Weisburger, J.H., H. Marquardt, N. Hirota, H. Mori, and G.W. Williams. 1980. Induction of cancer of the glandular stomach in rats by an extract of nitrite-treated fish. *J. Natl. Cancer Inst.* **64**:163.

COMMENTS

BRUNNEMANN: We did a study with 21 samples obtained from NIEHS people and found under 200 ng of NMOR/mouse treated with morpoline by gavage and NO_2 by inhalation. We consider that the NMOR was real because our NDMA/NMOR ratio varied from 0-2.1, with an average of 0.38. In Table 1 of Mirvish et al. (1981) a ratio of below 2 was used to indicate that the NMOR was not an artifact. Most of our points fail below this cut-off point and hence were considered to be real. Why did you choose just this cut-off point?

MIRVISH: We chose this point rather arbitrarily.

CONNEY: Well, I think it is important, in terms of what is real and what isn't real. Your results indicate there is a nitrosating agent if you extract the animals that have been exposed to nitrogen dioxide and then in vitro react it with a nitrosatable compound. Perhaps if one looked at other amines that are more rapidly nitrosated, one would have higher sensitivity. The data you have suggest that there is not in vivo nitrosation in animals that are exposed to nitrogen dioxide. Is that correct?

MIRVISH: That is correct, but we have only tried morpholine in vivo.

CONNEY: It would be interesting to look at it.

MIRVISH: Of course it would. The problem is only significant if nitrosamines or nitrosamides are produced in vivo from the NSA.

SEN: Couldn't you find any inhibitors, other than sulfamic and ascorbic acids, that would completely inhibit NDMA formation during the workup?

MIRVISH: We got a little NDMA, but not much. The point is that the agent producing NDMA is not nitrite but the NSA. The problem of whether the NSA is blocked by inhibitors is not the same as whether nitrite is blocked.

HOFFMANN: Back to your feeding studies of rats where nitrite was in the water and the morpholine was in the food. You got forestomach cancer but you were very cautious in your interpretation. Do you think the NMOR is formed while the food is in the forestomach, or while it's in the tissue? In general, NMOR doesn't induce forestomach tumors. So, when this is formed in the stomach, absorbed, and then metabolically activated in the forestomach, it could be a contact carcinogen. That would be of importance to esophogeal cancer.

MIRVISH: That is a good point that we hadn't thought about. The NMOR would be formed in the acidic glandular stomach, but there is some mixing so that some NMOR would move back to the forestomach.

TANNENBAUM: Morpholine is a very water-soluble amine. I think that, to get back to Dr. Conney's point, if you applied a lotion to the skin which contained amines and you have been exposed to nitrogen oxides then what your work suggests is that you have a very powerful nitrosation reaction taking place within the skin.

I think experiments should be done with different kinds of amines, not just morpholine.

MIRVISH: We intend to do that.

TANNENBAUM: I don't agree with your statement on the alkylureas. If you pick up any book that deals with naturally-occurring plant products, you find long lists of compounds which are alkylureas and alkylguanidines. I don't see where you come up with the statement that there are no naturally-occurring alkylureas.

MIRVISH: I said there were no alkylureas in the products that we analyzed. Firstly, we analyzed our dried fish and fried bacon samples for alkylureas without nitrosation and didn't find them. Secondly, Kawabata et al. (1979) surveyed 30 Japanese foods for alkylureas and did not find any (referred to in Mirvish et al. 1980).

TANNENBAUM: Yes, but that was by a sort of class test.

MIRVISH: In 1972, I reviewed the occurrence of ureas in plant products (Mirvish 1972). I agree with you, of course. However, MU has not been found.

TANNENBAUM: I agree.

PREUSSMANN: Nobody seems to be interested in the nitrosation of the peptide bonds, which astonishes me. Is it possible, and if so, what would be the chemical and the biological consequences?

MIRVISH: I know that Dr. S.J. Kubacki in Warsaw is working on them.

WEISBURGER: As you know, in my laboratory we have mutagens that came from the reaction of specific fishes and nitrite. With the help of Dr. Hoffmann and staff we hope to get the structure of this as-yet-unknown mutagen that has induced glandular stomach cancer (see Weisburger, this volume). It could be a nitroso-peptide.

FINE: Sid [Mirvish], have you considered the possibility in your NO_2 experiments with morpholine that what you are getting is a reaction of the surface of the hair, for example, much like you would get on charcoal or Tenax, where morpholine would be exhaled by the animal and the nitrosation is occurring entirely on the outside of the skin, not add in vivo?

MIRVISH: I think that's very likely, but remember there is no morpholine in vivo. The mice are just exposed to NO_2. We should separate the epidermis and dermis and see where the NSA is.

FINE: I think it's the large surface area of the hair.

MIRVISH: As you saw, the hair had by far the highest NSA concentration.

ARCHER: I find this experiment where you see, if not forestomach tumors, forestomach changes, with NMOR feeding. Maybe you are familiar with the fact that ascorbate in combination with transition metal ions can activate molecular oxygen. I wonder whether there is any chance that ascorbate in the stomach is actually activating the NMOR in this form. It's well known that you can take ascorbate and ferrous ion, for example, in the presence of molecular oxygen, and activate nitrosamines to form mutagens.

MIRVISH: We did a control experiment where we gave NMOR with and without ascorbate, and found no difference (Mirvish et al. 1976). Hans Stich in Vancouver has found some mutagenesis by ascorbate in the presence of heavy metal ions due to H_2O_2 liberation.

WEISBURGER: This is the Fenton reagent.

KIMBROUGH: I just wanted to mention that we have found at the Center for Disease Control an increased incidence of Kaposi sarcoma in a younger age group. This may be partially associated with virus infections. But one practice that many of these people have is that they use either amyl nitrite or isobutyl nitrite as a recreational drug, and inhale it, which somehow I think relates to this discussion of nitrous oxide, and the fact that you find these high concentrations in skin. I find that very interesting.

MIRVISH: According to Dr. Challis, simple nitrite esters are poor nitrosating agents.

CHALLIS: That's quite right. They themselves, unless they have substituents in them, do not react with amines. They have to release nitrous acid first. There is no difference between a chemical like butyl nitrite and sodium nitrite.

MICHEJDA: You mentioned the cocarcinogenic effect of sodium chloride. Are there actual experimental data?

WEISBURGER: Yes.

MICHEJDA: What is the nature of it, or is it just epidemiological?

WEISBURGER: MNNG followed by salt or together with salt was found to induce more glandular stomach cancers than when administered without salt (Tatematsu et al. 1975).

   Before that, Dr. Kinosita found with 4-nitroquinoline-*N*-oxide (4-NQO) that salt also enhanced the effect on the stomach. It seems to be a promoter.

   Professor Joossens and colleagues (1979) have data showing the association of salt use to hypertension, and if he plots hypertension versus gastric cancer, there is a relationship.

MICHEJDA: But, in that respect, it would be interesting, before one says that it's sodium chloride, to find out· whether other nucleophiles do the same thing, because these nitrosamides, nitrosoureas, and so on, can be transnitrosated.

WEISBURGER: True. But Tatematsu (1975) gave the salt afterwards and did an initiation promotion experiment.

MIRVISH: The point is that the animal experiments were done with a concentrated hypertonic salt solution. The idea is that this is an irritant causing hyperplasia in the stomach. It's not a chemical effect.

References

Joosens, J.U., H. Kesteloot, and A. Amery. 1979. Salt intake and mortality from stroke. *N. Engl. J. Med.* **300**:1396.
Kawabata, T., H. Ohshima, J. Uibu, M. Nakamura, M. Matsui, and M. Hamano. 1979. In *Naturally occurring carcinogens—mutagens and modulators of carcinogenesis* (eds. E.C. Miller et al.), p. 195. Japan Scientific Society Press, Tokyo University Park Press, Baltimore.
Mirvish, S.S. 1972. Studies on *N*-nitrosation reactions: Kinetics of nitrosation, correlation with mouse feeding experiments, and natural occurrence of nitrosatable compounds (ureides and guanidines). In *Topics in Chemical*

Carcinogenesis (eds. W. Nakahara et al.), p. 279. University of Tokyo Press, Tokyo.

Mirvish, S.S., A.F. Pelfrene, H. Garcia, and P. Shubik. 1976. Effect of sodium ascorbate on tumor induction in rats treated with morpholine and sodium nitrite, and with nitrosomorpholine. *Cancer Lett.* 2:101.

Mirvish, S.S., K. Karlowski, D.A. Cairnes, J.P. Sams, R. Abraham, and J. Nielsen. 1980. Identification of alkylureas after nitrosation-denitrosation of a bonito fish product, crab, lobster and bacon. *J. Agric. Food Chem.* 28: 1175.

Tatematsu, M., M. Takahashi, S. Fukushima, M. Hanouchi, and T. Shirai. 1975. Effects in rats of sodium chloride on experimental gastric cancers induced by *N*-methyl-N'-nitro-N-nitrosoguanidine or 4-nitroquinoline-1-oxide. *J. Natl. Cancer Inst.* 55:101.

Weisburger, J.H., H. Marquardt, N. Hirota, H. Mori, and G.M. Williams. 1980. Induction of cancer of the glandular stomach in rats by an extract of nitrite treated fish. *J. Natl. Cancer Inst.* 64:163.

A Kinetic Model for the Formation of Gastric N-Nitroso Compounds

---

BRIAN C. CHALLIS, STEVEN J. LOMAS, AND HENRY S. RZEPA
Department of Chemistry
Imperial College
London, SW7 2AZ, England

P. MICHAEL G. BAVIN, DAVID W. DARKIN, NICHOLAS J. VINEY,
AND PETER J. MOORE
Smith Kline and French Research Limited
The Frythe
Welwyn, Herts
AL7 1EX, England

Human exposure to exogenous N-nitroso compounds is well documented (National Academy of Sciences 1981), but less is known about exposure to those formed endogenously. Recent measurements show that N-nitroso compounds are usually absent from human blood (Eisenbrand et al. 1981), urine (Eisenbrand et al. 1981) and feces (Lee et al. 1981). Suitable conditions exist in the stomach, however, for the formation of N-nitroso compounds, and their presence in human gastric contents has been reported recently (Ruddell and Walters 1980; Bavin et al. 1981).

Much is known about the kinetics of nitrosation under acidic conditions in vitro and there is semi-quantitative evidence (Greenblatt and Mirvish 1973; Iqbal et al. 1980; Krull et al. 1980) that N-nitrosamine formation in mice follows similar equations. Further, the yields of N-nitrosoproline from ingested proline and nitrate found by Ohshima and Bartsch (1981) in humans compare favorably with those calculated assuming the reaction follows in vitro kinetics (Fine et al. 1981).

Recently, both pH values and nitrite concentrations of the gastric contents of eight humans on a normal diet have been monitored over 24 hours (Milton-Thompson et al. 1982). It is instructive to use these data to estimate the extent to which dietary constituents such as secondary amines and peptides are converted to their N-nitroso derivatives in the stomach.

METHODS

Yields of N-nitroso compounds are calculated by integrating the relevant differential rate equation over successive periods of 30 minutes. For example, for a hypothetical second order reaction between A and B following equation (1), the

$$d \, [\text{Product}]/dt = \bar{k} \, [\text{A}] \, [\text{B}] \tag{1}$$

yield of product over 30 minutes is given by equation (2), where $\bar{k}$ is the rate coefficient in units of $M^{-1} min^{-1}$ and [A] and [B] are the reactant

$$[\text{Product}] = 30 \, \bar{k} \, [\text{A}] \, [\text{B}] \tag{2}$$

concentrations at the start of the 30-minute period. Use of the differential rather than the integrated rate equation tends to overestimate the product yield, but the error is negligible when the extent of reaction is small as in the present case. The procedure is simple and readily accommodates changes in reactant concentrations (e.g., nitrite and pH) at 30-minute intervals. For convenience, the calculations are made from stoichiometric concentrations of nitrite and amino substrate.

The nitrosation of secondary amines in the stomach is assumed to follow the in vitro rate expression (equation 3), described by Mirvish (1975). Equation (3) uses stoichiometric concentrations of amine and nitrite but is derived from

$$d \, [R_2 NNO]/dt = \bar{k}_1 \, (\text{Amine})(\text{Nitrite})^2 \tag{3}$$

a rate-limiting reaction between $N_2 O_3$ and the unprotonated amine (equation 4). The rate coefficient $\bar{k}_1$ embodies equilibrium constants both for the

$$2HNO_2 \rightleftharpoons H_2 O + N_2 O_3 \xrightarrow[\text{slow}]{R_2 NH} R_2 NNO + HNO_2 \tag{4}$$

protonation of the secondary amine and the nitrite ion (NO_2^-), and for the formation of $N_2 O_3$. It is therefore pH dependent, passing through a maximum value at ca pH 3.4 (Mirvish 1975). To allow for this pH dependence, $\bar{k}_1$ values are related to the maximum at ca pH 3.4 by an empirical Gaussian function (equation 5), where Z is an adjustable parameter which is optimized to give good

$$\bar{k}_1 = \bar{k}_{1 \, max} \, \exp \, \left\{ -(\text{pH} - \text{pH}_{max})^2 / Z \right\} \tag{5}$$

agreement between calculated and experimental $\bar{k}_1$ values over the pH range 0.5 to 4. In practice, this agreement is not strongly influenced by small variations of the Z parameter, but optimum values are Z = 1.98 ± 0.20 for dimethylamine and Z = 1.09 ± 0.11 for N-methylaniline (MA).

The nitrosation of ureas and amides in the stomach is assumed to follow the in vitro rate expression (equation 6), also described by Mirvish (1975). Equation (6) is attributed to a rate-limiting reaction between the unprotonated

$$d \, [R'CON(R)NO]/dt = k_2 \, [R'CONHR] \, [HNO_2] \, [H^+] \tag{6}$$

$R' = \text{alkyl, } NH_2 \text{ etc; } R = \text{alkyl}$

amide or urea and the nitrous acidium ion (H_2ONO^+) as in equation (7). The rate coefficient $\bar{k}_2$ is defined in terms of actual (rather than stoichiometric)

$$HNO_2 + H_3O^+ \rightleftharpoons H_2ONO^+ \xrightarrow[\text{slow}]{R'CONHR} R'CON(R)NO + H_3O^+ \tag{7}$$

concentrations of the amino substrate and nitrous acid, and is independent of pH. For stoichiometric concentrations of the reagents, the reaction rate is defined by equation (8), where $\bar{k}_2 = k_2 \, [H^+] / \left\{ 1 + [H^+]/K_{SubH^+} \right\} \left\{ 1 + K_{HNO_2}/ [H^+] \right\}$ and K_{HNO_2} and K_{SubH^+} = acid dissociation constants of HNO_2 and

$$d \, [R'CON(R)NO] /dt = \bar{k}_2 \, (\text{Substrate})(\text{Nitrite}) \tag{8}$$

the protonated amine substrate, respectively. The rate coefficient $\bar{k}_2$ is, of course, pH dependent.

RESULTS

Mean values of gastric stoichiometric nitrite concentrations and pH for eight humans on a normal diet at 30-minute intervals over 24 hours (Milton-Thompson et al. 1982) are summarized in Figure 1. Time zero refers to 9:30 a.m. and food was normally consumed at time 9:31, 13:31, 17:31, and 21:31 hours. The subjects were allowed to take various beverages (including beer) at certain times and to smoke ad libitum. From these data and the literature values (Mirvish 1975) of rate coefficients $\bar{k}_1$ (equation 3) and k_2 (equation 6) summarized in Table 1, levels of N-nitroso compounds forming in the stomach can be calculated at 30-minute time intervals over a 24-hour period. The results obtained for four typical amino substrates, dimethylamine, MA, N-methylacetamide and N-methylurea at a constant concentration of 10^{-4}M are shown in Figures 2-5, respectively. Both separate 30-minute levels and their sum are plotted as a function of time. The 24-hour totals range from 1.6×10^{-14} mol/ℓ for N-nitroso-dimethylamine (NDMA) to 2.2×10^{-6} mol/ℓ for N-methyl-N-nitroso urea. For higher gastric concentrations of amino substrates, the calculated levels of N-nitroso product increase proportionately.

Table 1
Rate Coefficients at 25°C for the Nitrosation of Amino Substrates

Substrate	pK_A	$\bar{k}_1$ $(M^{-2} sec^{-1})$	k_2 $(M^{-2} sec^{-1})$
Dimethylamine	10.72	0.0017	—
MA	4.85	250[a]	—
MU	-0.9	—	10.5
N-Methylacetamide	-1.0	—	0.0025

Data from Mirvish (1975).
[a] At 0°C

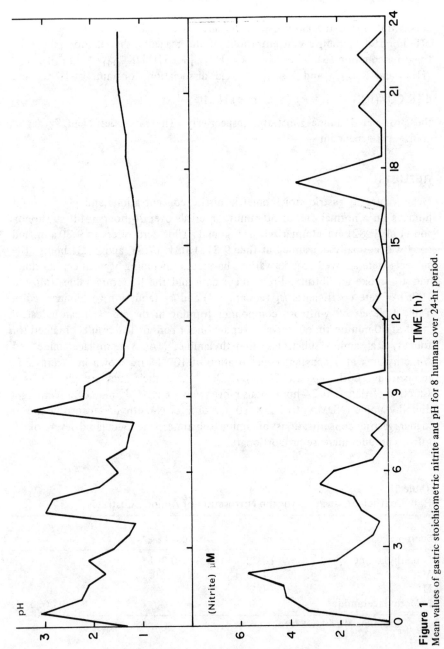

Figure 1
Mean values of gastric stoichiometric nitrite and pH for 8 humans over 24-hr period.

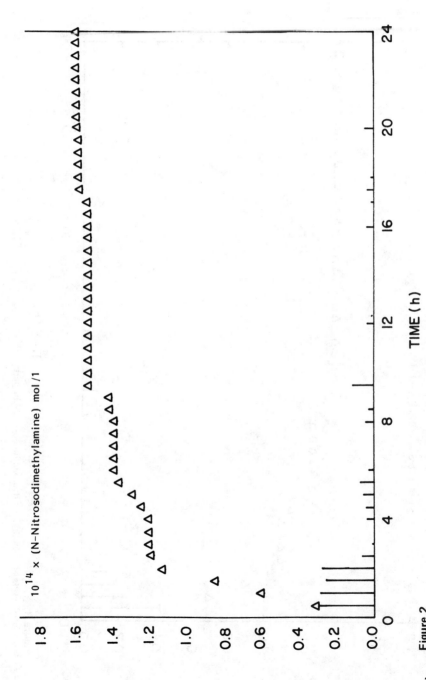

Figure 2
Calculated levels of *N*-nitrosodimethylamine over 24-hr period.

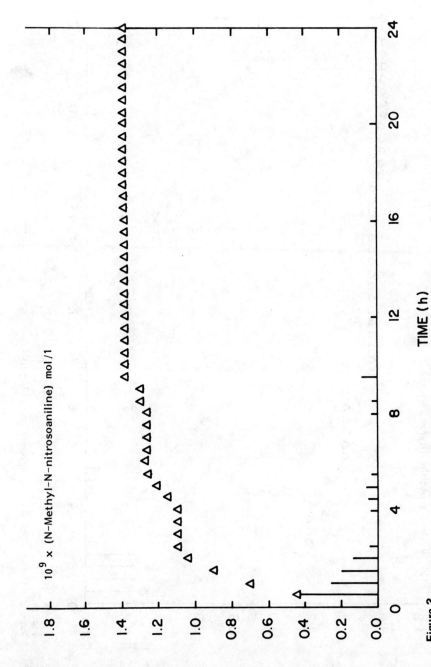

Figure 3
Calculated levels of *N*-methyl-*N*-nitrosoaniline over 24-hr period.

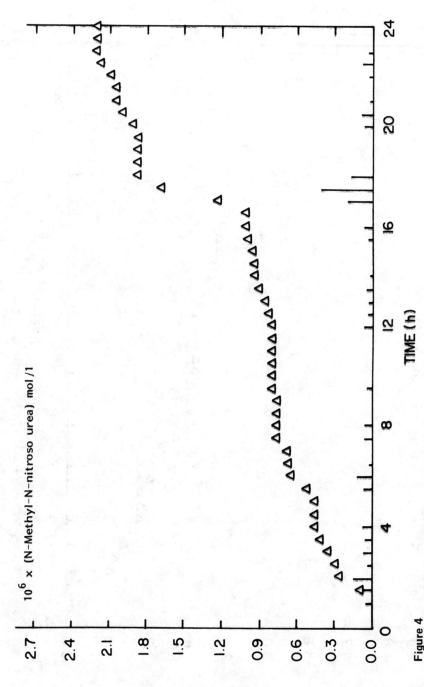

Figure 4
Calculated levels of *N*-methyl-*N*-nitrosourea over 24-hr period.

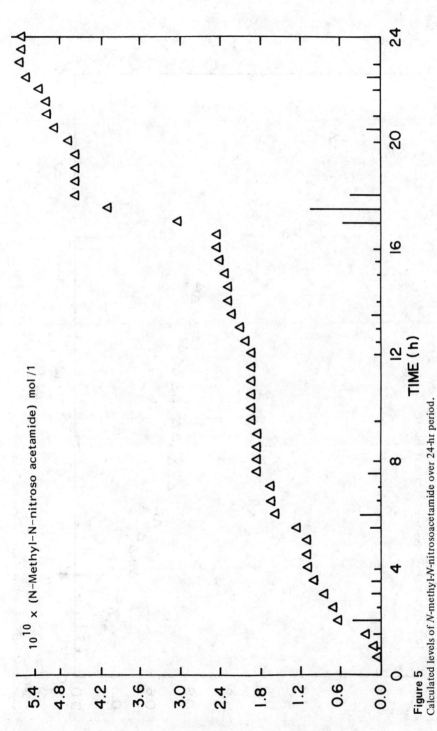

Figure 5
Calculated levels of *N*-methyl-*N*-nitrosoacetamide over 24-hr period.

250

DISCUSSION

The main aims of the present model are an estimate of the level at which N-nitroso compounds are synthesized in the stomach of healthy humans on a regular diet, and to identify the most reactive amino substrates present in these circumstances. The model is based on several assumptions some of which have been identified or discussed above. It is instructive to examine the probable consequences of these assumptions further.

1. N-Nitrosamine formation in the stomach follows in vitro kinetics

As noted at the beginning of this paper, this hypothesis is supported by a few experiments using relatively high nitrite concentrations where nitrosation in accordance with equation 3 is favored. At the low nitrite concentrations cited in Figure 1, it is conceivable that N-nitrosamine formation proceeds by pathways with only a first-order dependence on [Nitrite] and the yields of N-nitrosamine are therefore underestimated by the model. This caveat is particularly applicable in the presence of nucleophilic anions (e.g., SCN^-, I^-), thiols, and other potential nitrosation catalysts. Because suitable information is lacking, no allowance is made in the model for the kinetic effect of these catalysts, bacteria, and lipophilic media. We think it is unlikely, however, that the combinations of all these factors raises the N-nitrosamine yields by more than 100-fold.

2. N-Nitrosamide formation in the stomach follows in vitro kinetics

Although untested, this hypothesis is less questionable because N-nitrosamide formation has only a first-order dependence on [Nitrite] and is not accelerated by nucleophilic anions and other catalysts (Challis 1981).

3. Use of differential rather than integrated rate equations

As noted previously, any overestimation in yields of N-nitroso compounds arising from this approximation is negligible because the extent of the reaction over 30 minutes is so small.

4. Nitrite loss by absorption in the stomach and reaction with non-amino substrates (inhibitors)

Errors arising from these factors must be small, because experimental nitrite concentrations are used for each 30-minute interval. When the nitrite level decreases over the 30-minute period, the kinetic model overestimates the yields of N-nitroso compounds, but it underestimates the yield when the nitrite level increases. Over 24 hours these errors probably cancel out.

5. Amino substrate concentrations

The calculations assume a constant 10^{-4}M concentration for each amino substrate. Although arbitrary, this concentration roughly corresponds to that obtained from a 24-hour dietary intake of 1 kg containing 75 ppm of the amino substrate in total stomach contents of 7.5l. Few foods, however, contain secondary amine and amide levels as high as 75 ppm (Maga 1978; Smith 1981), so their gastric concentrations are likely to be lower than 10^{-4}M and the yields of N-nitroso compounds in Figures 2-5 are therefore overestimated.

Despite uncertainties arising from the above approximations, the results in Figures 2-5 suggest that only very small amounts of N-nitroso compounds are synthesized in the stomachs of healthy humans. This conclusion applies particularly to volatile N-nitrosamines, which have been the subject of considerable study and speculation. The detection of these compounds in normal human gastric contents should be regarded with circumspection unless some hitherto unknown, very efficient pathways exist for their formation.

If N-nitroso compounds are involved in gastric cancer, those derived from amides and related compounds must be prime contenders. N-Nitrosamides are direct-acting carcinogens (Magee et al. 1976), and the kinetic model suggests that gastric yields of N-nitrosamides are much higher than those of N-nitrosopeptides. The average daily protein intake is on the order of 110 g, which translates to an effective constant peptide group concentration of ca $0.2\,M$ for the kinetic model. Assuming the nitrosation kinetics and reactivity of the peptide N-atom is similar to N-methylacetamide, the concentrations of N-nitrosopeptides in the stomach over 24 hours could be on the order of 10^{-6} mol/l.

ACKNOWLEDGMENTS

One of us (SJL) thanks the Devon County Council for an Undergraduate Grant.

REFERENCES

Bavin, P.M.G., D.W. Darkin, and N.J. Viney. 1981. Total nitroso compounds in gastric juice. *IARC Sci Publ.* **41** (in press).

Challis, B.C. 1981. Chemistry of formation of N-nitroso compounds. In *Safety Evaluation of Nitrosatable Drugs and Chemicals* (eds. G.G. Gibson et al.) Taylor and Francis, London.

Eisenbrand, G., B. Spiegelhalder, and R. Preussmann. 1981. Analysis of human biological specimens for nitrosamine contents. *Ban. Rep.* 7:275.

Fine, D.H., B.C. Challis, P. Hartman, and J. van Ryzin. 1981. Endogenous synthesis of volatile nitrosamines: model calculations and risk assessment. *IARC Sci Publ.* **41** (in press).

Greenblatt, M. and S.S. Mirvish. 1973. Dose response studies with concurrent administration of piperazine and sodium nitrite to strain A mice. *J. Natl. Cancer Inst.* **50**:119.

Iqbal, Z.M., S.S. Epstein, I.S. Krull, E.U. Goff, K. Mills, and D.H. Fine. 1980. Kinetics of nitrosamine formation in mice following oral administration of trace-level precursors. *IARC Sci. Publ.* **31**:169.

Krull, I.S., K. Mills, G. Hoffman, and D.H. Fine. 1980. The analysis of N-nitrosocarbyl in whole mice. *J. Anal. Toxicol.* **4**:260.

Lee, I., M.C. Archer, and W.R. Bruce. 1981. Absence of volatile nitrosamines in human feces. *Cancer Res.* **41**:3992.

Maga, J.A. 1978. Amines in foods. *Crit. Rev. Food Sci. Nutr.* **10**:373.

Magee, P.N., R. Montesano, and R. Preussmann. 1976. N-nitroso compounds and related carcinogens. *ACS Monogr.* **173**:491.

Milton-Thompson, G.J., N.F. Lightfoot, Z. Ahmet, R.H. Hunt, J. Barnard, P.M.G. Bavin, R.W. Brimblecombe, D.W. Darkin, P.J. Moore, and N. Viney. 1982. Intragastric acidity, bacteria, nitrite and N-nitroso compounds, before, during and after cimetidine treatment. *Lancet* i:1091.

Mirvish, S.S. 1975. Formation of N-nitroso compounds: Chemistry, kinetics, and *in vivo* occurrence. *Toxicol. App. Pharmacol.* **31**:325.

National Academy of Sciences, Assembly of Life Sciences. 1981. The health effects of nitrate, nitrite and N-nitroso compounds. National Academy Press, Washington, D.C.

Ohshima, H. and Bartsch, H. 1981. Quantitative estimation of endogenous nitrosation in humans by monitoring N-nitrosoproline excreted in the urine. *Cancer Res.* **41**:3658.

Ruddell, W.J.J. and C.L. Walters. 1980. Nitrite and nitroso compounds in gastric juice. *Lancet* i:550.

Smith, T.A. 1981. Amines in food. *Food Chem.* **6**:169.

COMMENTS

WALTERS: You have tackled the job very well. I would like to add that, so far as the nonprotein nitrogen of fasting gastric juice is concerned, there is a value, which, if you assume 1 nitrogen per molecule, comes to a mean of 20 mmol, as compared with your suggested level of 0.1 mmol. This is in normal fasting gastric juice. In the case of pernicious anemia, that level is raised considerably.

CHALLIS: You did say 20 mmol?

WALTERS: The value given in the literature for nonprotein nitrogen is 20 mmol which obviously will contain a lot of nonnitrosatable peptides.

CHALLIS: That seems high and it would be useful to have the reference.

WALTERS: Yes. But bear in mind that there would be a lot of primary amino groups, and so forth, in that figure. Furthermore, they are precipitated proteins, so it would include peptides. We should be looking into the nitrosation of peptides (see Walters, this volume). Of the compounds that we observed in gastric juice, particularly under achlorhydrate conditions, at least 40% can be regarded as derivatives of simple peptides.

CHALLIS: I think the most interesting prediction by the model is that peptides should really dominate gastric nitrosation. However, we are at an early stage in the calculations and would like to examine the outcome when all the reactions are run in competition. Our expectations are that the peptides will react with all the available nitrous acid.

WEISBURGER: Total removal of nitrous acid by the peptides may actually be beneficial. Until we have some data on the mutagenicity of nitroso peptides, such reactions could be considered as a detoxifying process, rather than the reverse.

CONNEY: What is known about the biological activity of nitroso peptides? Has anyone looked at their biological activities?

CHALLIS: They have never been synthesized. They are not reported in the literature. We made the first one 3 days before I left for this conference and it is a fully-protected one. So we now have a nitroso peptide, specifically a nitroso dipeptide, and it is fully authenticated.

WEISBURGER: Are you going to do mutagenciity testing?

CHALLIS: If anybody would like to test the compound we would be delighted.

TANNENBAUM: About 10 years ago we published a paper (Fan and Tannenbaum 1973) which discussed pH-independent rate constants, mixed thiocyanate, and chloride reaction. In 1975, Sid Mirvish covered these considerations in kinetics.

Now, the problem with the model you presented is that we have also published data on nitrosation in human gastric juice samples (Tannenbaum et al. 1981). If one looks at the actual data and tries to predict, on the basis of all the things that you talked about, what the rate should be, one finds big differences from what one would predict and what we found—some gastric juice samples being much higher, and some being much lower. I think the reason for that is that there are a lot of factors that haven't been taken into consideration; like phenols or sulfhydryl compounds for example, of unknown structure, and maybe a lot of compounds that we don't even know about, that may participate in the reaction.

I think that in a sense it is a little premature to say that we can predict the amount that will be formed on the basis of measurements of just nitrite and pH in individuals over a period of time, because it could actually be much higher or it could be much lower. There may be huge individual differences. And it may be the individual differences which are really the most important factor in terms of carcinogenesis.

CHALLIS: I agree in general with what you say, and would make two comments.

First of all, catalysts may be there and may be important. Usually, it is assumed that thiocyanate is a very important catalyst; it is certainly one of the better ones. However we have shown that if you take an amine and thiocyanate and allow for the pH dependence, the pH profile for the thiocyanate-catalyzed reaction is reproduced very well and only very low levels of nitrosamine are predicted. The thiocyanate concentration that we use is the one reported by Boyland and Walker (1974).

Much has been said qualitatively about the effect of catalysts. When you do the calculations these expectations are not confirmed. You realize that the outcome is not quite what you think it is.

TANNENBAUM: I agree.

CHALLIS: The second comment is that you are quite right about individuals. Our calculations are made using averages. Subsequently, we have realized that this is undesirable because there is not "a standard" man. What we hope to do is the calculations for each individual patient. We have done

this for the three patients with the highest levels of nitrite and the nitrosamine and nitrosamide levels are not changed by more than a factor of
100.

WEISBURGER: May I suggest, as a last remark on this point, and these elegant
studies, that it could be for pickle foods, as they eat in Japan, and in some
other areas, that the potentially harmful materials exist preformed in the
food. The gastric synthesis of nitroso compounds that many of us are
thinking about may therefore be highly irrelevant to human disease risks.

CHALLIS: There is no need to comment on that.

References

Boyland, E. and S.A. Walker. 1974. Effect of thiocyanate on nitrosation of
amines. *Nature* **248**:601.

Fan, T.Y. and S.R. Tannenbaum. 1973. Factors influencing the rate of formation of nitrosomorpholine from morpholine and nitrite: Acceleration
by thiocyanate and other ions. *J. Agric. Food Chem.* **21**:237.

Mirvish, S.S. 1975. Formation of N-nitroso compounds—Chemistry, kinetics,
and in vivo occurrence. *Toxicol. Appl. Pharmacol.* **31**:325.

Tannenbaum, S.R., D. Moran, K.R. Falchuk, P. Correa, and C. Cuello. 1981.
Nitrite stability and nitrosation potential in human gastric juice. *Cancer
Lett.* **14**:131.

Carcinogenesis by Exposure to Nitrites and Amines

WILLIAM LIJINSKY
Chemical Carcinogenesis Program
NCI-Frederick Cancer Research Facility
Frederick, Maryland 21701

The possibility that human exposure to N-nitroso compounds could occur through formation of these compounds in vivo was discussed more than a decade ago (Druckrey et al. 1963; Lijinsky and Epstein 1970) and was given substantial support in the experiments of Sander and Bürkle (1969), who induced high incidences of tumors by feeding nitrite together with N-methyl-benzylamine or morpholine to rats. Following the report of Smith and Loeppky (1967) of the products of reaction of tertiary amines with nitrous acid, Lijinsky et al. (1972) suggested that tertiary amines as well as secondary amines could serve as a source of N-nitroso compounds for man.

There have been a large number of studies of the formation of N-nitroso compounds by reaction of both secondary and tertiary amines with nitrite under a variety of conditions, including gastric juice as the medium and short-term studies in vivo, in addition to purely chemical reactions. Large variations have been found in the rates of nitrosation between different amines, and the effects of accelerators of nitrosation, such as aldehydes (Keefer and Roller 1973) and thiocyanate (Boyland and Walker 1974), and of inhibitors of nitrosation, such as ascorbic acid (Mirvish et al. 1972), have been studied. The complexities of these reactions and the heterogeneous nature of the contents of stomachs make it virtually impossible to calculate the amount of N-nitroso compound formed from any particular amine in a human subject. It seems quite difficult to do this within several orders of magnitude even for animals in an experiment. All we are able to do at the present state of knowledge is to assume that some N-nitroso compound will be formed from an ingested secondary or tertiary amine, given that there is always nitrite in the saliva and that nitrite is present at considerable concentration in most cured meats, which are commonly eaten. There are also nitrosating agents other than nitrite which can react with amines, and these include nitrite esters and a number of N-nitroso compounds including aliphatic nitrosamines.

There is a natural reluctance to accept the results of chemical reactions in a laboratory as indicative of a risk to humans, even though laboratory experiments with negative outcomes are readily accepted as evidence of lack of risk to humans. Therefore, it seemed incumbent upon those of us concerned with a possible health risk in exposure to amines which could form carcinogenic *N*-nitroso compounds by nitrosation in vivo to demonstrate that tumors could be induced by concurrent feeding of amines and nitrite to experimental animals. The nature of carcinogenesis, as a response to a number of cumulative small risks, makes it difficult to simulate human experience lasting several decades in a rodent feeding study lasting only 2 years. The high toxicity of nitrite precludes the enormous exaggeration of dose considered necessary in a toxicity test in a small group of animals, yet the rate of formation of *N*-nitroso compounds is very dependent on the concentration of nitrite in the reaction mixture. Therefore, negative results in experiments in which amines and nitrite are fed to rodents for their lifetime can mean only that insufficient carcinogenic nitrosamine is formed (if the product of nitrosation is carcinogenic) to give rise to a significant incidence of tumors in the animals' lifetime. It is still possible that a risk to humans is posed by ingestion of the particular amine.

Studies of the induction of tumors by simultaneous feeding of amines and nitrite began with the experiments of Sander and Bürkle (1969), in which rats were the test animals. Most of the subsequent studies have used rats. There have been fewer studies using mice, which mostly have resulted in an increase in incidence of spontaneous tumors, such as lung adenomas or lymphomas, and which are therefore less informative. On the other hand, experiments in rats involving feeding of amines with nitrite have been numerous. The selection of rats as the test animal is propitious because rats appear to be more sensitive to the carcinogenic action of nitrosamines than are mice; that is, smaller doses give rise to tumors in a shorter time in rats than in mice.

Sander examined several amines in addition to methylbenzylamine and morpholine. These included dimethylurea, arginine, and methylguanidine, of which only dimethylurea and nitrite gave rise to a significant incidence of tumors. It is notable that both dimethylamine and diethylamine have failed to induce tumors when fed to animals together with nitrite. On the other hand, Shank and Newberne (1972), in an extensive set of experiments, demonstrated that morpholine at quite low concentrations gave rise to liver tumors when fed together with a sufficient concentration of nitrite to rats. The contrast between the effectiveness of morpholine and the ineffectiveness of dimethylamine and diethylamine is because of the strong basicity of the latter two amines, which reduces the rate of reaction considerably. Piperidine has not induced a significant incidence of tumors when fed with nitrite to rats, for the same reason.

There have been studies of the effect of feeding combinations with nitrite of several amines that are of only theoretical interest, because it is unlikely that man will be exposed to them, and something has been learned about the matter from them. For example, heptamethyleneimine with nitrite has given rise to lung tumors in Sprague-Dawley rats when fed in drinking water (Taylor and Lijinsky

1975a). This is of some relevance because much of the amines in tobacco smoke enters the stomach by being swallowed in the saliva. Methylurea and ethylurea have been shown to induce a high incidence of tumors when fed to animals with nitrite, including transplacentally.

Most of the efforts of a number of investigators have been devoted to studies of the interaction with nitrite of amines that are of practical interest, because humans are likely to be exposed to them. In this category of "important" secondary and tertiary amines are a large number of drugs and agricultural chemicals, and a few naturally occurring compounds. These amines invariably gave significant yields of N-nitroso derivatives in chemical reactions with nitrite at moderately acid pH (3-4), similar to that in a stomach during digestion of a meal, often at quite low concentrations.

Among the naturally occurring amines have been arginine, methyl-guanidine, citrulline, piperine, and trimethylamine-N-oxide, all of which gave negative results when fed to rats together with nitrite; that is, there was no significant incidence of tumors not seen in controls fed the amine and nitrite separately. Allantoin is a naturally occurring amine which has given rise to a small incidence of tumors under these conditions, but the effect is not very striking (Table 1).

The drugs which are secondary or tertiary amines have been of considerable interest, because they are often administered to people in quite large doses, and for long periods of time. The possible risk to these people of exposure to carcinogenic nitrosamines formed in vivo seems correspondingly greater than that of people exposed to traces of other amines in the environment. As examples, tolbutamide and tetracyclines are taken in doses of 500 mg, sometimes more. A large number of widely used drugs has been investigated from this point of view, as a consequence. Most of these experiments have not resulted in a significant incidence of induced tumors, which can quiet our anxieties that they pose any large risk of cancer through formation of N-nitroso derivatives. Among these are chlorpromazine, cyclizine, tolazamide, dipyrone, hexamethylenetetramine, quinacrine, lucanthone and methapyrilene; the last two compounds are carcinogenic themselves. In some cases the fact that the nitroso derivatives are not detectably carcinogenic provides reassurance that there is no carcinogenic risk from this source (as in the case of phenmetrazine and methylphenidate).

On the other hand, a number of commonly used drugs have, in such experiments, given rise to an incidence of induced tumors that is highly significant. Others have induced incidences of tumors that are of borderline significance. In the latter cases, duplication of the experiment, or studies on a larger scale might be justified to allay all anxiety about possible carcinogenic risks associated with taking these compounds. The most striking result has been obtained with aminopyrine (Pyramidon), which has induced essentially 100% incidences of tumors due to the formation of nitrosodimethylamine (NDMA) even after giving quite low concentrations of the drug and nitrite to animals

Table 1

Survival of F344 Rats Treated with Amines and Nitrite in Diet

Compound		Nitrite	Number of Survivors at Week									Number of Rats with Induced Tumors
			0	50	60	70	80	90	100	110	120	
Allantoin	0.2%	0	20 ♂	20	20	20	20	20	19	17	14	1 liver
	0.2%	0	20 ♀	19	19	19	18	17	16	10	9	2 liver
	0.2%	0.2%	20 ♂	20	20	20	20	19	17	13	9	1 liver, 5 forestomach
	0.2%	0.2%	20 ♀	20	19	19	18	18	14	12	9	6 liver, 3 forestomach
Thiram[a]	0.05%	0	24 ♂	24	24	24	23	22	19	16	14	1 tongue, 1 kidney
	0.05%	0	24 ♀	24	24	24	24	23	21	20	16	1 lung, 1 liver
	0.05%	0.2%	24 ♂	24	24	23	22	19	16	8	7	2 nasal cavity, 5 forestomach, 2 bladder, 1 kidney
	0	0.2%	24 ♀	24	24	23	22	19	14	12	10	4 nasal cavity, 2 forestomach, 1 liver, 1 tongue
	0	0.2%	48 ♂	48	47	46	45	43	37	20	16	
	0	0.2%	48 ♀	48	48	47	46	44	39	36	30	
	0	0	48 ♂	48	48	48	44	43	37	29	16	
	0	0	48 ♀	48	48	47	45	41	37	33	30	

[a]Thiram-treated and control groups have not been completely evaluated histologically.

(Taylor and Lijinsky 1975b). However, aminopyrine reacts exceedingly rapidly with nitrous acid, which explains its great biological activity in this type of experiment. Disulfiram (Antabuse) when fed to rats together with nitrite also gave rise to a high incidence of tumors, in this case esophageal tumors, due to the nitrosodiethylamine (NDEA) formed in vivo (Lijinsky and Reuber 1980). The remaining drugs studied gave results less striking, but nevertheless significant. A summary of the findings is given in Table 2, and shows that oxytetracycline and tolbutamide both gave significant incidences of tumors of the liver and forestomach, respectively. The results with chlordiazepoxide are equivocal, there being forestomach tumors in only one sex.

A number of other drugs are currently being tested and thus far have not shown evidence of tumors induced by formation of nitrosamines in vivo. They are chlorpheniramine, diphenhydramine, and hydrochlorothiazide, which are respectively two antihistaminics and an antidiuretic. All can theoretically give rise to N-nitroso compounds which are probably carcinogenic, and the N-nitroso derivative of hydrochlorothiazide has been shown to be mutagenic, but has not

Table 2
Feeding Tests of Amines with Nitrite in Rats

Amine	Duration of treatment	Tumors induced
Aminopyrine	30-50 weeks	liver angiosarcomas
Arginine	50 weeks	0
Chlorpromazine	50 weeks	0
Chlordiazepoxide	100 weeks	forestomach
Chlorpheniramine	100 weeks	U[a]
Cyclizine	80 weeks	0
Disulfiram	80 weeks	esophagus
Dimethyldodecylamine	80 weeks	bladder, forestomach
Dimethyldodecylamine Oxide	80 weeks	U
Diphenhydramine	100 weeks	U
Fenuron	50 weeks	0
Hexamethylenetetramine	50 weeks	0
Hydrochlorothiazide	100 weeks	U
Methylguanidine	50 weeks	0
Monuron	80 weeks	liver
Oxytetracycline	60 weeks	liver
Piperidine	50 weeks	0
Piperine	100 weeks	forestomach
Tolazamide	50 weeks	0
Tolbutamide	100 weeks	forestomach, liver
Thiram	100 weeks	nasal cavity, forestomach
Trimethylamine Oxide	50 weeks	0

[a]U = Unfinished

been tested for carcinogenic activity. None of these drugs, fed to rats at concentrations of 1000 or 2000 ppm. in the diet has led to any life-shortening, nor yet to any significant incidence of tumors, whether mixed with nitrite or alone. However, the majority of the animals in these experiments are still alive and no conclusions can be reached.

The other large group of amines studied are agricultural chemicals, many of which form N-nitroso derivatives which are powerful carcinogens, for example the insecticidal N-methylcarbamic acid esters. One of these, carbaryl, has been much studied and when given to pregnant rats together with nitrite failed to induce any tumors in the progeny (Lijinsky and Taylor 1977). This implied either that insufficient nitroso derivative was formed in vivo to give an effect or that nitrosocarbaryl does not cross the placenta of rats. In either case, the lack of response indicates that the risk of cancer from this source is very small. The substituted urea benzthiazuron was converted into its nitroso derivative. Although nitroso-benzthiazuron is a very potent carcinogen, tumors were not induced by feeding benzthiazuron with nitrite to rats (Ungerer et al. 1974). Similarly, the herbicide fenuron, which is a tri-substituted urea did not give rise to a significant incidence of tumors when given to rats together with nitrite for 50 weeks or more, while monuron gave a marginal tumor yield. In the experiment with thiram (the tetramethyl analog of disulfiram), however, a significant incidence of tumors of the forestomach and of the nasal cavity has been observed (Table 1) and more might be diagnosed later. One-third of the treated rats are still alive, and a few of those recently dead have not yet been examined histologically.

Another compound of some interest is the detergent builder dimethyl-dodecylamine-N-oxide, which is related to the antisuckering agent dimethyl-dodecylamine. The latter gave rise to a small incidence of tumors when fed to rats together with nitrite for more than a year; among the induced tumors were transitional cell carcinomas of the bladder, a tumor induced by feeding rats one of the products of nitrosation of this amine, nitrosomethyldodecylamine. The feeding study with the N-oxide is not yet complete and most of the rats are still alive. However, the rats that have died have not shown a significant incidence of induced tumors, and no conclusions can be drawn about this experiment.

The results so far suggest that there exists a real, but unquantifiable, risk in the ingestion of nitrosatable amines, particularly those susceptible to ready nitrosation, and that any increased carcinogenic risk therefrom can be reduced by limiting exposure to these amines or reducing the intake of nitrite or nitrite precursors.

ACKNOWLEDGMENT

This work was supported by Contract No. N01-C0-75380, with the National Cancer Institute, NIH, Bethesda, Maryland 20205.

REFERENCES

Boyland, E. and S.A. Walker. 1974. Effect of thiocyanate on nitrosation of amines. *Nature* 248:601.

Druckrey, H., D. Steinhoff, H. Beuthner, H. Schneider, and, P. Klärner. 1963. Prüfung von Nitrit auf chronisch toxische Wirkung an Ratten. *Arzneim.-Forsch.* 13:320.

Keefer, L.K. and P.P. Roller. 1973. N-Nitrosation by nitrite ion in neutral and basic medium. *Science* 181:1245.

Lijinsky, W. and S.S. Epstein. 1970. Nitrosamines as environmental carcinogens. *Nature* 225:21.

Lijinsky, W., L.K. Keefer, E. Conrad, and R. Van de Bogart. 1972. The nitrosation of tertiary amines and some biologic implications. *J. Natl. Cancer Inst.* 49:1239.

Lijinsky, W. and M.D. Reuber. 1980. Tumors induced in Fischer 344 rats by the feeding of disulfiram together with nitrite. *Food Cosmet. Toxicol.* 18:85.

Lijinsky, W. and H.W. Taylor. 1977. Transplacental chronic toxicity test of carbaryl with nitrite in rats. *Food Cosmet. Toxicol.* 15:229.

Mirvish, S.S., L. Wallcave, M. Eagen, and P. Shubik. 1972. Ascorbate-nitrite reaction: Possible means of blocking the formation of carcinogenic N-nitroso compounds. *Science* 177:65.

Sander, J. and G. Bürkle. 1969. Induktion maligner Tumoren bei Ratten durch gleichzeitige Verfütterung von Nitrit und sekundären Aminen. *Z. Krebsforsch.* 73:54.

Shank, R.C. and P.M. Newberne. 1972. Nitrite-morpholine-induced hepatomas. *Food Cosmet. Toxicol.* 10:887.

Smith, P.A.S. and R.N. Loeppky. 1967. Nitrosative cleavage of tertiary amines. *J. Am. Chem. Soc.* 89:1147.

Taylor, H.W. and W. Lijinsky. 1975a. Tumor induction in rats by feeding heptamethyleneimine and nitrite in water. *Cancer Res.* 35:812.

_____. 1975b. Tumor induction in rats by feeding aminopyrine or oxytetracycline with nitrite. *Int. J. Cancer* 16:211.

Ungerer, O., G. Eisenbrand, and R. Preussmann. 1974. Zur Reaktion von Nitrit mit Pesticiden. Bildung, chemische Eigenschaften und cancerogene Wirkung der N-Nitrosoverbindung des Herbizides N-Methyl-N'-(2-benzothiazolyl)-harnstoff (Benzthiazuron). *Z. Krebsforsch.* 81:217.

COMMENTS

MAGEE: Willie, you showed that thiram yields NDMA and produced forestomach tumors. Have you ever gotten forestomach tumors with NDMA by itself?

LIJINSKY: No. That's why I think our studies in the test-tube probably don't represent what really happens.

MAGEE: Is it conceivable that the nitrosation might be occurring within the gastric cell?

LIJINSKY: I suppose it's conceivable. I'm not sure that the thiram would get inside the gastric cell.

MAGEE: That's just a wild suggestion. This is something that is unexpected, isn't it?

LIJINSKY: Yes, it is. But, you see, there is a possibility you could cleave off one methyl group and put the nitroso group on the residue, which you can't isolate. I mean, you cannot isolate such a product. But it might form in vivo and exert its effect. That might be the source of the nasal cavity and the forestomach tumors. Our capacities as chemists are severely taxed in such reactions.

GRASSO: What about the weights that you give to these forestomach tumors? I don't think there is a forestomach at all in man.

LIJINSKY: No.

GRASSO: Secondly, as far as I know the forestomach is highly susceptible to irritation. We have had this big problem with benzo[a]pyrene.

There is a third element, which I am not sure is sufficiently appreciated. Recently, an experiment has been done in which ethylene oxide, propylene oxide, and beta-propiolactone was fed as his positive control. The beta-propiolactone produced squamous cell carcinomas which metastasize widely, whereas the other two did not. I just wonder, in effect, whether perhaps we are not giving too much weight, in terms of carcinogenic activity, to forestomach tumors. It's just a question.

LIJINSKY: Forestomach tumors are merely an index of carcinogenicity, as are the nasal cavity tumors in rodents. The nasal cavity tumors have no equivalent in man. Yet, we consider formaldehyde to be a human carcinogenic risk because of its importance in producing nasal cavity tumors. I think all of these lesions are indicators.

GRASSO: You know, other people may not regard formaldehyde in the same light, but we are not discussing that at the moment.

LIJINSKY: The point is this, we have no idea when we produce rat liver tumors that the compound, if it's a carcinogen for man, has liver as its target in man. It doesn't matter. All we do in our carcinogenicity experiments is rate risks. We say that one compound that induces tumors is probably a greater carcinogenic risk than one that doesn't. It's exactly the same outcome whether they're forestomach tumors or nasal cavity tumors or any other kind of tumor. I don't believe you can discount any malignancy or any neoplasm produced in an animal by a treatment at a significant level and say it doesn't matter, when we don't know enough to do that.

DURANT: Are you using 200 ppm nitrite in the water?

LIJINSKY: 2000 ppm.

DURANT: These are gross concentrations of nitrite.

LIJINSKY: Absolutely.

DURANT: How relevant is that? You say this represents carcinogenic risk or a potential carcinogenic risk. What is your basis for that assumption at that atypical nitrite concentration?

LIJINSKY: To do a carcinogenicity experiment, you have to exaggerate the risk to the animals, because we have millions of people who are at risk, and we only have 20 or 30 animals. I said any number of animals with tumors lower than four, that's a 20% incidence, I discount. Now, be fair. This is what we have to do.

DURANT: Yes. I just want to suggest that you're imbalancing the chemistry with these large concentrations.

LIJINSKY: Well, all right. All of those factors have to be considered. I mean, this is what we mean by doing toxicology. We do toxicology to the best of our ability. We try to represent human risk.

DURANT: Obviously, that goes without saying.

LIJINSKY: In fact, if I could give 5000 ppm nitrite I would do it. I can't give more than 2000 ppm because the animals die of methemoglobinemia. But, to give it the maximum chance to produce a result, I use the highest concentration I can get away with.

DURANT: Where do you go from there?

LIJINSKY: I have no next step. I am just rating the relative effect. Fortunately, I am not in business, and I'm not a regulator, so I don't have to have a next step. I want to get as much information as possible about human risks from exposures to nitroso compounds. My primary interest is how nitrosamines cause cancer in animals or man.

DURANT: Obviously, that's of interest.

LIJINSKY: But this is something I have chosen to do, and when I come to the end of it I will probably abandon it. In fact, Dr. Challis' calculations really bothered me, because maybe it's not fair to do what I do at all.

CASTONGUAY: Were the nasal cavity tumors from the olfactory duct?

LIJINSKY: They were mainly from the olfactory duct. There may have been squamous carcinoma, but I'm not sure.

ANDERSON: Were the amines included in the food?

LIJINSKY: Both nitrite and amines were included in the food. They were mixed together in the dry food once a week. Our assay showed that there was no nitrosamine formed in any case.

ANDERSON: Were all the amines at the same concentration?

LIJINSKY: No. It was usually 0.1 or 0.2%, depending on the quantity provided me by the parent company. Sometimes they sent me 1 kg or 2 kg. It was quite arbitrary.

ANDERSON: Did the rats eat the food very happily?

LIJINSKY: Absolutely.

ANDERSON: Did you measure the food consumption?

LIJINSKY: We measured the food consumption. It was about 30 gm/day for males, 20 gm/day for females. I didn't measure it throughout. Their weight gains were all reasonable, and the life expectancy was normal. So, all of these factors tell me that what we did was not terribly unphysiological.

SEN: Dr. Lijinsky, you mentioned there have been problems in people working with thiram?

LIJINSKY: Some people in Oregon have said that there was a higher incidence of tumors in forestry workers. I was asked this question when thiram was brought up as a prospective compound for the bioassay program, because there have been such reports. I never verified it. I just thought that was a good enough reason to test thiram.

TANNENBAUM: The hydrochlorothiazide question is very interesting, if it's a mutagen, because that drug is taken very extensively in pregnancy. There has been at least one epidemiological study that I know of that has raised it as a potential risk factor for nervous system tumors in children. So, I think it should be tested transplacentally.

LIJINSKY: That may be. Following Sid Mirvish's report, I expected early onset of tumors. The animals are now over 100 weeks in the experiment and there is no significant incidence of tumors yet.

MIRVISH: This compound is actually an alkylmethyl aniline, a secondary aromatic amine. It should form a nitrosamine extraordinarily readily.

LIJINSKY: Well, you showed it does.

DURANT: But how do you isolate it and characterize it?

LIJINSKY: Does it form one product?

MIRVISH: Yes.

DURANT: Well, why don't you just test that product?

LIJINSKY: I didn't test it because that wasn't part of my plan.

GARLAND: Have you looked at the effect of nitrite itself?

LIJINSKY: We get no significant incidence of any tumor. We get the fore-stomach tumor in nitrite-free animals, but I have about 300 animals treated with nitrite alone on test, and so far I have no indication that nitrite itself is a carcinogen in this protocol, I emphasize that. I have not done it transplacentally and I have not done multigeneration studies. But, in this protocol, I have not found any indications that nitrite is a carcinogen.

KIMBROUGH: Are there any other morphological changes in the forestomach in the animals where you don't find cancer?

LIJINSKY: Often hyperkeratosis occurs.

KIMBROUGH: Do you see that in animals where you just give nitrites?

LIJINSKY: Sometimes. There is often hyperkeratosis in the stomach, or irritation.

GRASSO: The problem with that model is really not that serious, but there is such a thing, which is quite well known in histopathology, called epitheliomatous hyperplasia. It has been mistaken in the past for squamous cell carcinoma. In view of the recent experiments of Dunkelbank (phonetic), I wonder whether we have not been misled into diagnosing these tumors assuming they are squamous cell carcinomas, whereas, in fact, they were not.

LIJINSKY: Most of these are papillomas, not carcinomas. I am very, very dependent upon my good pathologist friends to tell me what they find. I can't tell them.

GRASSO: I understand that.

MAGEE: Just a comment on what you have said. If I remember correctly, the Danish scientist Fibiger was awarded the Nobel Prize on the basis of misdiagnosis of these same lesions!

WEISBURGER: That occurred in 1913.

LIJINSKY: I am very unimpressed about any of these experiments in which only the forestomach tumor is a target. In fact, Librium was one in this experiment. I think it produced 5 or 6 forestomach papillomas, and possibly a couple of carcinomas, in only one sex. I am certainly not drumbeating for the results of that study, but the nasal cavity tumors are more significant.

HOFFMANN: I am a little surprised. We have never analyzed animal feed without finding traces of nitrosamines. You believe that adding nitrite will not mean anything? You didn't find any nitrosamines?

LIJINSKY: I didn't say I didn't find any, I said no significant amount. We find it perhaps at 0.2 ppm.

HOFFMANN: I think our data range 5-10 ppb in feed samples.

LIJINSKY: Well, in our experience it's 10-20 ppb.

HOFFMANN: At 20 ppb one might almost expect a biological effect.

LIJINSKY: What I meant was that there was no more nitrosamine than there was in the control—that is, without the amine and nitrite.

HOFFMANN: When one adds 0.2% of nitrite to the feed and when there is sufficient humidity, there is a possibility of a reaction.

LIJINSKY: We don't find significant quantities. Often we don't get any significant incidences of tumors. Remember, there are built-in controls in this experiment—every animal, every group, gets the same amount of nitrite.

HOFFMANN: I do not question your bioassay data. I am only reporting that we haven't found a feed which doesn't contain volatile nitrosamines.

LIJINSKY: I should have been more precise.

HARTMAN: What is the nitrite concentration in the stomachs of these animals, as compared with what has been found in humans?

LIJINSKY: I have no idea. I haven't measured it.

HARTMAN: Have you measured it under conditions of high gastric pH?

LIJINSKY: I never measured it.

HARTMAN: My guess is it is not a whole lot higher.

LIJINSKY: I think Sid Mirvish did an experiment that should tell you that.

MIRVISH: Actually, as I explained earlier, we fed nitrite, and the concentration in the glandular stomach, which is the acidic part, was one-ninth of the dose that we fed.

HARTMAN: But you gave it in water, didn't you?

MIRVISH: Water was mixed in the diet. We gave it in a meal. In those experiments, we gave the rats a meal containing nitrite.

Presence of Nitrosamines in Human Beings

DAVID H. FINE
New England Institute for Life Sciences
125 Second Avenue
Waltham, Massachusetts 02254

VOLATILE NITROSAMINES

In 1977 Fine et al. reported on the increased presence of nitrosodimethylamine (NDMA) and nitrosodiethylamine (NDEA) in the blood of a volunteer immediately after the ingestion of a meal consisting of bacon, bread, spinach, and beer. This was soon followed by other reports of the presence of volatile nitrosamines in human blood (Lakritz et al. 1980; Kowalski et al. 1980; Yamamoto et al. 1980) in normal urine of healthy volunteers (Hicks et al. 1977; El-Merzabani et al. 1979; Kakizoe et al. 1979; Tannenbaum 1981) and in the feces of healthy volunteers (Wang et al. 1978). Because the short half-life of NDMA in living animals was well known (Wishnok et al. 1978), these findings drew attention to the possibility that endogenous nitrosamines greatly exceeded those from exogenous sources (Tannenbaum 1980; Lijinsky 1980).

Despite the wealth of experimental evidence cited above, the analytical procedures had only been rigorously evaluated down to concentration levels of about 1 µg/kg (ppb). Levels in biological fluids were often one-tenth or one-hundredth of this amount. However, when proper analytical control protocols were developed and instituted, the experimental data base evaporated. Thus, Archer et al. (1982) showed that when a marker amine was added to fresh feces, the nitroso derivative of the marker amine was formed during the analytical work-up, indicative of artifact formation. Similarly, the inclusion of proper artifact controls demonstrated that volatile nitrosamines were absent from normal urine (Tannenbaum 1981; Spiegelhalder et al. 1982) and blood (Eisenbrand et al. 1981).

Spiegelhalder et al. (1982) did observe NDMA to be present in urine and blood, when it was co-administered with ethanol. In repeated experiments they showed NDMA excretion in humans after oral application of as little as 12 µg of NDMA in beer, and orange juice with 6% ethanol, but not in orange juice with added ethanol.

Volatile nitrosamines were reported to be present in vaginal secretions (Harrington et al. 1973). The result was determined using low resolution mass spectrometry of the parent ion at m/e 75 and the NO^+ ion at m/e 30, a technique which Gough et al. (1977) subsequently showed to be ambiguous. Artifact controls were also not carried out. Later analyses of samples from the same hospital were shown to be negative (D.H. Fine, unpubl. results).

Secondary amines, especially dimethylamine, piperidine, and pyrrolidine, are found in normal urine in levels as high as 6 mg/day (Drasar and Hill 1974). These amines are presumably formed by bacterial action on breakdown products of food in the intestine (Asatoor and Simenhoff 1965). Nitrosamines in concentrations of 2 to 3 µg/liter have been found in the urine of patients with *Proteus mirabilis* and *Escherichia coli* infections (Brooks et al. 1972; Radomski et al. 1978). Unfortunately, there were no adequate controls for possible artifactual formation of NDMA during analytical chemistry procedures. In the study by Brooks et al. (1972), urine was acidified to pH 2 and then extracted with chloroform. If amines and nitrite were present in the urine, NDMA could have been formed at this stage. In the study by Radomski et al. (1978) the urine was frozen prior to analysis without the inclusion of an artifact inhibitor.

NONVOLATILE NITROSAMINES

Ruddell et al. (1980) and Bavin et al. (1982) have reported the presence of compounds containing the *N*-nitroso moiety, using a chemical denitrosation technique. Unfortunately, the group analysis technique that was used was not capable of identifying the compounds giving rise to the positive response.

Recently Ohshima and Bartsch (1981) developed a technique for estimating the extent of in vivo nitrosamine formation in humans who have ingested proline with nitrate by assaying urine samples, collected for 24 hours following ingestion for nitrosoproline (NPRO), a nonvolatile nitrosamine. The approach is sensitive and practical for two reasons: NPRO is not carcinogenic in animals and it is not readily metabolized (80% is excreted in the urine within 24 hours). They reported a background NPRO level of less than 3 µg/liter or urine (3 µg/ person/day), which was not significantly increased by ingesting proline alone or nitrate alone. However, ingestion of red beet juice (containing up to 325 mg of nitrate) followed 30 minutes later by proline (500 mg) produced readily detectable levels of NPRO (0.16-0.030 mg).

The experimental data reported by Ohshima and Bartsch (1981) was compared with the calculated estimates of in vivo formation of NPRO from ingested proline and nitrate by Fine et al. (1982). They estimated the time-dependent nitrite build up in the stomach from studies of Spiegelhalder et al. (1976), taking into account absorption of nitrate through the gastrointestinal tract, the consequent nitrate build up in saliva, and its conversion to nitrite by oral cavity flora. Using the in vitro kinetic data of Mirvish (1975), the time-dependent build up of NPRO was calculated. The calculated NPRO values agreed with the experimental data within the limits of experimental error.

CONCLUSION

The finding of volatile nitrosamines in the body fluids of healthy human volunteers, who have not recently consumed alcohol, has not been substantiated—with one exception. Co-ingestion of ethanol apparently retards the metabolism of NDMA to make it detectable in volunteers who have recently consumed an alcoholic beverage.

There have been two studies on NDMA in urine of individuals with bacterial infections, but in neither of the studies were the artifact controls adequate. The data, therefore, remains ambiguous.

NPRO is the only N-nitroso compound whose presence in a body fluid (urine) has been able to withstand the critical test of properly designed artifact control protocols.

These are the end of the cold, hard facts. I would like to speculate a little bit though.

At the IARC meeting in Tokyo, we presented a speculative paper, based on Ohshima and Bartsch (1981). Two of the coworkers are in the audience, Brian Challis and Phil Hartman.

We used a simple kinetic model, a little bit cruder than the one Challis presented earlier. We took the Ohshima and Bartsch data, which are the circles, and broke the time zones into 1-hour intervals, using their nitrite intake and the amount of protein they were fed, using the Mirvish kinetics, and making some assumptions on the emptying time of the nitrate and the recirculation of the nitrate and formation of the nitrite, we were able to calculate what should have happened using a simple kinetic model; and also looked at what the variation would be from the mean. It gives a sort of bracket; a low value and a high value.

We decided to take the model one step further. Using some rather obvious kinetics and in vitro data. We could now predict the one good published experimental datapoint. Could we now use this model to estimate the amount of nitrosamines which were formed in vivo?

To proceed, we had to make a number of assumptions:

First, in the model, the hourly nitrite levels are important. We assumed that we had a reasonably good fit to the one good datapoint.

Second, was to assume that proline was a reasonably good amine to model. After all, in the environment we have been looking at only the volatile nitrosamines. Where does proline fall? The rate of nitrosation of proline is faster than dimethylamine, and it's a little bit slower than morpholine, so it seems to pretty well bracket the volatile nitrosamines that we have been looking at.

Third, in the absence of any real data on amine intake, we assumed that there were 4 gm proline/day intake, and divided it into two big meals a day. Then we also had to assume that NPRO was a reasonably good marker N-nitroso compound for the nitrosamines.

Fourth, the nitrite data we obtained from looking at average U.S. exposure and categorized the people to estimate what different population groups would be exposed to, in terms of nitrate and nitrite. We used the conversion of nitrate to nitrite, and then used the proline intake to try to estimate the range of NPRO values that people are being exposed to.

Fifth, this type of calculation had to take into account ascorbic acid. Most of the nitrate is coming from vegetables. It is getting into the bloodstream, and being converted in the saliva to nitrite. And we have to take into account that those vegetables also have ascorbic acid.

The details of this calculation are in the Academy report, and also presented at the meeting in Tokyo. It is this set of data that I want to look at.

We divided the U.S. population into five rather arbitrary population groups: an average diet, an average diet plus people who smoke 20 cigarettes a day, vegetarian, high-nitrate water, and very high meat diet. This is the range of NPRO levels that you would expect, based on this calculation.

The conclusion that we came to was that the levels here are not the height of the steeple compared to the exogenous exposure, as had been previously claimed, but instead they are about the same order. The persons with the highest nitrate exposure had the highest nitrosamine exposure.

We decided to go even further out on a limb and become even more speculative, just to see where it may lead. We combined all the known data on human exposure to nitrosamines: exogenous, plus calculated indogenous, plus the worker exposure, plus the cigarette smoker and we used the same U.S. population groups.

In order to determine risk assessment, we took the data of Terracini (Terracini et al. 1967), and extrapolated that to the low levels. This was carried out by John van Ryzin, a statistician (Fine et al. 1982). We used a low-dose linear extrapolation beyond 10^{-2} risk, and down to that level by means of the multi-hit model. We then assumed that all the nitrosamines we were calculating, in terms of our proline endogenous model and the exogenous human exposures, were as potent as NDMA, and that the animal data could be compared to man, and that man and the rat were behaving the same way. Again, this is probably a conservative estimate. Four arbitrary categories are considered here (an average, an average plus people who smoke, a high-risk group, and a low-risk group). In the U.S., for example, most of the people are in the average; with only a few people at high risk (totaling the maximum exogenous exposure and the maximum endogenous exposure, with worker exposure being the worst of everything). We come up with a total exposure, and compared this total exposure to the animal risk calculation.

What does that mean in terms of cancer incidence in the U.S.? The total comes to about 1,300-1,400 cases of cancer per year. The range of error is about half an order of magnitude. Thus, all known exposures to exogenous nitrosamines, plus worker exposure, plus the inclusion of calculated values for endogenous intake can only account for 1400 U.S. cancer deaths per year.

That conclusion really surprised us very much. For someone who has been in the research field for 8 years and has been measuring nitrosamines in the environment, it is a very humbling conclusion to realize that perhaps nitrosamines aren't as important a class of carcinogens as compared to the other nitroso compounds, as we had previously thought.

There is a major lesson to be learned here, by going back to the assumptions that were made and asking where could they have gone wrong by orders of magnitude to have underestimated things so badly? There are two possible explanations: We neglected the effect of catalysts. Maybe there are some catalysts we hadn't thought of which are really important and which we neglected. Probably, more importantly, we ignored the ureas, the amides and peptides, and materials like those. Why? Well, we knew from Mirvish's tables, which have been available for many years, that they nitrosated much faster than the amines that we've been looking at. But, being analytical chemists, we put on blinkers and just looked at the nitrosamines that we knew how to analyze. We ignored the nitroso compounds that were formed much faster than the nitrosamines just because we did not know how to measure them. For example, in that same calculation, if, instead of proline we had used methylurea, then we would have seen 10,000 times more of the nitroso compound than we calculated.

Are these other nonvolatile compounds present in the environment? No one has looked, so we don't know. We assume so.

Where I want to conclude is, reemphasizing Sid Mirvish's and Brian Challis' comments, that we should begin to really put the effort where it is most important, namely, in the nonvolatile compounds, like the amides and the ureas.

REFERENCES

Archer, M.C., L. Lee, and W.R. Bruce. 1982. Analysis and formation of nitrosamines in the human intestine. *IARC Sci Publ.* **41**:(in press).

Asatoor, A.M. and M.L. Simenhoff. 1965. The origin of urinary dimethylamine. *Biochim. Biophys. Acta* **111**:394.

Bavin, P.M.G., D.W. Darkin, and N.J. Viney. 1982. Total nitroso compounds in gastric juice. *IARC Sci Publ.* **41**:(in press).

Brooks, J.B., W.B. Cherry, L. Thacker, and C.C. Alley. 1972. Analysis by gas chromatography of amines and nitrosamines produced *in vivo* and *in vitro* by *Proteus Mirabilis. J. Infect. Dis.* **126**:143.

Drasar, B.S. and M.J. Hill. 1974. *Human intestinal flora.* Academic Press, New York.

Eisenbrand, G., B. Spiegelhalder, and R. Preussmann. 1981. Analysis of human biological specimens for nitrosamine contents. *Banbury Rep.* **7**:275.

El-Merzabani, M.M., A.A. El-Aasser, and N.I. Zakhary. 1979. A study on the aetiological factors of bilharzial bladder cancer in Egypt–1. Nitrosamines and their precursors in urine. *Eur. J. Cancer* **15**:287.

Fine, D.H., B.C. Challis, P. Hartman, and J. van Ryzin. 1982. Endogenous synthesis of volatile nitrosamines: Model calculations and risk assessment. *IARC Sci. Publ.* **41** (in press).

Fine, D.H., R. Ross, D.P. Rounbehler, A. Silvergleid, and L. Song. 1977. *In vivo* formation of volatile nitrosamines in man following ingestion of cooked bacon and spinach. *Nature* **265**:753.

Gough, T.A., K.S. Webb, M.A. Pringuer, and B.J. Wood. 1977. A comparison of various mass spectrometric and a chemiluminescent method for the estimation of volatile nitrosamines. *J. Agric. Food Chem.* **26**:663.

Harrington, J.S., J.R. Nunn, and L. Irwig. 1973. Dimethylnitrosamine in the human vaginal vault. *Nature* **241**:49.

Hicks, R.M., C.L. Walters, I. Elsebai, A.-B. El Aasser, M. El-Merzabani, and T.A. Gough. 1977. Demonstration of nitrosamines in human urine: Preliminary observations on a possible etiology for bladder cancer in association with chronic urinary tract infections. *Proc. R. Soc. Med.* **70**:413.

Kakizoe, T., T.-T. Wang, V.W.S. Eng, R. Furrer, P. Dion, and W.R. Bruce. 1979. Volatile N-nitrosamines in the urine of normal donors and of bladder cancer patients. *Cancer Res.* **39**:829.

Kowalski, B., C.T. Miller, and N.P. Sen. 1980. Studies on the *in vivo* formation of nitrosamines in rats and humans after ingestion of various meals. *IARC Sci Publ.* **31**:309.

Lakritz, L., M.L. Simenhoff, S.R. Dunn, and W. Fiddler. 1980. N-nitrosodimethylamine in human blood. *Food Cosmet. Toxicol.* **18**:77.

Lijinsky, W. 1980. Significance of *in vivo* formation of N-nitroso compounds. *Oncology* **37**:223.

Mirvish, S.S. 1975. Formation of N-nitroso compounds: Chemistry, kinetics, and *in vivo* occurrence. *Toxic Appl. Pharmacol.* **31**:325.

Ohshima, H. and Bartsch, H. 1981. Quantitative estimation of endogenous nitrosation in man by monitoring N-nitrosoproline excreted in the urine. *Cancer Res.* **41**:3658.

Radomski, J.L., D. Greenwald, W.L. Hearn, N.L. Block, and F.M. Woods. 1978. Nitrosamine formation in bladder infections and its role in the etiology of bladder cancer. *J. Urol.* **120**:48.

Ruddell, W.J.J., and C.L. Walters. 1980. Nitrite and nitroso compounds in gastric juice. *Lancet* i:550.

Spiegelhalder, B., G. Eisenbrand, and R. Preussmann. 1976. Influence of dietary nitrate on nitrite content of human saliva: possible relevance to *in vivo* formation of N-nitroso compounds. *Food Cosmet. Toxicol.* **14**:545.

———. 1982. Urinary excretion of N-nitrosamines in rats and humans. *IARC Sci. Publ.* **41** (in press).

Tannenbaum, S. 1980. A model for estimation of human exposure to endogenous NDMA. *Oncology* **37**:232.

———. 1981. Endogenous formation of *N*-nitroso compounds. *Banbury Rep.* **7**:269.

Terracini, B., P.N. Magee, and J.M. Barnes. 1967. Hepatic pathology in rats on low dietary levels of dimethylnitrosamine. *Br. J. Cancer* **21**:559.

Wang, T., T. Kakizoe, P. Dion, R. Furrer, A.J. Varghese, and W.R. Bruce. 1978. Volatile nitrosamines in normal human faeces. *Nature* **276**:280.

Wishnok, J.S., A.E. Rogers, O. Sanchez, and M.C. Archer. 1978. Dietary effects on the pharmokinetics of three carcinogenic nitrosamines. *Toxicol. Appl. Pharmacol.* **43**:391.

Yamamoto, M., T. Yamada, and S. Tanimura. 1980. Volatile nitrosamines in human blood before and after ingestion of a meal containing high concentrations of nitrate and secondary amines. *Food Cosmet. Toxicol.* **18**:297.

COMMENTS

PREUSSMANN: I want to make a general comment which is probably known to David Fine already. I am very suspicous of all these calculations and this risk assessment. It seems to be a contagious disease.

Just a moment ago you reported you had been working 8 years in the field and these data set you thinking. I have been working for 25 years, like some others in this field, and I simply don't believe so. I have no opposition to discussing such data at a meeting like this; that's perfectly justified. I am fully in favor of discussing it, looking at your assumptions, and discussing whether they are right or wrong.

But publishing such data with the assumptions is another thing. People may just look at your figures, of 50 or 200 cases of cancer. They only look at those figures, and say, "What fools are you that you are working for such a long time for such a low incidence?" That's my problem. In my country, we have had problems with such calculations—and they were, I think, on a firmer basis than these are.

HICKS: I was going to reemphasize your last remarks. It seems to me that it's like the man who loses his keys in front of his door and goes away and looks under the lamp post because that's the only place he can see.

There has been an enormous emphasis by the analysts on looking for NDMA because they can measure it, and for the volatile nitrosamines, generally, because they can measure them. You don't have to go just to amides. Take butylbutanolnitrosamine, which is a known bladder carcinogen. That also would not appear in your volatile fraction, it would appear in the nonvolatiles.

Your assertion, that as far as you can see, volatile nitrosamines are just not around in the body, may be true; but that doesn't mean to say that other nitrosamines and other N-nitroso compounds are not present. It seems to me that there has been a disproportionate emphasis on volatile compounds in all the discussions that have been given so far.

FINE: I agree with your comments very much.

TANNENBAUM: There is another really critical factor here, David. Your calculations are based on the results of the Ohshima and Bartsch experiment on one person. I think that maybe the critical point—and I'm not sure that Phil Hartman would agree with me on this—is that there are people who may be predisposed to forming much larger amounts of these compounds because of other conditions physiologically, such as intestinal metaplasia, which would lead to a much higher rate of formation. Bladder infections are another case. It may be that taking the normal person and extrapolating to the whole population is a big mistake, because the high-risk people are not necessarily the people who are exposed to a lot of nitrate. The high-risk people are the people who, for some reason or other, make a lot of nitrosating agent. We just don't know how to assess that yet.

LIJINSKY: But you can't average in this business.

MICHEJDA: That is exactly the point that I wanted to make. This type of model, and every model of this type, does not recognize hot spots. The fact is that this does not include occupational exposure, and it doesn't include a whole host of factors which we have all talked about—which you talked about, David.

FINE: The occupational exposure was included in that high-risk group. It is a small population group with a very high exposure. It included, for example, 250 μg/day exposure from five workers. Occupational exposure is very high, but only a relatively few workers are involved.

MICHEJDA: But you know very well that with the NDELA workers, people eat sandwiches in factories which are spraying out this stuff. I'm sure their intake of nitrosamine is much, much higher than even your high-risk exposure data would suggest. None of these things can be accounted for in a general kind of model.

FINE: But what would you suggest doing instead? We could stay where we are and not make a first step and not progress, or move on. What I am really trying to stress is we know from the in vitro data that there are other compounds which nitrosate much more rapidly. Why only stay with the ones which we can measure, when we know others are more important?

WEISBURGER: Perhaps. But what we need to do is to go back to realistic human environmental data.

MICHEJDA: I don't think this is real evidence against this. That's the point.

SEN: David, going back to the question of nitrosamines in human blood, the volunteers were on a high nitrogen diet including bacon and beer. We also had a diet with smoked meat containing high levels of NPIP—and in all of those cases, NPIR levels and NPIP amounts present in the diet was much more than NDMA in the beer or NDMA in the other diet. We never saw any NPYR or NPIP in the bladder, which will explain that they are probably metabolizing fast. Alcohol didn't seem to make any difference. The NDMA we saw in our case—we analyzed a total of 50 samples, and out of those 10 were positive at low levels. We don't know whether they are real or artifact. But we didn't see any NPIP or NPYR. Do you have any comments on that?

FINE: I think if alcohol is present, the resulting peak with a meal may be real. I think the background level that we showed before the meal, is probably not real. That's the point that I'm getting at, this background level is probably not real. That's the point that I'm getting at, this background level is probably not there—just because they are metabolized so fast.

SWANN: Isn't this really the critical point? If you accept that the levels you got with the alcohol were real—0.5 μg/liter of blood. The volume of distribution is roughly the same as the mass of the individual, that would give 0.5×70 μg/person, which by my rough calculation is about 10^{-7} moles. This differs from Brian Challis' calculation by a factor of 10^7.

It seems to me that there is something not quite resolved here. A factor of 2 or 10 is one thing; but 10^7 is something else.

CHALLIS: Just a few words about this averaging. In the SmithKline French data, they have individual patients. We took an average—although we really wanted to do a statistically balanced median variable. But it turns out that's impossible to do, because when you do it and take a proper statistical mean, all of the nitrite exposures end up being zero. So, what comes out of this is that you have to do it for each patient. If you now do it for each patient, or each subject, the differences in concentrations, the amount you produce, are about 100. In other words, we would raise our levels by a factor of 100. It's not an enormous figure.

There is no standard man therefore it's probably not worthwhile to try to do averages. You have to concentrate on each individual person.

WEISBURGER: Could you give us an idea whether there are any nitrosamine blood levels you have measured in China, Dr. Bartsch?

BARTSCH: It's too early to present these data.

FINE: Let me just go back to the point that Peter Swann raised. You are assuming in your calculation that the nitrosamine is evenly distributed throughout the body mass. I am not sure if that's a valid point. Based on Dr. Preussmann's urine excretion analysis, where nitrosamines in beer drinkers urine could be picked up. That wasn't based on the distribution throughout the body, was it? You had a lot of the nitrosamine collected in the urine, didn't you? Dr. Preussmann.

TANNENBAUM: It's valid. It's absolutely valid.

SWANN: The two things are not connected. I mean, Professor Magee showed 25 years ago that, although large doses of NDMA were distributed throughout the whole of the body water of the animal, 2-3% was excreted in the urine. Preussmann's data are 2%.

MIRVISH: I just want to emphasize the point that with the amides you get much more nitroso compound than for the amines because in the amides the nitrosation kinetics are proportional to nitrite; whereas, for the amines it is proportional to $[nitrite]^2$. Now, if there is a catalyst involved in the nitrosamine formation, it is proportional to nitrite. I believe this point was made before. It will become much more important at very low nitrite levels. I'm not sure we can discard the possibility of a catalyst at very low amine-nitrosamine levels.

MAGEE: I just wanted to comment. Toward the end of your talk, you remarked that if this had been methylurea and not proline, the nitrosation would have been very much more rapid. I think that methylurea is a compound that we really ought to be looking for, because, in terms of being a carcinogen, nitrosomethylurea is about the best one to explain any tumor you'd like to mention. On the list of organs of tumors caused by nitroso compounds, you could have just about said "by methylnitrosourea." It's just more versatile, in terms of organs, than any other nitrosamine.
    We don't really know whether methylurea does occur very much.

FINE: Kawabata has looked for it and has not found it.

TANNENBAUM: At least in food.

References

Kawabata, T., H. Ohshima, and M. Ino. 1978. Occurrence of methyl guanidine and agmatine, nitrosatable guanido compounds in food. *J. Agric. Food Chem.* 26:334.

Presence of Nitrosamines in Blood of Normal and Diseased Human Subjects

MICHAEL L. SIMENHOFF, STEPHEN R. DUNN,
AND R. GARTH KIRKWOOD
Division of Nephrology
Department of Medicine
Jefferson Medical College of
Thomas Jefferson University
Philadelphia, Pennsylvania 19107

WALTER FIDDLER AND JOHN W. PENSABENE
The Eastern Regional Research Center
United States Department of Agriculture
Philadelphia, Pennsylvania 19118

We have entered the nitrosamine field through an unusual route. Some years ago while investigating the biochemical aspects of uremic toxicity, using, at first, dinitrophenyl derivitization with reverse phase paper chromatography for primary and secondary amines (Simenhoff et al. 1963) and then gas chromatography (GC) to include trimethylamine (TMA) (Dunn et al. 1976), we found that the methylamines, dimethylamine (DMA) and TMA, were markedly raised in the blood of patients with chronic end-stage kidney failure. Subsequent investigation in the latter showed these compounds in tissues and biological fluids including cerebrospinal fluid (Simenhoff 1975). While investigating the origin of these we detected a significant exogenous and endogenous component—the former generated mainly via choline and lecithin which was then degraded by bacteria to give TMA; the TMA was then demethylated, probably in the liver, to DMA. The DMA, an end metabolite in man, was then excreted in the urine (Fig. 1) (Asatoor and Simenhoff 1965). Obviously in renal failure this metabolite would accumulate in the body fluids. We proceeded to demonstrate an increased generation of this compound in the intestinal fluid of patients with advanced renal failure coincident with marked bacterial overgrowth of both anaerobes and aerobes (Simenhoff et al. 1976, 1978). It then came to our attention that there seemed to be, from various reports, an increase in the incidence of cancer in patients with chronic renal failure particularly among those on dialysis (Matas et al. 1976; Miach et al. 1976; Sutherland et al. 1977; Lindner et al. 1981). Since the important N-nitrosodimethylamine (NDMA) precursor, DMA, was present in patients with renal failure in increased amounts and since bacterial overgrowth in the small bowel was present, the conditions seemed

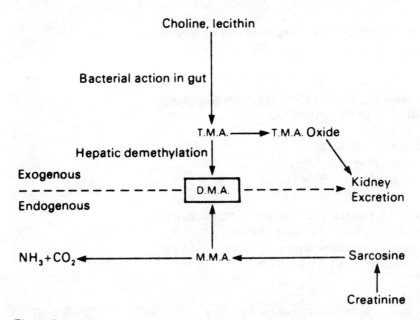

Figure 1
In vivo metabolic scheme for the methylamines not including possible bacterial transformations. (MMA) methylamine; DMA; TMA.

favorable for possible in vivo NDMA formation. Since reporting our NDMA results in blood of healthy subjects (Lakritz et al. 1980), we have extended the data in this category, as well as including blood NDMA concentrations in various diseased states.

EXPERIMENTAL PROCEDURES

Methods

The methodology for volatile nitrosamines was developed at the Eastern Regional Research Center of the United States Department of Agriculture, Philadelphia. Analyses were performed using modifications of current methodology that utilized gas liquid chromatography and a thermal energy analyzer (TEA) (W. Fiddler et al. unpubl. results). Selected samples were subsequently photolyzed to confirm the presumptive presence of NDMA, using the method of Doerr and Fiddler (1977). Selected pooled samples were also confirmed by either high-or low-resolution mass spectrometry (MS) (Kimoto et al. 1981; Kimoto and Fiddler 1982).

Patient Population

Information on 236 different blood samples involving 319 patients and the discrepancy between these two numbers relates to pooled samples and multiple samples in selected individuals.

The patient population discussed includes ambulatory subjects, hospitalized patients without renal failure, cancer patients, and patients with renal failure.

Dialysis Population

Additionally water was analyzed for NDMA at various sites in the hemodialysis purification system at 26 different dialysis centers in the Delaware Valley. Blood was drawn pre-dialysis, 15 minutes into dialysis, and immediately post-dialysis in 31 patients. The subjects were divided into Group I and Group II, the former consisting of those patients who were treated in dialysis units where water treatment did not contain a deionizer (DI) or a DI either with a preceeding carbon filter or followed by UV light downstream. Group II patients were from those units containing a deionizer but without carbon filter or UV light modules. The deionizer normally removes anionic and cationic compounds from the water because it contains mixed strong anionic and cationic resin. The anionic resin contains a quaternary ammonium group.

RESULTS AND DISCUSSION

Of 161 bloods analyzed for volatile nitrosamines by GC/TEA, 120 demonstrated NDMA to be present. In rare samples trace amounts of N-nitrosodiethylamine, N-nitrosopiperdine, and N-nitrosomorpholine were seen but not quantified. Figure 2 shows our results in normal subjects and hospitalized patients and especially in cancer and renal failure patients. These results suggest that there are small amounts of NDMA in the blood without significant differences between the groups with one qualification (see Fig. 3). This shows the differences in NDMA concentrations after the institution of additional control blanks and added ascorbic acid in the method of analysis, after 1978. The results on 38 of 58 subjects in 1978 were previously published (Lakritz et al. 1980) and with these procedural modifications we still demonstrate NDMA in normal blood, although at a lower mean level. The range now is from 0-0.8 μg/kg.

I would like to just digress briefly—in relation to that rather elegant presentation by Drs. Garland and Conney—and point out that we also do not usually find any NDMA in the blood with 8 ml samples. The critical point that I would like to emphasize for those who do not do these measurements, is that the work-up of the sample involving distillation and extraction procedures, and so forth, brings the sample down to 1 ml, no matter what sample size you start with. If you start with 8 ml blood the end result is 1 ml. If you start with 100 ml blood the end result is 1 ml. So, the size of the sample is critical in determin-

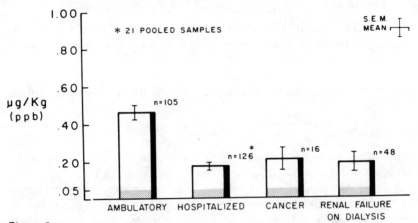

Figure 2
NDMA blood levels in healthy and diseased states. (▫) minimum detectable limit; (n) number subjects represented; (*) 126 patients; 21 pools of 6 patients each.

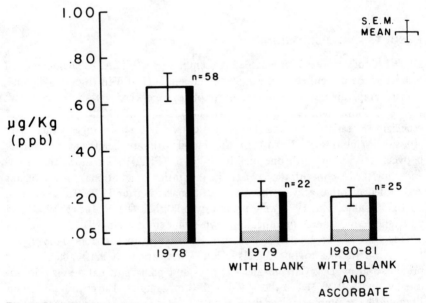

Figure 3
NDMA blood levels in ambulatory subjects. NDMA found in blank was subtracted from blood NDMA to give a true blood level. (▫) indicates minimum detectable limit; (n) number subjects represented. The blank used in 1979, 1980, and 1981 consisted of water in place of blood. 35-45 mg ascorbate was added to flask to inhibit possible nitrosamine formation during distillation.

ing how much you are going to measure. I want to emphasize that our samples were a minimum of 25 ml blood, and usually more. That is very important to realize.

Longitudinal Studies

Two subjects with blood samples over a 4-year span, are shown in Figure 4. Although there is a tendency for levels to decrease during the latter years when special blanks and ascorbate were added in the analyses, NDMA was low or absent within each time period, including 1978.

Cancer Patients

We examined blood from 16 cancer patients (Fig. 5) and separated those with severe liver metastases to identify possible differences in blood NDMA levels. A high level might indicate defective dealkylation of NDMA. Certain patients gave high levels but no trends were evident.

Renal Failure Patients

A series of renal failure patients is illustrated in Figure 6. Mean blood NDMA was lower in end-stage kidney failure patients on dialysis, compared to healthy

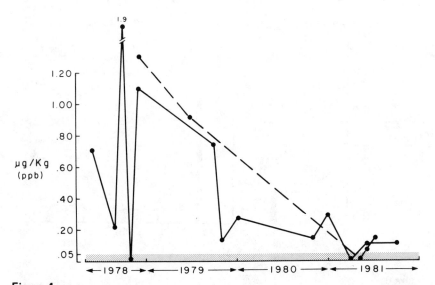

Figure 4
NDMA blood levels of two individuals during 4 years. Liver metastases was determined by isotopic scanning of liver. (◻) indicates minimum detectable limit.

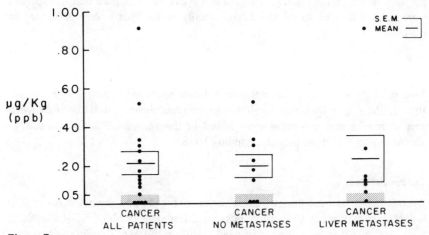

Figure 5
NDMA blood levels in 16 cancer patients. (□) indicates minimum detectable limit.

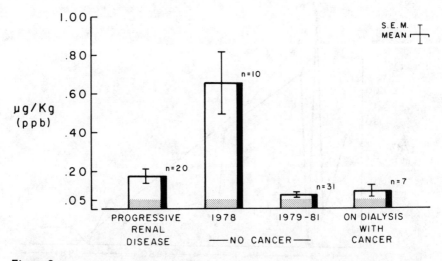

Figure 6
NDMA blood levels in renal failure. The 1978 determinations are distinguished from those in 1979-81 by use of blanks and ascorbate as in Figure 3. (□) indicates minimum detectable limit; (n) number subjects represented; (progressive renal disease) patients not on dialysis but with measurable decreased renal function of varying degree.

subjects (Fig. 7) being statistically significant at the 95% level using the Rank Sum Test. However, at such a low level of detection the question arises as to whether or not these differences are real. A subset of 7 patients was seen that had both uremia and cancer, but no increased level of blood NDMA was demonstrated as shown in Figure 6. Patients in early renal failure did not show this lower NDMA level, but the number of patients was too small to determine whether the degree of renal failure played a significant role.

True vs. Artifactual NDMA Measurements

Important considerations are whether the NDMA that we are measuring in the blood is due to artifact of the analytical method, or whether this represents authentic NDMA from reabsorption from external preformed sources, or from endogenous in vivo formation.

We feel artifactual formation has been largely eliminated by special reagent blanks and addition of ascorbate. The distillation should eliminate volatile nitrosating species. Further, the sequential acid followed by base back-washes (between the distillation and concentration procedures), eliminate amine and other aqueous substrates.

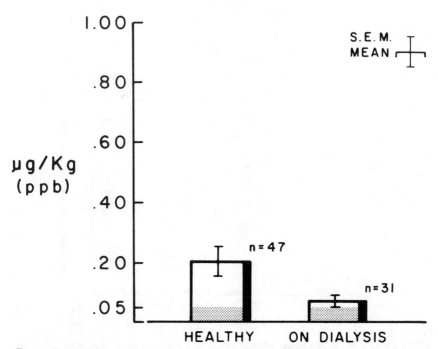

Figure 7
NDMA blood levels in healthy and dialysis patients. All determinations of NDMA included the use of blanks and ascorbate. (▣) indicates minimum detectable limit; (n) subjects represented.

NDMA Contamination in Renal Dialysis Units

During this time while we were investigating the presence of nitrosamines in the blood of patients with kidney failure from dialysis units in the Delaware Valley area, we stumbled upon an unexpected finding. Serendipity and discovery are among the oldest partners in history. The nurse forgot to take a pre-dialysis blood specimen from the patient and so obtained it about 15 minutes into dialysis—the NDMA level was high, especially for a uremic patient, and we thought it was an error. However, when repeated on the same patient at the same dialysis unit it was still high, but low in an analogous blood sample from a different unit. We then looked at the dialysis water of patients undergoing chronic hemodialysis.

Certain dialysate water contained large quantities of NDMA yet the municipal water prior to the purification system contained minimal to none (Fig. 8). On sampling from each module it was found that the deionizer was the source of the NDMA formation. It was clear, therefore, that these patients were being dialyzed against a water bath containing large amounts of NDMA. The results of blood NDMA levels for Group I and II patients pre-dialysis, 15 minutes into dialysis and post-dialysis are shown in Figure 9. There was a significant blood level of NDMA at 15 minutes and post-dialysis in Group II patients. Two patients with NDMA levels in dialysate as well as blood samples going to and

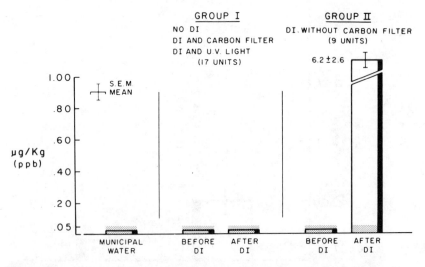

Figure 8
NDMA levels in water for hemodialysate before and after deionizer. Municipal water was collected from cold water tap. (DI) deionizer; (▨) indicates minimum detectable limit. (before) water prior to going to the DI; (after) water emerging from DI.

from the dialyzer coil are shown in Figure 10. The NDMA is being picked up in the blood going to the patient. The higher the NDMA was in dialysate, the higher it was in the blood.

Our survey of a number of dialysis units enabled us to obtain further samples in this way and we were able to clearly demonstrate that despite a significant intravenous load of NDMA, the blood NDMA levels disappeared very rapidly.

CONCLUSIONS

The conclusion that the blood NDMA concentration is a poor reflection of nitrosamine load from intravenous exposure might also apply to hepatic load from the digestive tract; and hepatic dealkylation of NDMA has been reported (Magee and Farber 1962; Montesano and Magee 1970).

In conclusion, we have shown low but measurable NDMA levels in the blood in a spectrum of health and disease, and that the level of blood nitrosamine does not necessarily reflect the body burden or load of NDMA.

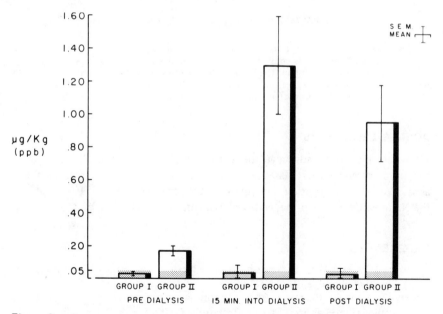

Figure 9
NDMA blood levels during hemodialysis. Pre-dialysis blood was drawn from the patient immediately before dialysis was begun. 15 min into dialysis, blood was again drawn from the arterial blood line. This line came directly from patient to the dialyzer coil. Post-dialysis arterial blood was drawn immediately after dialysis. Groups I and II are explained in Figure 8. (◘) indicates minimum detectable limit.

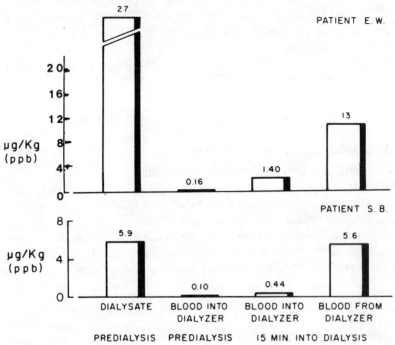

Figure 10
NDMA dialyzer levels. Blood into dialyzer is coming directly from patient (arterial blood line). Blood from dialyzer is coming directly from dialysis coil and will be returning to patient via the venous blood line. The blood in the dialyzer coil comes into equilibrium with the dialysate which is separated from the blood by a semi-permeable cupraphane or cellulose acetate membrane. (¤) indicates minimum detectable limit.

ACKNOWLEDGMENTS

We would like to acknowledge the assistance of Walt Kimoto, Ph.D. for mass spectrometry and Robert Gates, Steve Gorman, and Judith Foster for technical assistance. The investigation was supported by Grant No. CA 26571, awarded by the National Cancer Institute, National Institutes of Health, DHHS.

REFERENCES

Asatoor, A.M. and M.L. Simenhoff. 1965. The origin of urinary dimethylamine. *Biochim. Biophys. Acta* III:384.

Doerr, R. and W. Fiddler. 1977. Photolysis of volatile nitrosamines at the picogram level as an aid to confirmation. *J. Chromatog.* 140:284.

Dunn, S.R., M.L. Simenhoff, and L.G. Wesson. 1976. Gas chromatographic determination of mono-, di- and trimethylamines in biological fluids. *Anal. Chem.* 48:41.

Kimoto, W.I. and W. Fiddler. 1982. Confirmatory method for N-nitrosodimethylamine and N-nitrosoproline in food samples by multiple ion analysis with gas chromatography–low resolution mass spectrometry before and after U-V photolysis. *J. Assoc. Off. Anal. Chem.* (in press).

Kimoto, W.I., C.J. Dooley, J. Carré, and W. Fiddler. 1981. Nitrosamines in tap water after concentration by a carbonaceous adsorbent. *Water Res.* 15: 1099.

Lakritz, L., M.L. Simenhoff, S.R. Dunn, and W. Fiddler. 1980. N-nitrosodimethylamine in human blood. *Food Cosmet. Toxicol.* 18:77.

Lindner, A., V.T. Farewell, and D.J. Sherrard. 1981. High incidence of neoplasia in uremic patients receiving long-term dialysis. *Nephron* 27:292.

Magee, P.N. and E. Farber. 1962. Toxic liver injury and carcinogenesis. *Biochem. J.* 83:114.

Matas, A.J., R.L. Simmonds, C.M. Kjellstrand, T.J. Buselmeier, and J.S. Najarian. 1975. Increased incidence of malignancy during chronic renal failure. *Lancet* i:883.

Miach, P.J., J.K. Dawborn, and J. Xippel. 1976. Neoplasia in patients with chronic renal failure on long-term dialysis. *Clin. Nephrol.* 5:101.

Montesano, R. and P.N. Magee. 1970. Metabolism of dimethylnitrosamine by human liver slices *in vitro. Nature* 228:173.

Simenhoff, M.L. 1975. Metabolism and toxicity of aliphatic amines. *Kidney Int.* 7:S314.

Simenhoff, M.L., M.D. Milne, and A. Asatoor. 1963. Retention of aliphatic amines in uremia. *Clin. Sci.* 25:65.

Simenhoff, M.L., J.J. Saukkonen, J.F. Burke, L.G. Wesson, and R.W. Schaedler. 1976. Amine metabolism and the small bowel in uremia. *Lancet* ii:818.

Simenhoff, M.L., J.J. Saukkonen, J.F. Burke, L.G. Wesson, R.W. Schaedler, and S. Gordon. 1978. Bacterial populations of the small bowel in uremia. *Nephron* 22:460.

Sutherland, G.A., J. Glass, and R. Gabriel. 1977. Increased incidence of malignancy in chronic renal failure. *Nephron* 18:182.

COMMENTS

MIRVISH: I didn't understand something. An important finding from your results is how quickly NDMA disappears after dialysis. How quickly does it disappear?

SIMENHOFF: That's a good question. Unfortunately, patients aren't like rats. We tried to persuade the patient to stay for 1 hour after the dialysis so that we could get sequential blood samples. We obviously couldn't let the situation go on for very long. This is a very critical ethical problem. In fact, we only got one sample. We also went to the patients' homes to get blood from them, because after the dialysis they just don't want to stay around. It's very difficult to persuade them. You can't say, "Look, we have this cancer agent being infused into your blood and we really want you to stay so we can measure it."

So, unfortunately, we do not have good data on the follow-up. But I can say that within 6 hours or so, it's back to almost the pre-dialysis level.

SWANN: Yes, but you could calculate from the data you have.

SIMENHOFF: But, you see, there's a problem, because you're also dialyzing.

MIRVISH: No. You could calculate from the data you have.

SIMENHOFF: Well, I will tell you what the exposure is. We have actually estimated a range of 0.5-4.5 μg/min being infused into the patient. There are 3 dialyses a week. This leads to a range of exposure of 0.1-1.08 mg/week; and 1.4-12.9 mg/mo.; and over 150 mg/year.

TANNENBAUM: But do you have data as to how fast this is disappearing from the bloodstream? You have a reservoir which contains NDMA.

SIMENHOFF: It's not constant. It's within reason. For example, we had one value of 27. Another lower value was found, but I don't recall it. Unfortunately, it's not reproducible. I think when you have a value of 27 and you take a number of samples, it will reasonably be at that high level.

TANNENBAUM: It doesn't fall with time?

SIMENHOFF: With the same DI, the same municipal water, when you do it on 1 day it will be 27, on the next day it will be 5.6. It will always be high, but it won't be constant for a given DI and a given water system. That's part of the problem.

PEGG: What percentage of dialysis machines are involved in the set up that you described?

SIMENHOFF: I can't give you that number. I have a great deal of difficulty getting the information.

As I indicated before, in one of the units which had very high levels, within hours of putting a carbon filter on-line, the NDMA disappeared from the DI. There were not high nitrite levels and amine levels in the water. And, Kimoto has shown, at much lower levels, that if you boil the water you no longer form NDMA in the DI (Kimoto et al. 1981).

An additional interesting thing was that there was a high incidence of cancer in one group near Seattle, and they were dialyzing just with the DI. We asked them to send us water coming from that DI without these other qualifications, such as the carbon filters, UV, and so forth; and there was no NDMA.

So it looks like certain waters maybe have oxides of nitrogen or some of these other volatile nitrosating species that aren't related to the nitrite and to the amine. And the quaternary ammonium group in the DI provides some of that.

MONTESANO: It is correct that some of these dialyzed patients have signs of liver toxicity. This has been attributed to toluate. It could be that this level of nitrosamine can contribute.

SIMENHOFF: This is obviously an important point. The difficulty is that these patients are at risk from a number of hepatotoxic agents—Australia antigen—positive hepatitis is very common in the group. Many of the drugs they take are hepatotoxic and this factor was taken into consideration.

So you have such a background of at-risk factors for chronic liver disease, that it would be very difficult to evaluate this. But I agree with your point.

HOFFMANN: Are these data new?

SIMENHOFF: We presented this work at the International Congress on Nephrology in Greece in June.

HOFFMANN: But I assume these data will be available soon in the medical literature.

SIMENHOFF: Yes. You know, it's very interesting you raised that. People are not too anxious to publish it.

HOFFMANN: Therefore, that answers the question.

WEISBURGER: What is the average age of these patients?

SIMENHOFF: The ages vary from about 20-65. Some of them are younger; some of them are older. It's quite a wide range of age.

MONTESANO: You mentioned that DMA is not metabolized.

SIMENHOFF: As far as we know, aside from the microbiology literature, in man, DMA is an end metabolite. It is not metabolized.

MONTESANO: I did some experiments with tissue slices using C^{14} DMA, and I found a lot of activity in the guanine and adenine.

SIMENHOFF: I would be very interested in seeing that.

Monitoring of Excreted
N-Nitrosamino Acids as a
New Method to Quantitate
Endogenous Nitrosation in Humans

HIROSHI OHSHIMA, BRIGITTE PIGNATELLI, AND HELMUT BARTSCH
Programme of Environmental Carcinogens and Host Factors
International Agency for Research on Cancer
F-69372 Lyon Cedex 08, France

Human exposure to carcinogenic N-nitroso compounds may result from ingestion or inhalation of preformed compounds in the environment or from nitrosation of amino precursors in the body. Although limited data exist to quantitate human exposure, endogenous formation of N-nitroso compounds from ingested precursors may be the largest single source of exposure to these compounds for the general population (Coordinating Committee for Scientific and Technical Assessment of Environmental Pollutants 1978).

The formation of N-nitroso compounds in experimental animals in vivo has been demonstrated by identifying nitrosated products in the stomach contents (Sander and Schweinsberg 1972; Braunberg and Dailey 1973; Mirvish 1975) or in the whole animal (Rounbehler et al. 1977) after feeding relatively high doses of precursors. Formation in vivo has also been demonstrated in human subjects who ingested diphenylamine and nitrate, by detecting N-nitrosodiphenylamine (NDPhA) in their stomachs (Sander and Seif 1969). Although the endogenous formation of N-nitroso compounds from precursors has been proven, the extent to which nitrosation reactions occur in humans ingesting typical levels of nitrate, nitrite and nitrosatable compounds has not yet been determined. Moreover, any nitrosation reaction is influenced by many factors such as pH, amounts of precursors involved, basicity of the amine, and the presence of catalysts or inhibitors. Although these factors have been studied in in vitro systems, the lack of suitable methods for estimating endogenous nitrosation has hampered attempts to investigate them under in vivo conditions.

For all these reasons, we have recently developed a simple and sensitive method for the quantitative estimation of nitrosation reaction occurring in vivo (Ohshima and Bartsch 1981a; Ohshima et al. 1982a). It is based on our findings and reports in the literature (Dailey et al. 1975; Chu and Magee 1981) that certain N-nitrosamino acids, such as N-nitrosoproline (NPRO), are excreted almost quantitatively unchanged in the urine and feces.

Results obtained from the application of this method to study a number of factors affecting the nitrosation in vivo in rats as well as in humans, after administration of nitrosatable amino acids and nitrosating agents, are described. The utility of the method to carry out clinical and field studies in human subjects at high risk for stomach and esophageal cancer, is briefly discussed.

MATERIALS AND METHODS

Analysis of N-Nitroso Compounds in the Urine and Feces

Urine samples were spiked with N-nitrosopipecolic acid (NPIC) (as internal standard), and analysis for NPRO and N-nitrososarcosine (NSAR) was carried out according to a published procedure (Ohshima and Bartsch 1981a; Ohshima et al. 1982a) after conversion of the nitrosamines to their methyl esters by means of diazomethane (Kawabata 1974). The N-nitrosohydroxyproline (NHPRO) methyl ester was further converted to its O-acetyl derivative before chromatography.

A Tracor 550 gas chromatograph (Austin, TX) was used with argon carrier gas (20 ml/min) and interfaced to a Thermal Energy Analyzer (TEA 502, Thermo Electron Corp., Waltham, MA). The average recoveries of NPRO, NSAR, and NHPRO added to the urine samples at a concentration of 20 μg/l were 85, 82 and 43%, with minimum detectable levels of 0.5, 0.1 and 2 μg/l, respectively. Under these conditions, the peaks of the methyl esters of NPRO and NPIC were well resolved (retention times: 11.2 and 9.3 minutes, respectively), and no interfering peaks appeared on the chromatogram.

RESULTS

Monitoring of Excreted N-Nitrosamino Acids as a New Method to Quantitate Endogenous Nitrosation in Rodents and in Humans

Urinary and fecal excretion of orally administered N-nitrosamino acids and N-nitrosamines in rats was described by Ohshima et al. (1982a). Table 1 summarizes the urinary and fecal excretion of three N-nitrosamino acids and two aliphatic N-nitrosamines following their oral administration to fasting rats. N-Nitrosamino acids were found to be excreted almost quantitatively in the urine and feces per se within the first 24 hours. The excretion pattern in the urine and feces was dependent on the compound: ≥ 97% of the excreted amount of NPRO and NSAR was detected in the urine, whereas about 50% of the excreted NHPRO was found in both the urine and feces. On the other hand, when similar doses of N-nitrosodimethylamine (NDMA) and N-nitrosopyrrolidine (NPYR), both potent liver carcinogens, were administered orally to fasting rats, not even traces of the unchanged compound could be detected either in the urine or the feces (Table 1).

These results demonstrate that N-nitrosamino acids, when administered orally to rats, are excreted unchanged in the urine and feces almost quanti-

Table 1
Urinary and Fecal Excretion of N-nitroso Compounds Administered Orally To Rats (50-μg doses)

Compound	% Excretion[a]		
	Urine	Feces	Total
NPRO	96.5 ± 0.8	2.5 ± 0.9	98.9
NHPRO	46.8 ± 2.2	46.2 ± 3.2	92.9
NSAR	87.7 ± 2.4	0.07 ± 0.01	87.8
NDMA	<0.01	<0.01	<0.01
NPYR	<0.05	<0.05	<0.05

Reprinted, with permission, from Ohshima et al. (1982a)
[a]1 ml 0.9% saline containing an N-nitroso compound was gavaged to a group of 10 fasting rats. The urine and feces were collected separately for 24 hours. Values are means of 10 rats ± SD.

tatively. They have been reported to be weakly carcinogenic (NSAR) or non-carcinogenic (NPRO, NHPRO) (IARC 1978; Mirvish et al. 1980). The low carcinogenic potential of these compounds may probably be due in part to their high and fast elimination rates from the body, as conversion to their ultimate carcinogenic forms through α-c-hydroxylation appears to be blocked: the N-nitrosamino acids tested contain a carboxyl group at the carbon atom adjacent to the N-nitroso group.

A comparison of the yield of nitrosated product formed in vivo from proline, hydroxyproline, and sarcosine was carried out, as the formation of N-nitroso compounds is known to depend on the basicity of the nitrosatable amino compounds. Nitrosation in vivo of the amino acids, proline, and sarcosine was estimated from the amounts of N-nitrosamino acid excreted in the urine. Formation in vivo of NHPRO was determined from the total amount of NHPRO excreted in the urine and feces (Table 2). All the results were corrected for the excretion rates of the N-nitrosamino acids. After feeding an amino acid precursor and nitrite, the yield of N-nitrosamino acids formed in vivo and excreted increased in the order: NPRO < NSAR < NHPRO. The same order was seen when the nitrosation rates of the amino acids in vitro were compared. Thus, N-nitrosation in vivo in rats occurs via a similar mechanism to that observed in vitro. Monitoring of N-nitrosamino acids excreted in the urine and feces thus appears to provide a valuable index for endogenous N-nitrosation.

Effect of Single and Multiple Doses of Sodium Nitrite and Proline on NPRO Formation In Vivo in Rats

The effect on NPRO formation in vivo of a single dose of nitrite and proline was examined by measuring NPRO excreted in the 24-hour urine after oral administration of the precursors at various concentrations (Ohshima et al.

Table 2

Nitrosation In vivo and In vitro of Proline, Sarcosine, and Hydroxyproline

	N-Nitrosamino acid formed	
Compound	In vivo[a] nmol (relative yield)	In vitro[b] nmol (relative yield)
NPRO	24.0 ± 3.5 (1.0)[c]	101.8 (1.0)
NSAR	109.6 ± 21.3 (4.6)	428.8 (4.2)
NHPRO	174.3 ± 46.7 (7.3)	703.3 (6.9)

Reprinted, with permission, from Ohshima et al. (1982a)

[a]10 μmol amino acid in pH 3 buffer, was gavaged to groups of 10 fasted rats, followed by 10 μmol sodium nitrite in water. Formation in vivo of NPRO and NSAR was estimated from the amounts excreted in the 24-hr urine. Formation in vivo of NHPRO was estimated from a total amount of the NHPRO excreted in the urine and feces for 24 hours. All results were corrected for the excretion rate of the N-nitrosamino acid. Values are means of 10 rats ± SD.

[b]The reaction mixture consisting of 10 μmol amino acid in pH 3 buffer, and 10 μmol sodium nitrite in water were incubated at 37°C for 15 min (final pH 3). Values are means of two experiments.

[c]Ratio of the yield of the N-nitrosamino acid to that of NPRO are given in parenthesis.

1982a). The amount of NPRO excreted was found to be proportional to the dose of proline (the nitrite dose was kept constant) and to the square of the nitrite dose (the proline dose was kept constant). Thus, as shown in Figure 1, the nitrosation kinetics in rats were found to be of first order kinetics with respect to the proline dose and second order with respect to the nitrite dose. The results obtained in vivo were compatible with the kinetic data on the in vitro nitrosation of proline (represented by the dotted line in Fig. 1). At a dose of 10 μmol each proline and nitrite, the excretion of NPRO in the urine amounted to 3325 ng/24 hours, which is 136 times the background level. Considering the urinary excretion rate of NPRO to be 96.2% (mean recovery of two different doses), the amounts of NPRO formed in the rat in vivo can be estimated (3456 ng, 24.0 nmol). Thus, the yield of NPRO formed from 10 μmol each proline and nitrite in vivo was 0.24%.

A dose-response study on NPRO formation in rats in vivo was also carried out after concurrent administration of proline and nitrite to rats. Up to 50,000 ppm proline was given in the diet and up to 4,000 ppm sodium nitrite in the drinking water, in order to avoid any chemical interaction before ingestion. The total amount of NPRO excreted in the urine and feces was measured as an index of endogenous nitrosation of proline. Figure 2 shows a log-log plot of the amount of NPRO formed in vivo versus the precursor dose (proline) (nitrite)^2 which was calculated from the food and water consumption for each rat. Linear regression analysis yielded the following equation:

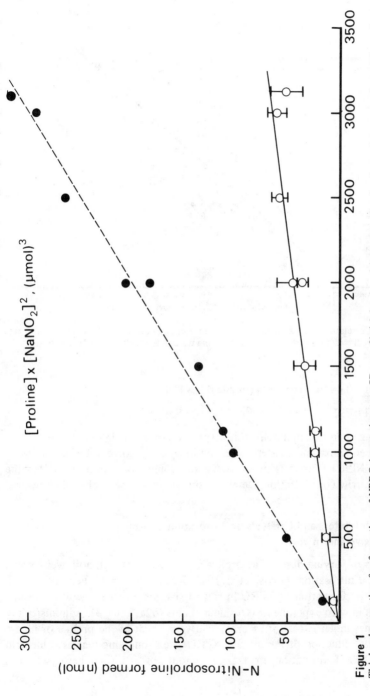

Figure 1

Third-order reaction for formation of NPRO in rats (mean ± SD; n = 3) (○) in vivo; (●) in vitro. In vivo formation was estimated from the amount excreted in 24-hr urine after administration of 0-30 μmol proline in pH 3 buffer, and pH 3 buffer containing proline (kept constant at 10 μmol), followed by 0-25 mol nitrite solution. Amounts of NPRO obtained in both experiments are plotted as a function of (proline) × (nitrite)². In vitro formation was determined by incubating the same precursor solutions used in the in vivo experiments at 37°C for 15 min (ph 3, final volume 1 ml). Mean values of 2 experiments are plotted. Reprinted, with permission, from Ohshima et al. (1982a).

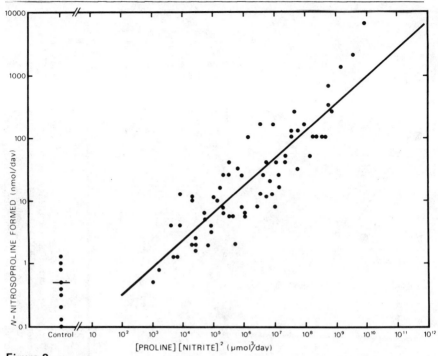

Figure 2

Dose-response relationship between NPRO formation and concurrent administration to rats of proline (in the diet) and nitrite (in the drinking water); for further details, see text.

$$\log(\text{NPRO}) = 0.44 \log [(\text{proline}) (\text{nitrite})^2] - 1.38 \qquad (1)$$

$$(r = 0.88; n = 79)$$

NPRO being expressed in nmol/rat/day; (proline) (nitrite)^2 in μmol^3.

   This equation is consistent with the kinetics for nitrosation of proline in vitro, i.e., NPRO formed is proportional to proline concentration and to the square of nitrite concentration. Details of this study will be published elsewhere.

Effects of Inhibitors and Catalysts on Nitrosation of Proline in Rats In vivo and In vitro

The effects of varying doses of ascorbic acid and α-tocopherol, both well-known inhibitors of nitrosation (Mirvish et al. 1972; Kamm et al. 1977; Pensabene et al. 1978), on the formation of NPRO in rats in vivo are compared with the results obtained in in vitro experiments (Ohshima et al. 1982a; Table 3). Administration of a 10-times molar excess of ascorbic acid versus that of the proline or nitrite resulted in a reduction of the urinary NPRO levels, implying that ascorbic acid inhibited NPRO formation in rats by about 98%. α-Tocopherol was less

Table 3

Effects of Ascorbic Acid and α-Tocopherol on In Vivo and In Vitro NPRO Formation

Compound	mol	In vivo		In vitro	
		NPRO formed nmol	Inhibition (%)	NPRO formed nmol	Inhibition (%)
Ascorbic acid	0	24.0 ± 3.5	0	101.8	0
	1	19.2 ± 7.6	20	85.6	15
	10	4.6 ± 0.8	81	3.8	96
	100	0.56 ± 0.04	98	0.2	99.8
α-Tocopherol	0	13.7 ± 5.1	0	9.7	0
	1	11.5 ± 1.7	16	5.4	44
	10	7.3 ± 2.2	47	4.8	51.5
	100	6.6 ± 0.6	52	4.2	57

Reprinted, with permission, from Ohshima et al. (1982a)

[a]Groups of 10 fasting rats were gavaged with pH 3 buffer containing 10 μmol proline and 0-100 μmol ascorbic acid, followed by 0.5 ml of 10 μmol sodium nitrite solution. In vivo formation of NPRO was estimated from the excreted amounts in the 24-hr urine. Values are means of 10 rats ± SD.

[b]The precursor solutions used in the in vivo experiments were incubated at 37°C for 15 min (final volume 1 ml). Values are means of two experiments.

[c]Groups of 10 fasting rats were gavaged first with 10 μmol proline in pH 3 buffer and 0.5 ml α-tocopherol (0-100 μmol) in ethanol, followed by 0.25 ml of sodium nitrite (10 μmol) solution.

[d]The precursor solutions used in the in vivo experiments were incubated at 37°C for 15 min (pH 3.6, final volume 1 ml).

effective, and only about 50% of the nitrosation of proline was inhibited by an excess amount.

After coadministration to rats of phenolic compounds together with proline and nitrite per os (Table 4), both catalysis (resorcinol, catechin, phenol, p-nitrosophenol) and inhibition (chlorogenic acid) of the nitrosation of proline were observed. Their modifying effects on in vitro nitrosation paralleled the results seen in vivo, although the magnitude was, in general, lower by 1/3 to 2/3 (Pignatelli et al. 1982).

Catechin, chlorogenic acid, and many flavonoids that contain a resorcinol moiety are abundant in beverages and edible foodstuffs, and their effect on endogenous nitrosation in man remains to be evaluated.

Endogenous Transnitrosation from NDPhA to Proline in Rats in the Presence or Absence of Thiocyanate

Transnitrosation reaction between NDPhA and amino compounds, which has been well studied in vitro (Singer et al. 1977), was further examined in vivo, using NDPhA and proline as a donor and receptor of a nitroso group, respec-

Table 4

Influence of Phenolic Compounds in the Nitrosation of Proline in vivo and in vitro

Experiment number	Ingredients[a] 10 μmol proline (I) + 20 μmol NaNO₂ (II) + phenolic compound (μmol)	NPRO formed			
		In vivo[b]		In vitro[d]	
		nmol/24 hr/rat mean ± SD	relative[c] yield	nmol/15 min at pH 4	relative yield
1	I + II	7.9 ± 1.5	1	28.9	1.0
2	I + II + resorcinol (5)	148.2 ± 42.2	18.7	1205	41.7
3	I + II + catechin (4)	60.7 ± 19.1	7.7	332	11.5
4	I + II + phenol (100)	31.4 ± 17.5	3.9	155.5	5.4
5	I + II + guaiacol (65)	8.4 ± 1.4	1.1	39	1.3
6	I + II + chlorogenic acid (50)	4.1 ± 0.6	0.5	8.6	0.3
7	I + II + p-nitrosophenol (10)	96.5 ± 36.2	12.2	526	18.2

[a]Groups of 9 rats each received 10 μmol proline and 20 μmol nitrite in pH 4 buffer. Groups of rats received either no phenolic compound (experiment 1) or a phenolic compound added to the proline solution at the dose indicated in parenthesis.

[b]24-hr urine of each rat was collected; NPRO excreted per rat (mean ± SD; n = 9) is given.

[c]Relative yield of NPRO was calculated taking the amount of NPRO in experiment No. 1 as 1.0.

[d]The solutions of precursors used in the in vivo experiments were incubated at 37°C for 15 min (pH 4, final volume 1 ml). Values are means of three experiments.

Table 5
Transnitrosation in vivo by NDPhA to Proline in Rats[a]

Experi-ment number	Reagent administered				nmol NPRO formed (mean ± SD)	Relative yield[b]
	NDPhA	Proline	Potassium thiocyanate	Nitrite		
1	0	0	0	0	0.17 ± 0.06	1
2	+	0	0	0	0.18 ± 0.03	1
3	0	+	0	0	0.15 ± 0.05	1
4	+	0	+	0	0.83 ± 0.19	5
5	0	+	+	0	0.24 ± 0.10	1.4
6	+	+	0	0	2.49 ± 1.46	15
7	+	+	+	0	145 ± 116	873
8	0	+	0	+	392 ± 47	2362

[a]Fasting rats were each gavaged with 50 μmol of the precursors, as indicated. Values are means of 5-20 rats ± SD.
[b]Relative yield is calculated taking NPRO formed in Experiment Numbers 1-3 as 1.

tively (Ohshima et al. 1982b; Table 5). A dose of either NDPhA or proline did not significantly increase the urinary levels of NPRO above the background. Coadministration of proline with NDPhA resulted in a 15-fold increase in NPRO excretion. In vivo coadministration of potassium thiocyanate together with proline and NDPhA resulted in a further 58-fold increase in the urinary levels of NPRO, confirming earlier reports that thiocyanate enhanced transnitrosation reaction in vitro (Singer et al. 1977; Singer 1978). The nitrosating capacity of NDPhA was compared with that of nitrite. The yield of NPRO through transnitrosation by NDPhA in vivo was about 160 times lower than that obtained by the reaction between nitrite and proline. Thus, endogenous transnitrosation by NDPhA was shown to occur in the body of rats although the yield of NPRO was lower when compared with that formed from N-nitrosation by nitrite. However, the catalyst thiocyanate was found to accelerate the reaction in vivo with similar efficiency, as reported in the in vitro system.

QUANTITATIVE ESTIMATION OF ENDOGENOUS NITROSATION IN HUMANS

Quantitative Excretion in Urine of Preformed NPRO After Ingestion from Foodstuffs

The quantitative excretion of preformed NPRO in the urine but not of other volatile nitrosamines after ingestion from foodstuffs was described by Ohshima et al. (1982b). On the basis of animal experiments (Tables 1 and 2), monitoring of urinary levels of N-nitrosamino acids such as NPRO appears to be a useful

Table 6
Urinary Excretion of NPRO, NDMA, NPYR in a Human Subject after Ingestion of Preformed Compounds Present in an Aqueous Extract from a Broiled Squid

Experiment	μg of N-nitroso compound		
	NPRO	NDMA	NPYR
Ingested amount (in 100 ml of the squid extract)	4.68	13.7	0.3
Excretion in the 24-hr urine after ingestion of 100 ml extract[a]	6.44 ± 0.48	<0.1[b]	<0.3[b]
Control 24-hr urine[c]	2.26 ± 0.66	<0.1[b]	<0.3[b]

[a]Values are means of 3 experiments ± SD.
[b]Below the limit of detection
[c]Control 24-hr urines collected during ingestion of low-nitrate diet were analyzed for the compounds; mean values of 5 experiments ± SD are given.

procedure for the quantitative estimation of nitrosation in vivo in man also. Therefore, the excretion pattern of NPRO as well as of some volatile N-nitrosamines (NDMA and NPYR) was studied in a human volunteer who had ingested trace amounts of these preformed N-nitroso compounds present in Japanese dried squid. The hot water extracts of the squid product contained NPRO, NDMA, and NPYR at concentrations of 0.3-13.7 μg/100 ml (Table 6).

Table 6 gives a comparison of the total amounts of preformed N-nitroso compounds recovered in the 24-hour urine after ingestion of the squid extract. Considering that about 2.3 μg NPRO are excreted daily in the urine as a background, the excretion of an additional 4.2 μg NPRO was attributable to ingestion of the preformed NPRO. Thus, the excretion rate of NPRO in the urine of a volunteer was estimated to be about 90%. However, no detectable levels of NDMA and NPYR were excreted in the urine, implying that in man these nitrosamines were completely metabolized in vivo. These results were in agreement with those obtained on the excretion rates of these N-nitroso compounds in rats (Table 1). Thus, monitoring of urinary NPRO seems to be more relevant than that of volatile nitrosamines to assess human exposure to N-nitroso compounds ingested in food or formed endogenously.

Endogenous Formation of NPRO in Man after Ingestion of Nitrate and Proline

The endogenous formation of NPRO in man after nitrate and proline were ingested is described by Ohshima and Bartsch (1981a) elsewhere. In the absence of adverse biological effects of NPRO (IARC 1978; Mirvish et al. 1980), a number of kinetic studies were carried out on the formation of NPRO in vivo in a human volunteer who had ingested vegetable juice (as a source of nitrate, 0-325 mg) 30 minutes later an aqueous solution of proline (0-500 mg) was ingested. The urinary excretion of NPRO was monitored. No food or beverages were taken for 2.5 hours after ingestion of proline; water was taken ad lib. Meals and other food and beverages taken on the day of the experiment were not standardized, but cured meat products and beer, which are presumed to contain preformed NPRO, as well as cigarette smoking, were avoided.

The typical pattern of excretion of NPRO in the urine after ingestion of 200 ml beetroot juice containing 260 mg nitrate, followed by 500 mg proline, is shown in Figure 3. The excretion pattern was similar to that obtained after ingestion of preformed NPRO in the squid extract (Fig. 3). NPRO appeared to be excreted into the urine as such, i.e., no formation of β-D-glucopyranosiduronic acid conjugate could be demonstrated.

Since 1) the urine analyzed before intake of precursors contained only trace amounts of NPRO (<3 μg/l), 2) the beet juice and proline used contained no detectable levels of preformed NPRO or nitrite, and 3) ingestion of either of the precursors alone did not increase urinary NPRO, the NPRO excreted in the urine is therefore most probably formed in the human body through the reaction of proline with nitrite. The formation of NPRO in vivo was found to be

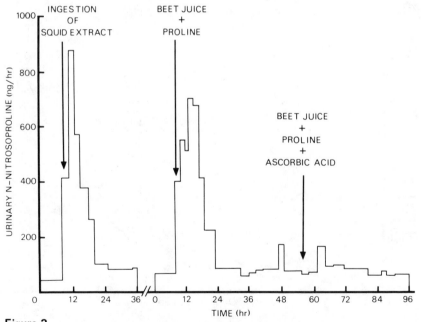

Figure 3
Urinary excretion of NPRO (ng/hour) in a human subject after ingestion of preformed NPRO, beet juice, and proline. The volunteer consumed 100 ml dried-squid extract containing 4.68 μg NPRO, or 200 ml beet juice (260 mg NO_3^-); 30 min later, 500 mg L-proline with or without 2 g ascorbic acid was ingested. (Details are given in the text.)

strongly dependent on nitrate intake: when less than 195 mg nitrate were ingested, a marginal or in most cases no increase in urinary NPRO was observed, as compared with that in a control experiment (no nitrate intake). However, when ≥ 260 mg nitrate was consumed, the excretion of NPRO increased exponentially with the dose of nitrate ingested (Fig. 4). It may be of relevance to note that Japan, which has one of the highest gastric cancer mortality rates, also has the highest average ingestion of nitrate (5.5 mmols or 341 mg/person/day) (Fine et al. 1982). This value is shown on the upper right-hand corner of the curve shown in Fig. 4.

As noted also in rats (Fig. 1), the formation in vivo of NPRO was shown to be proportional to the dose of proline ingested. These experiments show that in a healthy human subject, with the highest doses of nitrate (325 mg) and proline (500 mg) ingested, formation of NPRO ranged from 16.6-30.0 μg (mean 23.3) per 24 hours per person, corresponding to 0.002 and 0.004% of the ingested amounts of nitrate and proline, respectively.

Considering our results as a whole, the mechanism for NPRO formation in man appears to be as follows: the nitrate ingested in vegetable juice is re-

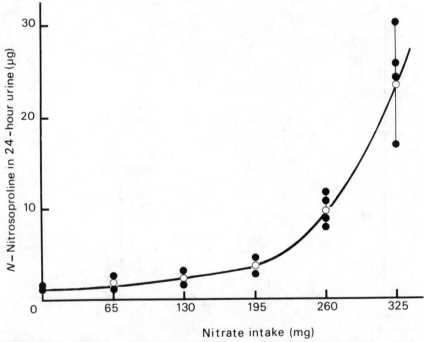

Figure 4
Effect of dose of nitrate ingested by a human subject on the formation of NPRO in vivo. (•) results from individual experiments; (○) arithmetic mean values plotted. (Details are given in the text.) Reprinted, with permission, from Ohshima and Bartsch (1981a).

secreted in the saliva, starting about 30 minutes after its ingestion, reaching a maximum after 1-2 hours (Ishiwata et al. 1975; Spiegelhalder et al. 1976; Tannenbaum et al. 1976). The resecreted nitrate is reduced to nitrite by the oral microflora. Proline ingested 30 minutes after intake of vegetable juice probably reacts with salivary nitrite to give NPRO under the acidic conditions prevailing in the stomach.

Inhibitory Effects of Ascorbic Acid (Vitamin C) and α-Tocopherol (Vitamin E) on the Formation of NPRO in Man In vivo

The effect of these inhibitors (ascorbic acid and α-tocopherol) was assessed quantitatively in experiments on a human subject (Ohshima and Bartsch 1981a, b; Table 7; Fig. 3). The amounts of NPRO excreted in the urine after ingestion of 325 mg of nitrate and 250 mg of proline ranged from 14.0-15.9 μg/24 hrs, with a mean value of 14.9 μg; the excretion rate was 5 to 7.5 times higher than that in control experiments in which either nitrate or proline alone were ingested. Intake of 1 g ascorbic acid simultaneously with the precursors was found to totally inhibit the nitrosation of proline in vivo. The amounts of NPRO detected were the same as those in the controls. α-Tocopherol (500 mg) was less effective and inhibited nitrosation in vivo only by about 50%. Similar effects were seen in rats (Table 3). The underlying mechanism is a reaction between vitamin C and nitrite to form nitric oxide and dehydroascorbic acid (Bunton et al. 1959); as a consequence, vitamin C competes with the nitrosatable amine for the available nitrite. Therefore, should it be demonstrated that the in vivo formation of N-nitroso compounds in the human body is a causative factor in certain human cancers, vitamin C would then appear to be effective in blocking N-nitrosation in vivo and thus play an important role from the point of view of primary cancer prevention.

POTENTIAL APPLICATION OF THE NPRO METHOD TO IDENTIFY HUMAN SUBJECTS AT HIGH RISK FOR STOMACH AND ESOPHAGEAL CANCER

Rationale of the Method and Practical Aspects

There is strong evidence to support the notion that in the human body carcinogenic N-nitroso compounds can be formed by the interaction of nitrosatable amino compounds and nitrosating agents (Correa et al. 1975; Ruddell et al. 1976; Fine et al. 1977; Tannenbaum et al. 1979; Schlag et al. 1980; Ohshima and Bartsch 1981a). The question that now requires clarification is whether the amounts of N-nitroso compounds formed endogenously correlate with an increased incidence of specific types of human cancer. However, the lack of suitable methods to estimate endogenous nitrosation in humans has hindered attempts to obtain such data. Monitoring NPRO excreted in the urine appears

Table 7
Effects of Ascorbic Acid and α-Tocopherol on the Formation of NPRO In vivo in Man

Experiment numbers	Material ingested (dose)	NPRO excreted in urine		
		μg/24 hours[b]	mean[c]	relative yield[d]
1	beet juice (250 ml containing 375 mg nitrate)	1.69; 3.44; 3.66	2.93	19.7
2	proline (250 mg)	1.05; 1.40; 3.42	1.96	13.2
3	beet juice (250 ml) + proline (250 mg)	14.0; 14.8; 15.9	14.9	100
4	beet juice (250 ml) + proline (250 mg) + ascorbic acid (1 g)	2.39; 2.96; 3.13	2.83	18.9
5	beet juice (250 ml) proline (250 mg) + α-tocopherol (500 mg)	8.17; 7.45; 6.16	7.26	48.7

Reprinted, with permission, from Ohshima and Bartsch (1981a).
[a] In the morning, the volunteer consumed the beet juice and then 30 min later, 10 ml of an aqueous solution of proline. Ascorbic acid (dissolved in water) and α-tocopherol (in wafer capsule) were taken at the same time as the proline. Urine was collected over 24 hr and analyzed for NPRO, as described in the text.
[b] Each value refers to individual experiment.
[c] Arithmetic means.
[d] Relative yield, taking NPRO excreted in experiment No. 3 as 100.

to be a useful method to estimate the extent of nitrosation in vivo in high-risk populations or human individuals. The rationale for applying this procedure in field or clinical studies is based on the following observations:

1. NPRO has been reported not to be carcinogenic and mutagenic (IARC 1978; Mirvish et al. 1980);
2. after gavage of rats with (^{14}C)-NPRO, the $^{14}CO_2$ production, and DNA alkylation were negligible (Chu and Magee 1981), but urinary excretion of NPRO (as the unchanged compound) was rapid and almost complete (Dailey et al. 1975; Chu and Magee 1981; Ohshima et al. 1982a);
3. urinary levels of NPRO in rats gavaged with proline and nitrite reflected well endogenous nitrosation of proline (Ohshima et al. 1982a);
4. in humans, preformed NPRO ingested in the aqueous extract of broiled dried squids was also rapidly and almost quantitatively eliminated in the urine within 24 hours after ingestion (Ohshima et al. 1982b).

Thus, the amount of NPRO excreted in the 24-hour urine sample was an indicator of daily endogenous nitrosation (Ohshima and Bartsch 1981a).

Additionally, it should be noted that application of the NPRO method to human subjects involves no risk to their health: It has been judged (Ohshima and Bartsch 1981a) that no carcinogenic risk to the human subject is involved when ingesting beetroot juice (as a source of nitrate) and proline, because: The experiments involved only an increased intake of commonly-occurring food ingredients; the absence of carcinogenic and mutagenic effects of NPRO is established; and, the natural occurrence of low levels of NPRO in many foodstuffs and in the urine of humans is known.

The experimental protocols described below would allow an estimation of the extent of endogenous nitrosation in individuals (groups of subjects) at high cancer risk in which endogenously formed N-nitroso compounds are suspected to be associated.

Evaluation of Human Exposure to N-nitroso Compounds and Nitrate in High-risk Areas of Esophageal Cancer

Epidemiological studies have associated an increased risk of stomach cancer and esophageal cancer with an elevated exposure to nitrate (Armijo and Coulson 1975; Coordination Group for Research on Etiology of Esophageal Cancer in North China 1975; Cuello et al. 1976; Fraser et al. 1980; Yang 1980). For example, in some provinces in Northern China, esophageal cancer is a prevalent disease, and a positive correlation has been reported between the cancer risk and the levels of nitrate (nitrite) in the drinking water, or the intakes of pickled vegetables and mouldy foods (Coordination Group for Research on Etiology of Esophageal Cancer in North China 1975; Yang 1980). In order to measure individual exposure to nitrate (nitrite) by monitoring excreted NPRO under conditions and dietary habits which may prevail in this high incidence area in

China, a series of experiments have been conducted in a human subject (Ohshima and Bartsch 1982).

Endogenous formation of NPRO was observed to occur in a human subject who ingested 100 g of pickled vegetables (Chinese cabbage prepared in France) as a source of nitrate and nitrite, followed one hour later by 100 mg of proline (Fig. 5). The pickled vegetable ingested (1 sample) contained about 750 ppm (mg/kg) sodium nitrate and 4.5 ppm sodium nitrite. Preformed NPRO was also detected in the pickled vegetable at a concentration of 35 ppb (μg/kg). Therefore, intake of the vegetable alone led to an increase in urinary NPRO (Fig. 5). When 100 mg proline was ingested 1 hour after intake of 100 g of the vegetable, urinary levels of NPRO were further increased (Fig. 5). These results support the notion that N-nitroso compounds can be formed in the body after simultaneous ingestion of nitrate (nitrite) containing vegetables and nitrosatable precursors, which can be present in foodstuffs or in the stomach.

In a high-incidence area for esophageal cancer such as exists in China, human subjects are more likely to be continuously exposed to nitrate and nitrite, which may be present in foodstuffs and drinking water or formed endogenously in the body. In order to investigate experimentally such a situation,

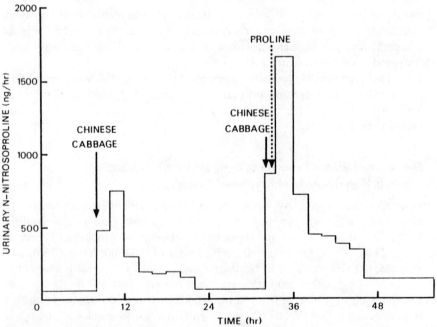

Figure 5

NPRO formation in vivo in a human subject after ingestion of pickled vegetable (Chinese cabbage) followed 1 hr later by L-proline. (For further details, see text.)

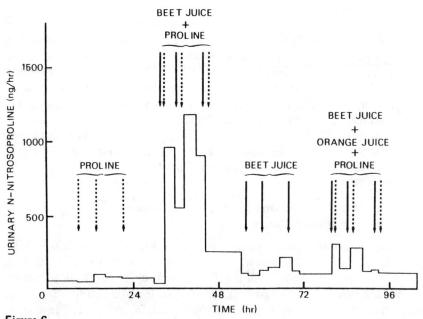

Figure 6
NPRO formation in vivo in a human subject after ingestion of multiple doses of beetroot juice and proline. (For further details, see text.)

where chronic exposure is involved, the following 4 series of experiments were conducted in one male volunteer (Fig. 6):

1. 3 times a day, 100 mg proline was taken 1 hr after each meal (consisting of a low nitrate diet), hereby, only trace amounts of NPRO were excreted in the urine (1.7 μg/24 hr/person);
2. nitrate-rich meals (low-nitrate diet plus 100 ml beetroot juice containing 130 mg NO_3^-) were taken 3 times a day together with 3 doses of proline; as a result, an increased amount of NPRO was excreted in the urine (13.4 μg/24 hr);
3. the intake of 3 nitrate-rich meals without proline did not significantly increase the urinary NPRO, as compared to experiment (1) (2.9 μg/24 hr);
4. when orange juice (a possible source of vitamin C) was taken at the end of each nitrate-rich meal, followed by proline, urinary excretion of NPRO was markedly suppressed (4.0 μg/24 hours versus 13.4 μg in experiment (2).

The results obtained from these experiments indicate that endogenous nitrosation may occur continuously in the body following chronic nitrate exposure. However, even when the amount of ingested nitrate was high enough to give rise to the formation of N-nitroso compounds in the human body, the presence of dietary vitamin C effectively inhibited nitrosation (Fig. 6). These results suggest that nitrosation in vivo may be modified by many factors such as the presence of catalysts or inhibitors in foods. Thus, in addition to data on individual exposure to nitrate, assessing of the extent of endogenous nitrosation may also be required to establish a possible causal relationship between the amounts of N-nitroso compounds formed and an increased incidence of specific types of human cancers. This can be achieved by collecting 24-hour urine specimens in, for example, subjects living in high- and low-incidence areas for esophageal cancer, following multiple ingestion of 100 mg proline (1 hour after each meal, 3 times a day). The levels of urinary NPRO can be compared with those in urine specimens collected from subjects without intake of proline. Such collaborative studies are in progress (IARC 1981).

Monitoring of Endogenous Nitrosation in Human Subjects at High Risk for Stomach Cancer

Endogenous formation of N-nitroso compounds has been associated with an increased risk of stomach cancer. For example, an elevated risk for stomach cancer has been observed in patients with chronic atrophic gastritis or pernicious anemia and in patients who have undergone gastric surgery such as Billroth-II gastrectomy (Blackburn et al. 1968; Stalsberg and Taksdal 1971; Cuello et al. 1976). It has been postulated that the achlorhydric stomach found in such patients may provide a suitable milieu for intragastric formation of N-nitroso compounds by the presence of a large number of bacteria, which may be involved in the conversion of nitrate to nitrite and subsequent nitrosation in vivo (Correa et al. 1975; Ruddell et al. 1976; Schlag et al. 1980). In fact, higher levels of N-nitroso compounds were more frequently found in fasting gastric juice samples of such patients than in those of normal subjects (Reed et al. 1981). However, the extent of endogenous nitrosation occurring in these individuals at high risk for stomach cancer has not been determined, but can now be estimated: The experimental protocol includes the ingestion of vegetable juice (as a source of nitrate), followed by a single dose of 500 mg L-proline. 24-Hour urine specimens can be analyzed for NPRO as an index for endogenous nitrosation. The results can be correlated with diagnostic findings on the presence of precancerous lesions and data on the gastric microenvironment such as the pH and bacterial flora. Such collaborative studies are under way (IARC 1981).

ACKNOWLEDGMENTS

We wish to thank Mrs. M.M. Courcier for secretarial help and Mr. J.C. Béréziat, Mlles. J. Michelon and M.C. Bourgade for technical assistance. The TEA detector was provided on loan by the National Cancer Institute under contract NOI CP-55715. The authors are grateful to the Délégation Générale à la Recherche Scientifique et Technique for financial support.

REFERENCES

Armijo, R. and A.H. Coulson. 1975. Epidemiology of stomach cancer in Chile—the role of nitrogen fertilizers. *Int. J. Epidemiol.* 4:301.

Blackburn, E.K., S.T. Callender, J.V. Dacie, R. Doll, R.H. Girdwood, D.L. Mollin, R. Saracci, J. Stafford, R.B. Thompson, S. Varadi, and G. Wetherly-Mein. 1968. Possible association between pernicious anaemia and leukaemia: A prospective study of 1625 patients with a note on t very high incidence of gastric cancer. *Int. J. Cancer* 3:163.

Braunberg, R.C. and R.E. Dailey. 1973. Formation of nitrosoproline in rats. *Proc. Soc. Exp. Biol. Med.* 142:993.

Bunton, C.A., H. Dahn, and L. Loewe. 1959. Oxidation of ascorbic acid and similar reductones by nitrous acid. *Nature* 183:163.

Chu, C. and P.N. Magee. 1981. The metabolic fate of nitrosoproline in the rat. *Cancer Res.* 41:3653.

Coordinating Committee for Scientific and Technical Assessment of Environmental Pollutants. 1978. *Nitrates: An Environmental Assessment.* National Academy of Sciences, Washington, D.C.

Coordination Group for Research on Etiology of Esophageal Cancer in North China. 1975. The epidemiology and etiology of esophageal cancer in North China, a preliminary report. *Chinese Med. J.* 1:167.

Correa, P., W. Haenszel, C. Cuello, S. Tannenbaum, and M. Archer. 1975. A model for gastric cancer epidemiology. *Lancet* ii:58.

Cuello, C., P. Correa, W. Haenszel, G. Gordillo, C. Brown, M. Archer, and S. Tannenbaum. 1976. Gastric cancer in Colombia. I. Cancer risk and suspect environment agents. *J. Natl. Cancer Inst.* 57:1015.

Dailey, R.E., R.C. Braunberg, and A.M. Blaschka. 1975. The absorption, distribution and excretion of (^{14}C)-nitrosoproline by rats. *Toxicology* 3:23.

Fine, D.H., B.C. Challis, P. Hartman, and J. Van Ryzin. 1982. Human exposure assessment of nitrosamines from endogenous and exogenous sources: Model calculations. *IARC Sci. Publ.* 41 (in press).

Fine, D.H., R. Ross, D.P. Rounbehler, A. Silvergleid, and L. Song. 1977. Formation *in vivo* of volatile *N*-nitrosamines in man after ingestion of cooked bacon and spinach. *Nature* 265:753.

Fraser, P., C. Chilvers, V. Beral, and M.J. Hill. 1980. Nitrate and human cancer: A review of the evidence. *Int. J. Epidemiol.* 9:3.

IARC. 1978. *Monographs on the Evaluation of the Carcinogenic Risk of Chemicals to Humans,* Vol. 17. International Agency for Research on Cancer, Lyon, France.

IARC. 1981. Annual Report, p. 91. International Agency for Research on Cancer, Lyon, France.

Ishiwata, H., P. Boriboon, Y. Nakamura, M. Harada, A. Tanimura, and M. Ishidate. 1975. Studies on *in vivo* formation of nitroso compounds. II. Changes of nitrite and nitrate concentrations in human saliva after ingestion of vegetables or sodium nitrate. *J. Food Hyg. Soc. Jpn.* 16:19.

Kamm, J.J., T. Dashman, H. Newmark, and W.J. Mergens. 1977. Inhibition of amine-nitrite hepatotoxicity by α-tocopherol. *Toxicol. Appl. Pharmacol.* 41:575.

Kawabata, T. 1974. Recent studies in Japan on the analysis and formation of *N*-nitroso compounds. *IARC Sci. Publ.* **9**:154.

Mirvish, S.S. 1975. Formation of *N*-nitroso compounds: Chemistry, kinetics and *in vivo* occurrence. *Toxicol. Appl. Pharmacol.* **31**:325.

Mirvish, S.S., L. Wallcave, M. Eagen, and P. Shubik. 1972. Ascorbate-nitrite reaction: Possible means of blocking the formation of carcinogenic *N*-nitroso compounds. *Science* **177**:65.

Mirvish, S.S., O. Bulay, R.G. Runge, and K. Patil. 1980. Study of the carcinogenicity of large doses of dimethylnitramine, *N*-nitroso-*L*-proline, and sodium nitrite administered in drinking water to rats. *J. Natl. Cancer Inst.* **64**:1435.

Ohshima, H. and H. Bartsch. 1981a. Quantitative estimation of endogenous nitrosation in humans by monitoring *N*-nitrosoproline excreted in the urine. *Cancer Res.* **41**:3658.

_____. 1981b. The influence of vitamin C on the *in vivo* formation of nitrosamines. In *Vitamin C (Ascorbic Acid)* (eds. J.N. Counsell and D.H. Hornig), p. 215. Applied Science Publishers, London and New Jersey, UK.

_____. 1982. Quantitative estimation of endogenous nitrosation in humans by measuring excretion of *N*-nitrosoproline in the urine. In *Environmental mutagens and carcinogens* (eds. T. Sugimura et al.), p. 577. University of Tokyo Press, Tokyo, Japan and Alan R. Liss, Inc., New York.

Ohshima, H., J.C. Béréziat, and H. Bartsch. 1982a. Monitoring *N*-nitrosamino acids excreted in the urine and feces of rats as an index for endogenous nitrosation. *Carcinogenesis* **3**:115.

_____. 1982b. Measurement of endogenous *N*-nitrosation in rats and humans by monitoring urinary and faecal excretion of *N*-nitrosamino acids. *IARC Sci. Publ.* **41**:(in press).

Pensabene, J.W., W. Fiddler, W. Mergens, and A.E. Wasserman. 1978. Effect of α-tocopherol formulations on the inhibition of nitrosopyrrolidine formation in model systems. *J. Food Sci.* **43**:801.

Pignatelli, B., J.C. Béréziat, I.K. O'Neill, and H. Bartsch. 1982. Catalytic role of some phenolic substances in endogenous formation of *N*-nitroso compounds. *IARC Sci. Publ.* **41**:(in press).

Reed, P.I., P.L.R. Smith, K. Haines, F.R. House, and C.L. Walters. 1981. Gastric juice *N*-nitrosamines in health and gastroduodenal disease. *Lancet* **ii**:550.

Rounbehler, D.P., R. Ross, D.H. Fine, Z.M. Iqbal, and S.S. Epstein. 1977. Quantitation of dimethylnitrosamine in the whole mouse after biosynthesis *in vivo* from trace levels of precursors. *Science* **197**:917.

Ruddell, W.S.J., E.S. Bone, M.J. Hill, L.M. Blendis, and C.L. Walters. 1976. Gastric juice nitrite: A risk factor for cancer of the hypochlorhydric stomach? *Lancet* **ii**:1037.

Sander, J. and F. Seif. 1969. Bakterielle Reduktion von Nitrat im Magen des Munschen als Ursache einer Nitrosamin-Bildung. *Arzneimittel-Forsch.* **19**:1091.

Sander, J. and F. Schweinsberg. 1972. Wechselbeziehungen zwischen Nitrat, Nitrit und kanzerogenen *N*-nitrosoverbindungen. *Zentralbl. Bakteriol. Parasitenkd. Infectionskr. Hyg., Abt.:Orig. Reihe.* **B156**299.

Schlag, P., R. Bockler, H. Ulrich, M. Peter, P. Merkle, and C. Herfarth. 1980. Are nitrite and *N*-nitroso compounds in gastric juice risk factors for carcinoma in the operated stomach? *Lancet* i:727.

Singer, S.S. 1978. Kinetics and mechanism of aliphatic transnitrosation. *J. Org. Chem.* **43**:4612.

Singer, S.S., W. Lijinsky, and G.M. Singer. 1977. Transnitrosation by aliphatic nitrosamines. *Tetrahedron Lett.* **19**:1613.

Spiegelhalder, B., G. Eisenbrand, and R. Preussmann. 1976. Influence of dietary nitrate on nitrite content of human saliva: possible relevance to *in vivo* formation of *N*-nitroso compounds. *Food Cosmet. Toxicol.* **14**:545.

Stalsberg, H. and S. Taksdal. 1971. Stomach cancer following gastric surgery for benign conditions. *Lancet* ii:1175.

Tannenbaum, S.R., M. Weisman, and D. Fett. 1976. The effect of nitrate intake on nitrite formation in human saliva. *Food Cosmet. Toxicol.* **14**:549.

Tannenbaum, S.R., D. Moran, W. Rand, C. Cuello, and P. Correa. 1979. Gastric cancer in Colombia. IV. Nitrite and other ions in gastric contents of residents from a high-risk region. *J. Natl. Cancer Inst.* **62**:9.

Yang, C.S. 1980. Research on esophageal cancer in China: A review. *Cancer Res.* **40**:2633.

Endogenous Nitrosoproline Synthesis in Humans

DAVID A. WAGNER, DAVID E. G. SHUKER, GORDANA HASIC,
AND STEVEN R. TANNENBAUM
Department of Nutrition and Food Science.
Massachusetts Institute of Technology
Cambridge, Massachusetts 02139

N-Nitrosamines are potentially important as causative agents in the induction of human cancer. Recently, there have been attempts to estimate the environmental exposure (Committee on Nitrite and Alternative Curing Agents in Food 1981) as well as attempts to predict endogenous synthesis of N-nitrosamines (Fine et al. 1982). None of these methods afford a direct measure of levels found in the human body and require significant assumptions for their predictions to be valid. However, direct measurement of N-nitrosamines in vivo has been characterized with many problems due to their rapid metabolism and ease of artifactual formation during analysis. For example, compounds like nitroso-dimethylamine (NDMA) are metabolized very rapidly after administration in animals (Heath 1962). Thus amounts which might be found in body fluids pose severe analytical problems. In our laboratory, we have developed analytical methodology for the measurement of 20 parts per trillion NDMA in urine and were unable to detect even that level in a large number of samples.

Recently, Ohshima and Bartsch (1981) reported that, after nitrate and proline administration, N-nitrosoproline (NPRO) formed in vivo in man, and could be quantitatively measured in urine. It has been shown that NPRO is not a carcinogen (Mirvish et al. 1980) and essentially unmetabolized in animals (Chu and Magee 1981). It is apparent, therefore, that NPRO excretion in urine could be used as a quantitative indicator of the amount of N-nitrosation in vivo.

We would like to report on an improved analytical method for the determination of NPRO in urine. This methodology was used to analyze formation of NPRO in six healthy young adults on a controlled dietary intake regimen.

METHODS

NPRO Analysis in Urine

Twenty-four hour urine collections were stored in prewashed 2 liter polyethylene bottles containing pure ethanol (100 ml), dibasic sodium phosphate (10 g), and sodium bisulphite (1.5 g) at 0°C to ensure that bacterial growth was inhibited and that artifactual nitrosamine formation was prevented.

An aliquot of urine (50 ml), to which N-nitroso-L-pipecolic acid (250 ng in 100 μl of methanol) was added as an internal standard, was eluted through a prewashed (water) column of strongly acidic cation exchange resin (2 cm x 10 cm, Dowex 50 W, 50 x 8-100, 50-100 mesh), to remove many interferences typically found in urine. The column was further washed with water (2 x 15 ml) and the combined eluates were concentrated to about 5 ml using a rotary evaporator with a water bath temperature of 55°C.

The concentrate was applied to a pretreated (15 ml ethyl acetate) Prep-Tube (Thermo Electron Corp., Waltham, MA) which is an improved medium for performing liquid-liquid extractions. After standing for 10 minutes, the Prep-Tube was washed with ethyl acetate (100 ml) and the organic phase was collected. The solvent was removed on a rotary evaporator at 35°C. The residue was extracted with methylene chloride (3 x 10 ml) and the solvent removed by rotary evaporation at 30°C. The residue was dissolved in methylene chloride (1 ml) and treated with diazomethane at 0°C until a yellow color persisted. After 10 minutes, the solution was transferred to a 1 ml Reacti-Vial (Pierce, Rockford, IL) fitted with a concentrating bulb. The reaction flask was washed with an additional 2 ml of methylene chloride. Samples were very slowly evaporated using a gentle stream of N_2 to a final sample volume of about 1 ml.

Aliquots of this solution (1-5 μl) were analyzed by a gas chromatography thermal energy analyzer GC/TEA (Thermo Electron Corp., Waltham). The retention times of N-nitroso-L-proline methyl ester and N-nitroso-L-pipecolic acid methyl ester were 5 minutes and 4 minutes, respectively, on a column packed with 3% OV-225 on 100/120 Supelcoport (Supelco, Bellefonte, PA) operating at 135°C isothermally with an helium flow rate of 25 ml per minute.

Diet samples were analyzed for NPRO similarly to urine samples but with the modifications described elsewhere (Sen et al. 1982).

NPRO Excretion in Human Subjects

Six subjects, three male and three female M.I.T. students, participated in this study. All subjects were judged to be healthy based on a thorough physical examination and routine blood and urine analysis. Subjects were fed a controlled, low nitrate diet consisting of a liquid soy and milk formula and egg omelette (Young et al. 1979). The liquid formula and egg omelette supply 2000 calories/day for a 70 kg man and the remaining calories are derived from protein-free cookies, cornstarch dessert, and sucrose beverages. Each subject consumed a diet to meet all energy requirements and vitamin and trace mineral requirements based on NAS/NRC recommendations.

The experimental protocol consisted of 5 day 24-hour urine collections on the low nitrate diet described above. The dietary intake of ascorbic acid during this part of the study was 60 mg. On the day 6, on a fasted stomach, subjects were administered orally 300 mg sodium nitrate in 10 ml distilled water, followed by 200 ml water. One hour later 500 mg L-proline in 10 ml water was administered. Urine was collected for 5 more days.

Results

Our method of analysis of NPRO in urine was efficient and sensitive. Adding NPRO in the range of 1-40 $\mu g/l$ to urine, showed an 85-100% recovery. A reliable and quantitable detection limit of NPRO was 0.5 $\mu g/l$. Photohydrolysis of a urine sample removed the GC/TEA peak of NPRO from the chromatogram. A blank control (i.e., distilled water in place of urine) gave no detectable NPRO peak. Addition of nitrite and proline to urine showed no artifactual formation of NPRO during the analysis.

For 5 days prior to the dose of nitrate and proline, the basal excretion of NPRO was relatively constant (6.9 ± 1.3 $\mu g/day$). Typical excretion patterns for three subjects are shown in Figure 1. Upon administration of nitrate and proline a significant rise in the excretion of NPRO was observed (12.2 ± 3.4 $\mu g/day$), as shown in Figure 1.

Analysis of the diet showed that approximately 3.5 μg NPRO/day was being consumed. This NPRO was all from the dried egg omelette mix. Since dietary intake was closely controlled for each subject, it was possible to quantitate the amount of NPRO consumed. The amount of NPRO endogenously synthesized per day was calculated by subtracting dietary intake from urinary excretion. The corrected endogenous synthesis in the absence of added nitrate or proline was found to be 3.4 ± 1.2 $\mu g/day$.

DISCUSSION

A basal excretion of significant levels of NPRO in urine, by subjects on a low nitrate diet cannot be accounted for by dietary intake alone. This indicates that endogenous biosynthesis of NPRO occurs in humans. The formation of this NPRO may be due to endogenous production of nitrate, previously reported by our group (Green et al. 1981). Nitrate produced in the body, recirculated to the salivary glands and reduced to nitrite by oral cavity bacteria, can expose the stomach to nitrite. Since proline is a common free amino acid it would then be available for nitrosation. The administration of nitrate followed by proline significantly increased the formation of NPRO.

Studies on the salivary concentrations of nitrate and nitrite in humans, following a dose of nitrate, have indicated that a maximum salivary concentration of nitrite is reached in the vicinity of 1 hour (Wagner et al. 1982). We therefore chose a time delay of 1 hour between nitrate and proline administration to maximize NPRO formation. Although the amount of NPRO formed is lower than previously reported (Ohshima and Bartsch 1981), their data is on one subject with a delay of ½ hour between nitrate and proline administration.

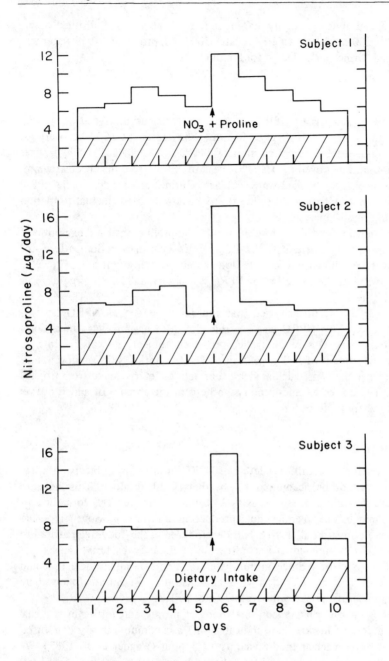

Figure 1
Typical urinary excretion patterns of NPRO (μg/day) in three human subjects on a controlled, low nitrate diet. (▨) dietary intake of NPRO. On day 6, subjects were administered 300 mg NaNO₃ and then, 60 min later, 500 mg L-proline. Details are given in the text.

We are currently carrying out studies to explore the nature of endogenous NPRO formation including the use of stable isotope labeled precursors.

ACKNOWLEDGMENTS

We thank Irene Baker and Walter Bishop for carrying out many of the analyses. This investigation was supported by PHS Grant Number NCI-1-P01-CA26731-03, awarded by the National Cancer Institute, DHHS.

REFERENCES

Chu, C., and P.N. Magee. 1981. The metabolic fate of nitrosoproline in the rat. *Cancer Res.* **41**:3653.

Committee on Nitrite and Alternative Curing Agents in Food. 1981. N-Nitroso compounds: Environmental distribution and exposure of humans. In *The Health Effects of Nitrate, Nitrite and N-Nitroso Compounds,* p. 7-1. National Academy of Sciences, Washington, DC.

Fine, D.H., B.C. Challis, P. Hartman, and J. Van Ryzin. 1982. Human exposure assessment of nitrosamines from endogenous sources: Model calculations. *IARC Sci Publ* **41**:(in press).

Green, L.C., K. Ruiz De Luzuriaga, D.A. Wagner, W. Rand, N. Istfan, V.R. Young, and S.R. Tannenbaum. 1981. Nitrate biosynthesis in man. *Proc. Natl. Acad. Sci. U.S.A.* **78**:7764.

Heath, D.F. 1962. The decomposition and toxicity of dialkyl nitrosamines in rats. *Biochem. J.* **85**:72.

Mirvish, S.S., O. Bulay, R.G. Runge, and K. Patil. 1980. Study of the carcinogenicity of large doses of dimethylnitramine, N-nitroso-L-proline and sodium nitrite administered in drinking water to rats. *J. Natl. Cancer Inst.* **64**:1435.

Ohshima, H., and H. Bartsch. 1981. Quantitative estimation of endogenous nitrosation in humans by monitoring N-nitroso-proline excreted in the urine. *Cancer Res.* **41**:3658.

Sen, N.P., S. Seaman, and L. Tissier. 1982. A rapid and sensitive method for the determination of non-volatile N-nitroso compounds in foods and some recent data on the levels of volatile nitrosamines in dried foods and malt-based beverages. *IARC Sci. Publ.* **41**: (in press).

Young, V.R., N.S. Scrimshaw, B. Torun, and F. Viteri. 1979. Soybean protein in human nutrition: An overview. *J. Am. Oil Chem. Soc.* **56**:110.

COMMENTS

TANNENBAUM: In relation to the effect of Vitamin E in lowering nitroso-proline, was that taken as a single dose?

BARTSCH: Yes, that's correct.

MIRVISH: Vitamin E was an emulsion?

BARTSCH: Vitamin E was taken inside of a small wafer capsule. We did the same experiment in rats, and we found identical inhibition figures for these two vitamins.

We were also interested in studying the effect of phenolic compounds which were already known to modify nitrosation in vitro, particularly because resorcinol has been shown to be very active as a catalyst. A lot of these compounds, flavonoids, carry the resorcinol moiety and are present in nature.

By applying this test, so far only done in rats, we were able to show catalysis of nitrosation of proline by resorcinol and by catechin—and you see here the relative increase is about up to 18-fold—and there was inhibition of chlorogenic acid of about 50%.

I think by further applying this method, it will be feasible now to study complex mixtures.

GARLAND: Did you try an experiment just giving nitrate? How did that change the background levels of NPRO?

TANNENBAUM: We had done a lot of experiments in the past with just nitrate. The background doesn't change very much.

GARLAND: It doesn't change.

TANNENBAUM: If it changed 10%, I couldn't tell you. Ohshima and Bartsch have similar data.

CONNEY: Helmut [Bartsch], I think in your data on the beet juice, it looked to me as if you had about a 50-75% increase in NPRO without giving the proline in addition.

Is that correct? And, if so, do you have any more data on whether giving just exogenous nitrate alone does anything?

BARTSCH: I don't think the increase was as much as you reported.

CONNEY: You think it was less than that?

BARTSCH: It was less than that. It was almost the same as the results you get for proline alone.

CONNEY: It looked as if there was an increase from the data you showed. I don't know how big it was, but maybe it was 50%.

SEN: Dr. Tannenbaum, this background NPRO you see, is that partially due to the diet?

TANNENBAUM: No, it is not all coming from the diet.

SEN: Is it formed due to nitrosation of peptides from the NPRO, and then stored in the body somewhere, breaking down later on?

TANNENBAUM: The proline could only be nitrosated if it was a free amino acid or an N-terminal amino acid. I can't exclude that possibility. I mean, the amount of proline in the daily diet is 4 or 5 gm. David [Fine] showed that.

SEN: You don't need much.

TANNENBAUM: Proline is one of the major amino acids in gastric juice. I think it is one of the most ubiquitous free amino acids in most body fluids. So there is always going to be some present. I don't think you have to assume that the nitrosation would have to take place in the protein to explain that.

HOFFMANN: You mentioned you have a standard diet. Do you control for coffee intake? We heard from Dr. Bartsch that he feels chlorogenic acid is catalyzing.

BARTSCH: Inhibiting.

HOFFMANN: So, you get 100-200 mg chlorogenic acid per cup of coffee. Did you control for coffee drinking?

TANNENBAUM: In our case, yes.

HOFFMANN: So the coffee is taken into account and that is an inhibitor. It's a great variable, when with each cup of coffee you get 100-200 mg chlorogenic acid. That should be considered.

HARTMAN: I just wanted to make a comment on the salivary recirculation of ascorbate. You mentioned that it wasn't recirculated. It was my impression that it is recirculated in all animals, including the human.

HARTMAN: In some animals, like the rat, you can inject it intravenously and then get out saliva, and the ascorbate concentration is elevated.

TANNENBAUM: My information comes from Harold Newmark (pers. comm.). He told me that studies had been done at Hoffmann-La Roche with labeled ascorbic acid. If it is recirculated, it is recirculated to a very small extent.

KIMBROUGH: Do you use a preservative when shipping the urine or do you freeze it? And, another question: if you want to do field studies would it be very impractical to collect 24-hr urine samples? Is there some other way you could take a sample?

TANNENBAUM: At the present time, I feel pretty strongly about 24-hr urine samples, because as you see from Helmut's [Bartsch] data, NPRO is excreted pretty rapidly. If you have a fractionated urine sample I don't think you'd have any idea how much was synthesized on a daily basis.
In our experience so far, the collection methods and the preservation methods we have worked out do not require immediate refrigeration or freezing, although we prefer to do that as soon as is practicable.

WEISBURGER: Is there any chance that some of the compound is formed at pH 6 in urine?

TANNENBAUM: No. We have an inhibitor and we have added morpholine. We know that under those conditions we would not have artifact formation.

WEISBURGER: I mean during bladder storage not in the urine.

TANNENBAUM: Well, we can only say what happens after the urine leaves the body.

WEISBURGER: Dr. Bartsch do you see any possibility that the urine components in the bladder could undergo nitrosation?

BARTSCH: We stabilize the urine by addition of alkali.

WEISBURGER: But I am asking whether there is a chance that some nitroso compound may form in the urinary bladder in normal humans, where the pH is about 6.

BARTSCH: I don't know. I think it's possible to collect 24-hr urine and stabilize it.

WEISBURGER: That's what you're asking, Dr. Kimbrough, isn't it?

KIMBROUGH: Well, I am asking how urines are collected. Do you put a preservative into the bottle?

TANNENBAUM: Yes. We prepare the collection vessels by cleaning them and adding a preservative to the bottle, so that the urine is introduced directly into the collection bottle.

SEN: What preservative do you use?

TANNENBAUM: We use isopropanol or ethanol, disodium phosphate, and sodium sulfite. It can be frozen, but we find that for NPRO it doesn't seem to matter.

CHALLIS: I think we should hear what Helmut does with his samples.

BARTSCH: We are using stabilization by sodium hydroxide. We use frozen aliquots which can be shipped. We need only about 50-ml aliquots. We have found that the patients are willing to cooperate so it is not so difficult to collect 24-hr urine samples.

CHALLIS: Steve, I believe in your dog study you mentioned that NDMA forms rapidly. Have you calculated whether it is significantly faster than you would expect from the in vitro work?

TANNENBAUM: The very first sample we can take, which is 3 minutes after adding the last ingredient, contains the highest concentration of NDMA we ever see. Apparently it is being rapidly absorbed through the stomach. We currently have too many degrees of freedom to be able to integrate those equations.

CHALLIS: You could just calculate as to what you would get after the 3 minutes.

TANNENBAUM: But we don't know the total content of the stomach.

CHALLIS: You could make a guess, can't you?

MICHEJDA: Don't you have a kind of a rate curve, a decay curve.

TANNENBAUM: No. That decay curve actually is arising from NDMA absorption. The reason NDMA is going down, the amount of stomach emptying over that period of time is minute, by the way, very, very small. But the thing that we didn't realize until we started to do these experiments is that NDMA would be absorbed through the stomach, because in the rat it is not. In the rat, NDMA is absorbed very, very slowly through the stomach. So we just can't do it.

BARTSCH: Dr. Conney asked about the administration of nitrate alone. I don't think the data were indicated. There were four sets of experiments: three doses of proline, and the excretion was 1.7 μg nitrosoproline/24 hours.

Beet juice plus proline ended up to be 13.4 μg. Beet juice alone was 2.9 μg. There was an increase. The triple treatment of beet juice, orange juice, and proline was something like 4.0 μg. The values of these experiments are: 1.7 μg proline; 13.4 μg beet + proline; 2.9 μg beet juice alone; and, 4.0 μg beet juice, orange juice, and proline.

CONNEY: Is the increase from 1.7 to 2.9 real?

BARTSCH: I'm not sure.

ELDER: Dr. Tannenbaum, you outlined the problem of keeping the ascorbic acid in the stomach. Since the well-known mechanisms of hypoosmotic solutions or fat solutions would delay gastric emptying. Just a comment: it might be worthwhile to look at the kinetics of nitrosation in hypoosmotic solutions or in solutions with low fat, because the duodenum brake mechanism controlling gastric emptying can be very easily manipulated within the physiological range. And I don't think you would have trouble keeping vitamin C in the stomach, but it might do something other than what you think.

WEISBURGER: Actually, there are low-release vitamin C tablets on the market, and I just learned from Dr. Conney that a slow-release study has been done.

MIRVISH: What about the background NPRO? If you take a 500-mg dose proline, what is the amount of proline in the stomach? Is it in proportion to the background?

TANNENBAUM: The background occurs during the period of time when they're not getting any proline.

MIRVISH: Yes. But how much proline is there in the gastric juice?

TANNENBAUM: The concentration of proline in gastric juice is in the micro-molar range of concentration. We don't have any data of our own on how much proline is in gastric juice. Perhaps that would be worthwhile to get. The fact that there is a background that is higher on our diet than on a natural diet, and that it's refractory to ascorbic acid is something that I only learned over the last couple of weeks. I haven't really digested the significance of it yet.

HARRIS: I have a question for both Steve and Helmut. You both mentioned a fairly large individual variation. Is there also an individual variation in base-line, and is there any correlation between baseline level and the amount of "induced level" when you administer the proline in beet juice? In other words, could you predict the individuals who would have a higher re-sponse by just determining baseline levels?

TANNENBAUM: I don't think we have done enough to be able to answer that. Between us, we have done probably less than a dozen.

CHALLIS: What is the range, though? Is it a factor of 10 or a factor of 5?

TANNENBAUM: On natural diets, we get numbers that are very similar to the ones that Helmut just reported—around 1 or 2. In fact, it's low enough to make you wonder.

CHALLIS: So they're really quite similar.

TANNENBAUM: Our numbers are quite similar. It was a great surprise to us that on our diet the numbers went up the way they did. But I think that the reason is it's simply a lack of inhibition. I think that natural diets probably contain a lot of inhibitors. That is my conclusion at the present time. I really can't say more than that.

BRUNNEMANN: Steve, since your diet does give an elevated background value, what do you think is significant about it? Why don't you stick to the natural diet? You would get a better baseline.

TANNENBAUM: Well, for two reasons. First of all, we have experiments in which the analysis is in progress; what I didn't tell you was that the nitrate that I gave was ^{15}N nitrate. In all of these studies, we have been doing nitrate pharmacokinetics in conjunction with looking at incorpora-tion of that ^{15}N nitrate into the nitrosoproline. Now, we have not yet finished the analyses on the ^{15}N content of the NPRO. So that is one of the critical things which I think will help us explain the experiment. So the reason we use that diet is to get a low-nitrate diet.

The other reason to use that diet was that we were concerned that we might have random contamination of the diet with preformed NPRO so that we would have problems interpreting the data.

I think this is a problem in the field collections. When you're collecting it from people, since it's not metabolized, if you find a lot, it's interesting. But I don't think you can say a priori whether it came from the diet or whether—for example, if you take the Chinese population, or if you take the Colombian population, it could have been in the food, as well as being formed.

BARTSCH: That's a plausible reason.

HECHT: If I have it right, your two methods differ some in that Steve uses a cation exchange column whereas Helmut uses only an extraction.

TANNENBAUM: We use a double extraction, but that is following the cation exchange.

HECHT: Why is it that the cation exchange column is necessary?

TANNENBAUM: We simply found that there were some urinary samples that could not be analyzed with the simple extraction procedure.

BARTSCH: We have the same experience. In some samples of urine, it is very difficult to analyze for NPRO. Normally, it's okay, but there are certain "dirty" urine samples which are difficult to analyze.

TANNENBAUM: We actually took this from a classical text on urine analysis in which, if you want to test anions, you take the urine sample and first put it through a strong cation exchange resin. Actually, it's interesting; it even takes out urea.

MAGEE: Is it an acidic condition?

TANNENBAUM: Yes, this was simply sort of a standard procedure that we adopted and we were not worried about artifact formation. There is an inhibitor but there is no artifact formation. We tested that first.

WEISBURGER: Do you think the ion exchange resin is going to work better, Dr. Bartsch?

BARTSCH: I think it gives you a guarantee; we have not seen this problem too often with some dirty urines which make problems.

WEISBURGER: Well, I am thinking in terms of recommendations to make to some other groups here that might like to go into this. Would you recommend the routine use of a column?

BARTSCH: Yes, I think so.

HOFFMANN: What is the inhibitor of your ion exchange?

TANNENBAUM: The inhibitor is sulfite.

HOFFMANN: Is it on the ion exchange?

TANNENBAUM: No, we have a high concentration of sulfite in the urine, which is converted essentially to H_2SO_3 by the column.

HECHT: Your technique sounds like a possible problem, if you have morpholine in it.

TANNENBAUM: Sulfite is an extremely effective inhibitor of nitrosation. In our hands, aside from azide we feel that sulfite is generally the most effective inhibitor.

SEN: I just want to make a comment about the methodology again. We used the direct extraction method, similar to Dr. Bartsch, but we used a column as we described at the Tokyo meeting. It has the advantage that we can also measure other compounds. You can do both the hydroxy and the carboxy at the same time, so you get a complete picture. It is quite rapid, too; you can do the whole test in maybe 2 hours.

ARCHER: Just a comment to Brian's [Challis] question. I was involved with Paul Newberne about 10 years ago in a similar dog experiment. We used pyrrolidine as the precursor, and similarly saw very rapid absorption in the stomach. In that experiment, an attempt was made to get the parameter you were talking about—the relative rate of nitrosation. I think it was a couple of orders of magnitude more rapid in the stomach than in vitro at the same pH. That does not allow for absorption by just taking the numbers we generated from the gastric juice itself. The reason is unknown, but it was very rapid in the stomach.

BARTSCH: Well, this is just opposite what we observed.

FINE: I wanted to follow up on the question which Dr. Weisburger asked earlier about holding time in the bladder. One of the variables you have here is how long the urine is held in the bladder before it's given up.

This could be used as a way of getting at perhaps whether there is any nitrosation in the bladder. Have either of you looked at the variability of how long it's held in the bladder, if it's being held for several hours or a longer time?

TANNENBAUM: Actually, that is an interesting question from a psychological point of view. When you ask someone to collect his urine for 24 hours, he or she urinates more frequently than they ordinarily do. If anything, I think our collection procedure is adequate. I am sure the same thing is true in Helmut's case where he is trying to get fractionated doses to get the kinetics. So, if anything, I think there has been less holding time in the bladder.

FINE: Have you looked at the effect of holding time?

KIMBROUGH: The only way you would be able to do that is to do it on patients that are being catheterized in the hospital. That's where you could get continuous urine samples.

TANNENBAUM: But they are generally on antibiotics.

KIMBROUGH: Then they are getting medication and problems like that. So I don't know whether that's relevant.
Are you checking the pH of the urine of the different patients. That can vary and there may be some correlation with that. That may be one way of looking at the variation.

TANNENBAUM: It's pretty stable. It takes a pretty extreme diet. The ascorbic acid drops the pH. In fact, that's why we did the sodium ascorbate experiment. The ascorbic acid drops the pH of the urine considerably. The reason we did the sodium ascorbate experiment was to check that we got the same data. We got exactly the same results with sodium ascorbate that we got with ascorbic acid. The pH of the urine was quite different in those two cases. But, of course, you've got ascorbic acid present in the urine.

HOFFMANN: But isn't it surprising that a vegetarian would have an elevated pH?

TANNENBAUM: Yes.

HOFFMANN: And do they have more ascorbic acid than we do as meat eaters?

TANNENBAUM: No. Probably Dr. Simenhoff could answer this—but it takes a considerable dose of ascorbic acid to lower the urine pH.

SIMENHOFF: You're right. Vegetarians often have pH changes.

HOFFMANN: Vegetarians get more ascorbic acid.

TANNENBAUM: But not enough to acidify the urine.

WEISBURGER: We really had a very good discussion about reliable and interesting nondestructive, noninterventionist methods to measure the potential of nitrite exposure. I think that will be a stepping stone for a future meeting. We thank Dr. Bartsch and Dr. Tannenbaum and the discussants for enlightening us in this very important field.

Now, we are still concerned with the exposure of humans to potential or actual nitrosamines. Those of you who are gastrointestinal physicians and scientists know that gastric and duodenal ulcers were important problems in men and women—mostly men—in the world, particularly in some areas of the world like northern Europe and Japan. In the past it made surgeons quite rich. However, in the last 5 or 10 years, the pharmaceutical industry came through with a number of products, among which cimetidine was found to be a very effective drug to relieve the effects of gastric and duodenal ulcers; and, indeed, it is one of the best drugs. A number of other houses came through with similar drugs, like ranitidine—a new product on the market. It didn't take long for some wise chemists in the oncology field to look at the structure of cimetidine and find that it had a structure that looked almost like methylguanidine. Those of us in the field almost automatically stick nitroso groups on these free hydrogens in these compounds, perform an Ames mutagenicity test and find them Ames-positive.

And so, a question arose as to possible carcinogenicity, especially since people that are prone to gastric ulcers are also somewhat at higher risk for gastric cancer.

Possible Role of Cimetidine
and its Nitrosation Products
in Human Stomach Cancer

JAMES B. ELDER, PROVASH C. GANGULI, CHRISTOPHER G. KOFFMAN,
STEPHEN WELLS, AND GEORGE WILLIAMS
University Departments of Surgery and Pathology
Manchester Royal Infirmary
Manchester M13 9WL

Of the fairly large numbers of preparations currently available to treat peptic ulcer disease in both the United States and in Britain, by far the most widely prescribed class of compounds are the H_2 blockers represented by cimetidine (CM) and ranitidine (Cocco and Cocco 1981; Schade and Donaldson 1981; *Lancet* 1982). CM (Fig. 1) blocks the H_2 receptor on the parietal cell and since its introduction in November 1976 to U.K. more than a million people have received it in that country and perhaps as many as 15 million patients world-wide. In a daily dose of 1 g/day^{-1} it is very effective in controlling gastric HCl secretion in duodenal ulcer (DU) subjects as is ranitidine (Table 1). It may also be given to patients where HCl may not be primarily involved such as those with gastric ulcer and reflux esophagitis. The acid-inhibiting effect of this compound can be compared with that of surgical vagotomy (parasympathetic denervation) but of course the advantage is that its effects are reversible on withdrawal of the drug. Symptoms are rapidly brought under control in up to 90% of the DU patients (less so with gastric ulcer) and because of this high clinical efficacy, patients are likely to continue treatment or even demand it. Maintenance dosage at night (400-800 mg orally) has been advocated on a long-term basis to prevent ulcer relapse, although clinically there is some doubt as to the efficacy in this case (Bardhan et al. 1982). Nevertheless, many patients have now been on maintenance therapy for some years. Clearly this method of exhibiting the drug would lead to its ingestion at a time when the pH of the stomach was acid, as opposed to treatment during full dosage when in some circumstances the intragastric pH may well be near neutral (McCloy and Baron 1981; Walt et al. 1981). Most such patients have antral gastritis (Morson 1979).

THE PROBLEM

The question may be asked why involve CM in issues concerning gastric cancer? In 1978, clinical circumstances arose in some patients where early gastric cancer

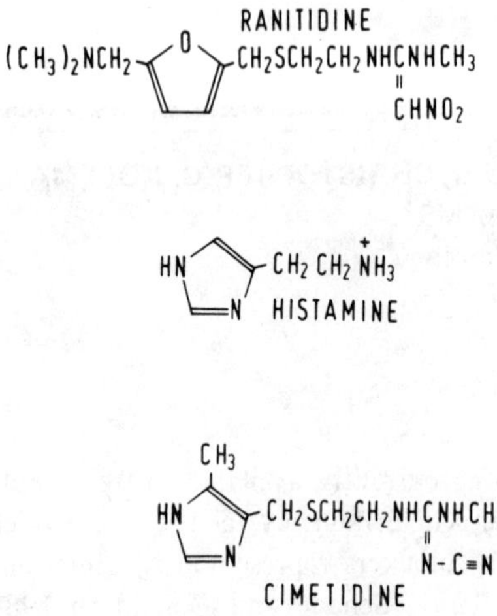

RANITIDINE

$(CH_3)_2NCH_2$ —[O]— $CH_2SCH_2CH_2NHCNHCH_3$
$\qquad\qquad\qquad\qquad\qquad \overset{\|}{C}HNO_2$

HN—[ ]—$CH_2 CH_2 \overset{+}{N}H_3$
$\qquad$ HISTAMINE

$\qquad CH_3$
HN—[ ]—$CH_2SCH_2CH_2NHCNHCH_3$
$\qquad\qquad\qquad\qquad \overset{\|}{N}-C\equiv N$
$\qquad$ CIMETIDINE

Figure 1
Molecular formulae: CM, histamine, and ranitidine.

Table 1
Mean Values of 24-Hour Intragastric Acidity

Treatment	Mean 24h H^+ activity (mmol/1)[a,b,c]	Percentage fall in H^+ activity	Mean intragastric pH
Placebo	41.8 ± 1.5	—	1.38
CM	21.6 ± 1.2^d	48	1.67
Ranitidine 150 mg bd	13.1 ± 1.0^e	69	1.88
Ranitidine 200 mg bd	12.1 ± 1.1^e	71	1.92

Data reprinted, with permission, from Walt et al. (1981).
[a] n = 10 DU male patients
[b] dose of CM 1 g/day
[c] ± S.E.M.
[d] p 0.001 compared with placebo
[e] p 0.001 compared with placebo and CM

was diagnosed unexpectedly while they were taking CM (Buck et al. 1979; Elder et al. 1979; Reed et al. 1979; Taylor et al. 1979; Hawker et al. 1980). In some, the primary diagnosis had been a DU, and in others a gastric ulcer or indeed no mucosal lesion was apparently present before using the drug. The early gastric cancers detected were antral or pyloric in location and although the diagnosis was made endoscopically, the stomach in two cases at operation appeared grossly normal. Jointly Dr. Reed and myself have details of 28 such cases where carcinoma of the stomach has been found after treatment of 6 months-2 years duration with CM. Undoubtedly we must consider the probability that malignant change was already present in some patients before CM treatment began, and that H_2 blockade masked the cancer. This is by no means the certain explanation in other patients. These cases are to be published and discussed in detail elsewhere but must nevertheless be regarded as anecdotal, however clinically disturbing.

INTRAGASTRIC MILIEU ON CIMETIDINE TREATMENT

Hypothesis A

There are at least two hypotheses why CM may possibly be implicated in the development of carcinoma of the stomach (Hypothesis A—Elder et al. 1979; Hypothesis B—Reed et al. 1981b). First, we must consider the available data on the intragastric conditions in patients on CM treatment. The data of Pounder et al. (1977); McCloy and Baron (1981); Walt et al. (1981 and Table 2) show clearly that the intragastric pH in virtually all patients given CM will initially be acid and then for some hours, particularly if it is given after a meal, the intragastric pH increases to more than 5 in 40-50% of patients. Concomitant with an increase in pH, intragastric nitrite levels have also been found to be elevated and to correlate with pH change in patients on CM (Bartholomew et al. 1980; Reed et al. 1981b; Stockbrugger et al. 1982). Direct nitrosation of the drug itself in

Table 2
Mean Values of Nocturnal Acid Output in 10 DU Patients (0100-0700hr)

Treatment	Mean nocturnal acid output (mmol h^{-1})[a]	Percentage fall in acid output	Percentage of samples with pH > 5.0
Placebo	6.1	—	0
CM	1.8[b]	70	39[d]
Ranitidine 150 mg bd	1.6[c]	90	54[d]
Ranitidine	0.7[c]	89	53[d]

Data reprinted, with permission, from Walt et al. (1981).
[a] $n = 10$
[b] $p < 0.01$ compared with placebo.
[c] $p < 0.01$ compared with placebo and $p < 0.05$ compared with CM.
[d] $p < 0.001$ compared with placebo (by x^2 analysis).

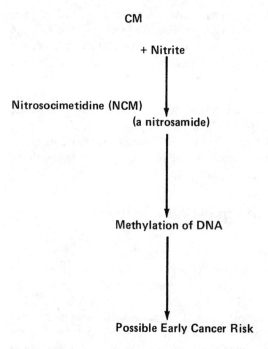

CM

+ Nitrite

Nitrosocimetidine (NCM)
(a nitrosamide)

Methylation of DNA

Possible Early Cancer Risk

Figure 2
Hypothesis A

the stomach with possible formation of N-monoNCM (Fig. 2) has been postulated and the similarity of part of the molecule to methyl-N-nitroso-guanidine (MNNG) noted (Fig. 3) (Elder et al. 1979). In vitro in acid conditions somewhat dissimilar to that proposed in the human stomach NCM is easily pre-pared (Foster et al. 1980; Bavin et al. 1980). The kinetics of this reaction under ideal chemical conditions have been studied by workers at SmithKline & French: At 37°C over physiologic pH range they have shown that the yield of NCM can reach up to 40% of drug substrate at pHl in 1 hour (Table 3). These con-ditions are somewhat extreme in terms of the nitrite concentrations used and did not involve catalysts of bacterial origin. However, some in vivo intragastric nitrosation is nonetheless likely if nitrite is available. The chemical activity of NCM is of the same order as the well known potent gastric carcinogen MNNG (Foster et al. 1980). NCM has been shown to cause DNA methylation both in vitro (Jensen and Magee 1981), and in human cell cultures (Jensen 1981); induction of DNA strand breaks (Schwarz et al. 1980); to cause toxicity towards cultured mammalian cells (Henderson and Basilio 1981); to cause inhibition of the cytochrome P-450 system in rat and man (Puurunen 1979; Puurunen and Pelkonen 1979) and is mutagenic in an Ames/Salmonella system

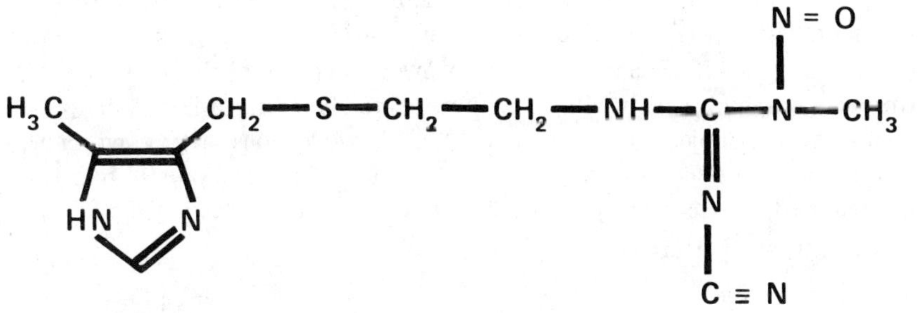

(a) nitrosocimetidine.

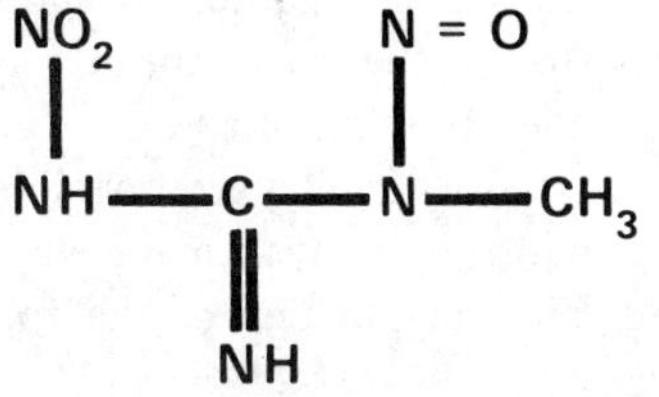

(b) N-methyl-N'-nitro-N-nitrosoguanidine.

Figure 3
Comparison of molecular formulae of NCM and *N*-Methyl-*N*-nitro-*N*-Nitrosoguanidine.

Table 3
In vitro Kinetics of the Nitrosation of CM at 37°C

pH	10^6 (initial rate) mol 1^{-1} s^{-1}	% Conversion into nitroso derivative after 1 hr	% Conversion into nitroso derivative after 4 hr
1.00	3.970	42.5	39.6
1.92	0.440	15.3	31.1
3.04	0.047	1.7	5.9
6.01	0.004	0.15	0.49

$[NaNO_2] = 0.04$ mol 1^{-1} [Cim] 0.01 mol 1^{-1}

Data from Bavin et al. (1980).

(Poole et al. 1979; De Flora and Picciotto 1980). Furthermore, NCM has recently been shown to induce chromosome aberrations in cultured Chinese hamster ovary cells. (Athanasiou and Kyrtopoulos 1981). All of these results point towards probable carcinogenic activity of NCM. Intragastric nitrosation is probably not a simple process and it has been suggested that the state of the gastric mucosa itself is important when considering intragastric nitrosation (Correa et al. 1975; Stemmerman and Mower 1981; Tannenbaum et al. 1981). Chronic atrophic gastritis with or without intestinal metaplasia may be present in many ulcer subjects receiving the drug. Two questions arise: First, is NCM formed in vivo? Secondly, is it carcinogenic? The first question still remains to be answered, but to provide data relevant to the second question the following experiment was performed.

METHODS

Four groups, each of 20 male Sprague-Dawley rats (weight 250 g), were prepared with an antro-fundic gastric mucosal wound using the method of Wong and Lowenthal (1976). Standard circular 5 mm diameter electro-cautery wounds of the gastric mucosa in this region of the rat stomach remain unhealed as chronic ulcers for 3-6 months, thus providing a parallel situation of an ulcerated area of mucosa with cell division and repair at its edge, crudely comparable to the human situation with a peptic ulcer. After allowing 7 days for recovery from the gastrotomy the animals were allocated randomly to one of the following groups;

1. Control group receiving $NaNo_3$ (3.75 g.1^{-1}) and $NaNo_2$ (0.75 g.1^{-1}) in deionized water (control solution).
2. Control solution containing 25 mg kg^{-1} (2.52 mg ml^{-1}) CM
3. Control solution containing (2.80 mg ml^{-1}) NCM equimolar to CM in group 2.
4. Control solution containing MNNG (1.47 mg ml^{-1}) equimolar to CM in group.

All animals received dosage by gavage in volumes of 1-1.4 ml for 6 months once daily for 6 days/week. The larger volumes were used towards the end of the study as the animals gained weight. A pilot kill of 5 rats from each group at 6 months did not reveal any evidence of carcinoma of the stomach, but rather dysplasia and hyperplasia near the edge of the chronic gastric wound largely in groups 1, 2, and 3. The remaining surviving rats were killed in ether at 14-15 months. After ligation of the pyloric sphincter each stomach was filled with 6-8 ml 10% Formalin by gavage tube. It was removed and placed in formal saline for 2 hours before being opened, rinsed gently with saline (0.154 M), and pinned out on cork boards. Specific search at postmortem was made for the presence or absence of an ulcer in the stomach and gross lesions in the mucosa. Microscopic examination of the mucosa of the stomach noting particularly adenomatous-hyperplasia, intestinal metaplasia, dysplasia, borderline lesions, and frank gastric carcinoma was performed by two of us (S.W. and G.W.) who were not aware of the groups to which the animals belonged.

Table 4

Histological Grading in Rat Experiment

Group	Antral dysplasia	Body dysplasia	Squamous metaplasia	Antro-fundic ulcer
Control (19)[a]	6	1	2	7
CM (20)	8	6	4	6
NCM (16)	4	1	2	3
MNNG (9)	1	3	3	3

[a]number in parentheses refers to number of patients in the group

RESULTS

No gross tumors of esophagus, lung, kidney, small bowel, adrenals, brains, or testicles were seen. The findings in the stomachs in each of the groups including those killed at 6 months are shown in Tables 4 and 5. Adenomatous hyperplasia in control rats was seen in the antrum in relation to the wounded area but no gastric carcinomas were found. Gastric carcinoma was found in those in the NCM and MNNG groups only and a borderline lesion in the CM group. All of these were at the edge of the experimental gastric wound. The low incidence of carcinomas in this study is probably related to the relatively small numbers in each group and to the dosage schedule employed which corresponds to the maximum dose of CM recommended clinically in man. Several rats in the MNNG group died of inanition or pneumonia between 6 and 15 months and acceptable histological examinations could not be obtained.

Table 5

Incidence of Dysplasia, Hyperplasia, and Gastric Carcinoma in Rat Experiment

Group	Adenomatous hyperplasia	Borderline lesion	Carcinoma
Control (19)[a]	6	0	0
CM (20)	4	1	0
NCM (16)	2	0	1
MNNG (9)	2	0	2

[a]Numbers in parentheses = number of subjects in the group.

Although adenocarinomas were seen in some rats in this study the data are not large enough for proper statistical analysis. Our results, however, suggest that, experimentally, if the gastric mucosa is exposed to NCM it can lead to the development of gastric carcinoma in the antrum. A further group of 50 rats of Sprague-Dawley strain from our Manchester University Animal House was similarly studied over the same time course and conditions as those in the above protocol, but they did not receive drugs. Detailed postmortem examinations of these 50 animals revealed no spontaneous tumors in the stomach on microscopic examination. It is germane to note that the other H_2-blocking drug available clinically in the U.K., ranitidine, has not been found to form an N-nitroso compound (Britain et al. 1981b). However, tiotidine, an H_2 blocker tested at I.C.I. England which has an identical side chain to CM (Fig. 4) gave rise to early antral carcinomas in the rat. (I.C.I. information on file).

Hypothesis B

The second hypothesis (Fig. 5) concerning CM or any other H_2 blocker and the possible development of gastric carcinoma depends on its pharmacological action (Britain et al. 1981a) on hydrochloric acid secretion. This hypothesis currently propounded by Reed et al. (1981b) draws heavily on the work of Correa et al. (1975). H_2 blockers as a group produce very effective inhibition of 70%-90% of maximal H-ion secretion clinically (Walt et al. 1981) but mean intragastric pH varies considerably throughout the day depending on

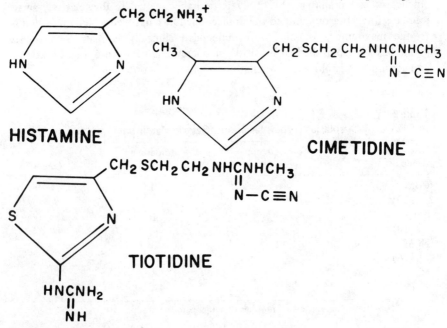

Figure 4
Molecular formulae; comparison of CM and tiotidine.

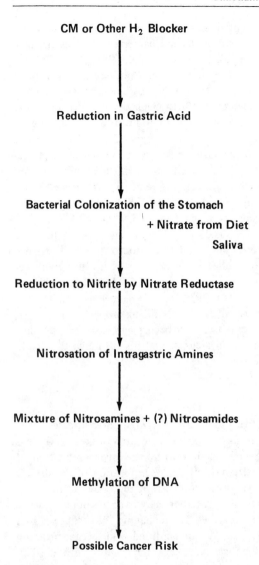

CM or Other H$_2$ Blocker

↓

Reduction in Gastric Acid

↓

Bacterial Colonization of the Stomach
+ Nitrate from Diet
Saliva

↓

Reduction to Nitrite by Nitrate Reductase

↓

Nitrosation of Intragastric Amines

↓

Mixture of Nitrosamines + (?) Nitrosamides

↓

Methylation of DNA

↓

Possible Cancer Risk

Figure 5
Hypothesis B

food ingestion and dosage times. Overall, the mean intragastric pH throughout 24 hours on H$_2$-blocking drugs in DU patients has been found to be between 1 and 2 (Table 1), but at night between 40-50% gastric juice samples in DU patients have been found to have pH values greater than 5 (Table 2; Walt et al. 1981). When 800 mg CM is taken before retiring the intragastric pH is often maintained close to neutrality throughout the night (Fitzpatrick et al.

1982). Several authors have documented that CM has been found to lead to increased levels of nitrite, N-nitroso compounds and bacteria in the gastric juice (Bartholomew et al. 1980; Ruddell et al. 1981; Reed et al. 1981b; Stockbrügger et al. 1982). Similar changes have been found in patients not on CM but who are known to be at risk of developing gastric carcinoma, or who are actually suffering from gastric carcinoma (Reed et al. 1981a; Schlag et al. 1981). The role of bacteria in catalyzing reactions between amines and nitrite at physiological pH has recently been reviewed with reference to Escherichia coli (Kunisaki and Hayashi 1979), and an enzymatic mechanism as well as nonenzymatic acceleration of formation of N-nitroso compounds was found. The bacteria commonly found in gastric juice after CM treatment are gram + ve cocci, enterococci, lactobacilli, and streptococcus salivarius (Ruddell et al. 1981). In this study the counts of nitrite reducing organisms increased from 1.3 ± 0.4 (SEM) $\log_{10}$ to $3.7 \pm 0.6 \log_{10}$ organisms ml^{-1} ($p < 0.01$, n = 23). Others disagree that CM treatment leads to increased nitroso compound formation or indeed to significant gastric colonization, but they studied small numbers of healthy volunteer subjects over short periods of time and found that the pH level seldom rose above 4 (Barnard et al. 1981; Muscroft et al. 1981). Thus in these studies it is likely that the gastric juice still retained its acid sterilizing properties. Recently, the importance of the gastric mucosa itself has been reemphasised in possible endogenous mechanisms of nitrosation in areas of gastritis, although this is still to be confirmed (Stemmerman and Mower 1981).

DISCUSSION

Given that H_2 blockers are effective inhibitors of hydrochloric acid secretion and that at least for several hours intragstric pH increases to 5 or greater, there is every possibility that intragastric colonization with consequent reduction of nitrate to nitrite will take place. Alternatively direct nitrosation of the drug is possible at acidic or near neutral pH, thus hypotheses A and B are not mutually exclusive. The mechanism of nitrosation whether enzymatic or nonenzymatic requires further investigation. Recent work by Tannenbaum (1981) suggests that there are factors in gastric juice as yet unidentified which can promote nitrosation. The extent to which the cascade, as shown in Figure 5, proposed by Reed et al. (1981b) may actually occur will depend on the individual patient, his sensitivity to H_2 blockers, the size of his parietal cell mass, the presence and severity of gastritis, and nitrite availability. Those patients with acid secretory capacity in the upper range of normal or frankly elevated secretory capacity (greater than 40 mM hr^{-1}) will be less likely to have reductions following H_2 blockade to acid levels which will reduce significantly the gastric acid sterilizing barrier. Others with gastric acid secretion in the low normal range or frank hyposecretion may well have their acid secretory capacities so markedly impaired following H_2 blockade that intragastric colonization will result. It appears likely that some patients with DU, two-thirds of whom fall in the normal gastric acid secretion range (Baron 1963), may well develop intragastric colonization on H_2 blockers. Depending on the extent of pH elevation and its

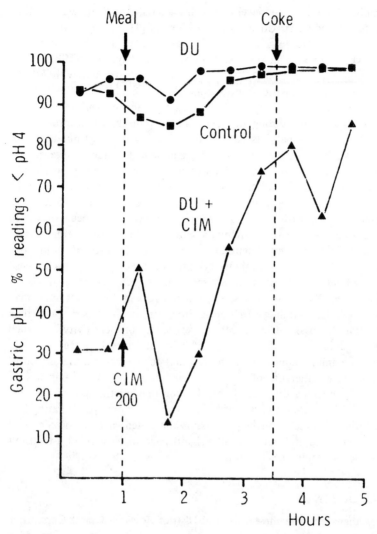

Figure 6
Mean gastric pH in 8 healthy controls, 10 patients with DU, and 5 of these patients on CM. Reproduced, with permission, from McCloy and Baron (1981).

time course in relation to drug ingestion these subjects may be at a higher risk than normal with respect to intragastric nitrosation and formation of N-nitroso compounds. Data is available on intragastric pH variation from McCloy and Baron (1981) using an intraluminal miniature glass electrode. They measured pH every 20 seconds for 1 hour before and 4 hours after a meal in 8 healthy subjects and 10 patients with DU. Five patients had paired studies while on 200 mg CM three times per day and 400 mg at night. Their results are summarized in Figure 6. In the 3½ hours after ingestion of 200 mg CM up to 87% of the pH readings were > 4, the level at which bacterial colonization is possible, and even after an acid drink (Coke pH 2.5) 14-36% of pH readings were still > 4. The importance of microorganisms in the response to a gastric carcinogen (MNNG) is well illustrated in the results of Sumi and Miyakawa (1981). They found experimentally that only 29% of germfree rats treated with MNNG (450 μg/rat) developed gastric tumors compared to an incidence of 93% in conventional similarly treated rats, indicating that the microflora might be exerting a significant promoting influence upon stomach tumor production. Recent evidence in DU patients suggested that as early as 60 minutes after ingestion of CM, gastric juice became mutagenic and detectable mutagenicity persisted for 3 hours but the gastric juice was not different from normal after 12 hours (Morris et al. 1982). Other groups whose intragastric pH may often be high, including post-vagotomy patients, post-gastrectomy patients, and those with chronic atrophic gastritis and intestinal metaplasia, have been shown to have an increased risk of gastric carcinoma. However, the question remains as to what proportion of nonoperated peptic ulcer patients on H_2 blockers in the long term are at risk. Conventional thinking about the time required for development of carcinomas holds that several years are required for their development. Nevertheless, experimentally, nitrosamines, and nitrosamides in 39 species other than man induce tumors, including carcinomas, in relatively short periods of time (Bogovski and Bogovski 1981). Man's resistance or sensitivity to such compounds is unknown, but it is very unlikely that he will prove to be exceptional in the animal kingdom and be resistant to the carcinogenic action of such compounds whether of endogenous or exogenous origin. Thus it may be said for the H_2-blocking drugs, as it has for the oral contraceptives, (Hoover and Fraumeni 1981), that millions of human beings are now participating in a clinical experiment which will help to assess the potential carcinogenicity of these compounds, but the public health significance of even small alterations in carcinogenic risk could be substantial.

ACKNOWLEDGMENTS

We wish to thank the Manchester Central District Research Grants Committee for financial support, Mrs. Ann Tomlin for expert technical assistance, and Miss Marlene Wray for typing the manuscript.

REFERENCES

Athanasiou, K. and S. Kyrtopoulos. 1981. Induction of sister chromatid exchanges and chromosome aberrations in cultured mammalian cells by N-nitrosocimetidine. *Cancer Lett.* 14:71.
Bardhan, K.D., J. Beresford, and R.F.C. Hinchcliffe. 1981. Low dose cimetidine maintenance treatment in duodenal ulcer: Intermediate term results. Paper presented at British Society of Gastroenterology. *Gut* 22:A879.
Barnard, J., D.W. Darkin, N.J. Viney, Z. Ahmet, N.F. Lightfoot, R.H. Hunt, and

G.T. Milton-Thompson. 1982. Effect of cimetidine on twenty-four intra-gastric pH, bacterial flora and concentrations of nitrite and nitroso-compounds. *Lancet* i:(in press).

Baron, J.H. 1963. The relationship between basal and maximal acid output in normal subjects and patients with duodenal ulcer. *Clin. Sci.* 24:357.

Bartholomew, B.A., M.J. Hill, M.J. Hudson, W.S.J. Ruddell, and C.L. Walters. 1980. Gastric bacteria, nitrate, nitrite and nitrosamines in patients with pernicious anaemia and in patients treated with cimetidine. *IARC Sci. Publ.* 31:595.

Bavin, P.M.G., G.J. Durant, P.D. Miles, R.C. Mitchell, and E.S. Pepper. 1980. Nitrosation of cimetidine [N″-cyano-N-methyl-N″- {2-[(5-methyl-midazol-4-Y1) methylthio] ethyl} guanidine] *J. Chem. Res.*(s) 212.

Bogovski, P. and S. Bogovski. 1981. Animal species in which N-nitroso-compounds induce cancer. Special Report. *Int. J. Cancer* 27:471.

Britain, R.T., D. Jack, and B.J. Price. 1981a. Recent development in histamine H_2 antagonists. *Trends Pharmacol. Sci.* 2:310.

Britain, R.T., D.M. Harris, L.E. Martin, D. Poynter, and B.J. Price. 1981b. Safety of ranitidine. *Lancet* ii:1119.

Buck, J.P., R.E. Murgatroyd, A.W. Boylston, and J.H. Baron. 1979. Perforation of gastric carcinoma (at site of previous benign ulcer) after withdrawal of cimetidine. *Lancet* ii:42.

Cocco, A.E. and D.V. Cocco. 1981. A survey of cimetidine prescribing. *N. Engl. J. Med.* 304:1281.

Correa, P., W. Haenszel, C. Cuello, S. Tannenbaum, and M. Archer. 1975. A model for gastric cancer epidemiology. *Lancet* ii:58.

De Flora, S. and A. Picciotto. 1980. Mutagenicity in nitrite-enriched human gastric juice. *Carcinogenesis* 1:925.

Elder, J.B., P.C. Ganguli, and I.E. Gillespie. 1979. Cimetidine and gastric cancer. *Lancet* i:1005.

Fitzpatrick, W.J.F., W.S. Blackwood, and T.C. Northfield. 1982. Bedtime cimetidine maintenance treatment: Optimum dose and effect on subsequent natural history of duodenal ulcer. *Gut* 23:239.

Foster, A.B., M. Jarman, and D. Manson. 1980. Structure and reactivity of nitrosocimetidine. *Cancer Lett.* 9:47.

Hawker, P.C., T.J. Muscroft, and M.R.B. Keighley. 1980. Gastric cancer after cimetidine in a patient with two negative pretreatment biopsies. *Lancet* i:709.

Henderson, E.E. and M. Basilio. 1981. Cellular DNA damage by nitroso-cimeti-dine: A comparison with N-methyl-N^1-nitro-nitrosoguanidine and x-irradiation. *Chem. Biol. Interact.* 38:87.

Hoover, R. and J.F. Fraumeni. 1981. Drug-Induced cancer. *Cancer* 47:1071.

Jansen, D.E. 1981. Deoxyribonucleic acid methylation in human cells exposed to nitrosocimetidine. *Biochem. Pharmacol.* 30:2864.

Jansen, D.E. and P.N. Magee. 1981. Methylation of DNA by nitrosocimetidine in vitro. *Cancer Res.* 41:230.

Kunisaki, N. and M. Hayashi. 1979. Formation of N-nitrosamines from secondary amines and nitrite by resting cells of *Escherichia Coli* B. *Applied and Environmental Biology* 37:279.

Lancet. 1982. Cimetidine and ranitidine. *Lancet* i:601.

McCloy, R.F. and J.H. Baron. 1981. Intragastric pH and cimetidine, fasting and after food. *Lancet* i:408.

Morris, D.L., D. Young, T.J. Muscroft, D.W. Burdon, and M.R. Keighley. 1982. Mutagenicity in gastric juice. Paper No. F41. Presented at the Spring Meeting of British Society of Gastroenterology, Norwich England. *Gut Abst.* (in press).

Morson, B.C. 1979. Gastritis. In *Gastrointestinal Pathology* (eds. B.C. Morson and Dawson), p. 107. Blackwell Scientific Publications, Oxford, UK.

Muscroft, T.J., D.J. Youngs, D.W. Burdon, and M.B. Keighley. 1981. Cimetidine is unlikely to increase formation of intragastric N-nitroso-compounds in patients taking a normal diet. *Lancet* i:408.

Poole, B.L., G. Eisenbrand, and D. Schmähl. 1979. Biological activity of nitrosated cimetidine. *Toxicology* 15:69.

Pounder, R., R. Hunt, S. Vincent, G.J. Milton-Thompson, and J.J. Misiewicz. 1977. Twenty-four hour intragastric acidity and nocturnal acid secretion in patients with duodenal ulcer during oral administration of cimetidine and atropine. *Gut* 18:85.

Puurunen, J. 1979. Cimetidine inhibits microsomal drug metabolism in man. Naunyu-Schmiedeberg's. *Arch. Pharm.* 308:Suppl. R24.

Puurunen, J. and O. Pelkonen. 1979. Cimetidine inhibits microsomal drug metabolism in the rat. *Eur. J. Pharm.* 55:335.

Reed, P.I., P. Cassell, and C.L. Walters. 1979. Gastric cancer in patients who have taken cimetidine. *Lancet* i:1234.

Reed, P.I., P.L.R. Smith, K. Haines, F.R. House, and C.L. Walters. 1981a. Gastric juice nitrosamines in health and gastroduodenal disease. *Lancet* ii:550.

_____. 1981b. Effect of cimetidine on gastric juice N-nitrosamine concentration. *Lancet* ii:553.

Ruddell, W.S.J., A.T.R. Axon, J.M. Findlay, B.A. Bartholomew, and M.J. Hill. 1981. Effect of cimetidine on the gastric bacterial flora. *Lancet* i:672.

Schade, R.R. and R.M. Donaldson. 1981. How physicians use cimetidine: A survey of hospitalized patients and published cases. *N. Engl. J. Med.* 304: 1281.

Schlag, P., R. Bockler, M. Peter, and C.H. Ilerfarth. 1981. Nitrite and N-nitroso-compounds in the operated stomach. *Scand. J. Gastroenterol.* 16:Suppl. 67, 63.

Schwarz, M., J. Hummel, and G. Eisenbrand. 1980. Induction of DNA strand breaks by nitrosocimetidine. *Cancer Lett.* 10:223.

Stemmerman, G.N. and H. Mower. 1981. Gastritis, Nitrosamines and gastric cancer. *J. Clin. Gastroenterology* 3:Suppl. 2, 23.

Stockbrügger, R.W., P.B. Cotton, N. Eugenides, B.A. Bartholomew, M.J. Hill, and C.L. Walters. 1982. Intragastric nitrites, nitrosamines and bacterial overgrowth during cimetidine treatment. *Gut* (in press).

Sumi, Y. and M. Miyakawa. 1981. Comparative studies on the production of stomach tumours following the intubation of several doses of N-methyl-N'-nitro-N-nitrosoguanidine in germ-free and conventional newborn rats. *Gann.* 72:700.

Tannenbaum, S.R., D. Moran, K. Falchuk, P. Correa, and C. Cuello. 1981. Nitrite stability and nitrosation potential in human gastric juice. *Cancer Lett.* 14:131.

Taylor, T.V., P. Lee, and A.G. Howatson. 1979. Gastric cancer in patients who have taken cimetidine. *Lancet* i:1235.

Walt, R.P., P.J. Male, J. Rawlings, R.H. Hunt, G.J. Milton-Thompson, and J.J. Misiewicz. 1981. Comparison of the effect of ranitidine, cimetidine and placebo on the 24 hour intragastric acidity and nocturnal acid secretion in patients with duodenal ulcer. *Gut* 22:49.

Wong, J. and J. Lowenthal. 1976. Chronic gastric ulcer in the rat produced by wounding at the antro-fundic junction. *Gastroenterology* 71:416.

The Effects of Cimetidine on
Intragastric Nitrosation in Man

PETER I. REED AND KAY HAINES
Departments of Medicine
Wexham Park Hospital
Slough, Berkshire SL2 4HL
and Royal Postgraduate Medical School
Hammersmith Hospital, London W12, England

PETER L. R. SMITH AND CLIFFORD L. WALTERS
Leatherhead Food Research Association
Leatherhead, Surrey, England

FRANK R. HOUSE
Department of Pharmacology
Guy's Hospital Medical School
London SE1, England

In 1968 Sander first demonstrated that bacteria could catalyze the N-nitrosation reaction, so that N-nitroso compounds could be formed in vivo whenever appropriate bacteria, nitrosatable amine, and nitrate or nitrite coexist in the body (Hill and Hawksworth 1972). The presence of nitrate-reducing bacteria and of N-nitroso compounds has been demonstrated in vivo in the human achlorhydric stomach (Sander et al. 1968; Ruddell et al. 1976; Ruddell et al. 1978), infected urinary bladder (Brooks et al. 1972; Hicks et al. 1977), colon (Hill 1979), and saliva (Tannenbaum et al. 1978).

It has also been demonstrated that elevated nitrite levels are found in the achlorhydric stomach (Ruddell et al. 1976; Tannenbaum et al. 1979), along with increased counts of total and nitrate-reducing bacteria. Such changes have been found in gastric cancer and in conditions predisposing to it, such as pernicious anemia (Ruddell et al. 1978), chronic atrophic gastritis with intestinal metaplasia (Jones et al. 1978), and after gastric surgery, including partial gastrectomy (Schlag et al. 1980; Muscroft et al. 1981) and vagotomy with drainage (Reed et al. 1982). Hitherto no systematic studies had been performed to correlate gastric juice N-nitrosamine concentration with the various parameters which may be affected by pH elevation in healthy subjects and especially in patients in whom the intragastric environment is altered by disease or treatment. However, such a study has been carried out prospectively by us recently in which we measured the pH, nitrite and N-nitroso compound concentrations, and cultured gastric juice for total and nitrate-reducing bacteria

Table 1
Patients Studied

Subjects	Number	Age range (yrs)	Number specimens
Male	160	18-81	186
Female	107	18-87	115
Total	267		301

obtained from fasting patients with various gastro-duodenal abnormalities, many also treated with the H_2-receptor antagonist, cimetidine (CM), as well as from healthy volunteers with no history of gastrointestinal disorders.

PATIENTS AND METHODS

The details of the methods employed have been reported elsewhere (Reed et al. 1981a; Reed et al. 1981b).

301 specimens of gastric juice were obtained from 267 untreated subjects, including 37 patients before starting CM treatment and 50 healthy volunteers acting as controls (Table 1). The diagnostic categories are listed in Table 2. In addition, 140 patients who were on CM treatment were studied, 216 gastric juice samples being obtained (Tables 3 and 4). The variables examined included age, sex, smoking habit, pH, presence of nitrite, N-nitrosamine concentration, and bacterial culture results. The data were subjected to computer analysis.

Table 2
Diagnostic Groups

Group	Subjects (n = 267)	Specimens (n = 301)
Duodenal ulcer	70	77
Vagotomy	24	26
Partial gastrectomy	14	16
Atrophic gastritis	13	14
Gastric ulcer	33	52
Pernicious anemia	16	17
Carcinoma of stomach	23	23
Reflux esophagitis	10	12
Miscellaneous-dyspepsia:		
endoscopy normal	14	14
Controls	50	50

Table 3
Patients Studied During CM Treatment

Subjects	Number patients	Age range (yr)	Number gastric juice samples
Male	103	18-80	156
Female	37	21-81	60
Total	140		216

Table 4
Groups Treated With CM

Group	Patients (n = 140)	Samples (n = 216)
Post-vagotomy	15	22
Post-partial gastrectomy	4	5
Duodenal ulcer	74	122
Atrophic gastritis	5	5
Gastric ulcer	24	40
Reflux esophagitis	7	8
Miscellaneous dyspepsia/ normal mucosa on endoscopy	11	14

RESULTS

The mean N-nitrosamine level in 50 healthy volunteers without gastrointestinal disease was 0.14 ± 0.07 μmol/1. In the untreated subjects a strong positive correlation was noted between a rise in N-nitrosamine concentrations and age ($p = 0.56 \times 10^{-4}$), gastric pH ($p < 10^{-6}$; Fig. 1), total bacterial growth ($p = 0.31 \times 10^{-5}$), nitrate-reducing bacterial growth ($p = 0.028$), and nitrite concentration ($p = 0.021$). There was a positive correlation between pH and age ($p < 10^{-6}$) and growth of nitrate-reducing bacteria ($p = 0.028$). A highly significant correlation was noted between N-nitrosamine concentration and pH in duodenal ulcer ($p = 0.91 \times 10^{-6}$), gastric ulcer ($p = 0.76 \times 10^{-5}$), post-vagotomy ($p = 0.40 \times 10^{-4}$), pernicious anemia ($p = 0.0052$), and gastric cancer ($p = 0.0061$). Those diseases which are known to be associated with reduced gastric acidity and raised pH were found to have higher mean N-nitrosamine levels (Fig. 2); these levels were significantly higher in male patients ($p = 0.0036$). Neither N-nitrosamine nor nitrite concentrations were affected by cigarette smoking.

In the CM-treated patients an equally strong correlation was demonstrated between pH and N-nitrosamine concentration (Fig. 3). Nitrosamine levels rose

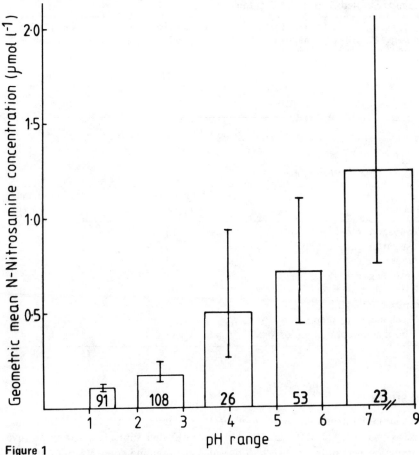

Figure 1

Relation between gastric pH and *N*-nitrosamine concentration. 301 samples tested. Base of histogram represents pH range. (I) 95% confidence limits.

progressively with pH elevation from a mean of 0.11 μmol/1 at pH 1-1.5 to a mean of 1.66 μmol/1 at pH 6.5-9 ($p < 10^{-6}$), compared with 0.10 μmol/1 and 1.20 μmol/1 respectively ($p < 10^{-6}$) in individuals not so treated. The pH levels were significantly higher during CM treatment (mean increase 0.5 pH units; $p = 0.0025$) as was the mean *N*-nitrosamine concentration ($p = 0.021$). In the higher pH range, especially when compared with untreated patients in the same diagnostic groups, *N*-nitrosamine concentrations were markedly elevated (Fig. 4). In those with a duodenal ulcer, correlation between pH elevation and *N*-nitrosamine levels was highly significant ($p = 0.0083$).

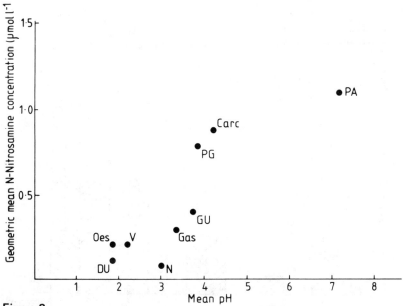

Figure 2
Gastric pH and N-nitrosamine concentrations in untreated groups. (N) normal controls; (DU) duodenal ulcer; (Oes) oesophagitis; (V) vagotomy; (Gas) chronic gastritis; (GU) gastric ulcer; (PG) partial gastrectomy; (Carc) carcinoma of stomach; (PA) pernicious anemia.

Serial studies were also carried out in 53 patients having CM treatment. In 30, the pretreatment state was compared with that after 3-9 weeks (mean 6 weeks) treatment, on daily doses of 0.8-1.6 g, usually 1 g (Fig. 5). Significantly higher levels were seen both in pH (mean rise from 2.3-4.1; p = 0.00048) and N-nitrosamine concentrations (geometric mean increase from 0.08-0.47 μmol/1; p = 1.9×10^{-6}).

In 23 patients gastric juice samples were obtained during CM treatment and again after stopping the drug. Treatment periods ranged between 1 and 48 weeks and samples were taken 1-40 weeks after CM was discontinued. Whereas treatment cessation resulted in a significant fall in pH (from 3.4 to 2.3; p = 0.0082), N-nitrosamine reduction was not significant (geometric mean fall from 0.30-0.16 μmol/l) (Fig. 6).

The gastric juice nitrite level rose and growth of nitrate-reducing bacteria increased with pH in the CM takers in a manner similar to that observed in patients with other causes of hypochlorhydria not so treated.

In the duodenal ulcer group, overall (n = 74), the N-nitrosamine concentrations were significantly higher during CM treatment (1.04 log units; p = 0083). However, in duodenal ulcer patients who smoked and were on CM

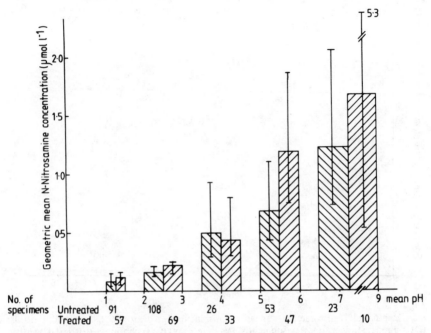

Figure 3
Relation between gastric pH and *N*-nitrosamine concentration in CM-treated patients. (Left-hand columns) untreated; (right-hand columns) CM-treated patients. (I) 95% confidence limits and base of histogram represents pH range.

treatment for recurrent symptoms after vagotomy *N*-nitrosamine concentrations (mean 2.37 log units; p = 0.031) were higher than *N*-nitrosamine levels in comparable preoperative duodenal ulcer patients (n = 41).

There were no significant differences in *N*-nitrosamine concentrations between the sexes during CM treatment.

DISCUSSION

The H_2-receptor antagonists were introduced into clinical practice because of their ability to reduce gastric acid output and while this effect is therapeutically beneficial it can also initiate other changes in the gastric milieu which might be potentially harmful. CM has been shown to inhibit basal and nocturnal acid output profoundly, as well as secretion stimulated by histamine, pentagastrin, and cholinergic mechanisms. Food stimulated acid secretion is inhibited by between 57 and 82% (Pounder et al. 1976; Walt et al. 1981) and when CM is

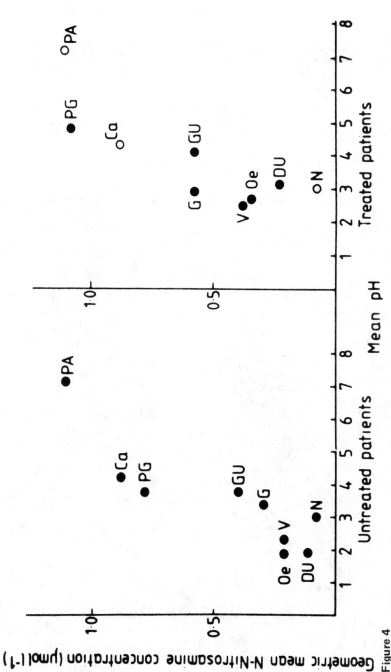

Figure 4

Gastric pH and *N*-nitrosamine concentrations in different diagnostic groups. Comparison between untreated and CM-treated patients. (●) treated groups, (○) untreated groups on right-hand side for comparison; (N) normal controls; (DU) duodenal ulcer; (Oe) oesophagitis; (V) vagotomy; (G) chronic gastritis; (GU) gastric ulcer; (PG) partial gastrectomy; (Ca) carcinoma of stomach; (PA) pernicious anaemia.

357

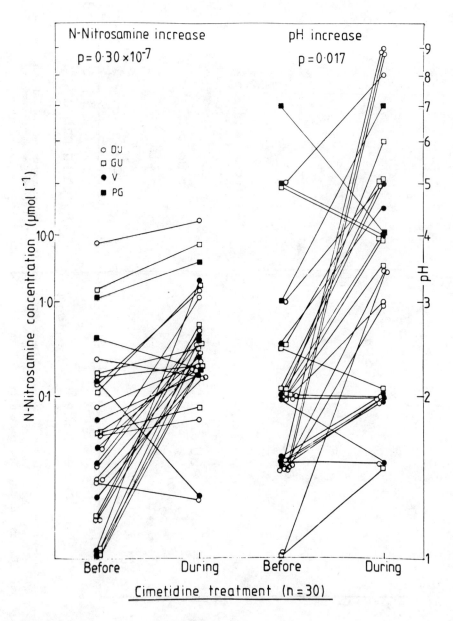

Figure 5
Gastric pH and *N*-nitrosamine concentrations before and during CM treatment.

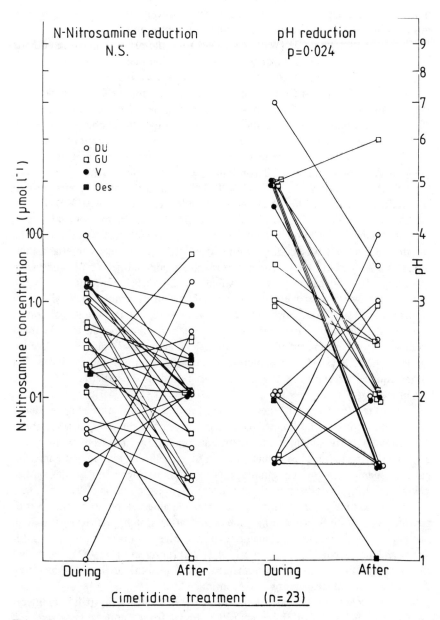

Figure 6
Gastric pH and *N*-nitrosamine concentrations during and after withdrawal of CM treatment.

given with food, blood levels of the drug are better maintained during the inter-digestive period when the buffering effect of the meal tends to fall and inhibi-tion of acid secretion is most desirable (Spence et al. 1976). It has also been shown that the intragastric pH first thing in the morning is greater than 5.0 in 40-50% patients taking CM (Walt et al. 1981) and the pH after meals in patients so treated is intermittently high for some hours (Pounder et al. 1975; Pounder et al. 1977). Furthermore, 24-hour studies have shown that CM treatment will raise gastric pH above 4-5 during 39-50% of the 24 hours (McCloy and Baron 1981; Walt et al. 1981). This, of course, is of value in either treating or pre-venting the formation of peptic ulcers, but a potentially undesirable by-product can be the encouragement to gastric bacterial growth. Several reports have con-firmed that a CM-induced rise in gastric pH can increase intragastric concentra-tions of fecal-type bacteria (Bartholomew et al. 1980b; Deane et al. 1980; Ruddell et al. 1980; Muscroft et al. 1981), as well as the nitrite concentration (Bartholomew et al. 1980a,b; Deane et al. 1980; Ruddell et al. 1980). For in-stance, in one study (Muscroft et al. 1981) 75% of aspirates from 44 fasting patients taking 1 gm CM daily were found to contain bacteria 2-4 hours after the last dose. Of 41 patients taking 400 mg at night, 34% still had bacteria in their aspirates 12-13 hours later. These writers also compared gastric pH and viable counts in those 44 patients and 51 patients with gastric carcinoma and the re-sults in the two groups were indistinguishable. Similar changes have also been confirmed by our data. Furthermore, detailed study of the individual results revealed that in some cases the N-nitrosamine concentration during CM treat-ment was up to a hundred times the normal value and of 74 duodenal ulcer pa-tients on CM 13 had N-nitrosamine concentrations and 24 had pH levels that either equaled or exceeded the mean levels found in 23 patients with gastric carcinoma.

The results from all these studies provide strong supporting evidence that in the hypochlorhydric stomach, especially when the pH is near or above 4, bacterial activity enhances intragastric nitrosation by increasing nitrite levels. The data from the studies quoted have also established that in patients with gastroduodenal disease, cimetidine treatment alters significantly the gastric milieu, resulting in increased pH and bacterial overgrowth and rises in nitrite and N-nitrosamine concentrations. The latter remained elevated in a number of patients in our study for a long time-period after stopping treatment, and in one patient for 34 weeks. Although unexpected, this finding is not unique to our study and has a parallel in the work of Stockbrügger et al. (1982) who found that mean N-nitrosamine levels remained raised in some of their patients even 2 months after CM treatment was discontinued.

Two recent studies carried out in a few normal healthy male volunteers have questioned some of the conclusions drawn from the previously reported data. In the first, (Muscroft et al. 1981) gastric pH, nitrite, total and nitrate-reducing bacteria were measured in 9 volunteers on a normal diet, 6 given 1 g CM for 3 weeks before being studied, with 5 subsequently taking a maintenance dose of 400 mg nocte for a further 3 weeks, when they were studied again. Nocturnal hypochlorhydria was infrequently achieved and only one subject in each group had a morning gastric juice of pH $\geq$ 3.5. Of the 48 aspirates from subjects on full treatment, 15 had a pH $\geq$ 3.5 and 12 of these had nitrate-reducing bacterial counts $\geq$ 10^4/ml. Similarly, of the 30 aspirates obtained during maintenance treatment only 5 had pH $\geq$ 3.5 and 4 had nitrate-reducing bacterial counts $\geq$ 10^4/ml. Nitrite concentrations were higher in juices of pH $\geq$ 4. While the authors postulate that the higher pH and bacterial counts seen after meals are due to swallowed saliva, even if true it must not be forgotten that N-nitrosation has been shown to occur in saliva. They concluded from this study that "nocturnal anacidity does not occur in normal subjects taking therapeutic doses of cimetidine and that such treatment does not predispose to bacterial colonisation in subjects on a normal diet." However, this paper has been heavily criticized (McCloy and Baron 1981; Ruddell 1981) and these authors question both the methodology employed and the conclusions drawn from the data. Ruddell concluded his letter by describing it as: ". . . an inadequate study which contributes nothing to our understanding of an unresolved problem."

The second, as yet unpublished study, was presented last September in summary form to the British Society of Gastroenterology (Barnard et al. 1981; Milton-Thompson et al. 1982). The effects of CM on the intragastric millieu were studied in 8 apparently healthy men, taking a standardized diet, throughout 24 hours on three occasions, namely before, at the end of 2 weeks CM 1 g daily and after 2 further weeks on 400 mg at night. Gastric juice was sampled once every 30 minutes daily and hourly overnight. However, bacteriological studies were carried out in only 4 subjects. Although 24-hour hydrogen ion concentration was decreased significantly by both treatments the gastric pH was rarely above 4 and then only isolated bacterial counts $\geq$ 10^5/ml were achieved. Unlike other workers (Ruddell et al. 1976; Ruddell et al. 1978; Tannenbaum et al. 1979) no correlation was seen between nitrite and bacterial counts and pH, neither was any relationship established between N-nitroso compounds and pH. Furthermore, wide variations in the data were observed. Until the full details become available a comprehensive critique is impossible, however, it must be stressed once again that healthy young sailors were studied and not subjects with gastroduodenal conditions in whom the intragastric environment is rather different. The diet was apparently purchased in bulk and prepacked and certain foods, including bacon, were excluded, though beer and cigarettes were allowed. Bacteriological data is available from only four men and the pH was > 4 in only 20% of samples. Unlike the method of Walters et al. (1978), the analytical method (Bavin et al. 1981) employed for the determination of N-nitroso compounds in this study would not have differentiated them from heat labile compounds potentially formed from nitrite such as pseudonitrosites and N-nitrosothiols. The claim made for this study (Brimblecombe 1982) that ". . . albeit in healthy volunteer subjects . . . a small number of subjects studied in detail give far more useful data than a large number of subjects studied at only one point in time . . ." is equally extravagant since the information was obtained from a small pool of normal subjects, rather than from those with mucosal disease. Furthermore, in a 24-hour study (McCloy and Baron 1981) (4320 readings) in a patient with *duodenal ulcer*, the pH was > 4 only 1% of the 24 hours off CM, but 50% of the 24 hours on 400 mg CM three times a day and 800 mg CM at night. This reinforces the point already made that in diseased patients CM often raises the gastric pH over a much longer part of the 24 hours.

While these studies provide information about the effect of CM in normal subjects, to infer similar conclusions for the diseased stomach or duodenum is not necessarily valid. Thus, those findings do not invalidate the conclusions drawn from the well documented and very extensive patient studies already reviewed. Therefore, it can be concluded that CM treatment in patients with gastroduodenal disease can frequently produce significant hypochlorhydria, with pH levels often > 4, thereby encouraging gastric bacterial overgrowth, including that of organisms able to reduce nitrate to nitrite, which in combination with dietary or pharmacological amine will probably form *N*-nitroso compounds in higher concentrations than in untreated patients or normal healthy men. The significance of these changes resulting from CM treatment will be discussed by James B. Elder (this volume).

ACKNOWLEDGMENTS

We thank the Cancer Research Campaign for financial support to P.L.R.S. and C.L.W., Sister D. Wheeler, and Mrs. A. Knott for technical assistance, Dr. H. Andrews for the bacteriological studies.

REFERENCES

Barnard, J., D.W. Darkin, N.J. Viney, Z. Ahmet, N.F. Lightfoot, R.H. Hunt, and G.J. Milton-Thompson. 1981. Effect of cimetidine on twenty-four-hour intragastric pH, bacterial flora and concentrations of nitrite and nitroso-compounds. *Gut* 22:A873.

Bartholomew, B.A., M.J. Hill, M.J. Hudson, W.S.J. Ruddell, and C.L. Walters. 1980a. Gastric bacteria, nitrate, nitrite and nitrosamines in patients with pernicious anaemia and in patients treated with cimetidine. *IARC Sci. Publ.* 31:595.

Bartholomew, B., R. Stockbrügger, N. Euginides, P. Mansell, M. Hill, and P.B. Cotton. 1980b. Gastric nitrate, nitrite and bacterial nitrate reductase in relation to gastric acid secretion. *Hepato-Gastroenterology* (suppl.), p. 108.

Bavin, P.M.G., D.W. Darkin, and N.J. Viney. 1981. Total nitroso compounds in gastric juice. *IARC Sci. Publ.* 41 (in press).

Brimblecombe, R.W. 1982. Cimetidine, nitrosation, and carcinogenicity. *Lancet* i:402.

Brooks, J.B., W.B. Cherry, L. Thaker, and C.C. Alley. 1972. Analysis by gas-chromotography of the amines and nitrosamines produced in vivo and in vitro by *Proteus mirabilis. J. Infect. Dis.* 126:143.

Deane, S.A., D.J. Youngs, V.A. Poxon, M.R.B. Keighley, J. Alexander-Williams, and D.W. Burdon. 1980. Cimetidine and gastric microflora. *Br. J. Surg.* 67:371.

Hicks, R.M., C.L. Walters, I. Elsebei, A.-B. El Aasser, M. Merzabani, and T.A. Gough. 1977. Demonstration of nitrosamines in human urine. Preliminary observations on a possible aetiology for bladder cancer in association with chronic urinary tract infections. *Proc. R. Soc. Med.* 70:413.

Hill, M.J. 1979. In vivo bacterial N-nitrosation and its possible role in human cancer. In *Naturally occurring carcinogens—mutagens and modulators of carcinogenesis* (eds. E.C. Miller et al.), p. 229. Japan Scientific Society Press, Tokyo, Japan/University Park Press, Baltimore, U.S.A.

Hill, M.J. and G. Hawksworth. 1972. Bacterial production of nitrosamines in vitro and in vivo. *IARC Sci. Publ.* 3:116.

Jones, S.M., P.W. Davies, and A. Savage. 1978. Gastric juice nitrite and gastric cancer. *Lancet* i:1355.

McCloy, R.F. and J.H. Baron. 1981. Intragastric pH and cimetidine, fasting and after food. *Lancet* i:609.

Milton-Thompson, G.J., N.F. Lightfoot, Z. Ahmet, R.H. Hunt, J. Barnard, P.M.G. Bavin, R.W. Brimblecombe, D.W. Darkin, P.J. Moore, and N. Viney. 1982. Intragastric acidity, bacteria, nitrite, and N-nitroso compounds before, during, and after cimetidine treatment. *Lancet* i:1091.

Muscroft, T.J., D.J. Youngs, D.W. Burdon, and M.R.B. Keighley. 1981. Cimetidine is unlikely to increase formation of intragastric N-nitroso compounds in patients taking a normal diet. *Lancet* i:408.

Muscroft, T.J., S.A. Deane, D. Youngs, D.W. Burdon, and M.R.B. Keighley. 1981. The microflora of the postoperative stomach. *Br. J. Surg.* 68:560.

Pounder, R.E., J.G. Williams, G.J. Milton-Thompson, and J.J. Misiewicz. 1975. Twenty-four hour control of intragastric acidity by cimetidine in duodenal ulcer patients. *Lancet* ii:1069.

Pounder, R.E., J.G. Williams, R.C.G. Russell, G.J. Milton-Thompson, and J.J. Misiewicz. 1976. Inhibition of food stimulated gastric acid secretion by cimetidine. *Gut* 17:161.

Pounder, R.E., R.H. Hunt, S.H. Vincent, G.J. Milton-Thompson, and J.J. Misiewicz. 1977. Twenty-four hour intragastric acidity and nocturnal acid secretion in patients with duodenal ulcer during oral administration of cimetidine and atrophine. *Gut* 18:85.

Reed, P.I., P.L.R. Smith, F.R. House, and C.L. Walters. 1982. The effect of vagotomy on gastric nitrosamine production. In *Verdict on Vagotomy*. (eds. J. Alexander-Williams et al.) Butterworths, London, England. (In press).

Reed, P.I., P.L.R. Smith, K. Haines, F.R. House, and C.L. Walters. 1981a. Gastric juice N-nitrosamines in health and gastroduodenal disease. *Lancet* ii:550.

_____. 1981b. Effect of cimetidine on gastric juice N-nitrosamine concentration. *Lancet* ii:553.

Ruddell, W.S.J. 1981. Cimetidine, gastric pH and nitrosation. *Lancet* i:784.

Ruddell, W.S.J., E.S. Bone, M.J. Hill, and C.L. Walters. 1978. Pathogenesis of gastric cancer in pernicious anaemia. *Lancet* i:521.

Ruddell, W.S.J., E.S. Bone, M.J. Hill, L.M. Blendis, and C.L. Walters. 1976. Gastric juice nitrite: A risk factor for cancer in the hypochlorhydric stomach? *Lancet* ii:1037.

Ruddell, W.S.J., A.T.R. Axon, J.M. Findley, B.A. Bartholomew, and M.J. Hill. 1980. Effect of cimetidine on the gastric bacterial flora. *Lancet* i:672.

Sander, J. 1968. Nitrosaminsynthese durch Bakterien. *Z. Physiol. Chem.* **349**: 429.

Sander, J., F. Schweinsburg, and H.P. Menz. 1968. Untersuchnung über die Entstehung cancerogener Nitrosamine im Magen. *Z. Physiol. Chem.* **349**:1691.

Schlag, P., R. Bockler, H. Ulrich, M. Peter, P. Merkle, and C. Herfarth. 1980. Are nitrite and N-nitroso compounds in gastric juice risk factors for carcinoma in the operated stomach? *Lancet* i:717.

Spence, R.W., D.R. Creak, and L.R. Celestin. 1976. Influence of a meal on the absorption of cimetidine—in a new histamine H_2-receptor antagonist. *Digestion* **14**:127.

Stockbrügger, R.W., P.B. Cotton, N. Euginides, B.A. Bartholomew, M.J. Hill, and C.L. Walters. 1982. Intragastric nitrites, nitrosamines and bacterial overgrowth during cimetidine treatment. *Gut* (in press).

Tannenbaum, S.R., M.C. Archer, J.S. Wishnok, and W.W. Bishop. 1978. Nitrosamine formation in human saliva. *J. Natl. Cancer Inst.* **60**:251.

Tannenbaum, S.R., D. Moran, W. Rand, C. Cuello, and P. Correa. 1979. Gastric cancer in Colombia. IV. Nitrite and other ions in gastric contents of residents from a high risk region. *J. Natl. Cancer Inst.* **62**:9.

Walt, R.F., P.J. Male, R.H. Hunt, G.J. Milton-Thompson, and J.J. Misiewicz. 1981. Comparison of the effects of ranitidine, cimetidine and placebo on the 24 hour intragastric acidity and nocturnal acid secretion in patients with duodenal ulcer. *Gut* **22**:49.

Walters, C.L., M.J. Downes, M.W. Edwards, and P.L.R. Smith. 1978. Determination of a non-volatile N-nitrosamine on a food matrix. *Analyst* **103**:1127.

COMMENTS

WEISBURGER: Let's have a brief question period on the methods and reserve the conceptual discussion for later.

HOFFMANN: Was it done with a thermal energy analyzer?

WALTERS: This was done on total extractable N-nitroso compounds. However, I will deal with this further in my presentation. (See Walters, this volume.)

HOFFMANN: I was a little startled that you did not find a difference between the nonsmokers and smokers. Does that include the tobacco-specific nitrosamines?

WALTERS: Only if they can be extracted from an acid milieu.

HOFFMANN: No, they would not be. So it does not include tobacco-specific nitrosamines.

REED: Interestingly, there was only one group of smokers in whom we identified significantly higher nitrosamine levels, namely in DU patients who previously had a vagotomy but subsequently developed recurrent ulcers for which they received CM treatment. However, the number studied was small.

CHALLIS: I have a question about this analysis. I think it would be very helpful if people knew how the gastric samples were handled and how they were stored. Did you include artifact inhibitors?

REED: Yes. The samples were obtained at endoscopy, after an overnight fast. The gastric juice pH was immediately measured, the presence of nitrite recorded, and an aliquot sent to the bacteriology laboratory for bacterial culture. The bulk of the juice was then treated with sulfamic acid to bring the pH below 2, and immediately frozen and subsequently transported to Dr. Walters' laboratory, in most cases within a few days of sampling.

GRASSO: Could you remind me what this Billroth II was?

REED: However, the Billroth I gastrectomy is one where the antrum and distal half of the body of the stomach have been removed and the gastric remnant and duodenum joined together.

Billroth II gastrectomy, a similar resection of the stomach is carried out, but it is joined to a loop of jejmum so there is no longer continuity with the duodenum, but a direct opening into the small intestine.

WEISBURGER: Dr. Grasso, if I might comment, Dr. Domellöf, a visiting surgeon in our department, has shown that the Billroth II gastrectomy is a procedure that shouldn't be done, because, while it is wide open for the gastric content to go down, the gastric stump is wide open for contents to reflux. Domellöf (Domellöf and Janunger 1977; Domellöf 1981) has data on patients who had undergone a Billroth II some 20-25 years ago almost invariably have gastric cancer in the region of anastamosis. We think it is both the anastamosis and the bile acids which are important factors. I wouldn't recommend that.

REED: I would just like to make one point, that this is not exclusive to the Billroth II gastrectomies. What is more, I recently had a patient who had a Billroth I gastrectomy less than 5½ years ago. He now has an early gastric cancer immediately proximal to the anastomosis. As this gastrectomy was performed for a gastric ulcer, it is probable that he had an atrophic mucosa for a good many years before.

CHALLIS: There is some work which was done I think by Teichmann in East Germany (Ziebarth and Teichmann 1980) which showed that sulfamic acid catalyzes nitrosamine formation at high pH and inhibits it at low pH. The break-even point is at about pH 4. I never really believed it, but he has reported it twice, over a period of 10 years. I don't know whether anybody else has any experience in this but sulfamic acid is not an effective inhibitor when the pH is above 4. I wondered whether you had considered this might be a problem because you see higher levels of nitrosamines at higher pH, and you may in fact be putting a catalyst in there when you store this.

WALTERS: The pH has always been below 2. We considered the low pH to be quite effective.

CHALLIS: Do you adjust the pH before you add the sulfamic acid?

WALTERS: There is sufficient sulfamic acid so that pH falls below 2 invariably. If you add nitrite to gastric juice treated with sulfamic acid, no additional nitrosation occurs.

DURANT: For the benefit of those who may not be completely familiar with these issues and in particular with the recent correspondence in *Lancet*, it should be added that this topic has been hotly debated. We have heard one view of this topic from Mr. Reed, but I would like to refer to the studies conducted by my colleagues Dr. Bavin and Mr. Darkin in conjunction with Dr. Barnard and several clinical collaborators including Dr. Milton-Thompson and coworkers at Portsmouth and Mr. Keighley and Muscroft at Birmingham. The results from these studies are at variance with those presented by Mr. Reed. The results from human volunteer studies have been accepted for publication (Milton-Thompson et al. 1982).

References

Domellöf, L. and K.G. Janunger. 1977. The risk for gastric carcinoma after partial gastrectomy. *Am. J. Surg.* **134**:581.

Domellöf, L., S. Ericksson, H. Mori, J.H. Weisburger, and G.M. Williams. 1981. Essect of bile acid gavage or sagotomy and pyloroplasty on gastrointestinal carcinogenesis. *Am. J. Surg.* **142**:581.

Milton-Thompson, G.J., N.F. Lightfoot, Z. Ahmet, R.H. Hunt, J. Barnard, P.M.G. Bavin, R.W. Brimblecombe, D.W. Darkin, P.J. Moore, and N. Viney. 1982. Intragastric acidity, bacteria, nitrite and N-nitroso compounds before, during and after cimetidine treatment. *Lancet* i:1091.

Ziebarth, D. and B. Teichmann. 1980. Nitrosation of orally administered drugs under simulated stomach conditions. *IARC Sci. Publ.* **31**:231.

Gastric Juice, Nitrite, and Nitroso Compounds

JOAN BARNARD, P. M. G. BAVIN, R. W. BRIMBLECOMBE,
DAVID W. DARKIN, GRAHAM J. DURANT
Smith Kline and French Research Ltd.
The Frythe, Welwyn, Herts, AL6 9AR

and

MICHAEL R. B. KEIGHLEY
Department of Surgery and Microbiology
The General Hospital
Birmingham, England

During the development of cimetidine (CM), two 2-year carcinogenicity studies have been carried out in Wistar rats, using 950 mg/kg/day as the maximum dose (Leslie et al. 1981), which is estimated to be 680 times the intraduodenal ID_{50} for inhibition of stimulated gastric acid secretion in the anesthetized rat. Beagles have also been dosed for 6 years at 144 mg/kg/day and examined at regular intervals by gastric endoscopy and biopsy of gastric mucosa (Crean et al. 1981). Evidence for carcinogenicity has not been found in any of these studies. Despite this, concern has been expressed based on plausible hypotheses and anecdotal case reports, that CM administration might be associated with the development of gastric carcinoma in man.

The first hypothesis is based upon the structural relationship between N-methyl-N'-nitro-N-nitroso-guanidine (MNNG) and the nitrosated derivative of CM: nitrosocimetidine (NCM). Several laboratories have studied the possible carcinogenicity of NCM by feeding studies with rats (Lijinsky and Habs et al., this volume) and mice (A. Giner-Sorolla, L.M. Anderson, and J.M. Budinger, unpubl. results), and by skin painting studies with mice (Lijinsky, this volume). The studies have shown that NCM, in marked contrast to MNNG, is either not carcinogenic or at most only weakly carcinogenic in these tests.

The second hypothesis is that reduced gastric acidity encourages bacterial colonization, leading to increased concentrations of nitrite in gastric juice from nitrate-reductase activity of the bacteria. In turn, the nitrite may lead to higher concentrations of potentially carcinogenic nitroso compounds in the stomach (Drasar et al. 1969; Ruddell et al. 1978). Such conditions are present in patients with pernicious anemia and after certain operations for peptic ulcer, and may be present after treatment with H_2-antagonists or antacids. The increased incidence of gastric cancer in pernicious anemia patients (Mosbech and Videbaek 1950)

369

and in patients after certain forms of gastric surgery (Nicholls 1979) has been attributed to raised concentrations of nitroso compounds.

AIMS AND METHODS

Bacterial Analysis

In investigating the second hypothesis we set several objectives. We wished to study the relationship between gastric pH and bacterial counts over 24-hour periods, since most previous studies have relied upon single samples in fasting subjects at endoscopy. Our results in volunteers show that high bacterial counts are usually found when the gastric pH is high, but that high counts may also occur after food intake. During acute or maintenance therapy with CM, episodes of high acidity occur regularly and are sufficient to destroy the bacteria. These studies have been reported (Milton-Thompson et al. 1982), and have been extended (M.R.B. Keighley, unpubl. results) to study healed duodenal ulcer (DU) patients, proximal gastric vagotomy, truncal vagotomy with pyloroplasty, and gastrectomy patients.

Nitrite Determinations

In order to measure nitrite in gastric juice reliably we have adapted the polarographic method of Chang et al. (1977). Each sample serves as its own control, by spiking with nitrite for calibration. Interference has only been found in samples of gastric juice containing beer. The method, which was reported in Tokyo (Bavin et al. 1981) has been checked by the chemiluminescent method for nitric oxide (Cox 1980) and by high pressure liquid chromatography (Thayer and Huffaker 1980) with satisfactory agreement. The method transfers nitrite to diphenylamine in acidic solution, so will not therefore distinguish nitrite esters from nitrite. Hence it measures the nitrosating potential of a sample, and this is the value of interest for the formation of N-nitroso compounds.

Nitrosamine Concentrations

Our third objective was to measure the total nitroso compounds in frequent small samples of gastric juice. For this, we needed a method which was specific for nitroso compounds, which had reasonable precision, and which was rapid, suitable for handling large numbers of samples. We wished particularly to measure the reactive N-nitroso derivatives of amides, ureas, and related compounds, as well as the unreactive N-nitrosamines. Prior destruction of nitrite was essential to avoid artifact formation.

A method (Walters et al. 1978), based on earlier work by Eisenbrand and Preussman (1970) was an obvious starting point. However, Walters employs sulphamic acid to destroy nitrite which is effective only in acidic media, below pH 2. Walters has reported adjusting the pH of gastric juice samples to less than 2, and making the solution 0.5% w/v with respect to sulphamic acid (Reed et al. 1981a). The hydrolysis of the N-nitroso derivatives of amides and related compounds is quite rapid at pH 2 (McCalla et al. 1968; Jensen and Magee 1981) and is, of course, irreversible in the presence of a nitrite trap. Furthermore, hydrolysis is expected to be much more rapid at pH 1 than pH 2 (McCalla et al. 1968). Gastric samples have been frozen, shipped, and thawed prior to analysis, (Reed et al. 1981a) and this analytical procedure also required an extraction, which is unsatisfactory for accurate and reproducible results. It seems likely that Walters measures only N-nitrosamines, most or all of the reactive nitroso compounds being destroyed.

In developing our procedure we have shown that hydrazine destroys nitrite very rapidly at pH 4, and at this pH, hydrolysis of nitroso compounds is very much slower than at pH 2 (McCalla et al. 1968). We have shown that, contrary to an earlier report (Walters et al. 1980), a small amount of water does not inhibit the denitrosation of compounds by hydrobromic acid in boiling ethyl acetate. These observations provided the basis for our method for measuring total nitroso compounds in gastric juice, which we reported in Tokyo (Bavin et al. 1981). Immediately after the sample of gastric juice is obtained the pH is measured. A portion of the juice is buffered with borax, frozen, and shipped to our laboratory for the determination of nitrite. An excess of hydrazine sulphate in water is added to the remainder of the juice and the pH is adjusted to 4 with alkali. The sample is then buffered with potassium hydrogen phthalate and an aliquot (1 ml) is injected into refluxing ethyl acetate containing hydrobromic and acetic acids. The nitric oxide evolved is measured with a chemiluminescence detector linked to a recording integrator. The total analysis time is less than 5 minutes, and the small volume of gastric juice required means that frequent sampling presents no problems. Values obtained in this way are referred to by us as "total nitroso compounds." We have also left additional samples of the gastric juice for 5-7 days in stoppered amber bottles for analysis for what we refer to as "stable nitroso compounds." Use of amber vials is essential because we have shown that light rapidly destroys low concentrations of nitroso compounds. Our values for stable nitroso compounds are comparable in magnitude with values reported by Walters (Reed et al. 1981a). They probably represent N-nitroso-alkylamines, stable to the hydrolytic conditions employed by Walters, and inert to nucleophilic attack by hydrazine under our conditions of analysis.

EVALUATING MEASUREMENTS FOR TOTAL
N-NITROSO COMPOUNDS

Our values for total nitroso compounds are very much greater than those for stable nitroso compounds and for Walters's method. Our method shows an excellent linear response for NCM down to a few nanograms and satisfactory reproducibility was obtained (±8-10%). Molar responses are shown in Table 1. The

Table 1
Results of Nitrosamine Analysis on Reference Compounds

Compound	Class	Molar Responses
N-Nitrosopyrrolidine	Nitrosoalkylamine	1.09
N-Nitrosoarcosine	Nitrosoamino acid	1.02
N-Nitroso-N-methylurea	Nitrosourea	0.92
N-Nitrosocimetidine	Nitrosoguanidine	1.00
2-(N-Nitroso-N-methylamino)-4-pyrimidinone	Nitrosoaralkylamine	1.18
N-Nitrosocarbazole	Nitrosoarylamine	0.55

low response from N-nitrosocarbazole appears to be due to its low solubility. In the absence of water it gives the expected unitary response as a sharp peak, unlike the broad one associated with the low response. The near unitary response from compounds of different structures and reactivities is good evidence for their stability during the period required for our analysis. We have examined the specificity of our method, using the range of compounds reported by Walters et al. (1978). The data are compared in Table 2, and are very similar. Nitrite esters are destroyed by hydrazine. The thionitrites derived from primary and secondary thiols are unstable (Rheinboldt 1926) but t-butyl and t-aryl thionitrites (Rheinboldt et al. 1931) can be isolated as stable liquids. However, t-

Table 2
Comparison of Results of the Present Method with those of Walters et al. (1978)

Compound	Class	Our Method	Walters et al.
isoPropyl nitrite	Nitrite ester	0.0	0.6[a]
Ethyl nitrate	Nitrate ester	–	0
2-Methyl-2-nitrosopropane	Aliphatic nitroso	0.03	0[b]
Nitroethane	Aliphatic nitro	0.05	0
2-Nitropropane	Aliphatic nitro	0.05	
Propionitrolic acid	Nitrolic acid	0.04	0.35
2-Nitronitroso-cyclohexane	Pseudonitrosite	0	very slow
2-Nitroso-2-nitropropane	Pseudonitrole	1.08	slow
t-Butyl thionitrite	Thionitrite	0.08	0
t-Butyl thionitrate	Thionitrate	0.51	0.25
Nitroguanidine	Nitroguanidine	0.02	0
N-Nitrodimethylamine	Nitramine	–	0
Cyclohexanone oxime	Oxime	0	0
3-Hydroxypyridine-N-oxide		0.02	0

[a] isopentyl nitrite
[b] under nitrogen

butyl thionitrite is also destroyed by hydrazine and it is very unlikely that thionitrites generally will interfere. Only t-alkyl thionitrates are stable enough to be isolated (Oae et al. 1979) and their occurrence in gastric juice seems unlikely. The formation of pseudonitroles from secondary nitroalkanes proceeds through the aci-form and requires special conditions (see Nygard 1946). Their presence in gastric juice is highly improbable. The specificity of our method seems, therefore, to be adequate.

Application of Methods: Early Results

In applying our methods to 24-hour studies, it quickly became apparent that the nature of the food had a marked effect on the levels of nitroso compounds. We therefore purchased prepackaged, frozen food in bulk, so that volunteers and patients had meals according to a standardized regime. Our method for total nitroso compounds is satisfactory in the presence of food. Smoking had no demonstrable effect on the levels of nitroso compounds.

Our results show that nitrite concentrations and the concentrations of total nitroso compounds vary markedly during a 24-hour period. Hence single sample studies do not reflect in any way what is, in fact, happening during 24 hours and under physiological conditions. In a recent study (Reed et al. 1981b) gastric analysis was reported in a highly artificial situation when CM was administered to fasted patients, leading to abnormally high gastric pH values and correspondingly high levels of "stable nitroso compounds."

In one of our recent studies (Muscroft et al. 1982) we have confirmed the relationship between pH and counts of nitrate-reducing bacteria. Nitrite concentrations > 5 μmol/l in gastric juice were significantly more common in samples of pH 4 and above. In another study (Milton-Thompson et al. 1982) the effects of CM on the intragastric milieu have been examined in eight healthy volunteers. This study consisted of five 24-hour periods: before treatment, after 2 weeks CM 1 g/day, after 2 weeks taking 400 mg at night, and after a further 5 weeks without taking CM. The subjects had a standardized diet. Gastric juice was sampled half-hourly during the day and hourly overnight for the measurement of pH, nitrite, and total and stable nitroso compounds. In addition, hourly samples from four of the subjects were examined for counts of total bacteria (aerobic and anaerobic), nitrate-reducing bacteria, and different species. The 24-hour hydrogen ion concentration was significantly decreased by both CM treatments but neither nitrite nor total and nitrate-reducing bacteria increased significantly with pH. This was attributed to failure of the bacteria to colonize the stomach. The bacterial species detected were those commonly found in saliva, rather than enteric organs. The concentrations of total nitroso compounds fluctuated markedly in relation to meals and overnight, but could not be correlated with pH, nitrite concentrations, bacterial counts, or with CM treatment. The concentrations of nitroso compounds in gastric juice were not significantly altered by treatment with CM.

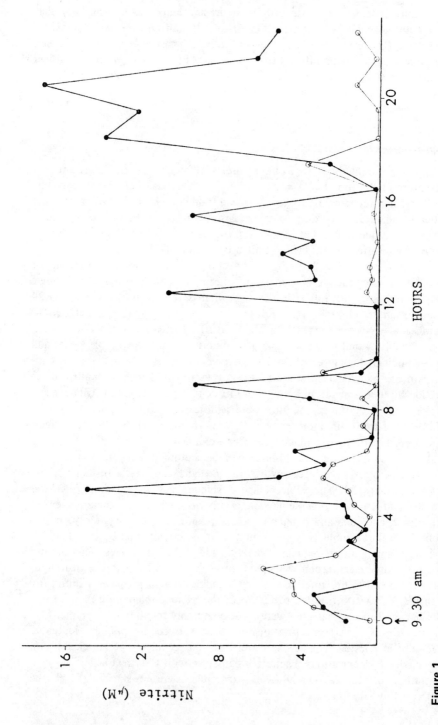

Figure 1
Mean nitrite concentrations of proximal gastric vagotomy and control groups. (●——●) PGV – 7 subjects; (○——○) control – 8 subjects.

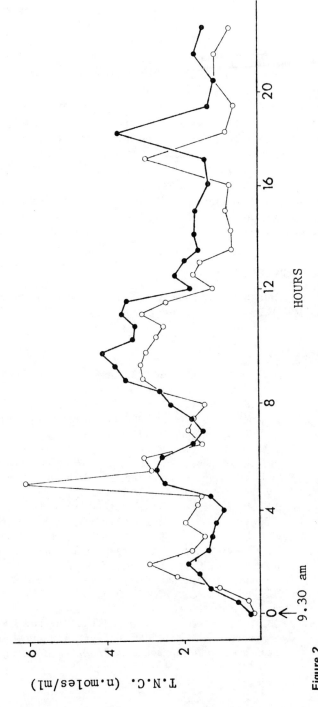

Figure 2
Mean total nitroso concentrations of proximal gastric vagotomy and control group. (●——●) PGV –7 subjects; (○——○) control–8 subjects.

Our results from patients having undergone successful proximal gastric vagotomy with healing of their DU at least 2 years earlier are particularly interesting. The concentrations of nitrite are much higher than those of the controls as shown in Figure 1. However, neither total nor stable nitroso compounds differ significantly from control values, p = 0.625 (see Fig. 2). Higher nitrite concentrations were found at higher pH values (5 and above). Total nitroso-compound concentrations showed no relationship with pH, nitrite concentration, or total bacterial count. However the concentrations of stable nitroso compounds were higher in the pH range 1.5-4.0, suggestive of the variation demonstrated by Mirvish (1970) for the rate of nitrosation of dimethylamine with pH. These results are consistent with the acid catalyzed formation of nitroso compounds, requiring substrate, nitrite, and an acidic medium. High nitrite concentrations do not necessarily lead to high concentrations of N-nitroso compounds. Furthermore, we conclude from both studies that neither CM therapy nor proximal gastric vagotomy increases the exposure of the stomach to N-nitroso compounds.

ACKNOWLEDGMENTS

We are grateful to Surgeon-Captain Milton-Thompson and Drs. N.F. Lightfoot and R.H. Hunt for their enthusiasm and facilities.

REFERENCES

Bavin, P.M.G., D.W. Darkin, and N.J. Viney. 1981. Total nitroso compounds in gastric juice. *IARC Sci. Publ.* **41** (in press).
Chang, S-K., R. Kozeniauskas, and G.W. Harrington. 1977. Determination of nitrite ion using differential pulse polarography. *Anal. Chem.* **49**:2272.
Cox, R.D. 1980. Determination of nitrate and nitrite at the parts per billion level by chemiluminescence. *Anal. Chem.* **52**:332.
Crean, G.P., G.B. Leslie, T.F. Walker, S.M. Whitehead, and F.J.C. Roe. 1981. Safety evaluation of cimetidine: 54 month interim report on long term study in dogs. *J. Appl. Toxicol.* **1**:159.
Drasar, B.S., M. Shiner, and G.M. McLeod. 1969. The bacterial flora of the gastrointestinal tract in healthy and achlorhydric persons. *Gastroenterology* **56**:71.
Eisenbrand, G. and R. Preussmann. 1970. A new method for colorimetric determination of nitrosamines by cleavage of the N-nitroso group by hydrogen bromide in acetic acid. *Arzneim. Forsch.* **20**:1513.
Jensen, D.E. and P.N. Magee. 1981. Methylation of DNA by nitrosocimetidine in vitro. *Cancer Res.* **41**:230.
Leslie, G.B., D.N. Noakes, F.D. Pollitt, F.J.C. Roe, and T.F. Walker. 1981. A two-year study with cimetidine in the rat: Assessment for chronic toxicity and carcinogenicity. *Toxicol. Appl. Pharmacol.* **61**:119.

McCalla, D.R., A. Reuvers, and R. Kitai. 1968. Inactivation of biologically active N-methyl-N-nitroso compounds in aqueous solution. *Can. J. Biochem.* 46:807.

Milton-Thompson, G.J., N.F. Lightfoot, Z. Ahmet, R.H. Hunt, J. Barnard, P.M.G. Bavin, R.W. Brimblecombe, D.W. Darkin, P.J. Moore, and N. Viney. 1982. Intragastric acidity, bacteria, nitrite and N-nitroso compounds before, during and after cimetidine treatment. *Lancet* i:1091.

Mirvish, S.S. 1970. Kinetics of dimethylamine nitrosation in relation to nitrosamine carcinogenesis. *J. Natl. Cancer Inst.* 44:633.

Mosbech, J. and A. Videbaek. 1950. Mortality from and risk of gastric carcinoma among patients with pernicious anaemia. *Br. Med. J.* ii:390.

Muscroft, T.J., D. Youngs, V. Poxon, D.W. Burdon, P.M.G. Bavin, D.W. Darkin, N.J. Viney, P.J. Moore, J. Barnard, and M.R.B. Keighley. 1982. Hypochlorhydria, bacteria, nitrite and nitrosamines in gastric juice. *Br. J. Surg.* 69:289.

Nicholls, J.C. 1979. Stump cancer following gastric surgery. *World J. Surg.* 3:731.

Nygard, E.M. 1946. U.S.P. 2,401,267.

Oae, S., K. Shinhama and Y.H. Kim. 1979. Reactions of t-alkyl thionitrates with p-aminophenols. *Chem. Lett.* 1077.

Reed, P.I., P.L.R. Smith, K. Haines, F.R. House, and C.L. Walters. 1981a. Gastric juice N-nitrosamines in health and gastroduodenal disease. *Lancet* ii:550.

——. 1981b. Effect of cimetidine on gastric juice N-nitrosamine concentration. *Lancet* ii:553.

Rheinboldt, H. 1926. Nitrosylmercaptides and thio-nitrites. *Berichte Der Deutsem Chemischem Geselschaft* 59:1311.

Rheinboldt, H., M. Dewald, and O. Diepenbruck. 1931. Actions of nitrosyl chloride on mercaptans and mercaptides-thionitrites. *Journal Fur Praktische Chemie* 3:130.

Ruddell, W.S.J., E.S. Bone, M.J. Hill, and C.L. Walters. 1978. Pathogenesis of gastric cancer in pernicious anaemia. *Lancet* i:521.

Thayer, J.R. and R.C. Huffaker. 1980. Determination of nitrate and nitrite by high pressure liquid chromatography: Comparison with other methods for nitrate determination. *Anal. Biochem.* 102:110.

Walters, C.L., R.J. Hart, and S. Perse. 1978. The breakdown into nitric oxide of compounds potentially derived from nitrite in a biological matrix. *Z. Lebensm. Unters. Forsch.* 167:315.

Walters, C.L., R.J. Hart, L.K. Keefer, and P.M. Newberne. 1980. The sequential determination of nitrite, N-nitroso compounds and nitrate and its application. *IARC Sci. Publ.* 31:389.

Walters, C.L., P.L.R. Smith, P.I. Reed, K. Haines, and F.R. House. 1981. N-Nitroso compounds in gastric juice and their relationship to gastroduodenal disease. *IARC Sci. Publ.* 41 (in press).

Factors Which Influence the In Vivo Methylating Potential of Nitrosocimetidine

DAVID E. JENSEN AND CHARLES T. GOMBAR
Fels Research Institute
Temple University School of Medicine
Philadelphia, Pennsylvania 19140

It has been shown that many compounds can become nitrosated at acid pH and in the presence of nitrite to become nitroso compounds which are proven carginogens in laboratory animal tests (Mirvish 1975; Magee et al. 1976; Lijinsky 1980). There is some evidence that such a nitrosation process can take place in the acid environment of the human stomach (Fine et al. 1977). The importance of this in vivo nitrosation in the etiology of human cancer, however, remains to be determined.

The report of Elder et al. (1979) made us aware that the very important drug cimetidine (Tagamet®) is a nitrosatable compound and that the chemical structure of its nitrosated derivative, nitrosocimetidine (NCM), is very similar to that of the gastric carcinogen N-methyl-N-nitroso-N'-nitroguanidine (MNNG; Fig. 1). Cimetidine (CM) is used in the treatment of gastric ulcers and other gastrointestinal disorders (Finkelstein and Isselbacher 1978). The success of this drug is reflected in the fact that worldwide sales of the compound have recently surpassed those of Valium. CM is available in 111 countries and, since its introduction about 6 years ago, approximately 20 million people have taken the drug. Typically the dose is in the range of 1 gm/day and treatment limited to 6-8 weeks. It has been reported that CM is nitrosatable in vitro in the acid pH range (Bavin et al. 1980) and there are indications that the compound can be nitrosated in isolated human gastric juice (DeFlora and Picciotto 1980). It remains to be demonstrated that CM is nitrosated in vivo.

Consistent with its chemical structure, NCM has been found to have many of the same effects on in vitro biological test systems as MNNG and the closely related compound methylnitrosourea (MNU). NCM is a direct-acting mutagen in the Ames test (Pool et al. 1979) and in cultured mammalian cells (Barrows et al. 1982). It demonstrates toxicity to mammalian cells in culture (Henderson et al. 1981), induces single strand DNA breaks (Schwarz et al. 1980; Henderson et al. 1981) and sister chromatid exchange (Athanasiou and Kyrtopoulos 1981), inhibits DNA synthesis, and also elicits increased DNA repair synthesis (Henderson et al. 1981). Subsequent to a report by Foster et al. (1980) that

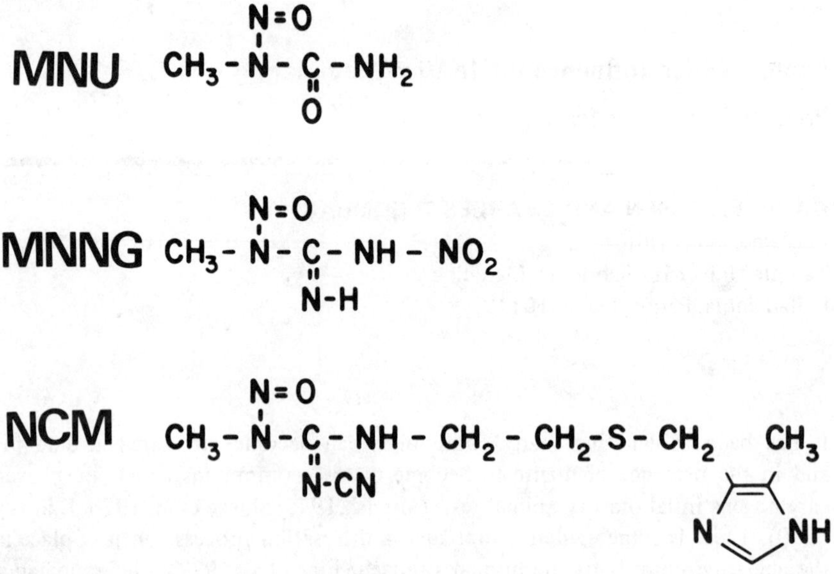

$$\text{MNU} \quad CH_3 - \overset{\overset{\displaystyle N=O}{|}}{N} - \underset{\underset{\displaystyle O}{\|}}{C} - NH_2$$

$$\text{MNNG} \quad CH_3 - \overset{\overset{\displaystyle N=O}{|}}{N} - \underset{\underset{\displaystyle N-H}{\|}}{C} - NH - NO_2$$

$$\text{NCM} \quad CH_3 - \overset{\overset{\displaystyle N=O}{|}}{N} - \underset{\underset{\displaystyle N\text{-}CN}{\|}}{C} - NH - CH_2 - CH_2 - S - CH_2 \quad \begin{array}{c} CH_3 \\ \text{(imidazole ring: } N \diagdown NH) \end{array}$$

Figure 1
Chemical structures of N-methyl-N-nitrosourea (MNU), MNNG, and NCM.

NCM is a methylating agent, we demonstrated that the compound will methylate DNA in vitro and in cultured human lymphoid cells to produce the same O^6 methyl G/7 methyl G product ratio as observed using MNNG and MNU (Jensen 1981; Jensen and Magee 1981). In most of these reported experiments CM was also tested and found to have no effect on the measured parameters.

In our work with direct-acting, methylating, nitroso compounds we have found that the factors which influence the rate and degree of compound degradation have a similar influence on the rate and degree of in vitro DNA alkylation by the agents. Apparently a methylating intermediate is a product of decomposition. We have discovered that NCM decomposes relatively slowly in neutral pH buffer solution. At 37° the half-life of the intact compound is about 50 hours compared to a value of approximately 3 hours for MNNG and 10 minutes for MNU. We have endeavored to determine to what degree the in vivo levels and distribution of tissue DNA methylation in the rat model system reflect the chemical stability of these nitroso compounds. In vitro, the decomposition rates of NCM and MNNG are markedly accelerated by thiol compounds. Unlike MNNG which demonstrates accelerated decomposition in the presence of any nucleophile, the enhanced decomposition rate of NCM appears to be thiol specific. Further, although thiols speed the rate at which alkylating intermediate is generated from NCM, the major pathway of decomposition is apparently denitrosation to produce the parent compound, CM. Our in vitro results indicate that this denitrosation occurs in blood. Dosing rats with NCM results in very low levels of tissue DNA alkylation relative to those observed using MNNG and MNU, suggests that denitrosation is a major pathway of NCM decomposition in vivo as well. Based on our experiments using rats we hypothesize that if NCM is formed by the nitrosation of CM in the stomach, the potential risk to human health may be considerably reduced by the propensity of this compound to denitrosate in the bloodstream.

In this paper we summarize our results on the in vitro characteristics of NCM, MNNG, and MNU decomposition and on tissue DNA methylation in rats dosed orally and i.v. with these compounds.

MATERIALS AND METHODS

A detailed description of the materials and methods used in these studies will appear in primary publications now in press (Gombar and Magee 1982) or in preparation; only a brief review will be given here. All chemicals and radio-labeled compounds were obtained from commercial sources except for ^{14}C-labeled and unlabeled NCM which were synthesized in these laboratories (Jensen and Magee 1981; Gombar and Magee 1982). CM and [^{14}C-methyl]-CM were kindly supplied by SmithKline and French Laboratories, Philadelphia, PA.

Nitroso compound decomposition rates were determined in aqueous buffered solutions, in whole rat blood, and in rat plasma by taking aliquots of the incubate at specified times, delivering the aliquot to a small volume of concentrated buffer for pH control and extracting this aqueous solution with a volume of octanol. The extraction and isolation of the octanol phase took less than 2 minutes. All of the compounds were relatively stable in octanol when kept in the dark and cold. The octanol phase was analyzed by high pressure liquid chromatography (HPLC) using a Microbondapac C-18 column, generally within 1 hour after extraction. MNNG and its denitrosated derivative and also NCM and CM were resolved by our chromatography. The elution of these compounds was detected by UV absorbance and concentrations quantified by measuring recorder chart peak heights. MNU elution was similarly detected by UV absorbance; its denitrosated derivative was invisible to our detector.

Six-week-old female Fischer 344 rats were used in our i.v. dosing experiments. ^{14}C-methyl nitroso compounds were used and dosing was via the tail vein. The animals were sacrificed and blood and various organs taken 4 hours after dosing. Globin was isolated from the blood following literature procedures described by Anson and Mirsky (1930); globin concentration determinations were based on UV absorbance (Waddell 1956) and the degree of globin methylation quantified by liquid scintillation counting. DNA was isolated from the frozen organs following a modified Kirby procedure (Swann and Magee 1968) and the degree of DNA methylation in mild acid-hydrolyzed samples determined using our published cation exchange HPLC technique (Jensen et al. 1981).

Fasted adult female Wistar rats were used in the studies in which ^{14}C-methyl nitroso compounds were dosed by gavage. In CO_2 exhalation experiments, animals were housed in metabolism cages and the amount of $^{14}CO_2$ trapped in an ethanolamine:ethoxyethanol solution was assessed at various times by liquid scintillation counting techniques. In other experiments the animals were sacrificed 12 hours after dosing with radioactive compound and various organs were taken for DNA isolation and quantitation of the degree of DNA methylation as described above.

RESULTS AND DISCUSSION

MNU, MNNG, and NCM, as well as the denitrosated products of the latter two compounds, can be reproducibly extracted from aqueous solution in fairly high yields with octanol. We have developed HPLC techniques which permit us to determine the concentration of each of these compounds in octanol. Thus by analyzing extracts of aliquots taken from aqueous incubates at specified times we can determine nitroso compound decomposition rates and, in the case of MNNG and NCM, what fraction of this decomposition yields the parent, denitrosated, compound.

Utilizing this methodology we have verified and extended the earlier work of Lawley and Thatcher (1970) which considered the decomposition rate of MNNG in buffer and in the presence of various nucleophilic compounds. In our experiments we observed the rate of disappearance of intact MNNG in pH 7.4 phosphate buffer, in the presence of a twofold excess of various amino acids or in the presence of a twofold excess of reduced glutathione. We believe that the several amino acids are representative of the kinds of nucleophilic chemicals likely to be encountered by nitroso compounds in a biological milieu. The results of this study are depicted in Figure 2. It was found that all of the nucleophiles caused, to a varying degree, an acceleration in the rate of MNNG decomposition relative to that observed in plain buffer. MNNG decomposed most quickly in the presence of the thiol-containing compounds, cysteine and reduced glutathione. The sulfur nucleophile is involved in the enhanced decomposition. This is evidenced by the observation that this rate is considerably reduced when the thiol moiety is blocked (i.e., in the presence of a twofold excess of S-methyl cysteine). . Our experiments also indicate that a fraction of MNNG decomposition in the presence of a twofold excess of thiol compound produces denitrosated product; 10% of the decomposition in the presence of glutathione produces N-methyl-N'-nitroguanidine (MNG) and 15% in the presence of cysteine. It is unknown what fraction of the decomposition of intact compound generates a methylating intermediate. However, based on our study of in vitro DNA alkylation by MNNG (Jensen and Magee 1981), it can be argued that the majority of the decomposition which does not proceed via a denitrosation pathway generates a DNA methylating species. Finally, less than 3% of the MNNG decomposition in the presence of amino acids other than those containing thiol or in plain phosphate buffer proceeds via a denitrosation pathway.

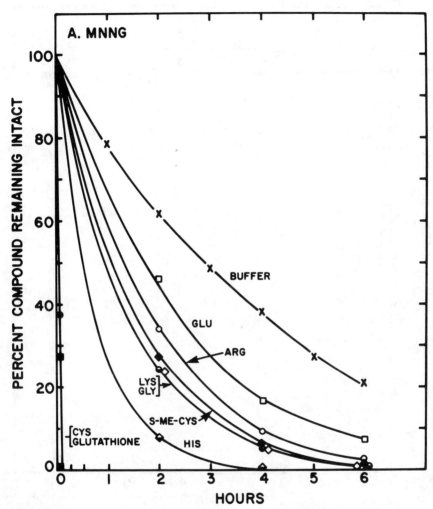

Figure 2
Degradation of MNNG at 37° in plain buffer and in the presence of a twofold excess of various L-amino acids or reduced glutathione as a function of time. Buffer, 50 mM KH_2PO_4, pH 7.4; nitroso compound, 3.5 mM; amino acids or reduced glutathione, 7.0 mM.

Using the same techniques we studied the in vitro decomposition characteristics of NCM; our results are summarized in Figure 3. In contrast to our findings with MNNG, we observed that only the thiol-containing nucleophiles, cysteine and reduced glutathione enhanced the rate of NCM decomposition. Consistent with our MNNG result, we find that when the thiol group in cysteine is blocked (i.e., S-methyl cysteine) the decomposition-accelerating principle is lost. We also discovered that the denitrosation of NCM by thiol compound is a

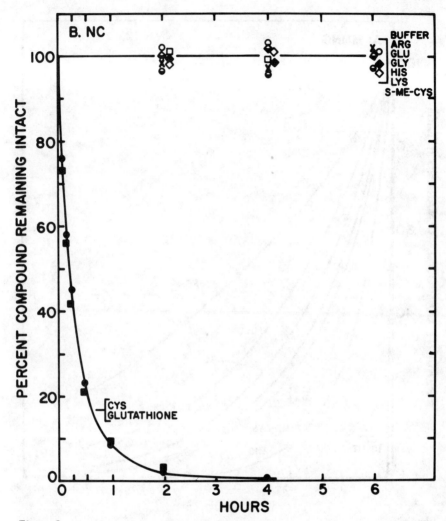

Figure 3
Degradation of NCM under same conditions as in Figure 2.

major decomposition pathway. At all of the time points assayed, about 30% of the decomposition of NCM in the presence of reduced glutathione resulted in the formation of CM and about 75% of the decomposition in the presence of cysteine produced CM.

We have also considered the decomposition rate of MNU by determining the rate of disappearance of intact compound. Consistent with the earlier report of Wheeler and Bowdon (1972), we found that excess cysteine had no detectable effect on the rate of degradation of this compound.

As a prelude to our in vivo experiments using MNU, NCM, and MNNG, we assessed the stability of these compounds in whole blood isolated from rats and in rat plasma. The results of these experiments are diagramed in Figures 4 and 5. The most startling finding was that obtained with NCM. At 37° the half-life of NCM in whole blood was in the range of 2.5 minutes, in sharp contrast to the approximately 50-hour half-life observed for NCM in neutral buffer at this

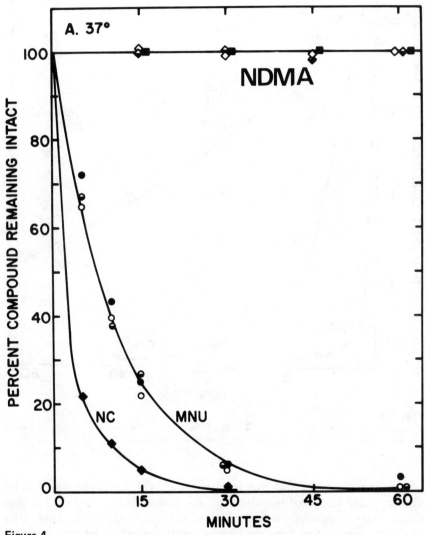

Figure 4

Degradation of NCM and MNU at 37° in whole rat blood (♦ ■ ● ●), in rat plasma (♦), or in phosphate-buffered saline (○ ◊) as a function of time. Nitroso compound, 3.5 mM.

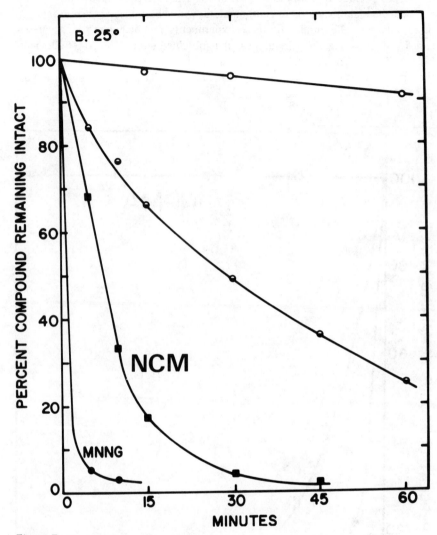

Figure 5
Degradation of NCM and MNNG at 25° in whole rat blood (■ ●), in rat plasma (◉), or in phosphate-buffered saline (○) as a function of time. Nitroso compound, 3.5 mM.

temperature. We also found that in plasma the NCM degradation rate was indistinguishable from that in buffer, an observation which suggested to us that the accelerating principle perhaps resides in red blood cells. In this same series of experiments we found that, at all time points assayed, about 65% of the decomposition of NCM in whole blood was via a denitrosation pathway to produce CM. MNNG decomposition in whole blood was also observed to be very rapid.

The data shown in Figure 5 were collected at 25°; at 37° the reaction was essentially completed during the time it took to do the octanol extraction (2 minutes). When MNNG degrades in whole blood at 37° approximately 35% of the decomposition produces the denitrosated product, MNG. Unlike NCM, MNNG was found to decompose at a more rapid rate in plasma than it does in buffer but still much more slowly than decomposition in whole blood. In plasma less than 3% of the MNNG decomposition produced denitrosated product. At 37° the rates of MNU decomposition in whole blood, in plasma and in buffer were indistinguishable (Fig. 4); the in vitro half-life was approximately 8 minutes.

We have done some experiments with isolated rat hemoglobin and have found that hemoglobin accelerates the rate of MNNG and of NCM decomposition relative to the degradation rate in neutral buffer, but has no effect on MNU decomposition. After the cysteine groups on hemoglobin have been blocked by modification with the thiol-specific reagent N-ethylmaleimide (EM), the hemoglobin completely loses its capacity to accelerate NCM decomposition. MNNG in the presence of EM-modified hemoglobin also decomposes more slowly than it does in the presence of unmodified protein but, unlike NCM, this degradation rate does not return to the rate characteristic of MNNG in buffer. This result is consistent with our previous observation that MNNG degradation is accelerated by any nucleophile and is not thiol specific as is the case for NCM.

In summary, our in vitro experiments indicate that, of the three compounds considered, MNU is least stable in neutral buffer but, as it turns out, is the most stable in whole blood with a half-life of about 8 minutes at 37°. MNU decomposition does not appear to be influenced by nucleophiles. In contrast, the MNNG half-life in whole blood is likely to be less than 1 minute. The MNNG decomposition rate is strongly influenced by all the nucleophiles tested and is most sensitive to thiols. Of the nucleophilic compounds considered, only those containing thiol appeared to promote significant MNNG denitrosation. The highest degree of MNNG denitrosation was observed to occur in whole blood where 35% of the decomposition produced MNG. NCM decomposition is exceedingly slow ($t_{1/2}$ ~50 hours) except in the presence of thiol-containing nucleophiles. The major degradation pathway in thiol-enhanced NCM decomposition results in compound denitrosation to produce CM. In whole blood in vitro the NCM half-life is approximately 2.5 minutes and about 65% of the degradation is denitrosation. Our experiments implicate hemoglobin cysteine residues as the thiols involved in NCM decomposition in blood.

We have treated rats with equimolar quantities of MNU, NCM, and MNNG, radiolabeled in the methyl group, dosed via the tail vein and have determined the degree of DNA methylation (i.e., μmole 7 methyl G/mole G) in several organs as well as the degree of hemoglobin methylation. The animals were sacrificed 4 hours after dosing. Our results are tabulated in Table 1. MNU methylated the DNA of all the organs considered to about the same degree, as

Table 1

Hemoglobin and Tissue DNA Alkylation in F344 Rats Dosed with $1.35 \cdot 10^{-4}$ moles/kg Nitroso Compound[a]

Agent	Hb methylation (pmole Ch_3/ mg globin)	DNA methylation (μmole 7 meGua/mole G)			
		liver	kidney[c]	lung[c]	brain[c]
MNU	16.0 ± 0.3[b]	113.8 ± 12.3[b]	128.3	104.4	107.9
MNNG	37.2 ± 4.3	3.8 ± 0.9	46.6	207.1	6.5
NCM	7.7 ± 0.5	3.9 ± 1.9	6.7	6.6	n.d.[d]

[a]Ether anesthetized rats were dosed via the tail vein at a rate of 0.5 ml vehicle/100 gm body weight. Vehicle: 10% DMSO in 0.9% sodium chloride.
[b]Standard deviation; three animals identically dosed.
[c]Combined tissue from three identically treated animals.
[d]No alkylation detectable.

previously noted in the literature (Swann and Magee 1968). The extent of DNA alkylation and of hemoglobin alkylation by this compound will be used as benchmarks against which to evaluate our results with MNNG and NCM. The short half-life of MNNG is perhaps reflected in the observed alkylation pattern. Hemoglobin labeling by MNNG was about twofold greater than that observed for MNU as was the methylation of DNA in the lung. Considerable decomposition of MNNG may have taken place in the bloodstream, and the lung is the first capillary mass encountered by i.v. injected compounds. Kidney, brain, and liver DNA methylation by MNNG were quite low relative to that observed for MNU; perhaps very little intact compound reaches these organs. Compared to MNU and even compared to MNNG, the tissue DNA and hemoglobin alkylation observed after dosing with NCM was low. Our in vitro results lead us to hypothesize that the low degree of methylation is due to the rapid conversion of a considerable fraction of NCM to CM upon interaction of the nitroso compound with thiols. Blood was drawn retroorbitally 10 minutes after dosing from a fourth rat treated with NCM in a manner identical to that of the three rats used to generate the data of Table 1. Immediate analysis of this blood by our octanol extraction and HPLC techniques indicated that 100% of the radioactivity recovered in this sample was CM, no radioactive NCM was detectable.

We have also determined the degree of tissue DNA alkylation in rats treated orally with radiolabeled MNNG and NCM. Before describing our findings, the results from two other in vitro experiments will be briefly mentioned.

The distribution of a compound between water and octanol (or other immiscible organic solvent) is often used to obtain a notion of the relative ability of a compound to pass from an aqueous environment to the lipoidal environment of a cellular membrane. We have determined the distribution of the nitroso compounds of interest between octanol and aqueous solution as a function of the aqueous phase pH. The results are summarized in Figure 6. It was found that NCM distributes preferentially into the aqueous phase in the acid pH range. Distribution into octanol is only observed when the pH of the aqueous phase approaches neutrality. This change in distribution is probably a reflection of the titration of the imidazole ring proton in NCM. MNNG and MNU distribute approximately equally between octanol and buffer at all pH values. We have assessed the stability of NCM, MNNG, and MNU in pH 2 buffer at 37°. The half-lives of MNNG and NCM are approximately 2 hours and 3.5 hours, respectively. MNU remains 90% intact after 6 hours of incubation at this pH.

When we initiated our oral dosing experiments, we did not know how rapidly NCM would be metabolized in the rat. We thus measured the amount of label expired as $^{14}CO_2$ as a function of time after dosing with ^{14}C-methyl-

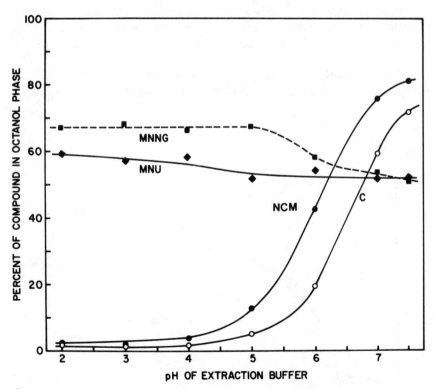

Figure 6

Distribution of nitroso compound between equal volumes of octanol and aqueous buffer as a function of buffer pH, 23°. Buffer was 50 mM sodium phosphate (pH 2, 7, and 7.5), sodium formate (pH 3 and 4), sodium acetate (pH 5), or sodium citrate (pH 6). Nitroso compound, 3.5 mM, was dissolved in octanol; the octanol was extracted with pH buffer and the concentration of compound remaining in octanol assessed by HPLC.

labeled MNNG, NCM or CM by gavage. The results are diagramed in Figure 7. Rats dosed with labeled MNNG expired labeled CO_2 for at least 12 hours; at this time the expired label accounted for about 12% of the administered dose. Rats treated with NCM expired about 4% of the label as CO_2 by 6 hours with very little expired after that time. CM-treated rats expired a very small amount of $^{14}CO_2$, about 0.4% of the dose, over a 12-hour period. Based on these results, 12 hours was chosen as the time after dosing at which animals would be sacrificed for our tissue DNA alkylation experiments. The results of these experiments are summarized in Table 2. We were unable to detect DNA methylation in any of the assayed tissues of rats treated with CM. Rats treated with MNNG by gavage had the greatest degree of DNA methylation in the stomach tissue. After being absorbed from the lumen of the stomach or the small intestine, compounds are carried by the bloodstream first to the liver. We observed some DNA methylation in the small intestine and a relatively high yield of DNA methylation in the liver. Very little DNA methylation was found in the lung, kidney, or the colon of MNNG-treated animals and none was found in the brain. Consistent with our i.v. dosing experiments, we find the highest levels of DNA alkylation by MNNG in those tissues which are first encountered by the compound.

The tissue DNA alkylation pattern produced by orally administered NCM was quite different from that produced by MNNG given at the same molar dose.

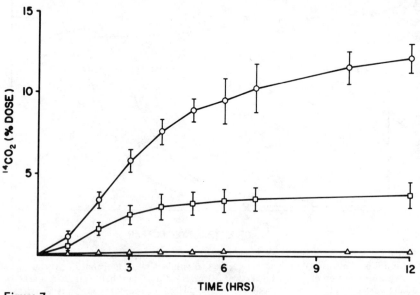

Figure 7
Expiration of $^{14}CO_2$ as a function of time after oral administration (gavage) of ^{14}C-methyl-labeled MNNG (o-o), NCM (□-□), or cimetidine (△-△).

Table 2

DNA Methylation in Organs of Rats Treated Orally with CM, NCM, or MNNG[a] (μmole 7 meGua/mole G)

Agent	Stomach	Small intestine	Colon	Lung	Kidney	Liver	Brain
CM	n.d.[b]	n.d.	n.d.	n.d.	–[c]	n.d.	–
NCM	8	45	n.d.	1	4	17	n.d.
MNNG	217	69	32	36	28	155	n.d.

[a]The doses administered were: CM 0.25 mmole/kg, 430 μCi; NCM 0.20 mmole/kg, 416 μCi; MNNG 0.20 mmole/kg, 45 μCi.
[b]n.d. = none detected.
[c]– = not performed.

Little alkylation was detectable in stomach and liver tissue and essentially none in the lung, kidney, colon, and brain. The highest level of DNA methylation by NCM was observed in small intestinal tissue and this was about 65% of that observed in the small intestine of MNNG-treated animals.

While the distribution and low levels of rat tissue DNA alkylation generated by orally dosed NCM are doubtlessly due to many factors, we propose that the two elucidated in our experiments may be predominant. First, NCM is apparently positively charged at acid pHs (imidazole ring proton) and thus will not readily pass from an aqueous acid to an organic environment. The failure of NCM to significantly alkylate stomach tissue DNA is perhaps a reflection of this condition. Second, our in vitro experiments indicate that a major fraction of NCM is rapidly denitrosated upon contact with blood. The very low levels of tissue DNA alkylation observed in rats treated i.v. via the tail vein with NCM corroborate this finding. Contact with the blood after absorption by the small intestine may similarly inactivate NCM as a methylating agent by denitrosation. NCM produces one-tenth of the liver DNA methylation generated by an equimolar dose of MNNG.

Since the two factors which we are considering are chemical, perhaps there is some justification in translating our results to the human problem by using the rat model system. The pK of NCM is apparently about 6; thus in environments more acid than pH 4.5-5, typical of the stomach, the charged state of the compound will predominate and passage into a cellular milieu might occur with low probability. There is no reason to anticipate that the rapid denitrosation of NCM in rat blood will not be a characteristic of human blood as well. We are currently testing this. If NCM is produced in vivo by the nitrosation of CM, our experiments suggest that the most likely consequence might be the alkylation of small intestinal tissue; significant methylation damage to other tissues in the body seems improbable.

ACKNOWLEDGMENT

The authors wish to thank Dr. Peter Magee for his interest and support throughout these investigations. This research was supported by grants CA-12227, CA-23451, and CA-31503 from the National Cancer Institute, NIH. C.T.G. is a postdoctoral trainee of the National Institutes of Health (CA-09214).

REFERENCES

Anson, M.L. and A.E. Mirsky. 1930. Protein coagulation and its reversal: The preparation of insoluble globin, soluble globin and heme. *J. Gen. Physiol.* 13:469.

Athanasiou, K. and S.A. Kyrtopoulos. 1981. Induction of sister chromatid exchanges and chromosome aberrations in cultured mammalian cells by N-nitrosocimetidine. *Cancer Lett.* 14:71.

Barrows, L.R., C.T. Gombar, and P.N. Magee. 1982. Mutation, DNA labeling and transformation of BHK-21/CL 13 cells by MNNG and nitrosocimetidine. *Mutat. Res.* (in press).

Bavin, P.M.G., G.J. Durant, P.D. Miles, R.C. Mitchell, and E.S. Pepper. 1980. Nitrosation of cimetidine. *J. Chem. Res. (Synop.)* 1980:212.

DeFlora, S. and A. Picciotto. 1980. Mutagenicity of cimetidine in nitrite-enriched human gastric juice. *Carcinogenesis* 1:925.

Elder, J.B., P.C. Ganguli, and T.E. Gillespie. 1979. Cimetidine and gastric cancer. *Lancet* i:1005.

Fine, D.H., R. Ross, D.P. Rounbehler, A. Silvergleid, and L. Song. 1977. Formation *in vivo* of volatile N-nitrosamines in man after ingestion of cooked bacon and spinach. *Nature* 265:753.

Finkelstein, W. and K.J. Isselbacher. 1978. Cimetidine. *New Engl. J. Med.* 299:992.

Foster, A.B., M. Jarman, and D. Manson. 1980. Structure and reactivity of nitrosocimetidine. *Cancer Lett.* 9:47.

Gombar, C.T. and P.N. Magee. 1982. DNA methylation by nitrosocimetidine and N-methyl-N'-nitro-N-nitrosoguanidine in the intact rat. *Chem. Biol. Interact.* 40:149.

Henderson, E.E., M. Basilio, and R.M. Davis. 1981. Cellular damage by nitrosocimetidine: A comparison with N-methyl-N'-nitro-N-nitrosoguanidine and X-irradiation. *Chem. Biol. Interact.* 38:87.

Jensen, D.E. 1981. Deoxyribonucleic acid methylation in human cells exposed to nitrosocimetidine. *Biochem. Pharmacol.* 30:2864.

Jensen, D.E. and P.N. Magee. 1981. Methylation of DNA by nitrosocimetidine *in vitro. Cancer Res.* 41:230.

Jensen, D.E., P.D. Lotlikar, and P.N. Magee. 1981. The *in vitro* methylation of DNA by microsomally-activated dimethylnitrosamine and its correlation with formaldehyde production. *Carcinogenesis* 2:349.

Lawley, P.D. and C.J. Thatcher. 1970. Methylation of deoxyribonucleic acid in cultured mammalian cells by N-methyl-N'-nitro-N-nitrosoguanidine. *Biochem. J.* 116:693.

Lijinsky, W. 1980. Significance of *in vivo* formation of N-nitroso compounds. *Oncology* 37:223.

Magee, P.N., R. Montesano, and R. Preussmann. 1976. N-nitroso compounds and related carcinogens. *ACS Monogr.* 173:491.

Mirvish, S.S. 1975. Formation of N-nitroso compounds: Chemistry, kinetics and *in vivo* occurrence. *Toxicol. Appl. Pharmacol.* 31:325.

Pool, B.L., G. Eisenbrand, and D. Schmähl. 1979. Biological activity of nitrosated cimetidine. *Toxicology* 15:69.

Schwarz, M., J. Hummel, and G. Eisenbrand. 1980. Induction of DNA strand breaks by nitrosocimetidine. *Cancer Lett.* 10:223.

Swann, P.F. and P.N. Magee. 1968. Nitrosamine-induced carcinogenesis: The alkylation of nucleic acids of the rat by N-methyl-N-nitrosourea, dimethylnitrosamine, dimethyl sulphate and methyl methanesulphonate. *Biochem. J.* 110:39.

Waddell, W.J. 1956. A simple ultraviolet spectrophotometric method for the determination of protein. *J. Lab. Clin. Med.* 48:311.

Wheeler, G.P. and B.J. Bowdon. 1972. Comparison of the effects of cysteine upon the decomposition of nitrosoureas and of 1-methyl-3-nitro-1-nitrosoguanidine. *Biochem. Pharmacol.* 21:265.

COMMENTS

MILO: Dr. Jensen shows, or interprets the data where he saw a fairly short half-life for MNNG in whole blood. How would this affect the distribution of the pharmacokinetics and the distribution of MNNG when you inject it i.v.? Would you expect to find it distributed equally throughout the tissues, since the half-life is very short?

JENSEN: No. It does seem to get to the lung first, and then after that it appears to be gone. We see very little of it hanging around.

SHANK: Is 7-meGua the only alkylated base you found from the DNA for NCM?

GOMBAR: In the in vivo work, yes, because the specific activity wasn't high enough to pick up the O^6. The levels we were looking at were not very high. The overall level of alkylation was pretty low.

PEGG: It is very important, when considering the potential carcinogenicity of compounds and the potential carcinogenicity of alkylation, to think that there may be differences in one's cell type even within an organ. I think it is really quite important to remember that, even with direct-acting alkylation agents, there can be very striking differences in the amount of alkylation in a particular cell type. I think the best example is streptozotocin, which, because of the glucose moiety, preferentially alkylates certain cells in the pancreas.

With something like NCM you know that there is a very high, or presumably high, affinity to certain cells. I'm not sure that you should just take some level of the parent CM—the affinity, I mean—or some level of alkylation that is measured in a whole tissue, because I don't think that is necessarily representative of the distribution of alkylation within the cells in that tissue.

WEISBURGER: MNNG was a positive control, so one has a reference to the data they obtained. But, sure, Dr. Pegg, your point is well taken.

PEGG: I don't see what MNNG has got to do with it really, because the level in particular cells might be very high—higher than the MNNG.

HECHT: Has anybody looked at the products of decomposition, other than the diazo hydroxide? What happens to the rest of the NCM?

JENSEN: I have only looked for CM itself as a product of decomposition. To my knowledge no one else has considered other NCM decomposition products.

WEISBURGER: That is a key point because, again, Kawachi and Sugimura showed that with MNNG the methyl group ended up on nucleic acid, but the guanidine group ended up on protein.

MIRVISH: Guttenplan showed that ascorbic acid reacts with MNNG. Have you tried ascorbic acid plus NCM?

JENSEN: No.

MIRVISH: I think he found it does not react with MNU, but it would be interesting to do that reaction.

DURANT: What does it do?

MIRVISH: Well, I think all he knows is that MNNG is unstable in the presence of ascorbic acid and reacts. I'm not sure he has done anything for the product. But I think that is of interest.

MICHEJDA: You said that NMU was stable for 6 hours in what?

JENSEN: pH 2 buffer.

References

Guttenplan, J.B. 1978. Mechanism of inhibition by ascorbate of microbial mutagenesis induced by N-nitroso compounds. *Cancer Res.* **38**:2018.

Kawachi, T., K. Kogure, Y. Kamijo, and T. Sugimura. 1970. The metabolism of N-methyl-N'-nitro-N-nitrosoguanidine in rats. *Biochim. Biophys. Acta* **222**:409.

Carcinogenesis Studies with Nitrosocimetidine

WILLIAM LIJINSKY
Chemical Carcinogenesis Program
NCI-Frederick Cancer Research Facility
Frederick, Maryland 21701

Nitrosocimetidine (NCM) is an analog of N-methyl-N'-nitrosoguanidine (MNNG) and might be expected to have similar properties. It is formed easily by nitrosation of cimetidine (CM) in acid solution and could, conceivably, be formed in the human stomach in vivo. Prior to investigations of the effect of chronic feeding of CM and nitrite to experimental animals, tests of NCM itself were desirable.

Since NCM would be expected to be a direct-acting carcinogen (it is known to be a direct-acting bacterial mutagen), a simple system for detecting carcinogenic activity is topical application to mouse. MNNG and a number of nitrosoalkylureas are very effective carcinogens when applied to mouse skin chronically (Takayama et al. 1971; Lijinsky and Winter 1981). Therefore, a test of NCM was undertaken in parallel with a test of MNNG, applying the compounds in measured doses of acetone solutions to the skin of Swiss mice and observing the appearance of skin tumors in the painted area.

A second system for studying the carcinogenicity of NCM was by chronic feeding to rats, which could be a measure of the possible risk in exposure of humans to NCM formed in the stomach from the drug and nitrite. Again, a parallel study in which MNNG was fed in drinking water solution to rats was carried out. MNNG induces gastric adenocarcinomas on chronic administration to rats (Sugimura and Kawachi 1973). In both the skin painting and the feeding study the concentrations of NCM were equimolar with those of MNNG in the positive control.

MATERIALS AND METHODS

NCM was prepared from the drug kindly supplied by SmithKline and French, Inc., by a method similar to that described by Pool et al. (1979). The precipitated salt of NCM was decomposed by stirring in aqueous solution with sodium carbonate and the generated free nitroso compound was a pale tan solid identical in all respects with a sample provided by Dr. Eisenbrand. The compound was soluble in acetone and fairly stable in aqueous solution; no significant change was observed in absorptivity of a solution in neutral deionized water kept in the dark at room temperature for a week. A solution of MNNG underwent 50%-70% decomposition under the same conditions. NCM and MNNG were completely stable in acetone solution kept in the dark and at 0°C for several weeks. MNNG was prepared according to the method of McKay (1949).

For the skin painting experiments NCM and MNNG were dissolved in distilled acetone at the concentrations shown in Table 1. 25 μl of the solution was applied from a calibrated pipette to the shaved interscapular region of each of a group of 20 female Swiss mice of the colony of the Frederick Cancer Research Facility, housed 10 to a plastic cage. The treatment was twice a week for 30 weeks with MNNG at both concentrations and twice a week for 110 weeks with NCM. The skin of each animal was examined for tumors and other lesions, which were charted on graph paper once a week. A group of acetone-treated and untreated control mice was maintained in parallel, but none of these developed tumors.

In the rat feeding study, NCM and MNNG were dissolved in dimethyl-sulfoxide and 5 ml of this solution was diluted each week to 2 liters with neutral deionized water. These solutions were administered as drinking water to groups of Fischer 344 rats, housed 4 to a cage, at the rate of 20 ml per day per rat, 5 days a week. On the remaining 2 days the rats were given tap water to compensate for any possible water deficiency. The stock solutions were prepared once in 5 weeks and were kept refrigerated. At the end of the treatments, which were 50 weeks for MNNG and 106 weeks for NCM, the animals were allowed to die naturally and were completely necropsied. All lesions and the major organs and tissues were fixed for histologic examination.

RESULTS AND DISCUSSION

The skin painting study is almost complete, with only a few animals remaining of the groups treated with NCM. Survival of the treated mice was excellent as shown in Table 1. In this very sensitive test system for direct-acting carcinogens, only a single skin tumor was found in an animal treated with the higher concentration of NCM, and that was a malignant lymphoma, not a tumor normally induced in skin by nitrosoalkylamides. It can be concluded that, under conditions of this test, NCM is not carcinogenic to mouse skin. In contrast, the analogous MNNG applied at equimolar concentration, but for a shorter time (Table 1), has induced skin tumors in 14 of 20 mice at the 0.02 M concentration and in 4 of 20 mice at the 0.008 M concentration. No tumors have been seen in either the acetone-treated controls or the untreated controls after more than 100 weeks observation.

The results, to date, of the rat feeding experiment with NCM are shown in Table 2. Again, a direct comparison is made with the known carcinogen MNNG, which was administered at equimolar concentration with NCM, but for 50 weeks

Table 1
Chronic Application of Nitrosocimetidine and MNNG to Mouse Skin

Compound	Concentration in acetone mg/ml (mM)	Length of treatment (wks)	Total dose mg (μmoles)	Number of mice	Week of first tumor	Number of skin tumor bearing mice	Number of survivors at 100 wks
NCM	5.6 (20)	110	31 (110)	20	60	1[a]	13
	2.2 (8)	110	12 (44)	20	–	0	18
MNNG	2.9 (20)	30	4.5 (30)	20	30	14	0
	1.2 (8)	30	1.8 (12)	20	60	4	15

[a]Malignant lymphoma

Table 2
Oral Administration of Nitrosocimetidine and MNNG to F344 Rats

Compound	Concentration in water mg/1 (mM)	Length of treatment (wks)	Total dose mg (mmoles)	Survivors at week					Number of rats with tumors		
				0	50	70	90	110	Stomach	Liver	Other
NCM	150 (0.53)	106	1600 (5.7)	♂20	20	20	19	12	0	2[a]	1 (myoblastoma) 1 (spleen hemangio-sarcoma)
	"		"	♀20	20	20	20	16	0	2[b]	1 (neurosarcoma) 1 (ear carcinoma)
MNNG	75 (0.51)	50	375 (2.5)	♂20	18	17	14	5	5[c]	0	1 (neurosarcoma) 3 (oligodendroglioma) 1 (jaw carcinoma)

[a] Hepatocellular carcinomas
[b] 1 hepatocellular carcinoma; 1 neoplastic nodule
[c] 5 with adenocarcinoma; 1 with forestomach papilloma also.

only, while NCM was given for more than 2 years. This study is not complete, being at week 110, and while most of the MNNG-treated rats have died, most of the rats treated with NCM are still alive. Five of the 15 rats that have died in the group treated with MNNG had adenocarcinomas of the glandular stomach. This is a somewhat lower incidence than has been reported by Sugimura and his colleagues (Sugimura and Kawachi 1973) in other strains of rat and perhaps represents the lower susceptibility of Fischer rats to this carcinogen. It is notable that there was only 1 animal with a tumor of the nonglandular stomach in this group, in contrast to the great susceptibility of the nonglandular stomach of Fischer rats to nitrosomethylurethane, which induced 100% incidence of carcinomas there after administration of a total dose of only 0.05 millimole.

NCM, even after a considerably larger dose than that of MNNG administered, has given rise to no tumors in the stomachs of the rats that have died. Because 70% of the rats given NCM are still alive, it is not possible to state conclusively that this compound does not induce stomach tumors in Fischer rats; however, even if some such tumors are found later, NCM is very much less effective than MNNG. Surprisingly, four of the animals treated with NCM, 2 males and 2 females, have liver neoplasms. One of these, in a female, was a neoplastic nodule, the remainder were hepatocellular carcinomas. Liver tumors are very rare in untreated control Fischer rats, an incidence of less than 1%. Until all of the NCM-treated rats are dead it will not be possible to speculate whether the finding of these liver neoplasms in the rats is significant. The numbers at this point are not statistically significant, and are merely troublesome. The dose of NCM received by the rats is large and the age at death with tumors is high, so that even were the liver tumors to be considered significant, the carcinogenic potency of NCM is very weak. Opinion about this must be reserved until completion of the study.

ACKNOWLEDGMENTS

This work was supported by Contract No. N01-C0-75380, with National Cancer Institute, NIH, Bethesda, Maryland 20215.

REFERENCES

Lijinsky, W. and C. Winter. 1981. Skin tumors by painting nitrosoalkylureas on mouse skin. *Cancer Res. Clin. Oncol.* 102:13.

McKay, A.F. 1949. The preparation of N-substituted N'-nitroguanidines by the reaction of primary amines with N-alkyl-N-nitroso-N'-nitroguanidines. *J. Am. Chem. Soc.* 71:1968.

Pool, B.L., G. Eisenbrand, and D. Schmähl. 1979. Biological activity of nitrosated cimetidine. *Toxicology* 15:69.

Sugimura, T. and T. Kawachi. 1973. Experimental stomach cancer. *Methods Cancer Res.* 7:245.

Takayama, S., N. Kuwabara, Y. Azama, and T. Sugimura. 1971. Skin tumors in mice painted with N-methyl-N'-nitro-N-nitrosoguanidine and N-ethyl-N'-nitro-N-nitrosoguanidine. *J. Natl. Cancer Inst.* 46:973.

Carcinogenesis Studies with N-Nitrosocimetidine

Part II: Oral Administration to Sprague-Dawley Rats

MICHAEL HABS, DIETRICH SCHMÄHL, GERHARD EISENBRAND,
AND RUDOLF PREUSSMANN
Institute of Toxicology and Chemotherapy
German Cancer Research Center
D-6900 Heidelberg
Federal Republic of Germany

The question of a direct correlation between cimetidine treatment and an increased risk for gastric cancer has been raised (Elder et al. 1979). Since cimetidine contains nitrosatable amino groups in the molecule, which can be nitrosated under simulated stomach conditions in the presence of nitrite, the endogenous formation of N-nitrosocimetidine (NCM) might be causally related to a carcinogenic effect. Since the nitrosation occurs exclusively at the N-methyl site of the guanidine residue of cimetidine, NCM behaves like a typical nitrosamide (Jensen and Magee 1981; M. Habs et al. unpubl. results) with some structural relationships to N-methyl-N'-nitro-N-nitrosoguanidine (MNNG), a known and potent carcinogen for the forestomach and glandular stomach in several animal species after oral administration (Sugimura and Fujimura 1967; Preussmann and Stewart 1982).

We therefore investigated the possible carcinogenicity of NCM in outbred Sprague-Dawley rats of both sexes (Habs et al. 1982). Two groups of 20 male and 20 female animals each received 500 and 50 mg/kg NCM respectively by gavage twice a week for 1 year with subsequent lifelong follow-up. NCM was dissolved in water by adding the necessary amount of hydrochloric acid to convert it to the soluble hydrochloride; this solution was near neutral and was stable under the used conditions of administration. Additionally 40 male rats were given 80 mg/kg MNNG for 3 months by gavage of an aqueous solution containing 20% alcohol. 50 male and 50 female animals served as untreated controls. All animals were observed for life or killed when moribund. In all the animals, stomach (forestomach as well as glandular stomach), duodenum, and those organs showing abnormalities macroscopically were investigated histologically after necropsy.

All MNNG-treated rats died with carcinomas of the forestomach after a median induction time (MIT) of 226 days (range: 126-286 days at 95% confidence). Out of 100 untreated controls 19 rats developed neoplasms including 7 rats with papillomas of the forestomach (MIT: 534 days, 95% range: 528-836 days).

No clearly treatment related tumors were detected in animals receiving NCM. Three rats of the high-dose group and one animal in the low-dose group developed papillomas of the forestomach. Further gastrointestinal tumors were not observed. In the 500 mg/kg NCM-group the following malignant tumors were recorded: 1 pheochromocytoma, 1 neurogenic sarcoma, and 1 skin carcinoma; in the 50 mg/kg NCM-group only one neurogenic sarcoma was noted. In both NCM-treated groups the median survival time was reduced. It was only 400 and 393 days respectively as compared to 630 days for untreated controls. No specific treatment-related causes of death could be established; animals that were not killed by a tumor died of infections (pneumonia, nephritis, enterocolitis, pyometria) like the controls. However, we had the impression of higher sensitivity towards infections in the treated groups.

In summary, the presented data of a pilot study investigating NCM after oral administration in one high- and one lower-dose group gave no evidence of carcinogenicity under the experimental conditions used. Although only a limited number of experimental animals was at risk and despite the reduced survival time in NCM-receiving rats it is concluded that NCM is either not carcinogenic or at least significantly less carcinogenic in comparison to MNNG. The results of the possible control experiment using MNNG demonstrates the sensitivity of the used rat strain against gastrocarcinogenesis.

The result of the present study is unexpected. In view of the structural similarities of NCM with other methylating N-nitrosamides, such as MNNG and methylnitroso-urea or methylnitrosourethane, both potent carcinogens, a carcinogenic effect would have been probable. However, the structural and chemical similarities should not be overemphasized. MNNG is a disubstituted nitrosoguanidine derivative, while NCM is a trisubstituted one. The effects of the cyano group on the carbimino moiety as well as that of the substituent on the N'-atom of the nitrosoguanidine moiety in NCM are difficult to predict, since similar structures have not yet been tested. It should be remembered that the imidazol ring in NCM can be protonated, and protonated NC might resorb badly through biological membranes. It should also be remembered that homologues of MNNG, such as those with higher alkyl chains (butyl-, isobutyl-, pentyl-, hexyl-) are noncarcinogenic on oral administration, although MNNG and its ethyl homologue are potent carcinogens (Preussmann and Stewart 1982).

However, it is also a fact that NCM, a methylating agent in vitro and in vivo, induces DNA breaks in vitro and is positive in at least some short-term tests (see Jensen and Gombar, this volume, for a summary). Therefore, it must be emphasized that the presently available results from carcinogenicity bioassays cannot rule out with certainty that NCM is not carcinogenic.

REFERENCES

Elder, J.B., P.C. Ganguli, and J.E. Gillespie. 1979. Cimetidine and gastric cancer. *Lancet* i:1005.

Habs, M., D. Schmähl, and G. Eisenbrand. 1982. Cimetidine, N-nitrosocimetidine and carcinogenicity. *Lancet* (in press).

Jensen, P.E. and P.N. Magee. 1981. Methylation of DNA by nitrosocimetidine
in vitro. *Cancer Res.* 41:230.

Preussmann, R. and B.W. Stewart. 1982. N-Nitroso carcinogens. *ACS Monogr.*
(in press).

Sugimura, T. and S. Fujimura. 1967. Tumor production in glandular stomach of
rat by N-methyl-N′-nitro-N-nitrosoguanidine. *Nature* 216:943.

The Question of Human Exposure to Nitrosamines

Discussion of Reports by

James B. Elder, Rudolf Preussmann, and William Lijinsky

JOHN H. WEISBURGER, CHAIRMAN

WEISBURGER: Perhaps we should look at Dr. Lijinsky's, Preussmann's, and Dr. Elder's reports. Dr. Elder's was a bit different from the straightforward testing Preussmann and Lijinsky did, insofar as he used the Wong-Lowenthal ulcer and promoter studies when those got tissue regeneration—thus, you have hepatitis-B aflatoxin interaction for liver cancer in man and perhaps in animals, and in other models. We know that it works better if the tissue is in regeneration.

MICHEJDA: Dr. Elder, did you say that there was a thiazole derivative of NCM which was a carcinogen?

ELDER: I said tiotidine has been shown to produce antral carcinomas in rats killed at 11 months after a 6-month exposure at about 8 or 10 times the recommended human dosage for that blocker.

MICHEJDA: That's curious, it is very similar.

CHALLIS: No, the chemistry and the electron binding is entirely different. When you nitrosate it, you attack the thiazole ring.

TANNENBAUM: The thiazole is going to be very reactive.

CHALLIS: It's a very, very reactive ring, and I don't think that one should draw the comparison across these data. It's very complicated.

MICHEJDA: Perhaps I'm misunderstanding then. It's the compound itself, not the nitroso derivative.

CHALLIS: It has nothing to do with the nitrosation.

ELDER: I'm not a chemist but I would like to hear the evidence that you have that the nitrosated derivative of tiotidine was not involved in experimental carcinomas. I have talked with people at ICI. They don't know whether the drug was nitrosated in the stomach of the rat or not. I think you've got to be careful as to what the actual carcinogen was with tiotodine. I don't know if it was the drug, but I don't know if it was the nitrosated product either. We don't know the actual molecule.

WEISBURGER: Let's review your results now.

REED: Dr. Preussmann, it seems unusual that in your rat population spontaneous tumors were observed. I would have expected an increased incidence in the NCM-treated rats as well. There seems to be a discrepancy. Can you explain it?

PREUSSMANN: The treated rats die earlier. The spontaneous tumors appear later in life.

REED: Why did they die earlier?

PREUSSMANN: This was at about 400 days vs 620 days—120 days shorter median-life expectancy.

GRASSO: Dr. Elder, did you do any biopsies on humans immediately after they started treatment on CM at the site where the carcinomas developed to determine whether there has been any irregularity in any of the tissue reaction?

ELDER: I have not biopsied human subjects. I have not had the opportunity. Carcinomas of the stomach have not been diagnosed at some variable time or even during treatment with H_2 blockers.

I have, however, patients I have biopsied before treatment was started, and others have such data. Then, we subsequently observed a carcinoma. But I don't think that means anything. Gastric biopsy is not very representative of the state of the mucosa.

GRASSO: I thought it was interesting to see if there was any abnormal hyperplastic process induced by the treatment, which wasn't existing before. This sort of follows Tannenbaum's suggestion that there may well be some hormonal reaction.

ELDER: I don't know.

WEISBURGER: Dr. Elder, were the neoplastic lesions you saw in the area of the ulceration?

ELDER: Yes.

WEISBURGER: Did you have an MNNG control with the ulcer?

ELDER: Yes, I did. The lesions were at the edge of the ulcer each time.

GRASSO: Did you actually diagnose the carcinoma?

ELDER: Yes with the operative specimen, but I have lymph node biopsies which pick that up.

HARRIS: We traditionally do carcinogenesis experiments in more than one species. Are there experiments going on in mice, and are there initiation-promotion experiments going on in mouse skin?

LIJINSKY: I can comment on my results. No, I don't find that there is initiation-promotion, since MNNG itself is a poor initiator for mouse skin. You need large doses, and you don't get many tumors.

HOFFMANN: Why do you say that? You just told us that we should be very cautious about the structure, and now you say MNNG isn't and therefore NCM isn't.

LIJINSKY: As an initiator.

MONTESANO: Usually in doing carcinogenicity studies, various bodies recommend that at least 50 animals per group be used. Why do you use only 20?

LIJINSKY: Because I'm short of money. Each animal that dies has to be processed.

MONTESANO: I think we are very much concerned with conclusive results. I don't find that justification useful.

LIJINSKY: Well, unfortunately, pathology on animals is very expensive. I reckon that each rat costs $400 in such an experiment, and I don't have that much money.

HARTMAN: Japanese workers have an ulcer model in which they get some intestinal metaplasia at some of the sites. This is a serosal low-temperature ulcer induction. That might be a good model system, since it will be more attuned to these human cases.

ELDER: How is the ulcer made, or what is the ulcerating mechanism?

HARTMAN: I think they just go in with a -7°C probe.

TANNENBAUM: There are two different ways of doing it. One is with a cold probe from the serosal side exposed by a laporotomy. The other way is to give a massive dose of sodium hydroxide and then immediately wash it out.

In a meeting which I just attended I learned that it is very difficult to get rodent models for chronic ulcers. In order to get a chronic ulcer, you have to give a really massive injury to the gastric mucosa. But, when you do, as Dr. Hartman just said, you wind up with a lot of intestinalized tissue at the border of the ulcer.

LIJINSKY: Could I make a comment? I think we should bear in mind that we are discussing the testing of NCM. If we were testing CM, that would be a different matter. Here we tested NCM at quite high doses. It seems to be negative. What more do we need to find out? NCM might be produced to some small extent from CM, which might or might not have an effect. I mean, we are getting down to the point of negligible risk.

MIRVISH: One could ask the question whether CM itself has been tested for carcinogenicity.

LIJINSKY: Of course.

DURANT: Exhaustive safety studies have been conducted including 2-year carcinogenicity studies with rats and long-term studies in dogs. No evidence for carcinogenicity has been found in any of these tests (see Barnard et al., this volume).

MAGEE: Dr. Preussmann's remarks drew attention, as several of the speakers have done, to the resemblance between MNNG and NCM. One was surprised that NCM, with all the in vitro tests proving so positive for mutagenicity, turned out apparently not to be carcinogenic. But I would like to suggest that the results reported by Dr. Jensen and Dr. Gombar from our laboratory, if you are prepared to look at them, might suggest just a possible explanation for this, if you believe in pharmacokinetics at all.

DURANT: I would agree with that, and in addition it could be added that with all the studies that have been done on CM itself, this adds up to a reasonably conclusive story for the safety of cimetidine.

WEISBURGER: This is an important subject. The question is whether a widely used drug is nitrosated and whether it is potentially a carcinogenic risk?

Might I suggest that my explanation is similar to Dr. Magee's. We have seen some biochemical data. We have seen the results of three animal experiments, including the results presented at this meeting. But may I say that, as a result of all the reports in journals, in the last few years on carcinogenic risk of NCM I get a bit edgy and I decided to comment on it. Based on Dr. Mirvish's seminal discovery in the Shubik's lab in 1972, where he accidentally found that ascorbic acid present in a commercial oxytetracycline formulation, as sold in the pharmacy, blocked nitrosation, I wrote a letter to the *Lancet* (Weisburger 1981) suggesting a sample solution, namely to formulate this drug, CM with Vitamin C, as are many other drugs. This would inhibit intragastric formation of NCM.

May I also suggest a more relevant question, in the light of Dr. Hoffmann's report on tobacco carcinogenesis, where literally tens of millions of people are now exposed to nitroso compounds at sizable levels, either in smoke or when they chew, and where it is reasonably certain that these nitrosamines do cause substantial neoplastic disease in man.

I say that since we are running short of money for cancer research we ought to concentrate on the aspects that really matter in terms of human disease. It is so simple to formulate drugs with Vitamin C, we will have to ask no questions, and we won't have to worry about any possible effects of NCM.

May I suggest that we really concentrate in the next 5 or 10 years on topics that are really important and which will give you a baseline for disease prevention in man.

REED: I feel I must make a final comment; I don't think we can leave Dr. Weisburger's comments as the last word on this subject. Over 15 million people have so far received CM worldwide—and it is estimated that that number is going to grow pretty dramatically over the years—I don't think, therefore, that it is necessarily such a small risk situation in comparison to tobacco. He was speaking of millions, and it is possible that of those 15 million there could well be some, perhaps only a handful, maybe eventually over a thousand, then that is a risk, and it is a preventable risk.

Although I agree that the formulation of CM with Vitamin C may be possible, we don't know what its effects might be if it were actually given, whether the drug, in fact, would behave in the same way. This thing cannot just be dismissed out of hand; even if the NCM effect remains unproven, I don't think we should forget about the pH effect which is real.

References

Weisburger, J.H. 1981. Cimetidine, nitroso compounds, and gastric cancer. *Lancet* i:1323.

SESSION V:

NITRITES AND AMINES

Overview:

Nitrite Load in the Upper Gastrointestinal Tract—

Past, Present, and Future

PHILIP E. HARTMAN
Department of Biology
The Johns Hopkins University
Baltimore, Maryland 21218

This brief overview will examine some factors involved in nitrate and nitrite flow and persistence in the upper gastrointestinal tracts of humans. Building upon this framework, the overview will then survey some elements that may be critical to esophageal and, particularly, to gastric cancer induction. Interplay of these same elements may possibly account for pronounced declines in gastric cancer mortality that have occurred in a number of countries over the past few decades. Some further actions that collectively could help to eradicate these two types of cancer will be mentioned. The underlying thesis which will be explicitly assumed is that both forms of cancer, except perhaps in cigarette smokers, are predominantly initiated by nitroso compounds formed in vivo by the interaction of persistent nitrite and nitrosatable substrates. Extensive literature citations documenting many of the assertions made below are to be found in two recent reviews (National Research Council 1981; Hartman 1982) to which this overview merely serves as a supplement. The area of endogenous synthesis of nitrite and nitrate will not be covered. Our knowledge in most areas of nitrate and nitrite "metabolism" in the human is still very limited; therefore, all of the literature values cited should be taken only as very crude estimates.

NITRITE AND NITRATE FLOW IN THE HUMAN

Detailed pharmacodynamic models are under development, but at the present time we can only outline some of the major features of the flow of ingested nitrate and nitrite in man. Ingested nitrate passes through the esophagus and stomach, and the vast majority of the nitrate reaches the plasma by transport through the mucosa of the upper small intestine. The nature of this rapid transport is completely uncharacterized but is amenable to ready analysis in laboratory animals utilizing labeled compounds coupled with techniques now standard in investigations of intestinal transport processes. Transport could be an active process, shared by iodide and thiocyanate ions, as found in some other tissues (Hartman 1982). The fate of low doses of ingested nitrite ions is unknown; some nitrite does reach the blood, possibly following damage to the gastric mucosa, when very high doses are present in the lumen. At low plasma concentrations, plasma nitrite is quantitatively converted to nitrate (Parks et al. 1981).

Plasma nitrate appears to equilibrate rapidly with some tissue compartments (Hartman 1982). Much of the residual plasma nitrate is excreted in the urine as a first-order process with a "plasma" half-life of 5 hours (National Research Council 1981). It has to be remembered that this "plasma" nitrate may include nitrate from other tissue compartments (Hartman 1982). Residual "plasma" nitrate is also secreted into saliva. Roughly 25% of ingested nitrate ends up in saliva, and roughly 20% of this recirculated nitrate is reduced to nitrite by oral bacteria (i.e., about 6.3 mole % of ingested nitrate) (Spiegelhalder et al. 1976; Eisenbrand et al. 1980; Stephany and Schuller 1980). Both thiocyanate and iodide compete for nitrate transport into saliva (reviewed in Hartman 1982). Thus, a salivary transport threshold for nitrate *that varies with plasma iodide and thiocyanate levels* is expected (Hartman 1982) and has been indicated as about 10 mg in one group of individuals given nitrate in water (Walters and Smith 1981).

There is a large variability from person to person in both salivary nitrate recirculation and in percent reduction (Hill 1979; Tannenbaum 1979; Eisenbrand et al. 1980; Walters and Smith 1981). Salivary iodide, which shares the nitrate transport system, has been observed to be several-fold higher in particular gastric cancer patients than in the normal subjects examined (Schiff et al. 1947; Honour et al. 1952). Thus, individual variations in salivary transport, combined with individual differences in indigenous microflora (Kraus and Gastron 1956; Richardson and Jones 1958; Hoffman 1966) may account for some of the heterogeneity observed in nitrate and nitrite contents of saliva. In any event, to examine if a threshold in nitrate transport exists, one needs to plot nitrate intake versus the sum of salivary nitrate and nitrite.

There is some evidence of nitrate recirculation from plasma into gastric juices, but quantitative aspects of this presumed transport are unknown. Several other parameters of nitrate flow (Hartman 1982) also lack quantitation. These parameters of nitrate flow need to be worked out before meaningful pharmacodynamic models can be developed.

NITRITE INGESTION AND ESOPHAGEAL CANCER

Daily nitrite ingestion in a high-risk area for esophageal cancer in Iran is given as 9 mg, and this is coupled with a low ascorbate intake (Joint Iran-International Agency for Research on Cancer Study Group 1977). A high salivary nitrite content also has been noted in persons of the high-risk area under certain conditions (Eisenbrand et al. 1980). In addition, a fibrous silica contaminant of flour has been indicated as a possible adjuvant in tumor induction in the high-risk region (O'Neill et al. 1980), and ascorbate intake is low there (Hormozdiari et al. 1975).

High levels of ingestion of nitrite and nitrate and low ascorbate intakes have been noted in high-risk esophageal cancer regions of Henan Province, China (Li et al. 1980; Li 1981). Table 1 presents some data regarding the measured contents in drinking water of nitrate, nitrite, and iodide in four contrasting regions of Henan Province (Chinese Academy of Medical Sciences 1980). Salivary nitrate is said not to vary between the high- and low-risk areas (Li 1981).

NITRATE INGESTION AND GASTRIC CANCER

Hill et al. (1973) suggested that there might be a link between high nitrate ingestion and gastric cancer mortality in a town in the United Kingdom. However, the increased mortality now has been attributed to other factors (Davies 1980). Nevertheless, data obtained in a number of additional epidemiological studies have served to keep alive the idea of a nitrate-gastric cancer relationship. One recent compilation indicates a correlation between age-adjusted gastric cancer mortality and levels of nitrate ingested in 11 countries for which both sets of data are available (Fine et al. 1982). This suggestive but very incomplete evidence needs to be filled out by similar examinations of total per capita nitrate intake in other high-risk countries such as those in Eastern Europe and in some very low-risk countries such as Australia and New Zealand. At present, the same correlation ($r = +0.88$) is found whether a linear or a nitrate-squared relationship is examined; more data might help determine the type of nitroso compound(s) involved in gastric cancer induction if, indeed, nitroso compounds are critical factors. Additionally, the linear plot (Fine et al. 1982) extrapolates close to zero dose of nitrate, whereas the nitrate-squared plot based on the same data extrapolates to roughly 30-40 mg nitrate/person/day.

Table 1
Nitrate, Nitrite, and Iodide in Drinking Water, Four Places in Anyang District, Henan Province, China

Region	1	2	3	4
Esophageal cancer (Age-adjusted death rate)	199.7	133.2	35.0	18.2
Population	118,588	119,194	128,718	129,828
Nitrate (mg/1)	16.4	18.1	14.4	3.2
Nitrite (mg/1)	0.053	0.016	0.055	0.017
Iodide (mg/1)	0.008	0.008	0.033	0.227
Number water samples assayed	59	57	54	32

Data from Chinese Academy of Medical Sciences (1980)

Table 2

Some Nitrite Scavengers and Nitrosation Enhancers

pH	Nitrite scavengers	Nitrosation enhancers
Low	urea[a], ascorbate	iodide, thiocyanate[a,b]
High	ascorbate (weak)[c]	phenols[d], aldehydes, alcohols, sulfhydryls

[a]No effect of added urea or of added thiocyanate on in vivo nitrosation of diethylamine or methylbenzylamine was found in the rat stomach (Schweinsberg 1974).

[b]In contrast to the results of Schweinsberg (1974)[a], a pronounced catalysis of in vivo nitrosoproline formation was observed in the rat upon thiocyanate addition (Ohshima et al. 1982). Thiocyanate does not facilitate nitrosation of amides at any pH in in vitro experiments (Hallett and Williams 1980).

[c]Ascorbate may have other effects near neutral pH. For example, Osawa et al. (1980) detected rapid degradation of the mutagen 1,4-dinitro-2-methylpyrrole to a non-mutagenic derivative in the presence of an 8-fold molar excess of ascorbate near neutral pH, but no inactivating effect of ascorbate was detected at pHs of 1.5 and 3.5.

[d]Phenol both increases the rate of nitrosation of a secondary amine and shifts the pH optimum to pH4-5 (Walker et al. 1979).

The correlation of Fine et al. (1982) is surprising since a number of factors in addition to levels of nitrate ingestion appear important in increasing and in diminishing formation of nitroso compounds (some examples in Table 2).

Not to belittle ascorbate which many studies have indicated is a molecule of high importance, one has to consider the impacts of an even more abundant molecule, urea (Table 3). Urea serves just as effectively as does ascorbate as a nitrite scavenger at pHs below 3 (Mirvish et al. 1975). Thus, urea is an effective nitrite scavenger in just that pH range where thiocyanate is most effective in catalysis of nitrosamine formation (Boyland et al. 1971; Fan and Tannenbaum 1973). Additional roles for thiocyanate and iodide that complicate interpretation of their possible effects on in vivo nitrosation are their competition for salivary transport of nitrate (Hartman 1982) and their roles as important antibacterial agents in saliva (Dogon and Andur 1970). Cigarette smokers generally have elevated salivary and gastric thiocyanate levels, and iodide (which is a better catalyst at low pHs than is thiocyanate) has been added to salt in the United States during the past 50 years. There is no evidence that enrichment of these nitrosation catalysts in substantial segments of the U.S. population has increased gastric cancer risk. In fact, gastric cancer mortality trends in the United States have been markedly decreasing over the past four decades (Devesa and Silverman 1978). It is quite possible that iodide and thiocyanate are not effective catalysts of nitrosation reactions under normal conditions in vivo due to their blockage of nitrate recirculation and the facile elimination of nitrite by ascorbate and by urea in the pH range where halide catalysis is effective. More attention needs to be given to catalysis of nitrosation reactions at higher pHs (i.e., above pH4) (Table 2).

Table 3
Urea and Ascorbate Concentrations in Some Biological Fluids Assuming Ascorbate Intake Approaches the RDA (60 mg) and Moderate Meat Ingestion

Fluid	Ascorbate	Urea	Urea:Ascorbate
Whole blood	0.035 mM	4.3 mM	120x
Plasma	0.025 mM[a]	4.5 mM[b]	180x
Saliva (children)	_c	4.6 mM	
Saliva (adults)	0.013 mM	3.5 mM[d]	300x
Gastric juice	_c	_c	
Urine	0.011 mM	600 mM	8200x
Milk	0.3 mM	13 mM	40 x
Milk (cow's)	0.06 mM 0.38 mM[e]	9.5 mM	25-160x

Values from Diem and Lentner (1970).
[a]This ascorbate value (and most others in the Table) is highly dependent upon intake:

Daily intake (mg):   0   5   10   20   50   70   600
Plasma value (mM): 0.002 0.003 0.006 0.006 0.02 0.03 0.06

[b]Plasma urea concentration is directly proportional to the amount of protein ingested and mainly a function of unutilized protein in the diet (Bodwell et al. 1978; 1979).
[c]No literature value located.
[d]75-90% of the blood concentration.
[e]Value from Pennington and Church (1980).

DECLINING INCIDENCE OF GASTRIC CANCER

Gastric cancer is decreasing in some countries but remaining relatively constant in others (recently reviewed in Devesa and Silverman 1978; Campbell 1980; Joossens and Geboers 1981). The decreases in age-adjusted mortality figures have been indicated as "linear" and as "exponential," and sometimes are presented both ways in the same paper. Stringent analyses of rates of decline may assist in deciphering the causal agents (e.g., nitrosamines *versus* nitrosamides). Also, it is of interest to determine among suspect factors what differences there are between, for example, Finland (where the decline in gastric cancer mortality is comparatively rapid) and Portugal (where an *increase* may be occurring). A number of factors are worthy of consideration under the nitroso compound theory (Table 4).

Cereals and Grains

Cereal and grain consumption has been tied to gastric cancer mortality (Hakama and Saxén 1967), an observation entirely compatible with the notion that nitroso compounds initiate gastric cancer (Table 5). Perhaps one surprise that came out of the National Research Council (1981) study is the magnitude of the direct dietary nitrate and nitrite contribution made by baked goods and

Table 4
Some Factors That May be of Consequence in the Declining Incidence of Gastric Cancer

1. Decreases in nitrite and nitrate contents of cured meats (see Tables 6, 7)
2. Decreases in per capita cured meat consumption (see Table 7)
3. Higher utilization of public water supplies with lower nitrate
4. Movement of vegetable industry to warmer, sunnier climates, leading to lower nitrate and higher ascorbate produce
5. Better marketing and refrigeration allowing lowered salt[a], aldehyde[b], and nitrite content of meats and lessening reduction of nitrate to nitrite in vegetables before consumption
6. Higher year-round ascorbate intake
7. Lower bacterial counts in foods
8. Decreased use of smoking as a meat preservative and, thus, lowered coingestion of nitrite with nitrosation catalysts such as phenols[c] and aldehydes
9. Utilization of iodized salt which maintains plasma iodide levels as a chief competitor of salivary and gastric nitrate recirculation
10. Decreased consumption of carbohydrates and increased total per capita meat consumption (see Table 5)

Adapted from Hartman (1982) with additions.
[a]An approximately 30% decrease between 1932 and 1979 (Cerveny 1980).
[b]Lowered aldehyde content due to less rancidity. Recent estimates of malondialdehyde content of foods indicate that fresh and cured meats are the major sources of ingestion (Shamberger et al. 1977; Siu and Draper 1978). While malondialdehyde is but a minor component of the total carbonyl content of meats, I calculate that current ingestion amounts to about 200-600 μg/person/day in the U.S. Malondialdehyde optimally catalyzes nitrosamine formation in the pH range of 3-5 (Kikugawa et al. 1980; Kurechi et al. 1980).
[c]Estimated deposition of up to 300 mg/kg of phenols on the meat matrix during smoking (Davies et al. 1978). A level of 7 mg/kg phenol has been detected in smoked summer sausage and about 29 mg/kg in smoked pork belly (Babich and Davis 1981).

Table 5
Some Persistent Physiological Effects of High-Carbohydrate, Low-Meat Diets[a]

1. Twofold induction of salivary amylase →
   a. products supply electron donors for bacterial nitrate reduction to nitrite
   b. monosaccharides slow gastric emptying
2. Decreased gastric acid secretion →
   a. increased activity of amylase and enzymes derived from intestinalized gastric mucosa
   b. decreased secretion of gastric mucins
   c. enhanced bacterial invasion of the stomach with increased opportunity for nitrate reduction to nitrite
   d. elimination of pH-dependent repression of bacterial nitrate reductase activity
3. Decreased production of urea (see Table 3)

Adapted from Hartman (1982) with additions.
[a]A possible role of "total calorie consumption" in determining the sex ratio of mortality from gastric cancer has been pointed out by Griffith (1968).

cereals when expressed in terms of the gastric nitrite load (Table 9, p. 424). Ingestion of carbohydrates has dropped by about 22% in the U.S. population over the years 1909-1974, and there has been a larger decrease (about 50%) in average daily consumption of starches, including both potatoes and cereal products (Gortner 1975).

Cured Meats

In the United States there have been substantial decreases in per capita cured meat consumption and in the nitrite content of cured meats (Tables 6 and 7). Given the values portrayed in Table 7, it is perhaps not surprising that ingestion of cured meats has been implicated in two retrospective studies of gastric cancer in the U.S. (Higginson 1966; Bjelke 1973). It is clear that decreases in nitrate and nitrite concentrations and decreases in cured meat consumption could well account for the decline in gastric cancer mortality noted in the United States in recent decades. Decreases in the cured meat contribution of nitrite and nitrate could have ensued well before 1926. In fact, Binkerd and Kolari (1975) mention a meat-pickling formula of 1894 that recommended addition of 1 part per 300 of saltpeter (potassium nitrate). A very broad range of nitrite and even of nitrate concentrations still persists in U.S. cured meats (American Meat Institute Foundation 1971; National Research Council 1981). Thus, key 1978 recommendations on nitrate and nitrite inputs and residuals in cured meats (Table 8) remain pertinent today in a U.S. industry that, except for bacon, still operates under regulations formulated in 1925 (Cerveny 1980).

A recent estimate proposes that cured meats now contribute about 9% of the gastric nitrite load in the average U.S. adult with normal gastric acidity (Table 9). Since the American Cancer Society (1981) estimates 13,800 U.S.

Table 6
Declining Nitrate and Nitrite Contents of Cured Meats at the Retail Level

Year	Nitrate (mg/kg)	Nitrite (mg/kg)	Number of samples	References
1926	340[a]	185	68	Kerr et al. (1926)
1937[b]	–	36	134	Kolari and Aunan (1972)
1972	170	17[c]	171	Panalaks et al. (1973); Fudge and Truman (1973)
1981	40	10	–	National Research Council (1981)

[a]Nitrate-cured products; estimated at twice the 1971-1972 level.

[b]Binkerd and Kolari (1975) present data from two surveys of U.S. cured meats performed in 1936-1937. An average nitrate concentration of 827 mg/kg and an average nitrite concentration of 56 mg/kg was observed in 130 samples of various products. However, it is not clear if these are concentrations of ions or of the sodium salts; the latter would require multiplication by a factor of about 0.7.

[c]An average value for 12 product categories involving 116 total samples assayed in U.S. products circa 1970 was 34 mg/kg nitrite (American Meat Institute Foundation 1971).

Table 7
Decreasing Contribution of Cured Meats to Gastric Nitrite Load

Year	Nitrate (mg/kg)	Nitrite (mg/kg)	Grams/person/day	Cured meats nitrate/nitrite (mg/person/day)		All other sources[a] nitrate/nitrite (mg/person/day)		Salivary nitrite[b] cured meats (mg/person/day)	Salivary nitrite[b] all other[a]	Total gastric nitrite load (mg/day)	Percent cured meat contribution
1926	340[c]	185	55[c]	18.7	10.2	74	0.47	0.9	3.4	15.0	74%
1936–1937	290[c]	36	55	16.0	2.0	74	0.47	0.8	3.4	6.7	42%
1971–1972	170	17	40[c]	6.8	0.68	74	0.47	0.34	3.4	4.9	21%
1981	40	10	30	1.2	0.3	74	0.47	0.06	3.4	4.2	9%

[a]For the present purposes, these values are assumed to be constant. Values taken from National Research Council (1981).
[b]5% of the nitrate ingested and assuming no thresholds for nitrate recirculation and salivary reduction to nitrite. Total nitrite load in the stomach would be lower if a threshold exists in salivary nitrate content, and the percentage contribution of cured meats would be increased.
[c]Crude extrapolates from other data in Table 6.

Table 8
Some Final Recommendations of the Expert Panel on Nitrites and Nitrosamines (1978) Regarding Establishment of Limits on Nitrites and Nitrates in Cured Meats

Product	Ingoing sodium nitrite (target level)	Ingoing sodium nitrate (target level)	Ingoing sodium ascorbate or isoascorbate (target level)	Maximum residual sodium nitrite at time of manufacture
Products which are canned, cured, and:				
Perishable (canned ham)	156 ppm	0	550 ppm	125 ppm
Shelf stable (corned beef)	156 ppm	0	550 ppm	125 ppm
Commercially sterile (deviled ham)	50 ppm	0	—[a]	<50 ppm
Bacon	120 ppm	0	550 ppm	80 ppm
Cooked sausages (frankfurters)	100 ppm	0	550 ppm	<100 ppm
Other pickle cured products (smoked ham)	156 ppm	0	—	125 ppm
Dry cured cuts (country ham)	100 ppm	300 ppm	—	—
Dry, semi-dry and fermented sausage (Lebanon bologna, pepperoni)	100 ppm	0	—	—
Infant, junior, and toddler foods	0	0	0	0

Various recommendations of the Expert Panel made through 1977 are summarized by Engel (1977).
[a] — = no recommendation formulated.

Table 9
Average Daily Gastric Nitrite Exposure in Adults in the United States Today with Normal Gastric Acidity (mg/person/day)

Source	Dietary nitrite	Dietary nitrate	Salivary nitrite[a]	Gastric nitrite	Percent contribution
Cured meats	0.30	1.2	0.06	0.36	9%
Fresh meats	0.06	0.6	0.03	0.09	2%
Vegetables	0.12	65	3.0	3.1	72%
Fruits, juices	0.01	4.3	0.2	0.21	5%
Baked goods and cereals	0.26	1.2	0.06	0.32	7%
Milk and milk products	0.01	0.2	0.01	0.02	<1%
Water	0.01	2.0	0.09	0.1	2%
TOTAL	0.77	75	3.5	4.2	

Table reprinted, with permission, from National Research Council (1981).
[a]Calculated by multiplying intake of nitrate by 6.3 mol % (0.05), according to Spiegelhalder et al. (1976) and Stephany and Schuller (1980).

gastric cancer deaths in 1982, a 9% contribution could still be of high relative importance. For comparison, although it is often argued that nitrate and nitrite additions to meats are necessary to prevent deaths from botulism, only three deaths due to botulinal toxins in commercially processed meats have been recorded in the United States in the past 55 years. This condition prevails in spite of the fact that the overwhelming majority of meats consumed in the U.S. contain nitrite levels below those necessary for inhibition of *Clostridium botulinum* outgrowth and toxin production (data in National Research Council 1981). Furthermore, even modest frying of bacon would inactivate any botulinal toxin possibly present.

Vegetables: Nitrate and Ascorbate

Vegetables constitute the major source of gastric nitrite arising from ingested nitrate and nitrite in normal U.S. adults (Table 9). Since vegetables are rich in nitrate, they assume even more importance under conditions of relative gastric anacidity. If the gastric pH rises above about pH 4.0, bacterial invasion occurs and results in intense and prolonged reduction of gastric nitrate to nitrite (Table 10). Relative gastric anacidity is a fairly prevalent condition, especially in the elderly; elevations in gastric pH also have been associated on numerous occasions with gastric carcinoma development in man (Hartman 1982). Intense reduction of gastric nitrate could account for the straightforward relationship between levels of nitrate ingestion and gastric cancer mortality (Fine et al. 1982), as noted above. (Otherwise, the relationship would depend on ingested nitrite + 5% ingested nitrate. Insufficient data are available to examine this latter possibility.)

Table 10

Projected Gastric Nitrite Load Under Conditions of Gastric Hypoacidity and Mixed Bacterial Invasion (mg/person/day)

Source	Nitrate	Nitrite	Percent total gastric nitrite
Ingested[a]	75	0.77	1%
Recirculated			
Salivary[b]	19	4	7%
Gastric[c]	19	54	92%
TOTAL	109[d]	59	

Table reprinted, with permission, from National Research Council (1981).

[a]See Table 9 for sources.

[b]Assumes 25% of nitrate is recirculated in saliva and 20% of this nitrate is reduced to nitrite, as footnote a, Table 9.

[c]Assumes recirculation of nitrate to stomach via active transport equals salivary recirculation and 50% of the total gastric nitrate is reduced to nitrite.

[d]Over a 24-hr period, 75 mg ingested nitrate reaches stomach, plus 15 mg recirculated from saliva (19-4 which is converted to nitrite), plus 19 mg which is recirculated directly to the stomach.

While rich in nitrate, vegetables also are a good source of the nitrite scavenger, ascorbate (Diem and Lentner 1970; Pennington and Church 1980). Ascorbate also inhibits mutagenesis by dimethylnitrosamine and by nitroso-guanidine (but not by methylnitrosourea) in a bacterial test system (Guttenplan 1977; 1978) and may have other beneficial effects (Cameron et al. 1979). The average U.S. daily consumption of ascorbate has been estimated to have remained relatively constant at about 110 mg/person over the years 1909-1974 while consumption of vegetable protein decreased about 48% (Gortner 1975). It is likely that there is a more balanced year round ascorbate intake in modern times, however.

Nitrate and ascorbate concentrations of single crops are inversely related in the few instances where both have been measured (Kilgore et al. 1964; Li et al. 1980). This relationship suggests that selection of conditions engendering a lowered nitrate content might lead to an increased ascorbate content and vice versa. The Chinese are successfully applying several simple means in an effort to increase the ascorbate: nitrate dietary balance in an esophageal cancer high-risk area (Li et al. 1980).

In the United States Maynard (1978) has indicated that the nitrate content of spinach can be reduced 73% by use of the proper strain, 34% by adjustment of fertilizer composition, and 27% by avoiding harvest in the early day while still maintaining optimal growth conditions. Breeding lines of vegetables with high-level ascorbate content exist (Table 11). Measurements of the nitrate contents of these breeding lines would be of interest. Such considerations are important since Senti (1974) has pointed out that the eating habits of elderly males and females (who are, after all, the individuals that contract gastric cancer) can

Table 11
Ascorbic Acid: Content in Breeding Lines and in Commercial Varieties of Some Vegetables (mg/kg)

Vegetable	Breeding lines	Commercial varieties	Average commercial
Cabbage	930	500-600	510 (fresh) → 420 (stored)
Muskmelon	30-610	300 (470)[a]	320
Tomato	>500	150-250 (500)[b]	230
White Potato	300	80-150	260 (fresh) → 120 (stored)

Compiled from Senti (1974) and Pennington and Church (1980).
[a]Recently released commercial variety "Planters Jumbo."
[b]Recently released commercial variety "Doublerich."

Table 12

Importance of Potatoes as an Ascorbate Source in Persons 65 Years and Older, North-Central United States, Spring, 1965

| | Percent eating per day | | Potatoes Quantity per day (g) | Percent ascorbate from potatoes | | Effect of a 2 1/2-fold increase in ascorbate content of potatoes | |
	Potatoes	Citrus fruits		Persons above RDA[a]	Persons below 2/3 RDA	Persons above RDA	Persons below 2/3 RDA
Males	62%	25%	70 g	19%	55%	39% → 56%	45% → 30%
Females	54%	33%	48 g	16%	48%	44% → 54%	45% → 36%

Adapted from Senti (1974)

[a]RDA = recommended daily allowance = 45 mg ascorbate at the time of study; thus, below 2/3 RDA = less than 30 mg ascorbate/day. (The RDA now has been raised to 60 mg ascorbate so that "2/3 RDA" actually means 1/2 RDA under present U.S. recommendations.)

vary between the sexes and that ascorbate intake can be relatively low in their diets (Table 12). As also indicated in the Table, utilization of just one high ascorbate vegetable, white potatoes, can substantially elevate the ascorbate intake, particularly in males who appear to be most deficient in this regard. That a deficiency exists is apparent if one compares the levels of ascorbate intake depicted in Table 12 with the plasma ascorbate concentrations noted at the bottom of Table 3. Other measurements indicate that about 100 mg ascorbate/day are necessary to saturate the body pools in 95% of a population of nonsmokers (Kallner et al. 1979). In terms of the balance between naturally occurring dietary nitrate and dietary ascorbate, it would appear that plant breeders and rather minor modifications in agricultural practices might be able to engender impressive results over a relatively short time-span.

ACKNOWLEDGMENTS

Publication No. 1177 of the Department of Biology, The Johns Hopkins University. This project was supported in part by BRSG Grant SO7 RR07041 awarded by the Biomedical Research Support Grant Program, Division of Research Resources, National Institutes of Health. Dr. Ya-Xian Su kindly translated the Chinese Academy of Medical Sciences (1980) reference.

REFERENCES

American Cancer Society. 1981. *Cancer facts and figures, 1982*. American Cancer Society, New York.

American Meat Institute Foundation. 1971. The use of nitrate and nitrite in the meat industry. *Meat Sci. Rev.* 2:1.

Babich, H. and D.L. Davis. 1981. Phenol: A review of environmental and health risks. *Regul. Toxicol. Pharmacol.* 1:90.

Binkerd, E.F. and O.E. Kolari. 1975. The history and use of nitrate and nitrite in the curing of meat. *Food Cosmet. Toxicol.* 13:655.

Bjelke, E. 1973. *Epidemiologic studies of cancer of the stomach, colon, and rectum; with special emphasis on the role of diet*, vol. 1-4. University of Minnesota, Minneapolis.

Bodwell, C.E., M. Womack, E.M. Schuster, and B. Brooks. 1978. Biochemical indices in humans of protein nutritutive value. II. Prosprandial plasma urea nitrogen. *Nutr. Rep. Int.* 18:579.

Bodwell, C.E., E.M. Kyle, E.M. Schuster, D.A. Vaughan, M. Womack, R.A. Ahrens, and L.R. Hackler. 1979. Biochemical indices in humans of protein nutritutive value. III. Fasting plasma urea nitrogen and urinary metabolites at a low protein intake level. *Nutr. Rep. Int.* 19:703.

Boyland, E., E. Nice, and K. Williams. 1971. The catalysis of nitrosation by thiocyanate from saliva. *Food Cosmet. Toxicol.* 9:639.

Cameron, E., L. Pauling, and B. Leibovitz. 1979. Ascorbic acid and cancer: A review. *Cancer Res.* 39:663.

Campbell, H. 1980. Cancer mortality in Europe. Site-specific patterns and trends, 1955 to 1974. *World Health Stat. Quart.* 33:241.

Cerveny, J.G. 1980. Effects of changes in the production and marketing of cured meats on the risk of botulism. *Food Technol.* **34**:240.

Chinese Academy of Medical Sciences, Department of Chemical Etiology and Carcinogenesis. 1980. Preliminary analyses of the distribution of esophageal cancer mortality rate, the geographic environment, and the chemical elements in foods and drinking water in Anyang District, Henan Province. A possible role for nitrate. *Zhonghua Zhongliu Zazhi* **2**:29.

Davies, J.M. 1980. Stomach cancer mortality in Worksop and other Nottinghamshire mining towns. *Br. J. Cancer* **41**:438.

Davies, R., M.J. Dennis, R.C. Massey, and D.J. McWeeny. 1978. Some effects of phenol- and thiol-nitrosation reactions on *N*-nitrosamine formation. *IARC Sci. Publ.* **19**:183.

Devesa, S.S. and D.T. Silverman. 1978. Cancer incidence and mortality trends in the United States: 1935-74. *J. Natl. Cancer Inst.* **60**:545.

Diem, K. and C. Lentner. 1970. *Scientific tables*, 7th ed. Ciba-Geigy Ltd., Basel, Switzerland.

Dogon, I.L. and B.H. Andur. 1970. Evidence for the presence of two thiocyanate-dependent antibacterial systems in human saliva. *Arch. Oral Biol.* **15**:987.

Eisenbrand, G., B. Spiegelhalder, and R. Preussmann. 1980. Nitrate and nitrite in saliva. *Oncology* **37**:227.

Engel, R.E. 1977. Nitrites, nitrosamines, and meat. *J. Am. Vet. Med. Assoc.* **171**:1157.

Expert Panel on Nitrites and Nitrosamines. 1978. *Final report on nitrites and nitrosamines*, U.S. Department of Agriculture.

Fan, T.-Y. and S.R. Tannenbaum. 1973. Factors influencing the rate of formation of nitrosomorpholine from morpholine and nitrite: Acceleration by thiocyanate and other anions. *J. Agric. Food Chem.* **21**:237.

Fine, D.H., B.C. Challis, P. Hartman, and J. van Ryzin. 1982. Endogenous synthesis of volatile nitrosamines: Model calculations and risk assessment. *IARC Sci. Publ.* **41** (in press).

Fudge, R. and R.W. Truman. 1973. The nitrate and nitrite contents of meat products. *J. Assoc. Public Anal.* **11**:19.

Gortner, W.A. 1975. Nutrition in the United States, 1900 to 1974. *Cancer Res.* **35**:3246.

Griffith, G.W. 1968. The sex ratio in gastric cancer and hypothetical considerations relative to aetiology. *Br. J. Cancer* **22**:163.

Guttenplan, J.B. 1977. Inhibition by *L*-ascorbate of bacterial mutagenesis induced by two *N*-nitroso compounds. *Nature* **268**:368.

———. 1978. Mechanisms of inhibition by ascorbate of microbial mutagenesis induced by *N*-nitroso compounds. *Cancer Res.* **38**:2018.

Hakama, M. and E. Saxén. 1967. Cereal consumption and gastric cancer. *Int. J. Cancer* **2**:265.

Hallett, G. and D.L.H. Williams. 1980. The absence of nucleophilic catalysis in the nitrosation of amides. Kinetics and mechanism of the nitrosation of methylurea and the reverse reaction. *J. Chem. Soc. Perkin Trans. II*, 1372.

Hartman, P.E. 1982. Nitrates and nitrites: Ingestion, pharmacodynamics, and toxicology. In *Chemical mutagens* (eds. F.J. deSerres and A. Hollaender), vol. 7, p. 211. Plenum Publishing, New York.

Higginson, J. 1966. Etiological factors in gastrointestinal cancer in man. *J. Natl. Cancer Inst.* **37**:527.

Hill, M.J. 1979. *In vivo* bacterial N-nitrosation and its possible role in human cancer. In *Naturally occurring carcinogens—mutagens and modulators of carcinogenesis* (ed. E.C. Miller et al.), p. 229. University Park Press, Baltimore, Maryland.

Hill, M.J., G. Hawksworth, and G. Tattersall. 1973. Bacteria, nitrosamines and cancer of the stomach. *Br. J. Cancer* **28**:562.

Hoffman, H. 1966. Oral microbiology. *Adv. Appl. Microbiol.* **8**:195.

Hormozdiari, H., N.E. Day, B. Aramesh, and E. Mahboubi. 1975. Dietary factors and esophageal cancer in the Caspian littoral in Iran. *Cancer Res.* **35**:3493.

Honour, A.J., N.B. Myant, and E.N. Rowlands. 1952. Secretion of radioiodine in digestive juices and milk in man. *Clin. Sci.* **11**:447.

Joint Iran-International Agency for Research on Cancer Study Group. 1977. Esophageal cancer studies in the Caspian littoral of Iran: Results of population studies—a prodrome. *J. Natl. Cancer Inst.* **59**:1127.

Joossens, J.V. and J. Geboers. 1981. Nutrition and gastric cancer. *Nutrition and Cancer* **2**:250.

Kallner, A., D. Hartmann, and D. Hornig. 1979. Steady-state turnover and body pool of ascorbic acid in man. *Am. J. Clin. Nutr.* **32**:530.

Kerr, R.H., C.T.N. Marsh, W.F. Schroeder, and E.A. Boyer. 1926. The use of sodium nitrite in the curing of meat. *J. Agric. Res.* **33**:541.

Kikugawa, K., K. Tsukuda, and T. Kurechi. 1980. Studies on peroxidized lipids. I. Interaction of malondialdehyde with secondary amines and its relevance to nitrosamine formation. *Chem. Pharm. Bull.* **28**:3323.

Kilgore, L., A.R. Stasch, and B.F. Barrentine. 1964. Relation of ascorbic acid to nitrate content of turnip greens and to methemoglobin formation. *Am. J. Clin. Nutr.* **14**:52.

Kolari, O.E. and W.J. Aunan. 1972. The residual levels of nitrite in cured meat products. In *Proceedings of the 18th meeting of meat research workers*, p. 422. Guelph, Ontario, Canada.

Kraus, F.W. and C. Gastron. 1956. Individual constancy of numbers among the oral flora. *J. Bacteriol.* **71**:702.

Kurechi, T., K. Kikugawa, and M. Ozawa. 1980. Effect of malondialdehyde on nitrosamine formation. *Food Cosmet. Toxicol.* **18**:119.

Li, M., P. Li, and B. Li. 1980. Recent progress in research on esophageal cancer in China. *Adv. Cancer Res.* **33**:173.

Li, M.-H. 1981. Studies on potential carcinogens in the diet of individuals at high risk for esophageal cancer. In *Cancer research in the People's Republic of China and the United States of America* (ed. P.A. Marks), p. 131. Grune and Stratton, New York.

Maynard, D.N. 1978. Potential nitrate levels in edible plant parts. In *Nitrogen in the environment*, (eds. D.R. Nielsen and J.G. MacDonald), vol. 2, p. 221. Academic Press, New York.

Mirvish, S.S. 1975. Formation of N-nitroso compounds: Chemistry, kinetics, and in vivo occurrence. *Toxicol. Appl. Pharmacol.* **31**:325.

National Research Council. 1981. *The health effects of nitrate, nitrite, and N-nitroso compounds.* National Academy Press, Washington, D.C.

Ohshima, H., J.-C. Bereziat, and H. Bartsch. 1982. Monitoring N-nitrosamino acids excreted in the urine and feces of rats as an index for endogenous nitrosation. *Carcinogenesis* 3:115.

O'Neill, C.H., G.M. Hodges, P.N. Riddle, P.W. Jordan, R.H. Newman, F.J. Flood, and E.C. Toulson. 1980. A fine fibrous silica contaminant of flour in the high oesophageal cancer area of North-East Iran. *Int. J. Cancer* 26:617.

Osawa, T., H. Ishibashi, M. Namiki, and T. Kada. 1980. Desmutagenic actions of ascorbic acid and cysteine on a new pyrrole mutagen formed by the reaction between food additives: Sorbic acid and sodium nitrite. *Biochem. Biophys. Res. Commun.* 95:835.

Panalaks, T., J.R. Iyengar, and N.P. Sen. 1973. Nitrate, nitrite, and dimethylnitrosamine in cured meat products. *J. Assoc. Off. Anal. Chem.* 56:621.

Parks, N.J., K.A. Krohn, C.A. Mathis, J.H. Chasko, K.R. Geiger, M.E. Gregor, and N.F. Peek. 1981. ^{13}N-Nitrite and ^{13}N-nitrate: Distribution and metabolism after intratracheal administration. *Science* 212:58.

Pennington, J.A.T. and H.N. Church. 1980. *Bowes and Church's food values of portions commonly used*, 13th ed. Harper and Row, N.Y.

Richardson, R.L. and M. Jones. 1958. A bacteriologic census of human saliva. *J. Dental Res.* 37:697.

Schiff, L., C.D. Stevens, W.E. Molle, H. Steinberg, C.W. Kumpe, and P. Stewart. 1947. Gastric (and salivary) excretion of radioiodine in man (preliminary report). *J. Natl. Cancer Inst.* 7:349.

Schweinsberg, E. 1974. Catalysis of nitrosamine synthesis. *IARC Sci. Publ.* 9:80.

Senti, F.R. 1974. Agricultural practices influencing vitamin-mineral content of foods and biological availability. In *Nutrients in processed foods: Vitamins, minerals*, p. 39. American Medical Association, Publ. Sciences Group, Inc., Acton, Massachusetts.

Shamberger, R.J., B.A. Shamberger, and C.E. Willis. 1977. Malonaldehyde content of food. *J. Nutr.* 107:1404.

Siu, G.M. and H.H. Draper. 1978. A survey of the malonaldehyde content of retail meats and fish. *J. Food Sci.* 43:1147.

Spiegelhalder, B., G. Eisenbrand, and R. Preussmann. 1976. Influence of dietary nitrate on nitrite content of human saliva: Possible relevance to *in vivo* formation of *N*-nitroso compounds. *Food Cosmet. Toxicol.* 14:545.

Stephany, R.W. and P.L. Schuller. 1980. Daily dietary intakes of nitrate, nitrite and volatile *N*-nitrosamines in the Netherlands using the duplicate portion sampling technique. *Oncology* 37:203.

Tannenbaum, S.R. 1979. Endogenous formation of nitrite and N-nitroso compounds. In *Naturally occurring carcinogens—mutagens and modulators of carcinogenesis* (ed. E.C. Miller et al.), p. 311. Japan Sci. Soc. Press, Tokyo.

Walker, E.A., B. Pignatelli, and M. Castegnaro. 1979. Catalytic effect of p-nitrosophenol on the nitrosation of diethylamine. *J. Agric. Food Chem.* 27:393.

Walters, C.L. and P.L.R. Smith. 1981. The effect of water-borne nitrate on salivary nitrite. *Food Cosmet. Toxicol.* 19:297.

COMMENTS

SEN: In calculating the decreased contribution of cured meats to gastric nitrite load, did you include salivary nitrite?

HARTMAN: Yes, that is in the calculations shown in Table 7. What is not there is endogenous synthesis, and there was no salivary threshold for nitrate transport considered in those estimates. If there is a salivary threshold, then the percentage cured meat contribution will rise.

TANNENBAUM: With regard to the data on the consumption of cured meats in the U.S., how do the years go on that again?

HARTMAN: 1926, mid-thirties, early seventies, and 1981.

TANNENBAUM: I'm just trying to figure out when we would have seen the effect of that.

HARTMAN: Well, there are no data that I know of that go back before 1926.

TANNENBAUM: No. I mean the people that you see with gastric cancer today, for example, and if you can make some estimate about it.

HARTMAN: There is generally considered to be a very long lag in gastric cancer induction that already has been mentioned at this meeting. Childhood exposure could be a very important component of gastric cancer. There are a dozen studies of immigrants that suggest this.

PETO: The question is whether these changes in nitrites are too recent to be relevant. Gastric cancer mortality is decreasing in the United States but the cancers already may have been in progress.

HARTMAN: Yes, okay. The figures in Table 7 indicate that there was a very big change between 1926 and the thirties, but we really don't know what happened before then. Some people think that there was already a large decrease occurring before 1926 (Binkerd and Kolari 1975), but I haven't seen any way to verify the actual change that might have occurred.

PETO: You really want the decrease during the end of the last century to produce the decreases in gastric cancer that you saw in the United States in the 1930s.

HARTMAN: Well, it just depends upon what ideas you have about generation of gastric cancer, i.e., whether nitrates are important just during the early period or if they are also important later in life. There could be some impact late in life. If you look at the immigrant studies, they're never right on the line of country of origin. There is always a shift, and that shift is actually, in some of the studies, fairly substantial. So there is, I think, maybe a role for nitrites later in life.

LIJINSKY: I recall hearing that nitrite wasn't used between 1906 and 1926 since Commissioner of Food and Drug thought it was a noxious compound and wouldn't allow it to be used?

HARTMAN: Yes, nitrate was used at very high concentrations. But it was reduced during the curing process to nitrite, so you ended up with 185 ppm nitrite in the average cured meat sample in the 1926 survey. Now average residual nitrite at market is down to 10 ppm (National Research Council 1981).

Right now there is still an enormous variation in the amounts of nitrates and nitrites in different cured meats. I think one thing we ought to do is try to get the high-level meat down to a reasonable level; you don't need that much to inhibit *Clostridium botulinum*.

SEN: Dr. Hartman, most of the gastric nitrites come from salivary nitrites which, in turn, are derived from nitrate in vegetables. Since nitrate levels in vegetables haven't dropped significantly during the last 30-40 years, I don't understand the results you showed indicating that there has been a significant drop of nitrate intake in the United States.

HARTMAN: I kept the vegetable contribution constant in Table 7 for that reason. There hasn't been a great change.

SEN: But, if vegetables contribute the most, and the nitrate levels haven't changed in vegetables, changes in meat won't change it that much.

HARTMAN: We were eating enormous amounts of nitrite in cured meats.

SEN: We were eating that much more?

HARTMAN: We also decreased our per capita consumption of cured meat by 45%, so there—

SEN: But that was only recently, in the last few years.

HARTMAN: I haven't back-tracked to 1926 but we are eating 45% less cured meat per capita right now than we did in the mid-fifties. But, then, the nitrate concentration of cured meats is now much lower.

SEN: Do you have some idea as to what happens to the nitrite concentration during cooking of vegetables?

HARTMAN: It depends upon how you cook the vegetable, and it varies with each vegetable. There are data on nitrate in the literature. In general, you tend to lose as much ascorbate as you do nitrate; nitrate leaches out.

MIRVISH: When we were writing the NRC/NAS 1981 report on "The Health Effects of Nitrate, Nitrite, and N-Nitroso Compounds" we referred to "nitrates and nitrites *in* the stomach," whereas, we should perhaps have referred to "nitrates and nitrites *entering* the stomach." There is a difference.

For example, I wonder how much of the nitrate in the saliva is reduced in the stomach after it's swallowed and before the gastric acid gets in and kills the bacteria. I wonder if maybe one of the gastroenterologists here could comment on how long food sits in the stomach before it becomes acidic.

HARTMAN: I don't know. There is some indication that there is some reduction of nitrate as it travels down the esophagus.

MIRVISH: Yes. But in the stomach it sits as a bolus of food for maybe 1/2 hour, maybe even longer.

KIMBROUGH: The time varies in different people.

PETO: There is one thing that worries me about the chief source of nitrates being vegetables. Insofar as one has any reliable knowledge about the causes of gastric cancer, the use of vegetables seems to be inversely associated. I don't see any recurrent positive association with the occurrence of any type of cancer. People have looked at vegetables because vegetables were, in fact, high in nitrate content. Whenever ingestion of vegetables was examined, there was either no particular association or sort of a moderate inverse association which could well be artifactual. In other words, the epidemiology with regard to vegetable consumption isn't reliable. It isn't like tobacco carcinogenesis. Insofar as one can say anything, vegetables appear to be protective. You can always say, "Yes, there are lots of other things in vegetables that are protective and that protective effect outweighs the nitrates." But I'm always rather unhappy with this discussion of nitrate. I just don't know how seriously to take it as a putative cause of human cancer.

HARTMAN: I can't really answer your question. I have thought about it. One thing that you generally find is that people such as vegetarians who ingest a large amount of vegetables also ingest a large amount of fruits rich in ascorbate. Pickled and improperly transported or stored vegetables contain much higher nitrite levels than do fresh vegetables. Also, different vegetables vary enormously in their nitrate contents (Corré and Breimer 1979; National Research Council 1981), and nitrate content varies inversely with ascorbate content of individual vegetables. Thus, the term "vegetables" applies to a very heterogeneous group of products. Epidemiologists need to score actual intakes of nitrate and nitrite as assayed in various food products and drinking water in high- and low-risk populations, as pointed out in my paper. Finally, gastric nitrite load as expressed in my talk (see Table 9) is for the U.S. today, a low-risk population that seems to have eliminated much of the nitrates and nitrites formerly ingested in cured meats and drinking (private well) water. In such a population, vegetables assume a high relative importance that may not apply to other populations and may not have even been true in the United States in earlier decades (as shown in Table 7).

References

Binkerd, E.F. and O.E. Kolari. 1975. The history and use of nitrate and nitrite in the curing of meat. *Food Cosmet. Toxicol.* **13**:655.

Corré, W.J. and T. Breimer. 1979. *Nitrate and nitrite in vegetables.* Literature Survey No. 39. Centre for Agricultural Publishing and Documentation, Wageningen, The Netherlands.

National Research Council. 1981. *The Health effects of nitrate, nitrite, and N-nitroso compounds.* National Academy Press, Washington, D.C.

Enhancement of Nitrate Biosynthesis by
Escherichia coli Lipopolysaccharide

DAVID A. WAGNER AND STEVEN R. TANNENBAUM
Department of Nutrition and Food Science
Massachusetts Institute of Technology
Cambridge, Massachusetts 02139

There is widespread concern for elevated exposure of nitrate from dietary and environmental origins and its potential risk to human health. The environment is not the only source of nitrate because long-term metabolic balance studies have demonstrated the biosynthesis of nitrate in healthy adult men consuming low, constant intakes of nitrate (Fig. 1). This is based on the finding that the excretion of nitrate in the urine is three-to fourfold greater than dietary intake of nitrate (Green et al. 1981a). Nitrate balance studies in other animal species has indicated more nitrate excreted than ingested (Table 1). Studies of nitrate balance in germ-free rats (Green et al. 1981b) have indicated that the bacterial flora are not involved, suggesting that nitrate biosynthesis is a mammalian process. The biochemical mechanisms responsible for the formation and regulation of nitrate appearance remain to be identified.

A potential stimulus for nitrate biosynthesis was observed by us during the course of a metabolic study. One human subject, on a low, constant intake of dietary nitrate, became ill with nonspecific intestinal diarrhea. It was found that nitrate excretion significantly increased during the illness (Fig. 2). Our initial hypothesis to explain this phenomenon was an increased generation of oxygen-free radicals derived from an activated immune system. Such oxidants could oxidize reduced nitrogen species to form nitrate. These oxidizing agents are produced by a number of different systems in the body, ranging from neutrophils and macrophages (the reticuloendothelial system); to mitochondria, when they are stimulated by excessive oxidative activity; to hyperbaric oxygen (oxygen toxicity); or indirectly through stimulation of peroxisomes and formation first of hydrogen peroxide.

Our initial attempts to explore the possibility that oxygen-free radical production is linked to nitrate biosynthesis are reported here. *E. coli* lipopolysaccharide endotoxin-induced fever was used as a tool to activate the reticuloendothelial system to examine the effect on nitrate biosynthesis.

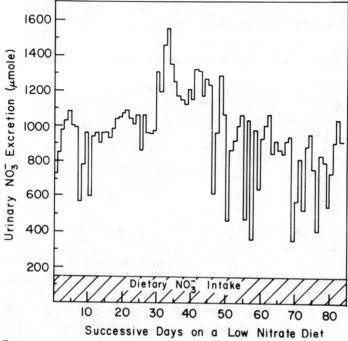

Figure 1
Urinary nitrate excretion in a human subject on a low nitrate diet for 84 days. Dietary intake of nitrate was 150 μmol/day.

Table 1
Comparison of Nitrate Biosynthesis in Various Animal Species on a Low Nitrate Diet for 5 Days

Species	Mean body weight	Dietary NO_3^- intake (μmol/day)	Urinary NO_3^- excretion (μmol/day)	NO_3^- biosynthesis (μmol/100 g b.w./day)
Rat (N = 6)	260 gm	$0.22 \pm .01$[a]	$5.03 \pm .40$[a]	$1.85 \pm .15$[a]
Rat (germ free) (N = 6)	242 gm	$0.18 \pm .02$	$4.85 \pm .61$	$1.93 \pm .32$
Hamster (N = 6)	115 gm	$0.11 \pm .04$	$1.47 \pm .65$	$1.18 \pm .53$
Man (N = 6)	71 kg	150 ± 26	860 ± 204	$1.00 \pm .25$

[a]Mean $\pm$ S.D.

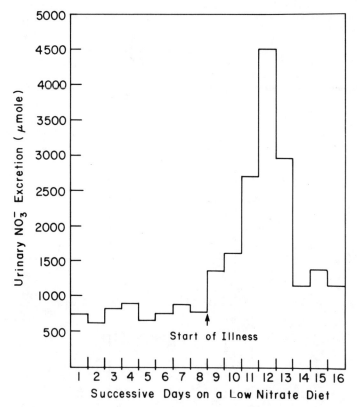

Figure 2
Urinary nitrate excretion in a human subject. On day 9, the subject contracted nonspecific intestinal diarrhea. Dietary intake of nitrate was constant at 120 μmol/day.

METHODS

Six adult Sprague-Dawley rats (200-250 gm) were housed in individual metabolic cages with food and water ad lib. The diet was low in nitrate and nitrite (7 μmoles/kg diet). After 1 week of urine collection, rats were injected i.p. with 1 mg/kg body weight *E. coli* lipopolysaccharide (Sigma Chemical Co.). Core rectal temperatures were measured 24 hours later (Yellow Springs Instrument Digital Thermometer) to show that a fever was induced. A control group of six rats was injected with 0.9% saline solution. Urinary nitrate was measured by an automated, modified Griess procedure (Green et al. 1982).

RESULTS AND DISCUSSION

Core rectal temperatures measured 24 hours after administration of lipopoly-saccaride revealed an increased temperature of 0.8 ± 0.1°C. Food intake during

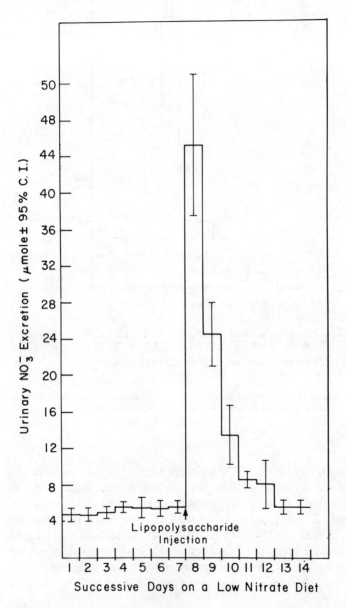

Figure 3

Induction of nitrate biosynthesis in the rat during an endotoxin-induced fever. On day 8, rats were injected i.p. with *E. coli* lipopolysaccharide. The mean urinary nitrate excretion for 6 rats ± 95% confidence interval is shown. Dietary intake of nitrate was less than 1 μmol/day.

the course of the fever was significantly reduced. Figure 3 shows that urinary nitrate excretion increased nine–fold (45 ± 6.3 μmol/day) during the first day of the fever compared to the average nitrate excretion during the control week (5.2 ± 0.13 μmol/day). The following days thereafter, as the fever subsided, nitrate excretion declined; nitrate levels returned to baseline 5 days after injection. Control rats injected with 0.9% saline solution showed no increase in nitrate excretion (data not shown).

We can conclude that activation of the reticuloendothelial system significantly increases nitrate biosynthesis. Since saline injection did not change nitrate output, we can rule out the possibility that stress to the animal was involved in the induction of nitrate biosynthesis. This is the first experimental evidence that nitrate biosynthesis can be modulated and suggests that it may be dependent upon oxygen radical formation, although other explanations cannot be ruled out at this time. Therefore, our current hypothesis for the pathway of nitrate biosynthesis is the oxidation of reduced nitrogen compounds, such as ammonia, by oxygen radicals generated within the body.

ACKNOWLEDGMENTS

This investigation was supported by PHS Grant Number NCI-1-P01-CA26731-03, awarded by the National Cancer Institute, DHHS.

REFERENCES

Green, L.C., K. Ruiz De Luzuriaga, D.A. Wagner, W. Rand, N. Istfan, V.R. Young, and S.R. Tannenbaum. 1981a. Nitrate biosynthesis in man. *Proc. Natl. Acad. Sci. USA* 78:7764.

Green, L.C., S.R. Tannenbaum, and P. Goldman. 1981b. Nitrate synthesis and reduction in the germfree and conventional rat. *Science* 212:56.

Green, L.C., D.A. Wagner, J. Glogowski, P.L. Skipper, J.S. Wishnok, and S.R. Tannenbaum. 1982. Analysis of nitrate, nitrite, and $^{15}NO_3^-$ in biological fluids. *Anal. Biochem.* (in press).

COMMENTS

SIMENHOFF: The important endogenous component you seem to be able to find when you gave the pyrogen to the rat—is that right?

TANNENBAUM: Yes.

SIMENHOFF: If you then repeated the experiment and gave the labeled nitrogen compound, wouldn't you be able then to see an increased incorporation of N^{15} into the nitrate pool?

TANNENBAUM: I'm sorry. I was rushing through, and I meant to say that. We have done that experiment. Not only do we get a tenfold induction of nitrate synthesis, we get a tenfold induction of N^{15} incorporation into the nitrate pool. Thank you very much.

FINE: How does the nitrogen oxide absorbed through the lung compare with the endogenous synthesis, in terms of quantity?

TANNENBAUM: Actually, Mike Archer should answer that question. I believe he has some data.

ARCHER: Again, I think it's too preliminary. We are going to have those numbers within the next couple of months.

FINE: Are they of the same order of magnitude?

ARCHER: We find that 1 ppm of nitrogen dioxide in the air per 24 hours leads to about half a milligram of nitrate in the urine.

TANNENBAUM: That's over and above what you find the animal making?

ARCHER: Yes. Over and above what he gets in his food or what he makes endogenously.

HOFFMANN: How much nitrate did the rats excrete in a day under normal conditions?

ARCHER: We'll have to get a comparison. I really can't answer that question quickly. I don't have all the data with me.

HOFFMANN: That would compare to 30-60 mg nitrate in man per day. For the rat it would be much less, I assume.

ARCHER: Yes.

SEN: Could we just have one more question or comment?

ARCHER: We have done some very rough preliminary calculations. Using a value of 0.1 ppm, which is a much more realistic concentration of NO_2, we calculate that this contributes about 2 mg nitrate/day to the human.

CHALLIS: Could that be significant for a smoker?

TANNENBAUM: Yes.

CHALLIS: What about NO itself, apart from NO_2?

TANNENBAUM: We haven't done that.

CHALLIS: That's the one that's really worth doing, because that's always much higher than NO_2.

MICHEJDA: Steve, you mentioned the reduced oxygen species. I take it you mean superoxide.

TANNENBAUM: Yes.

MICHEJDA: Is there any evidence that fever or infection induces a decrease in superoxide dismutase, or something of this nature? Are these things linked in some way?

TANNENBAUM: What happens is that, when you stimulate the reticuloendothelial system, you release neutrophils and macrophages, and they release large concentrations of these species in their immediate environment. Then superoxide dismutase comes in and gets rid of it.
    There are a lot of reactions now which are carried out by the whole cascade, which involves all those different oxidizing species as represented by the well-known Haber-Weiss reaction:

$$O_2^{-} + H_2O_2 \rightarrow OH^{\bullet} + OH^{-} + O_2 \text{ [From the blackboard]}$$

MICHEJDA: Is there any purpose to this thing?

TANNENBAUM: This is what lymphocytes use to kill bacteria.

Endogenous Amines in Human Gastric Juice

CLIFFORD LESLIE WALTERS AND PETER LEWIS ROLAND SMITH
Biochemistry Section
Leatherhead Food Research Association
Leatherhead Surrey, KT22 7RY, England

PETER IVAN REED
Gastrointestinal Unit
Wexham Park Hospital
Slough, Berkshire SL24HL, England

As long ago as 1931, Martin determined that the nonprotein nitrogen content of normal gastric juice ranged between 20-48 mg/100 ml, equivalent to a concentration of 14-34 mmoles 1^{-1} for compounds containing one nitrogen atom (Martin 1931). In simple achlorhydria and in pernicious anemia (PA) the corresponding ranges were 30-90 mg and 60-150 mg nonprotein nitrogen/100 ml gastric juice. These values would, of course, include nonnitrosatable compounds such as the majority of the amino acids.

As reported in Heathcote and Washington (1965), Washington compared the amino acid compositions of pooled normal human gastric juice with the mean values obtained for individual samples of juice from PA patients. Increases were observed in the concentrations of all amino acids quoted in the PA samples, the ratios of the mean PA levels to those within the normal pooled gastric juice ranging from 1.4-13.5. Of the potentially nitrosatable amino acids, arginine was observed in both normal and PA gastric juice at levels of 1.3 and 4.7 mg/100 ml respectively, equivalent to concentrations of 0.090 and 0.33 mmoles 1^{-1}. The corresponding values for proline were 0.3 and 1.3 mg/100 ml (0.026 and 0.11 mmoles 1^{-1} respectively). Of the four quantitative studies reviewed by Heathcote and Washington (1965) which compared the levels of amino acids in PA juices with those in normal subjects, two recorded a threefold increase in the concentration of total amino acids in the pathological condition. The third by Hiller and Bischof (1953) gave individual concentrations which were about one hundred times less than the values reported for normal gastric juice by other workers and must, therefore, be treated with reserve. The most recent investigation reviewed by Heathcote and Washington (1965) showed an increase of between four and five times the concentration of amino acids in PA gastric juice over the normal values. However, the volume of fasting juice in the stomach of the normal subject may be fifteen times that of the PA patient and hence it is likely that the overall amounts of some amino acids are greater in normal juices.

It has been established by Ruddell et al. (1978) that the nitrite levels in achlorhydric gastric juice associated with gastric cancer or obtained from a significant proportion of normal subjects without identifiable gastroduodenal lesions (Ruddell et al. 1976) or in PA (Ruddell et al. 1978) were significantly greater than those in normal acidic fasting gastric juice as were also the counts of both total and nitrate-reducing bacteria. A similar relationship was established by Tannenbaum et al. (1979) in hypochlorhydric patients from a region at high risk for gastric cancer and Schlag et al. (1981) in patients subjected to Billroth I and II partial resections. Thus, in considering the formation of N-nitroso compounds in relation to the possible induction of gastric cancer it is imperative to determine the nitrosatable amines and amides with which the nitrite could interact.

METHODS

Determination of N-nitroso Compounds as a Group

This was carried out in the manner of Walters et al. (1978) in which nitric oxide is obtained in sequence from heat labile compounds such as S-nitrosothiols and pseudonitrosites, then from inorganic and alkyl nitrites and finally from N-nitrosamines, -amides, -guanidines, -urethanes, and -sulfonamides. For the differentiation of N-nitroso compounds from other compounds potentially formed from nitrite it is therefore vital to release nitric oxide from the latter before the addition of hydrogen bromide to determine N-nitrosamines, -amides, etc. If this precaution is not adopted, it is likely that labile compounds releasing nitric oxide in refluxing ethyl acetate will be mistaken for N-nitroso compounds.

Determination of Individual N-nitroso Compounds

Volatile N-nitrosamines were determined by gas chromatography (GC) with a Thermal Energy Analyzer (TEA) as detector in the manner essentially that of Fine et al. (1975). Similarly the methylated products of gastric juices with and without deliberate nitrosation were separated by GC on a column of OV 225 on Chromosorb B with detection of the eluted N-nitroso compounds using a TEA. The temperature program usually involved 7 minutes at 140°C increasing thereafter by 2°C/minute to 230°C with argon as the carrier gas at a flow rate of 40 ml/min^{-1}.

Nitrosation of Gastric Juice and Peptides

The conversion of components of gastric juices and synthetic dipeptides into their N-nitroso derivatives was accomplished by treatment with nitrous acid (5-15 g l^{-1}) formed from sodium nitrite in dilute sulphuric acid at pH 2.0 at 4°C for periods ranging from 12-72 hours. Before extraction of N-nitroso compounds into ethyl acetate, the residual nitrous acid was removed from the products of nitrosation by treatment with sulfamic acid in excess.

RESULTS

Amines and Other Nitrosatable Compounds in Gastric Juice

Simple volatile N-nitrosamines can be obtained from the nitrosative cleavage of complex tertiary amines substituted with a dialkylamino group. Therefore, in studying the availability of precursors to N-nitroso compounds gastric juices have been subjected to nitrosation under optimal conditions and the products fractionated and studied as N-nitrosamines and N-nitrosamides.

The deliberate treatment of pooled acidic gastric juice with nitrous acid at pH 2.0 in the presence of thiocyanate has been found to produce only very small quantities of the conventional volatile N-nitrosamines. The predominant compounds of this type detected by GC with a TEA as detector were N-nitroso-dimethylamine (NDMA) and -pyrrolidine at concentrations approximating to 0.05 and 0.005 μmoles 1^{-1} respectively. However, much greater quantities of compounds responding as N-nitrosamines and (or) -amides, -guanidines, and -urethanes in the procedure of Walters et al. (1978) could be extracted into ethyl acetate from the products of nitrosation of a pooled gastric juice in which excess nitrous acid had been removed using sulfamic acid. In this manner, levels of putative N-nitroso compounds have been obtained equivalent to approximately 0.2 mmoles 1^{-1} in the original gastric juice. The assay adopted responds to all types of N-nitroso compounds tested and differentiates them from the great majority of other compounds potentially derived from nitrite in a biological matrix with the exception of nitrolic acids and S-nitrothiols. In addition, the products of the treatment of gastric juices with nitrous acid gave positive responses to the procedure of Eisenbrand and Preussmann (1970). After methylation with diazomethane, moreover, approximately 40% of the nitrosated gastric components could be converted into a form(s) which was amenable to GC during which at least 20 distinct peaks were observed with the TEA as detector in the manner of J.R.A. Pollock (pers. comm.).

A similar pattern of TEA-positive peaks was observed in GC from the methylated products of the nitrosation of an enzymic hydrolysate of the protein ovalbumin. In consequence, a number of dipeptides were treated with nitrous acid at pH 2.0. Excess nitrous acid was removed using sulfamic acid prior to the extraction of nitrosated products into ethyl acetate. The extents of nitrosation of the dipeptides under standardized conditions were generally low ($<$ 5% of theoretical for the amide linkage alone) except where a secondary amino group was present, as in prolylalanine, when determined by the method of Walters et al. (1978); this procedure is capable of differentiating N-nitroso from any C-nitroso or C-nitro compounds formed where phenyl residues are available. After methylation, with diazomethane, each product could be run in GC and detected by either the TEA or a mass spectrometer (MS). Only in the case of the product of nitrosation of alanylalanine, however, was a molecular ion observed at a mass/charge (m/z) ratio of 218. This and the predominant fragment ions were examined by GC coupled with high resolution (7000-8000) (MS), through the courtesy of Dr. P. Farmer, of MRC Toxicology Unit, Carshalton, Surrey, England. The precise m/z value found was 218.091, the nearest empirical formulae being $C_9H_{10}N_6O$ (m/s = 218.092), which would be most unlikely to be formed from alanylalanine, and $C_8H_{14}N_2O_5$ (m/z = 218.090). A major fragment ion occurred at m/z = 188.091 ($C_6H_{12}N_4O_3$ or $C_8H_{14}NO_4$), which is consistent with the loss of NO from $C_8H_{14}N_2O_5$. Other major fragment ions occurred at m/z = 159.076 (presumably loss of $-COOCH_3$ from $C_8H_{14}N_2O_5$) and m/z = 128.070 (presumably loss of NO and $-HCOOCH_3$).

Mutagenicity of the Product of Nitrosation of Alanylalanine

Through the courtesy of Dr. H. Bartsch, of the International Agency for Research on Cancer, Lyon, France, the mutagenicity of the product of nitrosation of alanylalanine has been studied.

Mutagenicity was established in *Salmonella typhimurium* TA100 without metabolic activation; at the level of 0.1 mg/assay, the number of revertants occurring was more than fivefold that of revertants occurring spontaneously. The high sensitivity of the TA100 strain as compared with the TA1535 indicates that most bacterial DNA adducts were not miscoding, but were repaired by an error-prone post-replicative repair system, thus increasing mutagenicity and decreasing the toxic effect. Furthermore, the lower sensitivity of the TA100NR strain, which is deficient in nitroreductase activity, as compared with the proficient nitroreductase TA100 strain suggests that bacterial nitroreductase may be involved in the activation of the nitrosated alanylalanine into a DNA damaging agent.

DISCUSSION

The fact that tertiary amines can react with nitrous acid is well illustrated by the facility with which NDMA is released by nitrosative cleavage from the analgesic aminopyrine (Lijinsky and Greenblatt 1972); similarly, nicotine can give rise on nitrosation to *N*-nitrosonornicotine. In assessing, therefore, the nitrosatable amines and amides occurring in human gastric juice it is necessary to include tertiary amine precursors. This can be achieved most readily by nitrosation under optimum conditions followed by the analysis of the resultant *N*-nitroso compounds.

Thus from these studies it would appear that the availability of precursors to NDMA in pooled human gastric juice is small. Nevertheless, dimethylamine itself has been shown to be present in fasting gastric juice in a study by S.P. Borriello and P.I. Reed (pers. comm.) and also Reed et al. (1981). Considerable variations in contents were seen in samples from normal controls with low pH ($<$ 5) and high pH ($>$ 5) as well as in fasting gastric juices from PA and hypogammaglobulinemia patients, the mean values being 0.26, 0.30, 0.22 and 0.30 mmoles 1^{-1} respectively. Trimethylamine was generally absent from or at low concentration in control gastric juice of both low and high pH but occurred in almost all gastric juices from PA and hypogammaglobulinemia patients with levels of 0.35 and 0.29 mmoles 1^{-1} respectively in the last two groups. The mean pH values for PA and hypogammaglobulinemia gastric juices were 7.3 and 8.1 respectively as compared with 1.9 and 7.6 for normal and achlorhydric controls.

The value found for total N-nitroso compounds extractable from normal acidic human gastric juices after nitrosation, namely 0.2 mmoles 1^{-1}, compares with that of 0.026 mmoles 1^{-1} quoted for proline levels by Heathcote and Washington (1965). The other nitrosatable amino acid reported in this source, namely arginine, would presumably not be extracted into an organic solvent from an acidified aqueous phase either before or after reaction with nitrous acid. The concentrations of α-amino nitrogen in normal gastric juice in a number of studies reviewed by Heathcote and Washington (1965) varied widely. Nevertheless, the mean value of 3.4 mmoles 1^{-1}, calculated on the basis of one nitrogen atom per molecule, is more than adequate to cover that found for nitrosatable precursors in normal gastric juice, although the majority of contributors to the α-amino content are presumably non-nitrosatable amino acids. Heathcote and Washington (1965) also reported the presence of a number of peptides in this biological fluid but no details were provided of their molecular weights or concentrations.

It is reported in an accompanying communication (Reed et al., this volume) that the availability of N-nitroso compounds in gastric juice increases with pH along with the nitrite concentration. This result would be expected also on the basis of the reported increase in nonprotein nitrogen in the hypochlorhydric gastric juices typical of PA (Heathcote and Washington 1965). Furthermore, the increase in total viable bacterial counts with pH would predispose to the formation of amines by such processes as decarboxylation or cyclization of amino acids. Nevertheless, it has similarly been reported that the volume of gastric juice produced in PA can be fifteen times less than that secreted by a normal individual in which case the difference in absolute amounts of nitrosatable precursor may not be borne out.

ACKNOWLEDGMENT

The financial support of the Cancer Research Campaign, London, is gratefully acknowledged.

REFERENCES

Eisenbrand, G. and R. Preussmann. 1970. Eine neue Methode zur Kolorimetrischen Bestimmung von Nitrosaminen nach Spaltung der N-Nitrosogruppe mit Bromwasserstoff in Eisessig. *Arzneim. Forsch.* **20**:1513.

Fine, D.H., F. Rufeh, D. Lieb, and D.P. Rounbehler. 1975. Description of the Thermal Energy Analyzer (TEA) for trace determination of volatile and non-volatile N-nitroso compounds. *Anal. Chem.* **47**:1188.

Heathcote, J.R. and R.J. Washington. 1965. Amino acids and peptides in human gastric juice with particular reference to pernicious anaemia: A review. *Nature* **207**:941.

Lijinsky, W. and M. Greenblatt. 1972. Carcinogen dimethylnitrosamine produced *in vivo* from nitrite and aminopyrine. *Nature* **236**:177.

Martin, L. 1931. Total nitrogen and non-protein nitrogen: partition of gastric juice obtained after histamine stimulation. *Bull. Johns Hopkins Hosp.* **49**:286.

Hiller, E. and H. Bischof. 1953. Uber den Protein und Aminosaure-Gehalt des Menschlichen Magensaftes Dargesellt Mittels Elektrophorese und Papier Chromatographie. *Medizinische* 1541.

Reed, P.I., P.L.R. Smith, K. Haines, F.R. House, and C.L. Walters. 1981. Gastric juice N-nitrosamines in health and gastroduodenal disease. *Lancet* **ii**:550.

Ruddell, W.S.J., E.S. Bone, M.J. Hill, and C.L. Walters. 1978. Pathogenesis of gastric cancer in pernicious anaemia. *Lancet* **i**:521.

Ruddell, W.S.J., E.S. Bone, M.J. Hill, L.M. Blendis, and C.L. Walters. 1976. Gastric juice nitrite. A risk factor for cancer in the hypochlorhydric stomach? *Lancet* **ii**:1037.

Schlag, P., R. Bockler, M. Peter, and Ch. Herfarth. 1981. Nitrite and N-nitroso compounds in the operated stomach. *Scand. J. Gastroenterol.* **16**:63.

Tannenbaum, S.R., D. Moran, W. Rand, C. Cuello, and P. Correa. 1979. Gastric cancer in Colombia IV Nitrite and other ions in gastric contents of residents from a high risk region. *J. Natl. Cancer Inst.* **62**:9.

Walters, C.L., M.J. Downes, M.W. Edwards, and P.L.R. Smith. 1978. Determination of a non-volatile N-nitrosamine on a food matrix. *Analyst* **103**:1127.

COMMENTS

WEISBURGER: Dr. Walters, I think it is important to realize that there are two kinds of gastric cancers, the intestinal type and the diffuse type. As it turns out, Dr. Munoz and others (Munoz et al. 1968), have related the PA blood group to the diffuse kind. We don't really know whether nitrosamines or what sort of nitroso compounds are involved in its etiology, and we need to look at this as a different sort.

WALTERS: Yes.

WEISBURGER: And, if I might also comment on Richard Peto's response to Hoffmann, relating the nitrate association with gastric cancer disease risk. Here again, we must be careful to discriminate between these very multifactorial elements that relate to any given disease risk or subclass. For example, Armijo et al. (1981) have shown that a high-risk population excreted less nitrate in the urine than the low-risk population. That is at variance with the hypothesis proposed by Dr. Correa and Dr. Tannenbaum. But it has to do with their nitrate coming from vegetables, and that is not related, because the vegetables have their built-in antidote, namely Vitamin C, as Richard Peto correctly said.

It is very complex. Unless we put the whole thing together in these multifactorial diseases, we are going to get hopelessly lost, especially if we are studying the wrong disease.

CORREA: You said that in PA the tumors are practically all in the intestinal tract. They do have this blood group A collection, but that is something different.

WALTERS: Well, that isn't clear yet, the way I read the literature.

HECHT: You said you get a lot more TEA-positive peaks after you methylate your extract; is that correct?

WALTERS: That is in gas chromatography.

SEN: Do you methylate it with diazomethane?

WALTERS: Yes.

HECHT: How do you generate the diazomethane?

WALTERS: From Diazald®, I believe.

HECHT: Isn't that a nitroso compound?

WALTERS: It is. It is a nitrososulfonamide.

HECHT: So could that be somehow producing some of your TEA positives?

WALTERS: No, you distill over the diazomethane. But the possibility is there.

HECHT: Is there a possibility of transnitrosation during your methylation?

WALTERS: No, because you produce the diazomethane by distillation.

HECHT: Okay. You distill the diazomethane?

WALTERS: Yes. Really, that would not give you a nitrosating agent that was volatile in GC. Diazald® is not volatile in GC.

HECHT: No. I was thinking of transnitrosation.

References

Armijo, R., A. Gonzalez, M. Orellana, A. Coulson, J.W. Sayre, and A. Detels. 1981. Epidemiology of gastric cancer in Chile: II-Nitrate exposure and stomach cancer frequency. *Int. J. Epidemiol.* **10**:57.

Munoz, N., P. Correa, C. Cuello, and E. Duque. 1968. Histologic types of gastric carcinoma in high- and low-risk areas. *Int. J. Cancer* **3**:809.

SESSION VI:

HUMAN EPIDEMIOLOGY

Nitrosamines as Possible Etiological Agents in Bilharzial Bladder Cancer

R. MARIAN HICKS
School of Pathology
Middlesex Hospital Medical School
London, England WIP 7LD

The schistosomes are Platyhelminth worms which are parasites for man in their adult sexual form, but have an obligatory larval phase in a specific molluscan host. Schistosomiasis affects approximately 250 million people in Asia, Africa, and South America and *Schistosoma haematobium* is responsible for vesical (bladder) schistosomiasis, otherwise known as bilharziasis in recognition of Theodor Bilharz who discovered the parasite (Bilharz 1852). The life cycle of the schistosomes has been reviewed elsewhere (Hyman 1951; Jordan and Webbe 1969), but in brief, after the worms have matured and paired in the intrahepatic vessels of human liver, they migrate to the wall of the urinary bladder and intestines where the females deposit many thousands of eggs. The majority of these are destroyed or immobilized by the host's defense mechanisms; they set up chronic inflammatory reactions in the bladder and gut wall, and many ova become calcified and remain within the wall which gradually becomes thickened and semirigid. A percentage of the eggs, however, survive and work their way through the bladder and gut epithelium to leave the body in the urine and feces. These viable eggs hatch in water to produce miracidiae which infect the secondary host, an amphibious snail of the *Bulinus* genus. Within the snail, sexually differentiated larvae develop which, when mature, are released into the water as cercariae, the free-swimming form of the trematode. These seek out and reinfect the primary human host by penetrating the skin of any portion of the anatomy exposed to the infected water source.

Bilharziasis is endemic in the Nile valley in upper and lower Egypt, and in other well-irrigated areas of the Middle East, and in east, west, southern, and central Africa. There is also an unusually high incidence of bladder cancer in Egypt; recent estimates vary from 15.8% of all cancers (About Nasr et al. 1962) to 27.6% (El-Sebai 1977), superimposed on the bilharzial bladder syndrome, and in general there is a good geographic coincidence between the incidence of bladder cancer and endemic schistosomiasis in those areas where the intensity and prevalence of the infection are high (Goebel 1905; Hashem 1961; Gillman and Prates 1962; Prates and Torres 1965; Brand 1979). A causal association between the parasite and bladder cancer was postulated (Ferguson 1911) and much effort has been expended, so far unsuccessfully, in attempting to either isolate a carcinogenic principle from the trematode and (or) its eggs, or to demonstrate unequivocally that infection with *S. haematobium* will directly cause bladder cancer in animal experiments. Further doubt is thrown on the direct causal role of *S. haematobium* in bladder carcinogenesis by the observation that in a few areas of endemic bilharziasis, including Zimbabwe (Southern Rhodesia), South Africa, and Uganda, there is no clear-cut association of an elevated bladder cancer risk with *S. haematobium* (Dodge 1962; Higginson and Oettle 1962; Houston 1964). Moreover, although the female *S. haematobium* worm deposits ova in the submucosa of the intestine as well as in the wall of the urinary bladder, no corresponding increase in the incidence of cancer of the bowel is associated with the infection, only an increase in bladder cancer.

In nonbilharzial infested populations throughout the world, the peak incidence of bladder cancer is in the sixth decade of life and only 12% of cases occur in people under the age of 50 (Payne 1959). In Egypt, by contrast, the mean age of incidence of bilharzial bladder cancer is 46 years (El-Bolkainy et al. 1972) and 73% of cases occur below the age of 50 (Aboul Nasr et al. 1962). The ratio of incidence in males to females is 5:1 (Ishak et al. 1967; El-Sebai 1978) which is probably attributable to the greater exposure of men to schistosome infection as a consequence of working in the irrigated fields. In man, bladder cancer can have a very long latent period between known exposure to an identified chemical carcinogen and the development of symptomatic tumors (Case 1966). The biogenesis of bladder cancer has been studied in experimental animals, and there is now good evidence that it is a multistage process involving early and late stages which can be influenced respectively by genotoxic and nongenotoxic carcinogens acting sequentially on the target tissue (Hicks 1980; 1982). Nonspecific irritants, which cause reparative hyperplasia of the urothelium and in so doing increase cell turnover, can act as late-stage carcinogens or propagating factors, and will accelerate the development of symptomatic bladder cancers from small, histologically undetectable foci of cancer cells in bladders previously exposed to initiating and other early-stage carcinogens. It thus seems possible that in areas where schistosomiasis is endemic and there is also an elevated bladder cancer incidence, the early stages of carcinogenesis in the bladder may be brought about by as yet unidentified carcinogens present in the environment, but that the unusual age-related incidence of the disease is the consequence of the schistosome acting as a late-stage carcinogen and accelerating the development of the cancers. According to this hypothesis, variations in bladder cancer incidence between different populations with endemic bilharziasis could be explicable in terms of variation in total exposure to early stage environmental or endogenous bladder carcinogens. Undoubtedly, low levels of unidentified bladder carcinogens are present in most environments and in Egypt, as in Europe and America, there is a low incidence of transitional cell carcinoma of the bladder which appears mainly in the older age groups in nonbilharzial infested individuals.

THE NITROSAMINE HYPOTHESIS

In Europe and America, a few people who develop bladder cancer are known to have been exposed to identified industrial carcinogens, and there is also epidemiological evidence that cigarette smoking is causally associated with bladder cancer. Some chemotherapeutic and immunosuppressive drugs are suspect, and there may be a very slightly increased risk associated with excessive use of artificial sweeteners and coffee drinking. The majority of bladder cancers, however, are of unknown etiology (Skrabanek and Walsh 1981).

Experimental studies have identified several compounds which are bladder carcinogens for rodents and (or) dogs, including the N-nitroso compounds N-nitrosomethylurea (MNU), N-butyl-N-(4-hydroxybutyl)nitrosamine (BBN) and N-nitrosomethyldodecylamine (NMDCA), (Druckrey et al. 1964; Hicks and Wakefield 1972; Lijinsky and Taylor 1975). Small amounts of nitrosamines are now known to be formed endogenously in the body by nitrosation of ingested or metabolically derived secondary and tertiary amines. In the bladder large quantities of N-nitroso compounds theoretically can be produced over a wide range of urinary pH during bacterial infections of the lower urinary tract. Many bacteria will reduce diet-derived nitrate in the urine to nitrite, and the production of N-nitrosamines by nitrosation of amine precursors has been demonstrated to occur in the urine of bacterially infected rats (Hill and Hawksworth 1972). Individual N-nitroso compounds are known to have different organ specificity in different species (Hirose et al. 1976; Lijinsky 1982) but as a class, they have been shown to be carcinogenic in all vertebrate and lower species in which they have been tested (Michejda et al., this volume). It thus seemed possible if secondary bacterial infections of the bladder are regularly associated with bilharziasis that endogenously produced nitrosamines in the bladder could act as early stage carcinogens and initiate the process of carcinogenesis in the urothelium (Hicks et al. 1977).

Advanced bilharzial bladder cancer is more often than not complicated by gross secondary bacterial infections, but for the nitrosamine hypothesis to be tenable, bacterial infection of the lower urinary tract would also have to be present many years before symptomatic bladder cancer developed. It was thus necessary to establish whether urinary bacterial infections and concomitant N-nitroso compounds were present in younger age groups in areas of endemic bilharziasis.

BACTERIAL INFECTION AND N-NITROSO COMPOUNDS IN THE URINES OF YOUNG EGYPTIAN MEN

Carter et al. (1970) had reported a relatively high level of bacterial infection of the urinary tract in adolescent village boys in Egypt, which varied between villages from 10%-37% and was related to standards of hygiene rather than levels of S. haematobium infection. They concluded that bacteriuria was more common in village boys than in adult males, and that the incidence of asymptomatic bacteriuria was more common in areas of poor hygiene than had been thought previously. More recently, a 5.1% incidence of bacteriuria was reported in Egyptian boys aged between 5 and 16 years in regions of endemic bilharziasis and this was 10 times greater than in areas nonendemic for *S. haematobium* infection (Laughlin et al. 1978). Despite these reports it is still not generally recognized that bacterial infections of the lower urinary tract are common in populations exposed to *S. haematobium*, for the usual symptoms of bacteriuria, namely haematuria and frequency, are automatically attributed to infestation with *S. haematobium*. Confirmatory studies were therefore undertaken.

In the first instance, in collaboration with Dr. C. Walters and Dr. T. Gough, and with Dr. Ismail El-Sebai and his colleagues at the Cairo Cancer Institute, urine samples were collected from hospitalized patients with advanced bilharzial bladder cancer, and analyzed to determine whether N-nitroso compounds were present in patients with heavy secondary bacterial infections superimposed on bilharziasis. The results were indeed positive and have been published (Hicks et al. 1977). We subsequently demonstrated the occurrence of nitrosamines in the urines of some British paraplegics and hemiplegics who also had urinary tract bacterial infections, but no nitrosamines were detected in the uninfected urines of healthy people with the exception of one Egyptian subject who could have had previous exposure to *S. haematobium* infection (Hicks et al. 1978).

More recently, with the collaboration of Dr. El-Alamy at the Centre for Field and Applied Research, Imbaba-Giza, the urines of adolescents and young adults in the Qalyub area of Egypt have been collected and analyzed. A full report of these experiments and results are in (Hicks et al. 1982).

Experimental Procedures

The urines of 82 male volunteers, aged between 10 and 25 years were collected and allocated to the following groups:

Group A: No infection of the urinary tract
Group B: *S. haematobium* ova but no bacteria in urine
Group C: Both *S. haematobium* ova and bacteria in urine
Group D: Urinary bacterial infection only

Since most of the people in the Qalyub area have bilharziasis, in order to have not less than 20 patients per group and to complete Group D, an additional 9 samples were obtained from an adjacent district and 2 of these were from young men aged 30 years. (One of these samples was lost in transit and so Group D comprised only 19 people.)

Morning samples of urine were collected into sterile bottles and immediately tested with N-labstix (Ames Co., Miles Laboratories Ltd., Stoke Poges, Slough, England) for pH, protein, glucose, ketones, blood, and nitrite. In those which gave a positive response for nitrite, it was assessed quantitatively by a colorimetric method. Egg counts of *S. haematobium* ova were made on 10 ml aliquots by the millipore filter technique of El-Alamy and Cline (1977).

The urines were then stabilized by addition to each sample of 3 g sulphamic acid, which lowered the pH below 2 and by removing residual nitrite prevented any artifactual formation of *N*-nitroso compounds from available precursors. The stabilized urines were frozen, stored at -30°C until being packed in dry ice and flown to England still frozen for further analysis.

For bacteriology, separate midstream samples were collected from the same patients, on the same day, and were cultured in the department of bacteriology at the Al-Azhar University Faculty of Medicine in Cairo, on MacConkey agar (oxoid), and blood agar plates. Colonies were identified and bacterial counts made using standard procedures.

Nitrate, volatile nitrosamines, and total *N*-nitroso compounds were analyzed in the stabilized urines by Dr. C. Walters. The nitrate content of the urines was estimated by the method of Cox (1980) in which nitric oxide produced by reduction of the urinary nitrate is determined in a Chemiluminescence Analyser.

Volatile *N*-nitrosamines were extracted with dichloromethane, with *N*-nitrosodi-n-propylamine added to the urine as an internal standard. They were estimated by combined gas chromatography (GC) and thermal energy analysis (TEA) (Fine et al. 1975). The level of detection was in the order of 0.2 μg/l (= ppb where b = 10^9).

The total *N*-nitroso compound content of the remaining urine was determined by the method of Walters et al. (1978). Ethyl acetate was used as the extractant of choice for the range of *N*-nitroso derivatives likely to be formed in urine from the more complex biological precursors. The method of analysis is based on that originally devised by Eisenbrand and Preussmann (1970) in which *N*-nitroso compounds are selectively denitrosated with hydrogen bromide to nitric oxide which is then determined in a Chemiluminescence Analyser. This method satisfactorily differentiates all types of *N*-nitroso compounds (*N*-nitrosamines, *N*-nitrosamides, *N*-nitrosoguanidines, *N*-nitrososulphonamides, etc.) from nitrite, nitrate, and the great majority of compounds potentially formed in a biological matrix with the possible exception of nitrolic acids and S-nitrothiols (Walters et al. 1979). The limit of detection was approximately 0.5 μg/l when expressed as micrograms of *N*-nitrosopyrrolidine (molecular weight = 100).

OBSERVATIONS

The prevalence of *S. haematobium* infection in the Qalyub area is known to be high and this was reflected by the results obtained. The volunteers came from villages where the only available treatment had been tartar emetic, and 78% either had *S. haematobium* ova in the urine on the day of collection or a recent history of infection. Furthermore there was a positive association of bacteriuria with active urinary schistosomiasis. Thus of the original batch of 82 urines collected in volunteers before their bacterial status was known, 30 samples (36%) proved to be contaminated by more than 10^3 bacterial organisms per ml, and 5 samples (6%) contained 10^5 or more organisms per ml. The level of urinary tract bacterial infection found in this sample of young men aged between 10 and 25 was thus in the same order as that reported in Egyptian village boys by Carter et al. (1970). Of the 5 boys with the highest levels of bacterial infection, 3 were aged 16, one was 19, and the fifth aged 22. It is of interest that in the 19 individuals eventually located who had bacteriuria but no *S. haematobium* infection, 8 had haematuria, which in areas of endemic *S. haematobium* infestation is automatically regarded as a symptom of bilharziasis. These observations show that a significant percentage of the young village men in Egypt living in areas where they are at risk for developing bladder cancer do indeed have *S. haematobium* infestation and concurrent bacterial infection of the urinary tract.

Despite the presence of bacterial infection in many urines, only 5 were found to be positive for nitrite by the Labstix test, and on quantitative analysis these samples ranged from 18-130 μg/l expressed as $NaNO_2$. This highlights the inadequacy of nitrite as an indicator of bacterial infection in the urine, but is hardly surprising considering the reactivity of nitrites and the presence in the urine of numerous nitrosatable compounds such as phenols, which may be expected to compete with the amine precursors of nitrosamines for any available nitrite formed. Nevertheless, *N*-nitroso compounds were found in all the Egyptian samples tested irrespective of the presence or absence of either bacteria or *S. haematobium* ova. This was unexpected, but has now been confirmed in urine samples from laboratory workers in England, and reflects the sensitivity of the analytical methods used.

The mean values for *N*-nitroso compound concentration in the four groups of urines is shown in Table 1. Those in the bacterially infected urines of Groups C and D were little higher than those in Group B, the uninfected group with *S. haematobium* infestation, though they were significantly higher than the

Table 1
Mean Urinary *N*-nitroso Compound Content of Young Egyptian Men Subdivided According to the Presence or Absence of *S. haematobium* Ova and Bacteria in Their Urines

Group	Number of urines	Presence or absence of *S. haematobium* ova	Presence or absence of bacteria	*N*-nitroso compounds (mean value) μg/l
A	22	−	−	12.87
B	21	+	−	20.81
C	20	+	+	26.02
D	19	+	−	22.91

Table 2
Mean N-nitroso Compound Content of Urines in Young Egyptian Men

Group	Number of urines	Presence or absence of S. haematobium	N-nitroso compounds mean value µg/l	Significance[a] p
		No bacterial infection		
A	22	–	12.87	
B	21	+	20.81	
		Infected with more than 10^3/ml nonnitrate reducing bacteria		
C'	9	+	13.78	C' v B N.S.
D'	9	–	14.91	D' v A N.S.
		Infected with more than 10^3/ml nitrate-reducing bacteria		
C"	11	+	36.04	C" v B 0.0005
D"	10	–	31.80	D" v A 0.025
				C" v C' 0.001
				D" v D' 0.01

[a]Students t-Test

levels in completely uninfected controls (p = 0.005). However, not all bacteria are nitrate reducing and when the groups were subdivided on the basis of the ability of their bacterial flora to reduce nitrate to nitrite a much higher mean level of N-nitroso compounds was present in those urines infected with nitrate-reducing than with nonnitrate-reducing organisms (Table 2). In people with no S. haematobium infection, the N-nitroso compounds were elevated from 13-32 µg/l (p = 0.025). In people who had S. haematobium infection, the elevation was from 21-36 µg/l which was highly significant (p = 0.0005) despite the small numbers involved. When more than 10^5 nitrate-reducing organisms per ml were present in the urine, the mean urinary N-nitroso compound level was 42 µg/l, a more than threefold increase over the uninfected control group and a twofold increase over the group with S. haematobium only. These results confirm the positive contribution from bacterial metabolism to the urine content of N-nitrosamines.

It has not yet been possible to characterize the individual N-nitroso compounds present in the urines. In urines which had been deliberately nitrosated approximately one-third of the N-nitroso compounds arising from the nitrosation of available precursors could be converted by methylation with diazomethane into forms amenable to gas chromatography. At least 20 TEA positive peaks were resolved, one of which corresponds in retention time with the methyl ester of N-nitrosoproline. Similar peaks were detected in the extract of the nonnitrosated urines used in this study. The only volatile N-nitrosamine detected in the whole series was N-nitrosodimethylamine (NDMA) which was found in three specimens at levels ranging from 0.4-3.3 μg/l. These specimens contained more than 10^5/ml nitrate-reducing organisms, although nitrite itself was detected in only one of the urines involved at a concentration of 44 mg/l. In these three urines, the formation of NDMA was accompanied by some of the highest values (48-190 μg/l) obtained for the total N-nitroso compounds. These results are reported in greater detail elsewhere (Hicks et al. 1982).

These observations suggest that everyone is exposed to low levels of urine-borne N-nitroso compounds though not, in the absence of bacterial infection, to detectable amounts of volatile N-nitrosamines such as NDMA. However, the metabolites of those nitrosamines which are known to be bladder carcinogens in experimental animals, e.g., BBN and NMDCA, if present would be in the nonvolatile fraction. The mean levels of N-nitroso compounds in Groups C" and D" (Table 2) underestimate the possible level of exposure for any individual within these groups, since the intensity of bacterial infection varies over a period of time. Judging from the amounts of nitrosatable precursors present in the Egyptian urines (Hicks et al. 1978, 1982) very much higher levels of exposure than those reported here are possible for short periods of time during acute infections of the bladder. Thus, in any population in which bacteriuria is common such as the Egyptian village population utilized for this study, there will be individuals who are exposed regularly and intermittently to above-normal levels of N-nitroso compounds in the urine, and the level of exposure will vary from person to person depending on the frequency and intensity of their bacterial infections. Whether or not the presence of such levels of N-nitroso compounds is causally related to the elevated incidence of bladder cancer in Egypt is still a matter for speculation in the absence of any direct evidence for the carcinogenicity of nitrosamines in man.

EVIDENCE THAT AN N-NITROSAMINE CAN INITIATE CARCINOGENESIS IN THE URINARY BLADDER OF ANOTHER PRIMATE SPECIES

While it is not possible to investigate directly the carcinogenicity of nitrosamines in human populations, it is possible to study these compounds in another primate species. A number, including MNU, ethylnitrosourea, nitrosodiethylamine, and nitrosopiperidine are carcinogenic in subhuman primates, usually after a long latent period following administration of high levels of the compound for a long time (evidence summarized in IARC 1978). The known bladder carcinogens BBN and NMDCA do not appear to have been tested in a primate species.

Since the baboon (*Papio sp.*) will substitute for the human host in the life-cycle of *S. haematobium*, rather than investigate BBN as a solitary carcinogen for the baboon bladder we set up an experiment to determine whether concurrent exposure to low doses of BBN and infection with *S. haematobium* could induce bladder cancer in this species. This was not designed as a classic initiation-promotion trial in which the initiating agent is given first and then followed later by a promoting regime. Instead, in order to simulate the human condition, the *S. haematobium* infection was established first and small pulses of the nitrosamine were administered throughout the experiment. There was thus concurrent exposure of the urothelium to the schistosome and to the urinary metabolites of BBN.

Experimental Procedures

Twenty-five young male baboons weighing 3-8 kg on arrival were divided into five experimental treatment groups:

Group 1: 5 animals were infected with *S. mansoni* to act as controls for the systemic effects of schistosomiasis.

Group 2: The 5 baboons in this group were given intramuscular injections of BBN and no other treatment. Three received 50 mg/kg BBN per week and the other 2 were given 5 mg/kg BBN per week.

Group 3: 5 baboons in this group were infected with *S. haematobium* (c. 1,000 cercariae).

Group 4: This was the main experimental group of 10 animals infected with 1,000 cercariae of *S. haematobium* and also given weekly injections of the lower dose of 5 mg/kg BBN. The injections were started 1 week after infection with the *S. haematobium* and continued until necropsy.

These baboons were kept for 2.5 years befsore necropsy with the exception of two animals which became moribund and were killed prematurely at 12 months and 14 months and another which died during the acute infection stage 3 months after exposure to *S. haematobium*. Further details of the experimental procedures are published by Hicks et al. (1980).

Observations

The urothelium in both bladders and ureters of baboons in Group 2, treated with BBN only, remained normal and neither the higher nor the lower dose produced any signs of cell death, hyperplasia, dysplasia, or loss of differentiation at the histological or subcellular level. Concurrent experiments with hamsters showed the same sample of BBN to be carcinogenic for the bladder of that species. Considering that the 3 baboons (average weight 8 kg) which received the higher dose of BBN had each been exposed to a total of approximately 50g BBN over the course of the experiment, it might be concluded that BBN is not carcinogenic for this primate species or alternatively, is not organotropic for the primate bladder. However, 2.5 years represents only a quarter or less of the normal lifespan of this animal. Primates are known to be relatively slow to respond to chemical carcinogens: It required 33 months for the first bladder cancers to develop in Rhesus monkeys treated with 2-naphthylamine (Conzelman et al. 1969), and the average latency before bladder cancer develops in man following exposure to 2-naphthylamine is 20 years (Case 1966). It is therefore possible that if the BBN-treated baboons had been permitted to survive for 5 years or longer bladder cancer could have developed in these animals also and negative findings after only 2.5 years must be regarded as inconclusive.

No deposition of eggs in the lower urinary tract was detected in the *S. mansoni*-infected control baboons of Group 1, and the 5 animals in this group had normal urothelia lining the bladders and ureters. In 4 of the 5 *S. haematobium*-infected animals of Group 3 there was egg deposition in the bladder wall and 4 baboons developed inflamed polyps of the bladder with mild polypoidal hyperplasia of the urothelium plus cystitis cystica. However, the urothelium remained well-differentiated as judged both by conventional histology and by electron microscopy. The most severe pathology seen was a single well-differentiated endophytic papillary process in the ureter of one baboon in which the infection was particularly heavy.

By contrast, in the 10 *S. haematobium*-infected baboons in Group 4 which had additionally received BBN, the lower urinary tract was grossly abnormal. Three developed gross adenomatous lesions of the bladder which, on the basis of their ultrastructure, appeared to be early adenocarcinomas. A fourth had a papillary carcinoma with invasion into the underlying lamina propria of the bladder wall. All but one of the remaining animals in this group had polypoidal hyperplasia and cystitis cystica of varying degrees of severity. In addition, five animals in this group had numerous, deep, endophytic urothelial processes which passed through the band of circular muscle deep in the ureter wall. In three of these, the degree of cell atypia was such that they were classified as early transitional cell carcinomas. There was thus a striking difference between the bladder pathology of the *S. haematobium*-infected animals in Group 3 which had received no further treatment, and those in Group 4 which had additionally received BBN (Table 3). The lesions are illustrated and described in detail elsewhere (Hicks et al. 1980).

CONCLUSIONS

In general, the total incidence of any cancer is directly proportional to the total dose of initiating (genotoxic) carcinogen received, and the latent period before symptomatic neoplasms develop is inversely proportional to the dose. The low total incidence and late age of peak incidence of bladder cancer in Europe and America, and in nonbilharzial-infested populations in the Middle East, could be consistent with endemic exposure in many parts of the world to low total doses of bladder carcinogens. In experimental multistage carcinogenesis models, the total number of tumors which can eventually develop is controlled by the dose of the initiating carcinogen but regular exposures to late-stage carcinogens

Table 3
Urothelial Pathology in the Bladders and Ureters of Baboons Infected with *S. haematobium* with and without Additional Treatment with BBN

Group	Number in group	*S. haematobium* infection	BBN treatment	Numbers of animals with bladder pathology	Numbers of animals with ureter pathology
3	5	+^{v}	nil	4 polypoidal hyperplasia plus cystitis cystica	1 endophytic papillary hyperplasia
				1 normal	4 normal
4	10	+^{v}	5 mg/kg/w	1 papillary carcinoma	3 papillary carcinomas
				3 early adenocarcinomas	5 hyperplasias, some papillary
				6 hyperplasias, mostly severe with cystitis cystica	1 normal
				0 normal	1 not examined

(promoters) will reduce the latent period before tumor growth commences, and thus increase the *age-related* incidence of neoplasms. The lowered age of peak incidence and the elevated age-related incidence of bladder cancer in some populations infested with *S. haematobium*, is consistent with bilharziasis acting as a late stage carcinogen.

The variation in the age-related bladder cancer incidence in different areas of *S. haematobium* infection could reflect either differences in the background levels of first stage carcinogens, or differences in duration and intensity of exposure to the accelerating (late stage) *S. haematobium* infection. We proposed the hypothesis that *N*-nitroso compounds in the urine could act as initiating carcinogens for bladder cancer. The elevated levels of nitrosamines found in the urines of young Egyptian men who are in an area of endemic bilharziasis at high risk for bladder cancer, are consistent with this thesis but do not exclude the possibility that other, as yet unidentified bladder carcinogens, are also present which could be quantitatively or qualitatively more important.

There is no *direct* evidence that any *N*-nitroso compound is carcinogenic for man, but other subhuman primates are susceptible to nitrosamine carcinogenesis. The experiments reported here suggest that BBN is carcinogenic for the baboon bladder and that cancer development is accelerated by concurrent infection with *S. haematobium*.

Neither the results of analysis of the urines of a village population of young men in Egypt, nor the results of the baboon study provide conclusive proof that nitrosamines and (or) their metabolites are causally related to human bladder cancer. However, they are consistent with this hypothesis, which goes some way to explaining the unusual age-related incidence of bladder cancer in areas where *S. haematobium* infection and concurrent bacterial infection of the lower urinary tract are endemic.

ACKNOWLEDGMENTS

The baboon studies were supported by grants from the Edna MacConnell Clark Foundation and the Ministry of Overseas Development through the Tropical Medicine Research Board of the Medical Research Council. The urine analyses and collection of samples in the Qalyub district of Egypt were supported by the UNDP/World Bank/WHO Special Programme for Research and Training in Tropical Diseases. I am most grateful to all my colleagues who have worked with me on the problem of bilharzial bladder cancer, and in particular to Dr. Cliff Walters for his enthusiastic cooperation over the last 6 years.

REFERENCES

Aboul Nasr, A.L., M.E. Gazayerli, R.M. Fawzi, and I. El-Sebai. 1962. Epidemiology and pathology of cancer of the bladder in Egypt. *Acta Univ. Int. Cancer* 18:528.

Bilharz, T. 1852. Fernere beobachtungen uber das die pfortader des menschen bewohnende Distomum haematobium und sein Verhaltnis zu gewissen pathologischen bildungen. *Z. Wiss. Zool.* 4:72.

Brand, K.G. 1979. Schistosomiasis-cancer: Aetiological considerations. *Acta Trop.* 36:203.

Carter, J.P., A.S. Diab, S. Nasif, W.R. Sanborn, L.E. Grivetti, and J.A. Davies. 1970. Bacteriological and urinary findings in adolescent Egyptian males with and without urinary schistosomiasis. *J. Trop. Med. Hyg.* 73:211.

Case, R.A.M. 1966. Tumours of the urinary tract. *Ann. R. Coll. Surg. Engl.* 39:213.

Conzelman, G.M., Jr., J.E. Moulton, and L.E. Flanders. 1969. Induction of transitional cell carcinomas of the urinary bladder in monkeys fed 2-naphthylamine. *J. Natl. Cancer Inst.* 42:825.

Cox, R.D. 1980. Determination of nitrate and nitrite at the parts per billion level by chemiluminescence. *Anal. Chem.* 52:332.

Dodge, O.G. 1962. Tumours of the bladder in Ugandan Africans. *Acta Unio. Int. Contra Cancrum* 18:548.

Druckrey, H., R. Preussmann, S. Ivankovic, C.H. Schmidt, H.D. Mennel, and K.W. Stahl. 1964. Selektive Erzeugung von Blasenkrebs an Ratten durch Dibutyl und N-Butyl-N-Butanol (4)-Nitrosamin. *Z. Krebsforsch.* 66:280.

Eisenbrand, G. and R. Preussmann. 1970. Eine Neue Methode zür Kolorimetrischen Bestimmung von Nitrosaminen nach Spactung der N-Nitrosogruppe mit Bromwasserstoff in Eisessig. *Arzneim. Forsch.* 20:1513.

El-Alamy, M.A. and B.L. Cline. 1977. Prevalence and intensity of Schistosoma haematobium and S. mansoni infection in Qalyub, Egypt. *Am. J. Trop. Med. Hyg.* 26:470.

El-Bolkainy, M.N., M.A. Ghoneim, and M.A. Mansour. 1972. Carcinoma of the bilharzial bladder in Egypt: Clinical and pathological features. *Br. J. Urol.* 44:561.

El-Sebai, I. 1977. Bilharziasis and bladder cancer. *Ca-Cancer J. Clin.* 27:100.

———. 1978. Cancer of the bilharzial bladder. *Urol. Res.* 6:233.

Fergusson, A.R. 1911. Associated bilharziasis and primary malignant disease of the urinary bladder with observations on a series of forty cases. *J. Pathol. Bacteriol.* 16:76.

Fine, D.H., F. Rufeh, D. Lieb, and D.P. Rounbehler. 1975. Description of the Thermal Energy Analyser (TEA) for trace determination of volatile and nonvolatile N-nitroso compounds. *Anal. Chem.* 47:1188.

Gillman, J. and M.D. Prates. 1962. Histological types and histogenesis of bladder cancer in the Portuguese East Africa with special reference to bilharzial cystitis. *Acta Unio. Int. Contra Cancrum* 18:560.

Goebel, C. 1905. Ueber die bei Bilharziakrankheit vorkommenden Blasentumoren mit bezonderer Beruchsichtigung des Carcinomas. *Z. Krebsforsch.* 3:369.

Hashem, M. 1961. The aetiology and pathogenesis of the bilharzial bladder cancer. *J. Egypt Med. Assoc.* 44:857.

Hicks, R.M. 1980. Multistage carcinogenesis in the urinary bladder. *Br. Med. Bull.* 36:39.

———. 1982. Promotion in bladder cancer. In *Carcinogenesis* (eds. E. Hecker et al.), Vol. 7, p. 139. Raven Press, New York.

Hicks, R.M. and J.St.J. Wakefield. 1972. Rapid induction of bladder cancer in rats with N-methyl-N-nitrosourea. I. Histology. *Chem.-Biol. Interact.* 5:139.

Hicks, R.M., T.A. Gough, and C.L. Walters. 1978. Demonstration of the presence of nitrosamines in human urine: Preliminary observations on a possible etiology for bladder cancer in association with chronic urinary tract infection. *IARC Sci. Publ.* 19:465.

Hicks, R.M., C. James, and G. Webbe. 1980. Effect of Schistosoma haematobium and N-butyl-N-(4-hydroxybutyl)nitrosamine on the development of urothelial neoplasia in the baboon. *Br. J. Cancer* 42:730.

Hicks, R.M., C.L. Walters, I. Elsebai, A.B. El-Aasser, M. El-Merzabani, and T. Gough. 1977. Demonstration of N-nitrosamines in human urine. *Proc. R. Soc. Med.* 70:413.

Hicks, R.M., M.M. Ismail, C.L. Walters, P.T. Beecham, M.F. Rabie, and M.A. El Alamy. 1982. Association of bacteriuria and urinary nitrosamine formation with Schistosoma haematobium infection in the Qalyub area of *Egypt. Trans. R. Soc. Trop. Med. Hyg.* 76:(4):519.

Higginson, J. and A.G. Oettle. 1962. Cancer of the bladder in the South African Bantu. *Acta Unio. Int. Contra Cancrum* 18:579.

Hill, M.J. and G. Hawksworth. 1972. Bacterial production of nitrosamines in vitro and in vivo. *IARC Sci. Publ.* 3:116.

Hirose, M., S. Fukushima, M. Hananouchi, T. Shirai, T. Ogiso, M. Takahashi, and N. Ito. 1976. Different susceptibilities of the urinary bladder epithelium of animal species to three nitroso compounds. *Gann* 67:175.

Houston, W. 1964. Carcinoma of the bladder in Southern Rhodesia. *Br. J. Urol.* 36:71.

Hyman, L.H. 1951. The invertebrates: Platyhelminthes and Rhynchocoela. *The Acoelomate Bilateria.* McGraw-Hill, New York.

IARC 1978. Some N-Nitroso Compounds. *IARC Monogr. Carcinog. Risk Chem. Hum.* 17.

Ishak, K.G., O.C. Le Golvan, and I. El-Sebai. 1967. Malignant bladder tumours associated with bilharziasis, a gross and microscopic study. In *Bilharziasis* (ed. F.K. Mostofi), p. 67. Springer-Verlag, New York.

Jordan, P. and G. Webbe. 1969. *Human Schistosomiasis.* Heinemann Medical Books, Ltd., London.

Laughlin, L.W., Z. Farid, N. Mansour, D.C. Edman, and G.I. Higashi. 1978. Bacteriuria in urinary schistosomiasis in Egypt. A prevalence survey. *Am. J. Trop. Med. Hyg.* 27:916.

Lijinsky, W. and H.W. Taylor. 1975. Induction of urinary bladder tumors in rats by administration of nitrosomethyldodecylamine. *Cancer Res.* 35:958.

Payne, P. 1959. In *Tumours of the bladder* (ed. D.M. Wallace), p. 285. E. and S. Livingstone, Edinburgh and London.

Prates, M.D. and F.O. Torres. 1965. A cancer survey in Lourenço Marques, Portuguese East Africa. *J. Natl. Cancer Inst.* 35:729.

Skrabanek, P. and A. Walsh. Eds. 1981. Bladder cancer. *UICC Tech. Rep. Ser.* 60:118.

Walters, C.L., R.J. Hart, and S. Perse. 1978b. The breakdown into nitric oxide of compounds potentially derived from nitrite in a biological matrix. *Z. Lebensm Unters. Forsch.* **167**:315.

Walters, C.L., M.J. Downes, M.W. Edwards, and P.L.R. Smith. 1978a. Determination of a non-volatile N-nitrosamine on a food matrix. *Analyst.* **103**: 1127.

COMMENTS

WEISBURGER: I simply want to say that that is an elegant study, showing that in human, as well as other diseases, promotion can be the determining element, whether or not cancers erupt rapidly.

PARSA: Adenocarcinoma is a rarity in the human bladder. What is the origin of those cells?

HICKS: The origin is the urothelium. As you know, in the West the main form of bladder cancer in man is transitional cell carcinoma; in Egypt in man it is mainly squamous, but different species react to the same carcinogen in different ways. For example we can take a carcinogen such as BBN and give it to a rat and get slow-growing exophytic papillary carcinomas; the same carcinogen given to a particular mouse strain gives slow-growing exophytic squamous cell carcinomas; given to another strain of mouse, it produces flat invasive transitional cell carcinomas. So the actual cell type produced in response to a particular carcinogen may be species- or strain-related. So I am not too worried about the fact that baboons developed adenocarcinoma rather than squamous cell carcinoma.

GRASSO: Is it not possible that the adenocarcinoma could have originated from the gut and then invaded the bladder?

HICKS: No, there is no sign of gut contamination and mucous metaplasia is quite a common occurrence in the urothelium.

FINE: When you collected the urine samples and did the analysis, did you add a marker amine to see if there had been any artifact formation?

WALTERS: No, not at that stage. The procedure was that the nitrite estimations and the microbiology were done in Egypt. The sulfamic acid was added to bring the pH down below 2, and at that stage we did not add a marker amine. If you add nitrite to urine containing sulfamic acid, you do not get additional nitroso compound formation. In fact, we examined all the samples by GC and TEA, and only in three specimens were there any volatiles. In each of these three urines there was a nitrate-reducing bacterial population in excess of 10^5. The only volatile that was seen was NDMA, at levels up to 10 μg/liter.

KIMBROUGH: Did you measure nitrosamine levels in the urine of the baboons? And were the urine samples that you collected in Egypt 24-hour samples or grab samples?

HICKS: They were grab samples, taken midmorning.

KIMBROUGH: Did you adjust for specific gravity in your calculations?

HICKS: No, we didn't. And we didn't do the nitrosamine analysis in the baboons. Baboons are not that easy to handle, and for that reason also, we administered the carcinogen in a very unusual way. Normally, you give BBN in the diet or by gavage. For this experiment the baboons were held in a crush cage so that they could be pushed up to one end, and they were given the BBN by intramuscular injection. This is a very unusual route of administration, but it seemed to work in the long run. BBN is a compound which is known to be specific for the bladder only, and it and its metabolites are excreted via the urinary tract.

Possible Relationship of Nitrosamines in the Diet to Causation of Cancer in Hong Kong

LOUISE Y. Y. FONG
Department of Biochemistry
Faculty of Medicine
University of Hong Kong
Hong Kong

As compared with other parts of the world, Hong Kong is defined as an unusually high incidence area for nasopharyngeal carcinoma (NPC) (Ho 1967, 1972, 1975), a high incidence area for primary liver cancer (Gibson and Chan 1972), and cancer of the esophagus (Doll 1969; Fong 1982). The age-standardized adjusted rates to the world per 100,000 for males are: 41.5 for NPC, 39.8 for primary liver cancer, and 22.0 for esophageal cancer (Cancer Registry 1978). The high risk for the three forms of cancer in question is not associated with the mongoloid race per se but rather with the basic elements of life such as the diet, because even among Chinese in China, there are regional differences (Kaplan and Tsuchitani 1978). This is in line with the widely accepted theory that most human cancers have environmental factors in their etiologies (Higginson 1969; Miller 1978).

The discovery of the highly carcinogenic aflatoxins prompted the speculation that liver cancer in the tropics might be caused by ingestion of nuts and grains contaminated with *Aspergillus flavus* as a result of improper harvesting and storage. Estimations of the aflatoxin actually ingested by the inhabitants of certain localized regions in Thailand (Shank et al. 1972a) and in Africa (Alpert et al. 1971) have shown that there is an approximately quantitative relationship between unusually high levels of ingestion of aflatoxin and the very high local incidences of hepatocellular carcinoma. Such a clear-cut relationship however seems to be rare. Though aflatoxin contamination of food probably plays a part in causing hepatocellular carcinoma, it does not appear to be the only factor concerned. Thus in Hong Kong, Shank et al. (1972b) found that, in general, aflatoxin contamination of foods bought in the market was less frequent and at lower levels than in Thailand. Rice, the staple food in both areas, was seldom contaminated and then only at low levels.

Nitrosamines are a group of potent chemical carcinogens within which compounds with different structures cause tumors in different organs of the experimental animals (Magee et al. 1976). Furthermore, nitrosamines may be generated in foods in the course of preparation or even within the stomach from ingested precursors. In considering the possibility that the high incidence of NPC, liver, and esophageal cancer in Hong Kong might be due to nitrosamines, a more complex train of events than that exemplified by aflatoxin contamination must be sought. This paper presents data to show ways in which one of the local practices of food preparation (i.e., the salted fish) might lead to the ingestion of nitrosamines, and how, in an animal model, nutritional deficiency as exemplified by dietary zinc deficiency might influence esophageal carcinogenesis by methylbenzylnitrosamine (MBN), and by its precursors.

SALTED FISH AND NPC

The incidence of NPC has been noted to be high among southern Chinese for about 60 years (Todd 1921; Shanmugaratnam 1971; Ho 1972). Ho (1971) first suspected that salted fish might be a causative factor because it was a favorite item of food among Cantonese in Hong Kong and Southeast Asia. Support for Ho's hypothesis was found in the following studies. Topley (1973) reported that salted fish was commonly fed to infants in Hong Kong in the weaning and post-weaning period in the form of a salted fish-congee, a mushy form of rice. The ingestion of salted fish from early childhood might explain the sudden rise in the age-specific incidence curves for both sexes after the age of 19-24 (Ho 1975). More recently, Anderson et al. (1978) conducted a case-control study on 24 young NPC patients in Hong Kong. All 24 patients were found to have been fed salted fish from weaning. The consumption of salted fish during weaning was determined by multivariate analysis to be a risk factor in the development of NPC. This was independent of traditional lifestyle which was itself a risk factor (Geser et al. 1978).

Traditional Way of Preparation of Salted Fish

The common practice of preparing salted fish is to place the fish in pickle brine containing 20-30 parts rock or sea salt per 100 parts fish without cleaning or removal of the gut and gills (McCarthy and Tausz 1952). This would allow a sort of "benign decay" and produce a gamey flavor which is relished by most southern Chinese palates. Salted fish is dried in the sun. Since the average relative humidity in Hong Kong is around 85% in the summer and 72% in the winter months it is obvious that at no time of the year would it be physically possible to completely dry the fish. The sun-dried fish is then sold in the market. According to demand and weather, the fish may finally be consumed months after it is first pickled. Therefore, the fish, which in the first place may not be well preserved because salting may be too light and secondly, may not be well dried, is likely to undergo chemical and bacterial denaturation.

Nitrosamines in Salted Fish

Since the first report of human toxicity arising from the use of dimethylnitros-aming (NDMA) in an industrial laboratory (Barnes and Magee 1954) and that of NDMA as a potent carcinogen (Magee and Barnes 1956), a considerable length of time had elapsed before the possible occurrence of nitrosamines in situations other than the industrial environment was suspected. The possibility first emerged rather dramatically in Norway. NDMA at levels as high as 30-100 ppm was found to be the toxic principle in the fish-meal feeds (Ender et al. 1964; Sakshaug et al. 1965) responsible for the sudden outbreak of toxic hepatosis in sheep in Norway (Koppang 1964). This report sparked off the search for nitrosamines in foods for human consumption. In the subsequent years, low levels of NDMA were reported in a number of processed meat and fish (Ender and Ceh 1968; Howard et al. 1970; Sen et al. 1970; Fazio et al. 1971; Crosby et al. 1972; Sen 1972; Wasserman et al. 1972).

In 1971 we began to investigate whether nitrosamines are present in Cantonese salted fish and if so what are the conditions that led to their forma-tion. Using gas chromatography (GC), we found NDMA at levels between 0.6-9 ppm in all nine species of salted fish studied, including white herring, yellow croaker, croaker, anchovies, and pomfret (Fong and Walsh 1971). In the following 2 years, as more samples of market salted fish were analyzed, we found that there was a considerable variation in NDMA content among different batches of salted fish. Significant amounts of this compound, usually in the 0.05-0.3 ppm range were detected by GC and were confirmed by gas chromatography-mass spectrometry (GC/MS). Also, up to 40 ppm residual nitrate and negligible amounts of nitrite were detected in the salted fish. Crude salt commonly used for pickling was always found to contain nitrate as an impurity, and this nitrate was a precursor of NDMA. Salted fish prepared in the laboratory with crude salt containing 17-40 ppm nitrate but not more than 1 ppm nitrite was thus shown to contain 40 times more NDMA than the same fish pickled with chemically pure NaCl (Fong and Chan 1973a).

As far as nitrosatable amines are concerned, marine fish is a far richer source than freshwater fish. The degree of N-nitrosation detected (expressed as μmols N-nitroso derivatives/kg fish, on the basis of one nitrosatable group/mol amine) ranged from 45-443 and from 4-34 for three species of marine and fresh-water fish, respectively. The level of NDMA in marine fish (1.7-45 ppm) following N-nitrosation reaction was also much higher than that (0.02-0.4 ppm) in freshwater fish (Fong and Chan 1976).

We have also obtained viable culture from salted fish on salt agar of nitrate-reducing *Staphylococcus aureus* and halobacteria. We were able to demonstrate an increase in NDMA in fish broth innoculated with the *S. aureus* originally isolated from salted fish obtained from the market (Fong and Chan 1973b). The results for this experiment are shown in Figure 1. A homogenate of salted fish was made with water and divided into three equal portions—A,

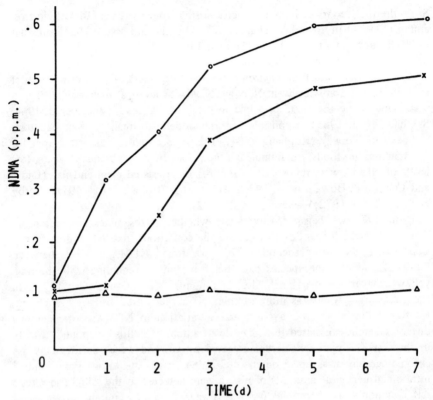

Figure 1
Concentration of NDMA in fish broth after incubation at 37°C, (Δ) Portion A, sterilized; (O) portion B, inoculated with 10^9 S. aureus per lot; (X) portion C, untreated. Reprinted, with permission, from Fong and Chan (1973b).

B, and C. Portion A was sterilized by heating in a water bath at 70°C for 1 hour daily. Portion B was similarly sterilized on O day and then 10^9 S. aureus in 1 ml was added. Portion C was untreated. The samples were incubated at 37°C for a total of 7 days. There was no change in NDMA content of the sterilized fish broth A, while B and C showed progressive increases with the curve flattening towards the end of the 7-day period. This experiment demonstrates the important role of the S. aureus originally isolated from salted fish in the production of NDMA from its precursors in the fish. The amount of NDMA present would thus seem to be dependent on the storage condition, degree of contamination by nitrate-reducing bacteria, and the amount of precursors present.

Attempts were therefore made to inhibit the formation of nitrosamines in salted fish (Fong and Chan 1976). Benzoic acid was found to be more effective in reducing the rate of nitrosamine formation than the tetracyclines, which actually increased its production. Salting with chemically pure NaCl produced less NDMA than that using crude salt which commonly contained nitrate. From these data, it seems likely that the possible levels of NDMA in salted fish could be reduced in three ways, namely, by limiting the concentrations of NDMA precursors (amine and nitrate or nitrite), by reducing the level of bacterial contamination which could be brought about by improving on drying, packaging, and storage procedures, and by adding antimicrobial preservatives with the pickling salt.

Rats Fed Salted Fish Have Mutagenic Urine

Urine was collected from 5-month old experimental rats that were fed daily with steam-cooked salted fish since weaning, and from matched control rats fed Purina rat chow. Urine from rats on the salted fish diet was found to exhibit mutagenic activities by the Ames mutagenicity assay (Ames et al. 1975). Furthermore, it was demonstrated that the level of such activities decreased markedly when the experimental rats were transferred from a salted fish diet to Purina rat chow (Fig. 2). These data suggest that the mutagenic activities of

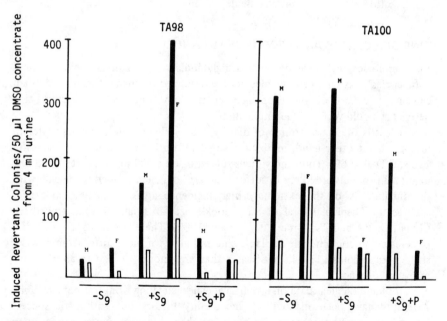

Figure 2
Mutagenic activities of urine from male and female rats fed regularly with salted fish and after such feeding had been suspended. Induced revertant colonies: colonies counted minus spontaneous colonies. (■) induced revertant colonies while rats were being fed with salted fish; (□) induced revertant colonies after the rats were transferred from a salted fish diet to Purina rat chow. Reprinted, with permission, from Fong et al. (1979).

their urine were derived from the consumption of salted fish (Fong et al. 1979). Our data are also in support of the long-term salted fish feeding experiments of Huang et al. (1978) which described the induction of carcinomas in the nasal and maxillary sinus of 4/20 inbred WA rats after an experimental period of 12-24 months.

Nitrosamines in Other Chinese Preserved Foodstuffs

Low levels of NDMA (1-15 ppb) and N-nitrosopyrrolidine (2-37 ppb) were detected and confirmed by GC/MS in a number of commonly consumed Chinese food products including dried shrimps, shrimp sauce and paste, oyster sauce, fish sauce, Chinese sausages, and dried squids (Fong and Chan 1977). The levels of NDMA were significantly lower than the levels of 50-300 ppb reported for salted fish (Fong and Chan 1973a). There are three possible reasons for this. The sauces and pastes being in fluid or semi-fluid forms contain lower concentrations of nitrosatable amines. On the other hand, solid foods such as dried shrimps and squids provide a less favorable environment for bacterial growth than do salted fish because they can be dried more efficiently. Lastly, benzoate is routinely added to these sauces to inhibit microbial growth and hence possible N-nitrosation reactions might also be depressed.

ZINC DEFICIENCY AND ESOPHAGEAL CANCER

Epidemiological evidence has increasingly indicated that dietary excesses and deficiencies play important roles in the etiology of many forms of human cancer. In cancer of the esophagus apart from other factors, dietary zinc deficiency could very well be implicated.

Meat is the major source of dietary zinc while phytate and a high calcium intake, on the other hand, inhibit intestinal absorption of the mineral (Heekstra 1964; O'Dell 1969). Thus, individuals subsisting on a diet high in cereals and low in animal products are likely to suffer from zinc deficiency. Such is the case with the inhabitants of the extremely high incidence areas of esophageal cancer such as the Caspian littoral of Iran (Cook-Mozaffari et al. 1979) and northern China (Kaplan and Tsuchitani 1978; Yang 1980). These people eat a staple diet of cereals that contain little available zinc and many of them suffer from diseases such as tuberculosis and liver diseases that are known to lead to an excessive excretion of zinc.

Epidemiological data on esophageal cancer in Hong Kong are not available. Attempts have been made to define dietary history but with little success beyond observations that many such esophageal cancer patients consumed traditional Chinese diets (Lin et al. 1977) and were fond of locally made alcoholic spirits. Traditional Chinese foods are often contaminated with nitrosamines as described earlier and Lee and Fong (1979) reported that 17/27 of the traditional Chinese alcoholic spirits analyzed exhibited mutagenic activities by the Ames *Salmonella* assay (Ames et al. 1975). Furthermore, we also found lower levels of zinc in the blood, hair, and esophageal tissue of patients with esophageal cancer than in matched control subjects or matched patients with other forms of cancer (Lin et al. 1977). The reduced serum levels of zinc were accompanied by an increased serum level of copper and such changes have been observed in humans under conditions ascribed to zinc deficiency (Prasad et al. 1963; Hambidge et al. 1972).

In the experimental animal, dietary zinc deficiency has been shown to induce parakeratosis, hyperkeratosis in the esophagus of the rat (Follis 1966; Diamond and Hurley 1970). Since cell proliferation and hyperparakeratosis are considered to be involved in cancer initiation, these data appeared to suggest that nutritional zinc deficiency would, in fact, render the esophagus more vulnerable to the development of neoplasm in situ.

Zinc Deficiency and Esophageal Carcinogenesis by MBN in the Rat

The data in Table 1 clearly suggest that zinc deficiency enhances the induction of esophageal cancer in the rat. With a total of 8 doses of MBN at 2 mg/kg body weight, administered intragastrically, 79% of the zinc-deficient rats versus 29% of the controls developed tumors; size and multiplicity of tumors were greater in the deficient group. With a total of only four doses of MBN; 21% of the zinc deficient and none of the control rats developed tumors in the esophagus (Fong et al. 1978). When higher doses of MBN (17 or 24 doses) were used, invasive carcinoma of the esophagus appeared, again with the incidence significantly higher in the zinc-deficient animals (Fong et al. 1978).

Zinc Deficiency and Esophageal Carcinogenesis by Precursors of MBN in the Rat

Male Sprague-Dawley rats (Laboratory Animal Unit, University of Hong Kong) were used in this study. They were fed the respective zinc-deficient and sufficient-control diets for 5 weeks before they were administered drinking water containing freshly mixed N-methylbenzylamine (NMBA) and sodium nitrite (Fong et al. 1982). Table 2 shows that after an experimental period of 37 weeks, significantly higher incidence of invasive carcinoma of the esophagus and forestomach was observed in the deficient as compared to the sufficient rats (X^2 test: $p = 0.05$).

The mechanism by which zinc deficiency enhances esophageal carcinogenesis by MBN or its precursors is still largely unknown. On one hand, zinc deficiency by itself produces parakeratosis in the rat esophagus (Follis 1966; Diamond and Hurley 1970). This is characterized by thickening of epithelium and deranged keratinization, thus rendering the lining more sensitive to an esophageal carcinogen such as the MBN. On the other hand, as compared to control animals, zinc-deficient animals including mice and rats were reported to

Table 1

Incidence of Esophageal Tumors Induced by Low Doses of MBN in Male Charles River CD Rats Fed Control and Zinc-deficient Diets

Group	Diet	MBN[a] (mg/kg b.w.)	Time to killing from first dose (days)[b]	Tumor incidence[c]	Number of tumors/esophagus				Tumor size (2x2 mm)
					1	2	3	5	
III	Control, pair-fed	16	63	14/48 (29)	10/48	2/48	2/48	—	7/48
	Zinc-deficient, ad libitum	16	63	34/43 (79)	3/43	7/43	8/43	16/43	25/43
IV	Control, pair-fed	8	75	0/40 (0)	—	—	—	—	—
	Zinc-deficient, ad libitum	8	75	9/43 (21)	8/43	1/43	—	—	5/43

Data, reprinted with permission, from Fong et al. (1978).
[a]Dose was 2 mg/kg b.w. twice weekly.
[b]First dose was given at 7 wk. of age, 4 wk after the rats were started on the experimental diet.
[c]Numbers in parentheses are percent incidence.

Table 2

Incidence of Tumors in the Esophagus and Forestomach Induced by MBA and $NaNO_2$ in Rats Fed Zinc-deficient and Sufficient Diets

Group	Diet	Experimental period (weeks)	Tumor Incidence[a]	
			carcinoma	papilloma
I	0.05% MBA + 0.5% $NaNO_2$	16	2/33 (6)	24/33 (73)
	Zinc-deficient, ad libitum	16	2/33 (6)	24/33 (73)
	Zinc-sufficient, pair-fed	16	0/25 (0)	7/25 (28)
II	0.25% MBA + 0.5% $NaNO_2$	37	7/9 (78)	9/9 (100)
	Zinc-deficient, ad libitum	37	7/9 (78)	9/9 (100)
	Zinc-sufficient, ad libitum	37	2/7 (28)	7/7 (100)

Data, reprinted with permission, from Fong et al. (1982).
[a]Numbers in parentheses are percent incidence.

show depressed immunocompetence as indicated by a number of criteria such as reduced lymphoid tissues and ability to undergo blast transformation after exposure to mitogens etc. (Hass et al. 1976; Frost et al. 1977; Gross et al. 1979a,b). This again may sensitize the animals to subsequent carcinogenic insults.

CONCLUSIONS

Apart from genetic variations, two factors must be considered in the etiologies of the three forms of cancer that occur with high frequency in Hong Kong. Contamination of foodstuffs with a carcinogen or carcinogens and nutritional deficiencies of one kind or another. Salted fish has been shown by epidemiological data to be a possible factor for the development of NPC in Hong Kong. We have demonstrated a mechanism whereby NDMA could be formed in salted fish and that the ingestion of salted fish by rats could lead to excretion of mutagenic urine. Dietary deficiency as exemplified by zinc deficiency was shown to enhance esophageal carcinogenesis in the rat. Epidemiological evidence shows that the combination of such a deficiency and food contamination with nitrosamines are in fact operating in northern China, and probably in Hong Kong as well.

REFERENCES

Alpert, M.E., M.S.R. Hutt, G.N. Wogan, and C.S. Davidson. 1971. Association between aflatoxin content of food and hepatoma frequency in Uganda. *Cancer* 28:253.

Ames, B.N., J. McCann, and E. Yamasaki. 1975. Methods for detecting carcinogens and mutagens with the *Salmonella*/mammalian-microsome mutagenicity test. *Mutat. Res.* 31:347.

Anderson, E.N., M.L. Anderson, Jr., and J.H.C. Ho. 1978. Environmental backgrounds of young Chinese nasopharyngeal carcinoma patients. *IARC Sci. Publ.* 20:231.

Barnes, J.M. and P.N. Magee. 1954. Some toxic properties of dimethylnitrosamine. *Br. J. Ind. Med.* 11:167.

Cancer Registry. 1978. Institute of Radiology and Oncology, Medical and Health Department of Hong Kong.

Cook-Mozaffari, P.J., F. Azordegan, N.E. Day, A. Ressicaud, C. Sabai, and B. Aramesh. 1979. Esophageal cancer studies in the Caspian littoral of Iran: Results of a case-control study. *Br. J. Cancer* 39:293.

Crosby, N.T., J.K. Foreman, J.F. Palframan, and R. Sawyer. 1972. Estimation of steam-volatile N-nitrosamine in food at the 1 μg/kg level. *Nature* 238: 342.

Diamond, I. and L.S. Hurley. 1970. Histopathology of zinc-deficient rats. *J. Nutr.* 100:325.

Doll, R. 1969. The geographical distribution of cancer. *Br. J. Cancer* 23:1.

Ender, F., G. Havre, A. Helgebosted, N. Koppang, R. Madsen, and L. Ceh. 1964.

Isolation and identification of a hepatotoxic factor in herring meal produced from sodium nitrite preserved herring. *Naturwissenschaften* **51**:637.

Ender, F. and L. Ceh. 1968. Occurrence of nitrosamines in foodstuffs for human and animal consumption. *Food Cosmet. Toxicol.* **6**:569.

Fazio, T., J.N. Damico, J.W. Howard, R.H. White, and J.O. Watts. 1971. Gaschromatographic determination and mass spectrometric confirmation of N-nitrosodimethylamine in smoked processed marine fish. *J. Agric. Food Chem.* **19**:250.

Follis, R.H., Jr. 1966. The Pathology of zinc deficiency. In *Zinc metabolism* (ed. A.S. Prasad), p. 129. Charles C. Thomas, Springfield, Illinois.

Fong, Y.Y. and E.O.F. Walsh. 1971. Carcinogenic nitrosamines in Cantonese salt-dried fish. *Lancet* ii:1032.

Fong, Y.Y. and W.C. Chan. 1973a. Dimethylnitrosamine in Chinese marine salt fish. *Food Cosmet. Toxicol.* **11**:841.

_____. 1973b. Bacterial production of dimethylnitrosamine in salted fish. *Nature* **243**:421.

_____. 1976. Methods for limiting the content of dimethylnitrosamine in Chinese marine salt fish. *Food Cosmet. Toxicol.* **14**:95.

_____. 1977. Nitrate, nitrite, dimethylnitrosamine and N-nitrosopyrrolidine in some Chinese food products. *Food Cosmet. Toxicol.* **15**:143.

Fong, L.Y.Y., A. Sivak, and P.M. Newberne. 1978. Zinc deficiency and methylbenzylnitrosamine induced esophageal cancer in rats. *J. Natl. Cancer Inst.* **61**:145.

Fong, L.Y.Y., J.H.C. Ho, and D.P. Huang. 1979. Preserved foods as possible cancer hazards, WA rats fed salted fish have mutagenic urine. *Int. J. Cancer* **23**:542.

Fong, L.Y.Y. 1982. Environmental carcinogens and dietary deficiencies in esophageal cancer in Asia. In *Carcinoma of the esophagus–an international review* (ed. C.J. Pheiffer), CRC Press Inc., Florida. (In Press)

Fong, L.Y.Y., J.S.K. Lee, W.C. Chan, and P.M. Newberne. 1982. Zinc deficiency and the induction of esophageal tumors in rats by methylbenzylnitrosamine. *IARC Sci. Publ.* **41** (in press).

Frost, P., J.C. Chen, I. Rabbani, J. Smith, and A.S. Prasad. 1977. The effect of zinc deficiency on the immune response. In *Zinc metabolism: Current aspects in health and disease.* (eds., G.J. Brewer and A.S. Prasad), p. 211. Alan R. Liss, New York.

Gibson, J.B. and W.C. Chan. 1972. Primary carcinomas of the liver in Hong Kong: Some possible aetiological factors. In *Recent results in cancer research* (eds., E. Grundmann and H. Tulinius), vol. 39, p. 107. Springer-Verlag Berlin, New York.

Geser, A., N. Charnay, N.E. Day, H.C. Ho, and G. de Thé. 1978. Environmental factors in the etiology of nasopharyngeal carcinoma: Report on a case-control study in Hong Kong. *IARC Sci. Publ.* **20**:213.

Gross, R.L., N. Osdin, L. Fong, and P.M. Newberne. 1979a. Depressed immunological function in zinc-deprived rats as measured by mitogen response of spleen, thymus, and peripheral blood. I. *Am. J. Clin. Nutr.* **32**:1260.

_____. 1979b. In vitro restoration by levamisole of mitogen responsiveness in zinc-deprived rats. II. *Am. J. Clin. Nutr.* **32**:1267.

Hambidge, K.M., C. Hambidge, M. Jacobs, and J.D. Baum. 1972. Low levels of zinc in hair, anorexia, poor growth and hypogeusia in children. *Pediatr. Res.* **6**:868.

Hass, S., P. Fraber, and R.W. Luecke. 1976. The effect of zinc deficiency on the immune response of A/J mice. *Fed. Proc. Fed. Am. Soc. Exp. Biol.* **35**: 659.

Heekstra, W.F. 1964. Recent observations on mineral interrelationships. *Fed. Proc. Fed. Am. Soc. Exp. Biol.* **23**:1068.

Higginson, J. 1969. Present trends in cancer epidemiology. *Can. Cancer Conf.* **8**:40.

Ho, J.H.C. 1967. Nasopharyngeal carcinoma in Hong Kong. *UICC Monogr. Ser.* **1**:29.

_____. 1971. Genetic and environmental factors in nasopharyngeal carcinoma. In *Recent advances in human tumor virology and immunology* (ed. W. Nakahara et al.), p. 275. University of Tokyo Press, Tokyo.

_____. 1972. Current knowledge of the epidemiology of nasopharyngeal carcinoma—A review. *IARC Sci. Publ.* **2**:357.

_____. 1975. Epidemiology of nasopharyngeal carcinoma. *J. R. Coll. Surg. Edinb.* **20**:233.

Howard, J.W., T. Fazio, and J.O. Watts. 1970. Extraction and gas chromatographic determination of N-nitrosodimethylamine in smoked fish: Application to smoked nitrite-treated chub. *J. Assoc. Off. Anal. Chem.* **53**:269.

Huang, D.P., J.H.C. Ho, D. Saw, and T.B. Teoh. 1978. Carcinoma of the nasal and paranasal regions in rats fed Cantonese salted marine fish. *IARC Sci. Publ.* **20**:315.

Kaplan, H.S. and P.J. Tsuchitani. 1978. *Cancer in China.* Alan R. Liss, New York.

Koppang, N. 1964. An outbreak of toxic liver injury in ruminants. *Nord. Veterinaermed.* **16**:305.

Lee, J.S.K. and L.Y.Y. Fong. 1979. Mutagenicity of Chinese alcoholic spirits. *Food Cosmet. Toxicol.* **17**:575.

Lin, H.J., W.C. Chan, L.Y.Y. Fong, and P.M. Newberne. 1977. Zinc levels in serum, hair and tumors from patients with esophageal cancer. *Nutr. Rep. Int.* **15**:635.

Magee, P.N. and J.M. Barnes. 1956. The production of malignant primary hepatic tumours in the rat by feeding dimethylnitrosamine. *Br. J. Cancer* **10**:114.

Magee, P.N., R. Montesano, and R. Preussmann. 1976. N-Nitroso compounds and related carcinogens. *ACS Monogr.* **173**:491.

McCarthy, J.P. and J. Tausz. 1952. *Salt fish industry in Hong Kong*, p. 6. The Government Printer, Hong Kong.

Miller, E.C. 1978. Some current perspectives on chemical carcinogenesis in humans and experimental animals: Presidential address. *Cancer Res.* **38**: 1479.

O'Dell, B.L. 1969. Effect of dietary components upon zinc availability. A review with original data. *Am. J. Clin. Nutr.* **22**:1315.

Prasad, A.S., A. Miale, Z. Farid, H.H. Sandstead, A.R. Schulert, and W.J. Darby. 1963. Biochemical studies on dwarfism, hypogonadism and anemia. *Arch. Intern. Med.* **111**:407.

Sakshaug, J., E. Sognen, M.A. Hansen, and N. Koppang. 1965. Dimethylnitrosamine: Its hepatotoxic effect in sheep and its occurrence in toxic batches of herring meal. *Nature* **206**:1261.

Sen, N.P., D.C. Smith, L. Schwinghamer, and B. Howsam. 1970. Formation of nitrosamines in nitrite-treated fish. *J. Inst. Can. Technol. Aliment.* **3**:66.

Sen, N.P. 1972. The evidence for the presence of dimethylnitrosamine in meat products. *Food Cosmet. Toxicol.* **10**:219.

Shanmugaratnam, K. 1971. Studies on the etiology of nasopharyngeal carcinoma. *Int. Rev. Exp. Path.* **10**:361.

Shank, R.C., N. Bhamarapravati, J.E. Gordon, and G.N. Wogan. 1972a. Dietary aflatoxins and human liver cancer. IV. Incidence of primary liver cancer in two municipal populations of Thailand. *Food Cosmet. Toxicol.* **10**:171.

Shank, R.C., G.N. Wogan, J.B. Gibson, and A. Nondasuta. 1972b. Dietary aflatoxins and human liver cancer. II. Aflatoxins in market foods and foodstuffs of Thailand and Hong Kong. *Food Cosmet. Toxicol.* **10**:61.

Todd, P.J. 1921. Some practical points in the surgical treatment of cervical tumours. *Chin. Med. J.* **35**:21.

Topley, M. 1973. Cultural and social factors relating to Chinese infant feeding and weaning. In *Growing up in Hong Kong* (eds., C.E. Field and F.M. Barber), p. 56. Hong Kong University Press, Hong Kong.

Wasserman, A.E., W. Fiddler, R.C. Doerr, S.F. Osman, and C.J. Dooley. 1972. Dimethylnitrosamines in frankfurters. *Food Cosmet. Toxicol.* **10**:681.

Yang, C.S. 1980. Research on esophageal cancer in China, a review. *Cancer Res.* **40**:2633.

Nitrosamines and Other Etiological Factors in the Esophageal Cancer in Northern China

CHUNG S. YANG
Department of Biochemistry
University of Medicine and Dentistry of New Jersey
New Jersey Medical School
Newark, New Jersey 07103

Cancer of the esophagus is not a common disease in most Western countries but is widely occurring in many developing countries. The largest population group that is at high risk to this cancer is in the Taihang Mountain range area in northern China. The national annual mortality rates of esophageal cancer (EC) in China are 19.60 and 9.85/100,000 for males and females, respectively (Li et al. 1980; Yang 1980). EC accounts for 22.34% of the total cancer deaths, ranking second in prevalence below stomach cancer (23.03%) and above liver cancer (15.08%). In Linxian and several other nearby counties in the provinces of Henan, Hebei, and Shanxi, the mortality rate is above 100/100,000. As is the case with many high incidence areas, the male to female ratio of EC incidence is low, 1.6, in this area. Extensive research work has been performed during the past 15 years. The results indicate that smoking or drinking is not an etiological factor. The cancer is believed to be closely related to environmental and dietary factors (Li et al. 1980; Yang 1980). This belief is also supported by the discovery of pharyngeal and esophageal cancers in chickens (CICAMS 1976) who share the same environment and dietary sources with the population. In the effort to identify the causative factors, nitrosamines and their precursors have received a great deal of attention.

NITROGENOUS COMPOUNDS IN DRINKING WATER

In the mountainous regions of Linxian and other areas, water supply has historically been a serious problem. Traditionally the majority of people in Linxian relied on water from "dry wells" or man-made ponds which were used to collect rain water for use throughout the year. The water was said to be infested with microorganisms and frequently contaminated with refuse from human and domestic animals. Water was also stored in the home for several days for family use in large ceramic jars (known as "gang") which were not cleaned often. It has been observed that the nitrite content in "dry well" and pond water was much higher than in spring and well water. In certain cases, the

Table 1
Nitrate and Nitrite Contents in Well Water[a]

Season	Nitrates (mg/l)	Nitrites (mg/l)
Spring	12.33 ± 1.20	0.021 ± 0.021
Summer	12.65 ± 6.09	0.052 ± 0.101
Autumn	8.39 ± 3.20	0.036 ± 0.060
Winter	8.84 ± 3.56	0.047 ± 0.030

[a]Water samples were taken during 1976-1977 from 495 wells in 49 production brigades of Yaocun Commune (annual EC mortality rate 187.85/100,000) in Linxian, Henan. Results are expressed as mean ± S.D.

source of water has been considered as an important factor in determining the incidence rate of EC (TPTRGHP 1977). In a study in 1976 and 1977, nitrates and nitrites were found in most drinking water samples (CICAMS 1978). The average concentrations of nitrates and nitrites for the year were 10.55 (0-75) and 0.039 (0-2.63) mg/liter, respectively. The concentration was especially high in the summer with averages of 12.65 and 0.052 mg/liter for nitrates and nitrites, respectively (Table 1). In the 49 brigades surveyed, using the brigade as a unit, the average concentrations of nitrates and nitrites in well water were reported to have a positive correlation with the incidence rates of carcinoma and marked epithelial hyperplasia of the esophagus. Moreover, the nitrites in drinking water were found to increase during storage or heating (Table 2). They could reach 0.5-0.7 mg/liter in stored warm water or in gruel. In families with EC patients, the average nitrite nitrogen in "gang" water (29 samples) was 0.106 mg/liter and the ammonia-ammonium nitrogen content was 0.567 mg/liter, 7 and 30 times higher, respectively, than samples from families with no EC patients (TPTRGHP 1978). Contamination by microorganisms has been suspected as the reason for the high nitrite and ammonia contents in water. This type of correlation study is very interesting. More extensive studies with better analytic tools and sampling methods would be extremely useful in elucidating the roles of nitrosamines in this human cancer.

Table 2
Increase in the Nitrite Concent of Drinking Water During Storage[a]

Sample	Nitrite content (mg/l)	
	I	II
Well water	0	0.004 (109)
"Gang" water	0.074 ± 0.25 (60)	0.014 (129)
Warm water in iron pots	0.512 ± 0.74 (135)	
Gruel	0.695 ± 1.38 (76)	

Studies I and II are two different surveys.
[a]The results are expressed as mean ± S.D. (number of samples).

Table 3
Salivary Nitrites of Inhabitants in Linxian and Xinyangxian

Subject	Salivary nitrites (mg/l)
I.[a] Normal	3.17 ± 3.23 (45)
Mild epithelial hyperplasia	4.50 ± 4.20 (43)
Marked epithelial hyperplasia	6.00 ± 6.60 (33)
Cancer	5.06 ± 5.50 (38)
II.[b] Normal, Linxian	4.57 ± 4.80 (216)
Normal, Xinyangxian	5.74 ± 6.30 (51)

Results are expressed as mean ± S.D. (numbers of subjects).
[a]Study I dealt with subjects from Linxian who were grouped according to lesions of the esophagus.
[b]Study II dealt with normal subjects from Linxian (high EC incidence area) and Xinyangxian (low EC incidence area). Data, reprinted with permission, from Li et al. (1980).

Nitrates and nitrites were detected in human gastric juice and saliva in Linxian (Table 3). The salivary nitrites in patients with marked epithelial hyperplasia or carcinoma of the esophagus were significantly higher than the normal controls (CICAMS 1978). The salivary nitrite contents of persons in Linxian, however, were not higher than those in Xinyangxian, a low incidence area of EC.

There are preliminary reports concerning the presence of nitrosamines in drinking water, but the result remains to be confirmed. One possible complication in this work is the possible presence of a trace amount of dimethylnitrosamine (NDMA) in the solvent (methylene chloride) used.

NITROSAMINES AND THEIR PRECURSORS IN FOOD SAMPLES

Food samples from Linxian (high-incidence area of EC) and Fanxian (low-incidence area of EC), both in Henan Province, were analyzed for nitrosamines by thin layer chromatography (TLC) (LRTPTEC 1978a). The samples analyzed were wheat, corn, millet, rice, millet bran, dried sweet potato, and vegetables (Table 4). Of the 124 food samples from Linxian, 29 were "positive" in the nitrosamine assay, whereas only one out of 86 samples from Fanxian was positive. The presence of NDMA and diethylnitrosamine (NDEA) in some of the food samples was confirmed by gas chromatography (GC). Levels of secondary amines, nitrites, and nitrates in 7 varieties of grain and vegetable samples from these counties were also compared (Table 5). The samples from Linxian generally contained more nitrites and secondary amines than the corresponding samples from Fanxian. Such a difference, however, was not observed in the nitrate content (LRTPTEC 1978b). These samples had been oven-dried before the analysis. It is known that the nitrite content of vegetable samples changes drastically during storage. It would be useful if the actual dietary intake of nitrites, nitrates, and secondary amines could be measured in future studies.

Table 4

Nitrosamines in Food Samples[a]

	Linxian		Fanxian	
Sample	sample number	positive	sample number	positive
Eggplant	9	0	6	0
Pumpkin	9	0	6	0
Dried sweet potato	16	0	14	0
Wheat	20	6	14	0
Corn	22	10	13	1
Millet	19	4	14	0
Rice with hull	14	2	10	0
Bran of millet	15	7	9	0
Total	124	29	86	1

[a]Samples were collected during August 1972 and May 1973, analyzed by TLC and sprayed for nitrosamines.

Table 5

Contents of Nitrites and Secondary Amines in Food Samples[a]

	Nitrites		Secondary amines	
Sample	Linxian	Fanxian	Linxian	Fanxian
Eggplant	90.20 (9)	27.60 (6)	3.08 (9)	2.44 (6)
Pumpkin	29.33 (9)	17.66 (6)	2.12 (11)	1.59 (6)
Corn	2.44 (18)	2.18 (14)	1.82 (20)	2.12 (13)
Rice with hull	0.68 (8)	0.74 (7)	1.90 (14)	1.59 (12)
Millet	3.32 (18)	1.33 (15)	1.54 (17)	1.54 (12)
Dried sweet potato	3.55 (14)	3.05 (14)	2.66 (14)	1.71 (17)
Wheat	2.78 (29)	1.85 (11)	1.83 (19)	1.11 (14)

[a]Samples were collected during August 1972 to May 1973 from Linxian (high-EC incidence area) and Fanxian (low-EC incidence area). Data are expressed in mg/kg "dry weight" with sample numbers in parentheses.

PICKLED VEGETABLES

Pickled vegetables have traditionally been a popular food in some high-EC incidence areas in China. They were prepared each autumn by placing chopped, blanched Chinese cabbage, turnip leaves, soybean leaves, sweet potato leaves, sesame leaves, and other vegetables in a large ceramic container. The vegetables were pressed, covered with water, and allowed to ferment for several months. The products were usually covered with white mold. The vegetables and juice were consumed either uncooked or cooked in gruel. In some families, the pickled vegetables were eaten daily for as long as 9-12 months a year as an important part of the diet. Using the commune as a unit, a positive correlation between EC-mortality rate and the frequency of pickle consumption was found in 1973. That is, in communes where more people ate pickled vegetables or ate pickled vegetables for a greater portion of the year, the EC-mortality rates were higher (CICAMS 1977). In order to study the carcinogenicity of this substance, the extracts and concentrated liquid of pickled vegetables from Linxian were fed to Wistar rats. Among 29 rats fed for 330-730 days, one developed adenocarcinoma of the glandular stomach, one had angioendothelioma of the thoracic wall, four had fibrosarcoma of the liver, and many had epithelial dysplasia lesions in the esophagus and the forestomach. No tumors were noted in the 10 control rats (Li et al. 1980). Mice fed intragastrically with concentrated fluid of pickles developed papillomas in the forestomach after 143 days of treatment (Li et al. 1980). The extract of the pickled vegetables was mutagenic in *Salmonella typhimurium* TA100 and TA98 (Takahashi et al. 1979; Lu et al. 1981). It induced mutations in V79 cells and increased sister chromatid exchanges in V79 cells and Syrian hamster embryo cells. The extract also induced transformed foci in Syrian hamster embryo cells and in 3-methylcholanthrene initiated C3H/10T1/2 cells (Cheng et al. 1980). The active principles of the extract have not been identified. No nitrosamine has been isolated, but a nitroso compound, Roussin's red methyl ester, has been isolated from the ethereal extract of pickled vegetables. This compound is a weak mutagen for tester strain TA100 but not a mutagen for TA98. In experiments with mice, Roussin's red, when administered ig induced epithelial hyperplasia of the esophagus and forestomach and papilloma of the forestomach in 194-269 days (Li et al. 1980).

FORMATION OF NITROSAMINES IN MOLDY FOOD

In areas where EC is prevalent, foodstuffs are frequently contaminated with fungi. The most common species are *Fusarium moniliforme, Geotrichum candidum, Aspergillus versicolor, A. flavus, Penicillium chrysogenum,* and *Cladosporium herbarum.* In order to simulate these conditions, steamed corn bread was kept at room temperature or 26-30° for 3-5 days. The corn bread usually became moldy. During this process, the concentration of secondary amines increased fourfold and the contents of nitrates and nitrites also rose (Miao et al. 1978b). Furthermore, nitrosamines were detected in the stomach contents of rats fed moldy corn bread, but not in those fed unmoldy corn bread (Miao et al. 1978b). Inoculating cornmeal with pure cultures of several strains of fungi isolated from grains in Linxian also increased the nitrite and secondary amine contents as well as the synthesis of nitrosamines (Miao et al. 1978a,b). The greatest increase in the content of secondary amines, 17-fold, was with *F. moniliforme.* When sodium nitrite was added to the moldy corn bread, NDMA, NDEA, and methylbenzylnitrosamine (NMBA) were produced (Table 6) (Li et

Table 6
Nitrosamines in Fungi Infested Corn Bread after Nitrosation[a]

Fungi	TLC		GC-MS				
	Number of experiments	Positive	Number of experiments	NDMA	NDEA	NMBA	MAMBNA
Fusarium moniliforme Sheld	39	34	27	1	0	2	24
Aspergillus flavus Link	9	6	3	1	2	0	0
A. Terreus Thom	4	4	2	0	0	0	2
A. niger v. Tiegh	2	2	2	1	1	0	0
Geotrichum candidum Link	1	1	1	0	0	0	1
Mixed fungi[b]	4	4	4	2	2	0	0
Control	10	1	1	1	0	0	0

[a]$NaNO_2$ (1 mg/g) was added to the corn bread sample after 8 days of incubation with fungi.
[b]Mixed fungi: *F. moniliforme* Sheld, *A. flavus* Link, *A. niger v.* Tiegh, *Penicillium cyclopium* Westl., and *P. oxalicum* Currie et Thom. (from Li et al. 1980).

al. 1979). A new compound, N-1-methylacetonyl-N-3-methylbutylnitrosamine (MAMBNA), was found to be present at 0.2-0.3 ppm (Lu et al. 1979). It is mutagenic to *S. typhimurium* strains TA1535 and TA100 (Lu et al. 1980). The carcinogenicity of this nitrosamine is under active investigation. Papillomas of the forestomach were induced in mice fed N-1-methylacetonyl-N-3-methylbutylamine together with $NaNO_2$ for 5 months (Li et al. 1980).

CARCINOGENICITY OF FUNGAL PRODUCTS

In order to investigate the carcinogenicity of fungi, cultured *G. candidum* Link, a fungus found in most pickled vegetables in Linxian, was fed to rats and mice. After 20 months, epithelial dysplasia and precancerous lesions of the forestomach were found in a large percentage of rats and mice. Nevertheless, only a few cases of epithelial dysplasia and precancerous lesions of the esophagus were found.

In other studies, cornmeal was inoculated with fungi and incubated at 26°C for 6-8 days. The moldy cornmeal was mixed with uncontaminated cornmeal and fed to Wistar rats. *F. poae (peck)* Wr. infested cornmeal was found to induce papillomas of the stomach, carcinoma of the forestomach, and other cancers; whereas, *A. flavus* Link infested cornmeal did not induce any tumor (Liu et al. 1978). Cornmeal infested by *F. moniliforme* with or without the addition of $NaNO_2$ was found to induce papillomas, early carcinomas, and squamous cell carcinoma of the forestomach and tumors on several different tissues. Carcinoma of the esophagus was not observed, but epithelial hyperplasia of the esophagus was induced (Li et al. 1980; Liu et al. 1978). The possible synergism between moldy food and nitrosamines has also been studied. In a preliminary study, NMBA was given at a dosage of 0.75 mg/kg/day to 30 rats maintained on fungi-infested cornmeal. After 176 days, about 65% of the rats developed esophageal carcinoma as compared to 15% of the control group with unmoldy cornmeal (TRTRGHP 1975). These studies suggest that fungal contamination can be an important factor in carcinogenesis. The results, however, may not be solely due to nitrosamines. The involvement of mycotoxin is also worth considering.

NUTRITIONAL FACTORS

Diet and nutrition have been implicated as contributing factors to EC in many parts of the world (Warwick 1973). The lack of fresh fruits and vegetables or deficiencies in vitamin A, riboflavin, and ascorbate have been suggested as a common feature for high-risk populations. Even in economically developed countries, nutritional deficiency is also found among high-EC risk subpopulations; for example, the urban black males in the United States (Ziegler et al. 1981). The diet in Linxian, and probably in other high-EC incidence areas of China, is extremely simple, consisting mainly of grains and tubers such as corn,

Table 7
Food Allowance of Peasants in Chengguan Commune, Linxian, Henan[a]

Food	Average	Range
Cereals[b]	564	369-762
Sweet potatoes	496	127-1187
Legumes, dried	15	0-51
Vegetables[c]	685	353-1141
Fruits	2.1	0-21
Nuts	1.0	0-16.6
Pork	4.2	2.1-8.3
Vegetable oil	3.3	0.2-7.8

[a]Data are expressed as g/day/person. They were obtained in 1980 from 18 production teams in 15 brigades with a total population of 3491.
[b]Wheat, corn, millet, and rice amount to 46, 43, 9, and 2%, respectively.
[c]Mainly Chinese cabbage, radishes, pumpkins, and eggplants.

wheat, millet, rice, sweet potato, and some seasonal vegetables (Table 7). The diet is extremely low in animal products and fat. Consumption of vegetables and fruits is low. It was estimated that 80% of the calories was from grains, 12% from tubers, 7% from beans and other plant products, and less than 1% from animal products. Of the total caloric intake, 81% was from carbohydrates, 11% from proteins, and 8% from fats. Only 0.5% of the protein and 9% of the fat were from animal sources. Food preparation is very simple. Often, a pot of millet gruel containing some vegetables is simmered for hours on a coal stove. This is usually the sole food for a meal.

As shown in Table 8, the supply of calories and protein was marginal. Lower levels of ascorbate intake and deficiencies in calcium and riboflavin were indicated. In a survey carried out in 1980, the average plasma retinol level of the adults was 0.27 μg/ml with about 20% of the individuals having levels

Table 8
Energy and Nutrient Allowance (Daily per Person)[a]

Energy[b]	2835 kcal	Iron	24.6 mg
Protein[c]	73 g	Carotene	9.12 mg
Fat	28 g	Thiamine	3.13 mg
Carbohydrate	573 g	Riboflavin	0.96 mg
Calcium	0.56 g	Niacin	17.3 mg
Phosphorus	1.71 g	Ascorbate	51 mg

[a]Calculated from the result of the same survey shown in Table 7.
[b]Sources: cereals, 70.6%; sweet potato, 21.5%; dried legumes, 2.0%; vegetables 3.9%; animal products, 0.9%; refined carbohydrates, 1.1%.
[c]Sources: cereals, 71.9%; dry legumes, 6.1%; vegetables, 21.4%; animal products, 0.6%.

< 0.2 µg/ml (Yang et al. 1982). The average plasma ascorbate level was 5.7 µg/ml with about 23% of the individuals having levels < 2.0 µg/ml. The results indicate that a portion of the population has a low or marginal nutritional status with regard to these two vitamins. Retinoids have been suggested to inhibit the promotion phase of carcinogenesis and probably also tumor cell growth (Sporn and Newton 1979). Ascorbate is known to inhibit the possible in vivo formation of nitrosamine via nitrosation (Mirvish et al. 1972). This aspect is of special importance in Linxian because the dietary intake of nitrites and secondary amines can be rather high. Almost 90% of the people surveyed had a glutathione reductase activation coefficient > 1.2 indicating a widely occurring riboflavin deficiency. The effect of riboflavin deficiency on carcinogenesis remains to be investigated. Riboflavin deficiency together with iron deficiency has been implicated in Plummer-Vinson disease which bears a correlation with EC (Wynder and Bross 1961; Larson et al. 1975). It has been demonstrated in animals that riboflavin deficiency enhanced liver carcinogenesis by azo dyes (Griffin and Bauman 1948; Mulay and O'Gara 1968). During recovery from riboflavin deficiency, mice are more prone to skin tumor induction by 7,12-dimethyl-benz[a]anthracene (Wynder and Chan 1970).

Riboflavin is a precursor of flavin mononucleotide (FMN) and flavin adenine dinucleotide (FAD) which are coenzymes of NADPH-cytochrome P-450 reductase. Being a component enzyme of the mixed-function oxidase system, this enzyme plays key roles in the activation and detoxification of carcinogens. Generally, the deficiency would decrease the oxidase activity and a low rate of hepatic metabolism may prolong the biological half-life of an esophageal carcinogen, thus increasing the exposure of the target tissue to the carcinogen. A low protein diet is also expected to have such an effect. In an agrarian society like Linxian, riboflavin deficiency is expected to be more severe in winter than in the growing seasons. There are possible mechanisms by which a seasonal or cyclic deficiency may enhance carcinogenesis. Recovery from riboflavin deficiency may cause a temporary "overshoot" of mixed-function oxidase system above the normal level (Yang 1974). This may enhance carcinogen activation in the esophagus. The changes in the rate of cell proliferation during the deficiency and recovery states may also enhance the initiation or progression phase of carcinogenesis. These possibilities are being tested in my laboratory. Alternatively, nutritional deficiency may also increase the rate of carcinogenesis by affecting the immunosurveillance or DNA repair systems. Although nutritional deficiency can be an important contributing factor to the high-EC incidence in Linxian, it is probably not the primary causative factor of the cancer because similar nutritional deficiencies can also be observed in some low incidence areas.

CONCLUDING REMARKS

Some of the possible primary causative and contributing factors to the EC in the high incidence areas in northern China are summarized in Figure 1. Nitros-

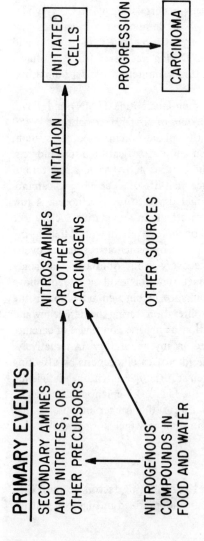

Figure 1
Primary events and contributing factors in esophageal cancer.

amines are the primary suspects in causing the cancer. Nitrosamines can be synthesized either in vivo or in vitro from secondary amines and nitrites. Both precursors can be derived from nitrogenous compounds in food and water through the action of fungi or other microorganisms. Low molybdenum content in the soil may be an indirect contributing factor because it increases the amount of nitrates (nitrites) in crops and decreases the vitamin C content in vegetables. Nutritional deficiencies may be an important factor in enhancing carcinogenesis. Polycyclic hydrocarbons may play a role as cocarcinogens or promoters. Poor oral hygiene and undesirable eating habits may enhance carcinogenesis by increasing microbial production of nitrites or nitrosamines (Hsia et al. 1981) and by continuously injuring the epithelium of the esophagus. Although fungal infection is not a prerequisite for EC, the fungi may contribute to carcinogenesis by producing carcinogens or promoters at the infection sites or by inducing hyperplasia. Defects in the DNA repair and immune defense mechanisms may also increase the susceptibility to cancer. The roles of these factors in EC remain to be elucidated.

In conclusion, although nitrosamines are the most probable carcinogens for EC in northern China, there is not enough evidence to firmly establish this. It is very important to continue studying the nitrosamines and other carcinogenic factors in the environment. More definitive data may be obtained now because the research environment and methodology have improved. At the same time, the diet and living standards of the peasants are changing. It would be useful to collect data at different time periods so that changes in dietary carcinogens and nutritional status may be correlated with changes in the incidence rate of EC in the future.

ACKNOWLEDGMENTS

I thank the colleagues in the esophageal cancer research groups in Beijing and Henan who made their results available to me. This work was supported by the International Union Against Cancer, U.S. National Academy of Sciences (Research in China Program), and U.S. National Cancer Institute Grant CA-16788.

REFERENCES

Cheng, S.-J., M. Sala, M.-X. Li, M.-Y. Wang, J. Pot-Deprun, and I. Chouroulinkov. 1980. Mutagenic, transforming and promoting effect of pickled vegetables from Linxian, China. *Carcinogenesis* 1:685.

CICAMS (Cancer Institute of the Chinese Academy of Medical Sciences). 1978. *Collection of research papers 1958-1978* (in Chinese), p. 63 and p. 70, Beijing, China.

CICAMS, Department of Epidemiology and other research groups. 1977. Preliminary investigation of the epidemiological factors of esophageal cancer in China. *Res. Cancer Prev. Treat.* 2:1.

CICAMS, Department of Pathology. 1976. Epidemiological and pathological morphology of pharyngeal and esophageal cancers in domestic fowls. *Acta Zool. Sin.* 22(4):319.

Griffin, A.C. and C.A. Bauman. 1948. Hepatic riboflavin and tumor formation in rats fed azo dyes in various diets. *Cancer Res.* 8:279.

Hsia, C.-C, T.-T. Sun, Y.-Y. Wang, L.M. Anderson, D. Armstrong, and R.A. Good. 1981. Enhancement of formation of the esophageal carcinogen benzylmethylnitrosamine from its precursor by *Candida albicans. Proc. Natl. Acad. Sci. U.S.A.* 78:1878.

Larson, L., A. Sandstrom, and P. Westling. 1975. Relationship of Plummer-Vinson disease to cancer of the upper alimentary tract in Sweden. *Cancer Res.* 35:3308.

Li, M.-X., P. Li, and B.-R. Li. 1980. Recent progress in research on esophageal cancer in China. *Adv. Cancer Res.* 33:173.

Li, M.-X., S.-X. Lu, C. Ji, M.-Y. Wang, S.-J. Cheng, and C.-L. Jin. 1979. Formation of carcinogenic N-nitroso compounds in corn-bread inoculated with fungi. *Sci. Sin.* 22:471.

Liu, G.-T., C. Miao, Y.-Z. Zhen, J.-Z. Zhang, and others. 1978. Studies on the relationship between fungi and cancer. *Med. Ref.* (Special issue on Cancer) (2):27 and 34.

LRTPTEC (Linxian Research Team for the Prevention and Treatment of Esophageal Cancer). 1978a. Nitrosamines and related compounds in food from Linxian and Fanxian. In *CICAMS Collection of research papers 1958-1978*, p. 38. Cancer Institute of the Chinese Academy of Medical Sciences, Beijing, China.

―――. 1978b. Secondary amines, nitrites, and nitrates in food samples of Linxian and Fanxian. In *CICAMS Collection of research papers 1958-1978*, p. 46. Cancer Institute of the Chinese Academy of Medical Sciences. Beijing, China.

Lu, S.-H., A.-M. Camus, L. Tomatis, and H. Bartsch. 1981. Mutagenicity of extracts of pickled vegetables collected in Linxian, a high-incidence area for esophageal cancer in northern China. *J. Natl. Canc. Inst.* 66:33.

Lu, S.-H., A.-M. Camus, C. Ji, Y.-L. Wang, M.-Y. Wang, and H. Bartsch. 1980. Mutagenicity in *Salmonella typhimurium* of N-3-methylbutyl-N-1-methyl-acetonylnitrosamine and N-methyl-N-benzylnitrosamine, N-nitrosation products isolated from corn-bread contaminated with commonly occurring moulds in Linxian, a high incidence area for esophageal cancer in Northern China. *Carcinogenesis* 1:867.

Lu, S.-X., M.-X. Li, C. Ji, M.-Y. Wang, Y.-L. Wang, and L. Huang. 1979. A new N-nitroso compound, N-3-methylbutyl-N-1-methylacetonyl-nitrosamine, in corn-bread inoculated with fungi. *Sci. Sin.* 22:601.

Miao, C., M. Guang, and G.T. Liu. 1978b. Relationship between fungi and nitrosamines: 1. Mold growth on foods. *Med. Ref.* (Special issue on cancer) (2):39.

Miao, C., F.-C. Guo, J.-Z. Zhang, G.-T. Liu, Y.-Z. Zhen, T.-J. Wei, and G.-Y Feng. 1978a. Relationship between fungi and nitrosamines: 2. The action of fungi isolated from grains in Linxian. *Med. Ref.* (Special issue on Cancer) (2):46.

Mirvish, S.S., L. Wallcave, M. Eagen, and P. Shubik. 1972. Ascorbate-nitrite reaction: Possible means of blocking the formation of carcinogenic N-nitroso compounds. *Science* **177**:65.

Mulay, A.S. and R.W. O'Gara. 1968. Enhancing effects of a riboflavin analog on azo-dye carcinogenesis in rats. *J. Natl. Cancer Inst.* **40**:731.

Sporn, M.B. and D.L. Newton. 1979. Chemoprevention of cancer with retinoids. *Fed. Proc.* **38**:2528.

TPTRGHP (Tumor Prevention, Treatment, and Research Group of Henan Province). 1975. Studies on the relationship between fungi and esophageal cancer. *Res. Cancer Prev. Treat.* (3):201.

TPTRGHP and other research groups. 1977. Determination of nitrate, nitrite, ammonia, and organic matters in Linxian of Henan Province. *Anti-cancer Commun.* (December):13.

———. 1978. Nitrogenous compounds in the drinking water of Chengguan Commune in Linxian. *Med. Ref.* (special issue on Cancer) (7):6.

Takahashi, Y., M. Nagao, T. Fujimo, Z. Yamaizumi, and T. Sugimura. 1979. Mutagens in Japanese pickle identified as Flavonoids. *Mutat. Res.* **68**:117.

Warwick, G.P. 1973. Some aspects of the epidemiology and etiology of esophageal cancer with particular emphasis on the Transkei, South Africa. *Adv. Cancer Res.* **17**:81.

Wynder, E.L. and I.J. Bross. 1961. A study of etiological factors in cancer of the esophagus. *Cancer* **14**:389.

Wynder, E.L. and P.C. Chan. 1970. The possible role of riboflavin deficiency in epithelial neoplasia. II. Effect of skin tumor development. *Cancer* **26**:1221.

Yang, C.S. 1974. Alterations of the aryl hydrocarbon hydroxylase system during riboflavin depletion and repletion. *Arch. Biochem. Biophys.* **160**:623.

———. 1980. Research on esophageal cancer in China: A review. *Cancer Res.* **40**:2633.

Yang, C.S., J. Miao, W.-X. Yang, M. Hung, T.-Y. Wang, H.-J. Xue, S.-H. You, J.-B. Lu, and J.-M. Wu. 1982. Diet and vitamin nutrition of the high esophageal cancer risk population in Linxian, China. *Nutr. Cancer* **4** (in press).

Ziegler, R.G., L.E. Morris, W.J. Blot, L.M. Pottern, R. Hoover, and J.F. Fraumeni. 1981. Esophageal cancer among Black men in Washington, D.C. II. Role of nutrition. *J. Natl. Cancer Inst.* **67**:1199.

COMMENTS

HOFFMANN: How do you determine secondary amines? Is this the nitrosatable portion?

YANG: A colorimetric method was used for the determination of secondary amines.

LIJINSKY: Dr. Singer in my laboratory has tried, using Chinese cornmeal, to repeat some of this, and he found that the chances of artifacts are very high. In fact, the values of NDEA, for example, he found are possibly 100 times lower than have been reported from China, using the same sort of cornmeal. I wonder how reliable some of these data are. I am not saying that ours are reliable either, but I am—

YANG: I think they had their share of artifacts in China also, since they did not have much resource for research. One possibility is that the cornmeal is different.

LIJINSKY: We got Chinese cornmeal since the American cornmeal is different (it is mold-resistant).

YANG: Another factor that I think is very important is that the situation is changing. Dr. S.-X. Lu has repeated some of the early experiments. Even with similar types of samples, and the same type of procedure, some of the contents of nitrosamines and nitrite are decreased. Therefore, this is a very difficult problem to resolve.

HARRIS: What mycotoxins have been identified?

YANG: I don't know of any. Dr. M.-X. Li is actively working in that area, but they haven't identified any specific compound yet.

CHALLIS: Did you say that some of the foods were oven-dried before analysis?

YANG: Yes, for the nitrite determination.

CHALLIS: Do you know how that oven was heated? Gas, coal, electric?

YANG: Coal or gas, probably.

CHALLIS: I wonder whether those results mean anything. There is quite a bit of evidence that direct drying processes add nitrogen oxides and then nitrite.

YANG: That is quite possible, yet there were differences between the samples from the high- and low-incidence areas.

HOFFMANN: You said riboflavin plays a role?

YANG: I am speculating that riboflavin might play a role, because we can postulate several mechanisms by which riboflavin deficiency might enhance carcinogenesis.

HOFFMANN: When riboflavin was deficient, did you see this type of cancer more in women than in men?

YANG: No, that is not the case. There was a correlation in the Plummer-Vinson disease in Swedish women only.

In animal studies, azo dye carcinogenesis is known to be enhanced by riboflavin deficiency. Drs. Wynder and Chan have shown that in the DMBA initiated skin carcinogenesis in mice, the incidence was enhanced if DMBA was applied during the recovery period. We are working on animal model systems to test the hypothesis that riboflavin deficiency may enhance the carcinogenicity of nitrosamines in the esophagus.

Gastric Cancer: An Etiologic Model

GAIL CHARNLEY AND STEVEN R. TANNENBAUM
Department of Nutrition and Food Science
Massachusetts Institute of Technology
Cambridge, Massachusetts 02139

PELAYO CORREA
Department of Pathology
Louisiana State University Medical Center
New Orleans, Louisiana 70112

Gastric cancer, while declining in recent years, remains a significant cause of death in a number of areas in the world. As recently as a few decades ago, gastric carcinoma was near the top of the list in the United States for lethal cancers; it now ranks fifth as a cause of cancer deaths (U.S. Dept. of Health and Human Services 1981). Incidence rates (new cases per year) exceed death rates by only 11%, due to the high mortality from the disease; in fact, only roughly 5% of patients survive for 5 years. Countries reporting high incidence rates include Japan, Chile, the USSR, Austria, Finland, Iceland, Israel, several other countries in central and eastern Europe, and Costa Rica; the lowest incidence rates were recorded in the United States, Australia, Canada, and New Zealand (Logan 1976). Cancer of the stomach preceded that of the lung as the leading cause of death from cancer among males in Chile, Japan, Italy, Norway, Portugal, and Sweden. Among females, stomach cancer preceded breast cancer as the leading cause of cancer mortality in Chile, Japan, Austria, Finland, Federal Republic of Germany, Italy, and Portugal. It is clear that gastric carcinoma, though little publicized and therefore not in the public limelight, is a significant cause of death in many areas of the world.

Race by itself does not explain this geographic distribution. Sedentary Japanese have several times the incidence rate of people of Japanese extraction living in Hawaii, especially the second generation. Whites in eastern and northern Europe have considerably higher rates than whites in New Zealand and the United States. Chinese in Singapore have incidence rates approximately five times greater than those of Chinese in Hawaii. Blacks in Jamaica and Louisiana have rates much higher than those of African blacks.

These observations clearly indicate that the disease is determined mostly by the environment and not by the race of the population. Since the geographic environment per se is ruled out, it seems that the cultural environment is the one that matters. The most obvious component of the cultural environment is the diet, which may explain the interpopulation distribution.

There have been many attempts to characterize the diets of populations at high gastric cancer risk and of patients with gastric cancer (Haenszel and Correa 1975). No individual food item has been found to be universally associated with gastric cancer. This probably should have been anticipated when considering dietary habits in high-risk areas as dissimilar as those of England, Finland, Japan, Iceland, Hawaii, and Latin America. The similarities among these diets can only be described in general terms. Most diets associated with high gastric cancer risk have the following characteristics (Correa and Tannenbaum 1981):

1. They are low in animal fat and animal protein
2. They are high in complex carbohydrates
3. They obtain a substantial part of their proteins from vegetable sources, mostly grains
4. They are low in salads and fresh, green, leafy vegetables
5. They are low in fresh fruits, especially citrus
6. They are high in salt content

Exactly how this type of diet predisposes to gastric cancer has not been determined. Its high bulk obviously influences the gastric microenvironment, and its low fat content probably interferes with the absorption of lipid-soluble substances such as vitamin A and vitamin E. The scarcity of fresh, green, leafy vegetables and of citrus fruits may also indicate some vitamin deficiencies. The high salt content may damage the mucous barrier that protects the mucosa from food items as well as from the acid-pepsin secretions.

There are many populations in the world with high bulk diets and low gastric cancer rates. In some populations such as Finland, the gastric cancer rate has been steadily declining without apparently drastic changes in the bulk or the vegetable content of the diet. The epidemiologic observations suggest that in some populations a protective factor is being added to the diet.

Another ingested substance which has been linked to the diet is nitrate (Hartman 1982). It has been found that in some, but not all, populations at high gastric cancer risk the ingestion of nitrates in the food and drinking water is higher than in similar populations with lower risk (Cuello et al. 1976). The correlation of nitrate intake and gastric cancer rates is not observed in some other populations. This is not unexpected since nitrate by itself has not been implicated in carcinogenesis. Nitrate is reduced to nitrite in the saliva and may then be ingested into the stomach. Ingested nitrate is probably not reduced to nitrite to any significant degree in the gastric cavities of normal individuals. In patients with chronic gastritis, however, a significant amount of nitrite is detected in the gastric juice, especially when the pH is above 5.

The role of dietary factors in the etiology of gastric cancer is obscure at this point; except for the apparent "protective" effect of some foods, no firm conclusions can be drawn from the available data. The interactions are no doubt subtle and complex, requiring substantial additional investigation to identify the common factors.

Wynder and coworkers (1963) presented a hypothesis which provides a possible explanation for the ability of carcinogens to penetrate the normally well protected gastric mucosa. They suggested that there are two levels of defense in the gastric mucosal cells: The first barrier is mucus, and the second defensive layer is the mature mucus-producing cells. Where gastric lesions are present, carcinogens which penetrate the mucus encounter a layer of primitive transition cells rather than the mature mucus-producing cells. Such conditions may allow a more facile carcinogenic transformation (Wynder et al. 1963).

The implications of this suggestion are several: Some agent or condition must exist which in some way reduces or eliminates the protective mucus layer that coats the gastric epithelium. A number of agents are known to have this effect, including hard grains and other physically abrasive agents, high salt concentrations, surfactants, drugs such as aspirin, and some acids. A carcinogen passing through the mucus layer (or in the absence of that layer) is then faced with a second defensive layer—the mature mucus-producing cells. In the case of a defective mucosa, however, such as in atrophic gastritis, ulceration, etc., this second defense is compromised, so that the carcinogen encounters primitive transitional cells, which may be more susceptible to the action of the carcinogen.

While this is a possible explanation for the ability of a carcinogen to reach the mucosa, it does not address the multitude of other questions posed by the gastric cancer problem. The causal significance of dietary components remains uncertain. Formation of an etiologic hypothesis for gastric carcinogenesis requires investigation and correlation of the microecology of the gastric mucosa, observations of the epidemiology of gastric cancer and the precancerous conditions which accompany it, as well as the identification of dietary carcinogens.

MULTISTAGE MODEL

Figure 1 depicts how pathological, biochemical, histopathological, and histochemical observations associated with gastric carcinogenesis may fit into the framework of a multistage model of carcinogenesis.

A multistage model of carcinogenesis suggests that for cancer to occur, there must be several changes, each of which is necessary but not sufficient to cause cancer. Normal cells may first undergo a process of "pre-initiation" or sensitization during which cellular proliferation is increased as a result of an injury or inflammatory reaction. Anti-inflammatory agents which prevent cell proliferation, such as dexamethasone, have been shown to inhibit experimental carcinogenesis (Slaga 1980). Proliferating cells may provide a suitable condition for a process of successful initiation of carcinogenesis to occur. Initiation is thought to be a process during which mutation of genetic material occurs to produce a heritable alteration in a cell's ability to control its own state of differentiation and proliferation. Initiation can be caused by modification of DNA by chemical carcinogens. A number of considerations support the view that DNA is a critical target of chemical carcinogens:

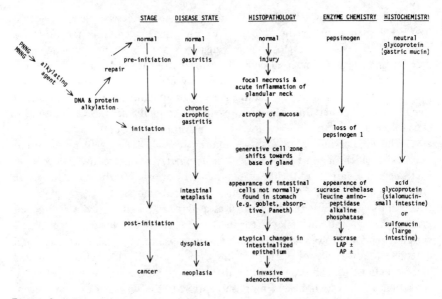

Figure 1
Continua of changes associated with the process of gastric carcinogenesis. (MNNG = *N*-methyl-*N'*-nitro-*N*-nitrosoguanidine; PNNG = *N*-propyl-*N'*-nitro-*N*-nitrosoguanidine)

1. Many carcinogens react covalently with DNA
2. Many carcinogens are also mutagens
3. Defects in DNA repair such as xeroderma pigmentosum predispose to cancer development
4. Most, if not all, cancers display chromosomal abnormalities and aberrant gene expression.

Once initiation has occurred, a process of "post-initiation" or cell selection occurs in which a successfully initiated cell becomes phenotypically expressed and proliferates to form a tumor. The characteristic features of cancer are such that normal pathways of terminal differentiation are blocked, and the cell is permitted to express altered phenotypes and increase mitosis, eventually multiplying logarithmically and becoming invasive. This post-initiation or promotional phase of carcinogenesis raises some basic questions with regard to an initiated or transformed cell's ability to express its neoplastic phenotype: First, how do initiated cells persist in tissues? This question is of particular importance in the gastrointestinal tract, which has a very high rate of cell turnover.

Secondly, what factors operate to keep dormant initiated cells from becoming overt tumors, and how are these factors modified during post-initiation, permitting tumors to appear? The ultimate fate of initiated cells appears to depend more on the combined influence of modifying agents, both endogenous and exogenous, than with chemical carcinogens themselves. In the case of gastric cancer, diet is an obvious candidate as a supplier of both initiating agents (via ingested chemicals) and modifying or promoting agents (e.g., dietary salt).

EPIDEMIOLOGY OF GASTRIC CANCER

Marked contrasts in the geographic distribution of gastric cancer incidence rates have been recognized for a long time. Figure 2 depicts the rank order of magnitude of the incidence rates for populations throughout the world (Correa and Tannenbaum 1981). The geographic distribution of areas of high gastric cancer risk (of the so-called epidemic or intestinal type) coincides with that of high risk for environmental chronic gastritis (Correa 1980). This type of gastritis is referred to as environmental as it is probably related to the diet (an important component of the environment) and is distinguished from the types of gastritis which accompany pernicious anemia or duodenal peptic ulcer. It is now recognized that environmental chronic gastritis and gastric carcinoma are part of the same etiologic complex (Correa 1980).

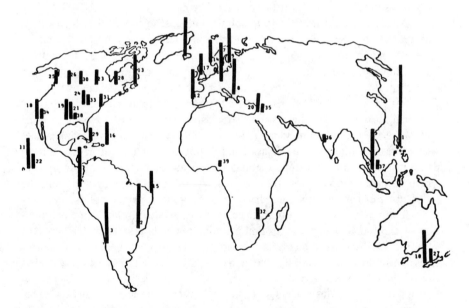

Figure 2
Map showing the ranks of the age-adjusted (world population) incidence rates for gastric cancer. The following regions are represented by more than one racial group: Singapore (Chinese rank 5, Malay rank 37); New Zealand (Maori rank 10, non-Maori rank 27); Hawaii (Japanese rank 11, Caucasian rank 22); California Bay area (black rank 18, white rank 34); New Mexico (Indian rank 19, Spanish rank 21, other white rank 38). Reprinted, with permission, from Correa and Tannenbaum (1981).

Many studies of populations at high gastric cancer risk in different parts of the world have focused on the role of chronic gastritis as a gastric cancer precursor (e.g., Nakahara 1978). The first evidence of injury to the gastric mucosa begins early in life, usually around the second decade. By the age of 20-25 years, those individuals who will later develop chronic gastritis already have histologic indications of the beginning of the process (Correa et al. 1976). In populations where gastric cancer is infrequent, the proportion of chronic gastritis is usually less than 20% while in high-risk populations that proportion is usually 70% or higher (Correa et al. 1976). Autopsy studies, for example, have shown that individuals who died from gastric cancer had an atrophic gastric mucosa significantly more frequently than did those who died of other causes (Guiss and Stewart 1943). A series of follow-up studies in Finland has revealed that of 116 patients with atrophic gastritis, 8% died of gastric cancer within 10-15 years, while none of the 261 matched controls died of gastric cancer in that time period (Siurala et al. 1966). If chronic atrophic gastritis precedes the development of gastric cancer, then the age of onset of atrophic gastritis may be highly significant (Chatterjee 1976). In the United States, chronic atrophic gastritis is very rare among persons under age 40 (Robbins 1974); in parts of Colombia, however, chronic atrophic gastritis is present in 50% of the people less than 40 years old (Correa et al. 1976).

A correlation of intestinal metaplasia with gastric cancer is also apparent. The natives of Java and Sumatra, for example, have a very low incidence of intestinal metaplasia, while their Chinese immigrant neighbors demonstrate a high incidence; similar differences are observed in concurrent rates of gastric cancer among these two groups (Bonne 1935). People in the highland areas of Colombia, who are at a high risk for gastric cancer, display a high incidence of intestinal metaplasia; on the coast, where gastric cancer rates are low, intestinal metaplasia is correspondingly rarer. Morson (1955) found foci of malignancies within areas of intestinal metaplasia, and estimated that 30% of gastric tumors develop from sites of intestinal metaplasia. Indeed, the areas of the stomach in which adenocarcinomas most frequently arise (i.e., the lesser curvature and the pyloric antrum) are also the most frequent sites of intestinal metaplasia.

It is worth mentioning that no sex differences were noted in the presentation of chronic atrophic gastritis and intestinal metaplasia, a result inconsistent with the twofold male excess in incidence of newly diagnosed gastric cancer cases. This raises the possibility that some transitional event may occur later that shows the same sex differential as that observed for gastric cancer incidence. Development of dysplastic changes in the metaplastic gastric mucosa is a possible candidate. This question has been studied in gastric biopsies from patients in Nariño, Colombia not suspected to have stomach cancer. The biopsies showed the prevalence of metaplasia with dysplastic changes to have the typical male preponderance found in case series (Cuello et al. 1979).

A crucial observation concerning the distribution of gastric cancer has been that populations migrating from a high-risk area (such as Russia, Norway,

Japan, and Latin America) to a low-risk area (such as the United States or Australia) keep their original high risk in the host country (Haenszel 1961). They continue to have high rates of incidence and mortality in spite of the fact that they live practically all of their adult lives in a country whose indigenous population displays low rates. This migration effect cannot be explained adequately by dietary patterns, and it has led to the idea that gastric cancer is the result of forces set in motion many years before cancer becomes clinically evident.

The Hawaiian Japanese, who exhibit two distinct food styles (Japanese and Western), present a situation particularly favorable for observation. Migrants from the high-risk Japanese prefectures continue to be at excess risk in Hawaii, though their offspring do not demonstrate this effect (Haenszel et al. 1972). These nativity distinctions are consistent with inferences from earlier reports on migrants with respect to the critical nature of exposures in childhood. The major diet effects for the Hawaiian Japanese were elevated stomach cancer risks for users of salt-pickled vegetables and dried/salted fish; a dose-response relationship was suggested by higher risks for users of larger amounts of these foods (Haenszel et al. 1972). Since no associations were found for raw fish and unprocessed vegetables, their methods of preparation appeared to be implicated. Low risks were also described for some vegetables (i.e., lettuce, celery, and corn) but the latter appeared to be independent of the findings for pickled Japanese foods, thus raising the possibility of protective effects. A companion case-control study conducted in Japan did not reproduce the elevated risks reported for the Hawaiian Japanese; presumably, the homogeneous background of food habits in early life operated against their detection (Haenszel et al. 1976). However, it is interesting to note that the controls in Japan did report greater frequency of use of lettuce, thus lending credence to the concept of protective food effects.

A marked inverse relationship exists between income and gastric cancer risk. In the United States, there is a 50% excess of stomach cancer incidence for the lowest socioeconomic classes relative to the highest classes (Dorn and Cutler 1959). This excess holds for whites and for nonwhites in this country. It is even more apparent in England (Haenszel 1958), and holds in Norway (Torgerson and Peterson 1956) and Denmark as well (Clemmeson and Nielsen 1951). These class differences do not appear to be due to inaccuracy of diagnosis or incompleteness of reporting; they seem to reflect real differences in incidence of the disease.

Urban excess, so pronounced in diseases linked to industrial causes, is slight, if not insignificant (Doll 1956). There appears to be a slight urban excess in this country, while in England and Wales, there is, if anything, a rural excess (Stocks 1947). Since gastric cancer rates reflect exposures early in life, urban-rural gradients mostly depend on the origins of people who migrate to cities. Migrants from rural areas will increase the risk of a city if they come from high risk areas but will decrease it if their homeland displays low risk.

Table 1

Gastric Cancer: Average Age-adjusted (1970 Standard) Annual Incidence Rate per 100,000 Population for Males Only, by Race

Location	All Races	Whites	Blacks	Other
Connecticut 1973-1977	14.7	14.3		
Detroit 1973-1977	15.1	14.1	20.5	
Iowa 1973-1977	10.1	10.1		
Atlanta 1975-1977	9.8	7.4	18.0	
New Orleans 1974-1977	15.0	9.8	29.0	
New Mexico 1973-1977	15.9	15.0		30.9 (American Indian)
Utah 1973-1977	10.4	10.1		
Seattle-Puget Sound 1974-1977	10.1	11.4		
San Francisco-Oakland 1973-1977	15.7	14.7	24.9	
Hawaii 1973-1977	30.2	15.6		51.4 (Hawaiian)
Puerto Rico 1973-1977	28.4			

Data from U.S. Dept. Health and Human Services

In the United States, the overall incidence rate of gastric cancer has been steadily declining (Everson 1969) and now ranks ninth in order of frequency among tumor sites (U.S. Dept. Health and Human Services 1981). However, variations among regions and races within a country make overall incidence rates deceptive. For example, Table 1 shows age-adjusted incidence rates of gastric cancer among males by race and for all races combined, for different locations throughout the U.S. It is clear that if only the incidence rates for whites or all races combined are considered, the two- to threefold greater incidence rates among blacks will be overlooked, along with the much higher rates for American Indians and Hawaiians. Table 2 shows incidence rates for gastric cancer for different populations in Los Angeles County. Blacks and Japanese have rates two and four times greater, respectively, than that of whites, while Hispanic immigrants have rates which increase relative to the more southerly location of their place of birth. Thus, while gastric cancer may not be a leading cause of death among white Americans, it is a greater problem for other ethnic groups within the United States.

Table 2

Gastric Cancer: Average Age-adjusted Annual Incidence Rate per 100,000 Population for Males Only, by Race, in Los Angeles County

Population	Incidence Rate
White	12
Spanish-surname (born in U.S. or Canada)	19
Mexican-born	24
Central American-born	34
South American-born	46
Black	23
Japanese	46

Data from S. Preston-Martin (pers. comm.)

DISEASE STATES

Observation of the natural history of gastric cancer in high-risk populations indicates that several precancerous disease states precede or accompany the actual tumor formation. The first to appear is gastritis. As mentioned in the discussion of gastric cancer epidemiology, chronic atrophic gastritis (CAG) develops in 70% or more of populations where gastric cancer occurs frequently (Correa et al. 1976). CAG is assumed to represent the failure of the mucosa to respond adequately to repeated acute injuries (superficial gastritis) and is reflected as focal necrosis and regenerative hyperplasia (Correa 1980). As the chronicity of the condition develops, atrophy of the mucosa (loss of parietal and zymogen cells) becomes apparent (Correa 1980). The lost cells are replaced by cells that are normally found in the intestine but are not present in the normal stomach. This phenomenon constitutes intestinal metaplasia. It is characteristically a focal process, starting around the union of the antrum and corpus of the stomach, but gradually expanding until extensive areas of the surface are covered (Correa 1980). Metaplastic glands have been classified as "complete," that is, possessing all the characteristics of normal adult small intestine cells, or "incomplete," resembling crypts of the large intestine, but recent studies have shown that metaplasia is of a more heterogeneous nature, combining characteristics of both the small and large intestines (Ming 1982). These changes are detectable biochemically and histochemically. In some patients, however, groups of metaplastic glands appear which become less mature, lose some of their intestinal enzymes, and become dysplastic. Dysplasia includes distortions of the architecture of the glands, and as it progresses it begins more and more to resemble cancerous tissue (Cuello et al. 1979). Finally, the dysplastic cells lose their dependency on surrounding tissues and become invasive, and a malignancy is formed.

The process of gastric carcinogenesis, therefore, appears to be a continuum of changes which turns areas of normal gastric mucosa first into metaplasia and later into progressive dysplasia, and finally cancer. The changes usually take several decades in man, and the change from one disease state to another does not seem obligatory. The changes seem to reflect sequential alterations of phenotypic expression.

HISTOCHEMISTRY AND BIOCHEMISTRY

The morphological changes which occur during gastric carcinogenesis are accompanied by profound histochemical alterations, especially with regard to glycoproteins and cytoplasmic enzymes. The normal surface epithelial cell of the stomach mucosa accumulates in its cytoplasm multiple drops of a neutral glycoprotein which constitutes the gastric mucus (Lev 1965). Metaplastic cells, on the other hand, accumulate in their cytoplasm a large globus (goblet) of acid glycoproteins (mucin). The mucin may resemble small intestinal mucin and be classified as a sialomucin (Spicer 1965), or it may resemble that of the colon and therefore correspond to sulfomucin (Abe et al. 1974).

The chief or zymogen cells of normal gastric pits principally secrete pepsinogen. One of the earliest detectable changes in experimental gastric carcinogenesis is the loss of one of the three pepsinogen isozymes, pepsinogen 1 (Furihata et al. 1975). Loss of pepsinogen 1 occurs only as a result of exposure to gastric carcinogens, such as MNNG, and does not follow exposure to other types of carcinogens, such as dimethylnitrosamine (Furihata et al. 1981). The loss of this zymogen represents an irreversible, heritable, phenotypic change caused by a gastric carcinogen.

Conversely, intestinal metaplasia brings a variety of previously undetected enzymes to the stomach. In small intestinal metaplasia, sucrase, trehalase, leucine aminopeptidase, and alkaline phosphatase are present; in large intestinal metaplasia, sucrase but not trehalase is present in the surface, leucine aminopeptidase is found in the tissue sections, and alkaline phosphatase is present only in small amounts (Matsukara et al. 1980).

Thus the biochemical and histochemical changes which accompany gastric carcinogenesis reflect the morphological changes that occur and represent phenotypic changes that result from the altered expression of normal gastric mucosal DNA.

CELL KINETICS

A gastric pit and gastric gland of the fundic and pyloric mucosa constitute an inseparable unitary tubular structure (see Fig. 3). The pit and neck of the gland form a smooth-surfaced, simple tubular structure, while the glandular portion is irregularly branched in the pyloric mucosa and unbranched in the corpus and fundus. The generative cells, that is, the cells which actively incorporate

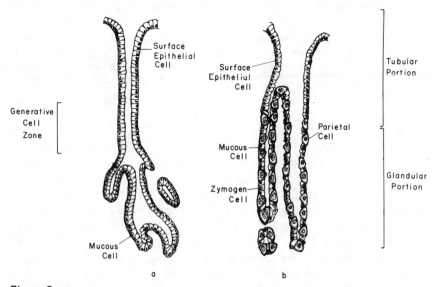

Figure 3
Diagram of gastric pits in the pyloric (a) and fundic (b) regions of the mucosa. The generative cells are restricted to the middle third of the pits. The pyloric gland shows marked branching, while the fundic gland is more tubular in shape.

[3]H-TdR, are confined to the lower part of the tubular portion (Fujita and Hattori 1977). Normal proliferation occurs in undifferentiated precursor or stem cells referred to as mucous neck cells. Proliferation and growth are balanced by cell loss through exfoliation of surface cells, so that under normal conditions cell populations are maintained at a steady state. Insufficient cell production or increased cell loss may result in ulceration or atrophy. Increased cell production or the prolonged life of certain cell types may result in hyperplasia. Due to the rapid turnover rates of most of the cell populations, therefore, any alteration in the processes regulating growth is likely to produce functional changes (Johnson 1981).

The mucous neck cells actively proliferate and differentiate into surface epithelial cells as well as into glandular cells. Most newly produced cells migrate rapidly to the surface while differentiating into mucus-producing epithelial cells. Surface epithelial cells migrate in a continuous and regular manner to be sloughed off into the gastric lumen. Their life span is 4-8 days in normal human stomach (Bell et al. 1967). Glandular cells migrate downward in a somewhat less regular manner. Their life spans have been estimated to be 200 ± 100 days in hamster fundic mucosa, 14 days for mucin-producing cells, and 60 days for endocrine cells in the pyloric mucosa (Hattori and Fujita 1976). Most studies agree that parietal cells are unable to divide (e.g., Ragins et al. 1968), and that some newly formed cells slowly migrate down the gland to differentiate into acid-producing cells (Willems et al. 1972). Parietal cells in the mouse have been shown to survive for 90 days, which is also the time it takes for migration to the bottom of the glands to occur (Ragins et al. 1968). Zymogen cells have been observed to originate from undifferentiated cells after injury (Lawson 1970), but they are replaced by mitosis in normal adult mucosa (Ragins et al. 1968). The mechanism by which gastrin-producing cells (G cells) replicate is not clear, with both mitosis (Lehy and Willems 1976) and differentiation (Fugimoto et al. 1979) reported.

In atrophic mucosa, shorter pit lengths result from the atrophy of the mucosa and epithelial cells consequently experience a life span as short as 2 days in human stomach (Bell et al. 1967). The generative region widens into the lower gland region, and some otherwise apparently normal epithelial cells at the luminal surface incorporate ^{3}H-TdR as well (Deschner et al. 1972). This expansion of the compartment of proliferating cells and incorporation of ^{3}H-TdR at or near the luminal surface continues during intestinalization of the mucosa (Winawer and Lipkin 1969).

In fully developed intestinalized mucosa, as in the normal intestine, the generative cells are confined to the lowest portion of the gland (Fujita and Hattori (1977). The shape of the intestinalized gland is that of a simple tube without branching. The highest frequency of metaplasia occurs in the pyloric region of the stomach, with the branched pyloric glands reforming into a simple tubular type of gland while the generative zone shifts downward.

In less complete intestinal metaplasia, pits have ^{3}H-TdR-incorporating cells and increased protein and RNA syntheses in surface cells as well as at the base of the crypts (Deschner et al. 1972). This shift in generative zones is an abnormality which has been demonstrated in precancerous diseases of human and animal colon (Deschner and Lipkin 1975; Chang 1978) and cervix (Hasegawa et al. 1976) as well as stomach (Deschner et al. 1979). Thus, during the development of neoplasms in other organs as well as in the stomach, persistent DNA synthesis occurs in cells that normally would be terminal or end cells, while associated pathological changes lead to atypias, dysplasias, and malignancy.

As has been described, kinetic studies of normal as well as intestinalized gastric mucosa have revealed that a complete renewal of almost all the mucosal cells occurs within a relatively short period of time. The question arises, then, as to how an initiated cell can remain in the mucosa for several years or more of latent growth, escaping from the flow of regular turnover of the surrounding normal cells. One would expect an initiated cell to be sloughed off together with its neighbors (see Fig. 4a,b). However, if the cell is caught during the process of progressive intestinalization a scenario may be imagined in which the cell is captured in a cystic, isolated glandular structure, as is depicted in Figure 4b,c,d. During intestinalization of the pylorus, only one of the glandular branches is utilized when intestinal conversion of a gland takes place. The rest of the branches must be isolated from the main branch during this process. Most would

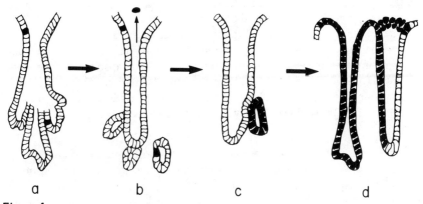

Figure 4
So-called well-differentiated carcinoma. If cancer cells arise in the proper fundic or pyloric glands, they do not stay in the mucosa for a long time because of the sloughing-off mechanism of cell renewal. If cancer cells happen to be captured in the cystic, isolated glandular structures, they can stay in the mucosa for a long enough time to develop into an incipient cancer. (Adapted from Fujita and Hattori 1977).

be expected to undergo complete atrophy because they contain only non-dividing, mature glandular cells with a limited life span. If, however, generative cells are trapped in isolated branches, as is frequently seen in flash-labeled autoradiographs of human gastric mucosa undergoing progressive intestinalization, the structure could persist indefinitely as the generative cells continue to proliferate. If an initiated cell were included in such an isolated yet persistent structure, the cell would be protected from normal sloughing-off mechanisms and would have ample opportunity for latent growth. The process of progressive intestinalization is concluded to be an important factor in the etiology of stomach cancer, since it may provide an opportunity for initiated cells to escape destruction and develop into stomach tumors (Fujita and Hattori 1977).

ETIOLOGIC MODEL

In 1975 we proposed an etiologic hypothesis linking high rates of gastric cancer with atrophic gastritis, intestinal metaplasia, and progressive microenvironmental changes leading to conversion of nitrate to N-nitroso compounds (Correa et al. 1975). This hypothesis was later refined, in light of increasing experimental evidence, to two potential nonexclusive variations (Tannenbaum et al. 1977):

1. An agent in the environment, or formed by a combination of factors in the environment, leads to gastritis. Gastritis can then be naturally followed by intestinal metaplasia and finally cancer. These stages are parallel but appear at different times due to varying latencies for phenotypic expression and differences in cell kinetics for different types of gastrointestinal stem cells. A key

factor is the inception of gastritis at a sufficiently early age to allow for the relatively long induction period of gastric cancer.

2. The conditions of gastritis and metaplasia, caused by any of several possible environmental factors, lead to elevation of the pH of the stomach and, concomitantly, to the establishment of a microbial flora capable of nitrate reduction. This process in turn leads to a steady formation of carcinogenic N-nitroso compounds over a long time period, which leads ultimately to gastric cancer. The susceptible cells may be intestinalized stem cells.

The current version of our working model is illustrated in Figure 5. The essential characteristic of this model is that it proposes a chain of events which lead from the normal stomach to gastric cancer, and that interruption of any part of the sequence leads to a reduced risk for gastric cancer. In other words, the model provides a scientific framework for risk factors identified through epidemiological investigations, and in addition it suggests possible modes for intervention in high-risk populations.

In Phase 1 of Figure 5, an injury occurs to the gastric mucosa which leads to elevation of the pH of the stomach (Phase 2). The nature of the injury does not appear to be important as long as there is a permanent loss of gastric glands. Some examples of such injuries which have an elevated risk are indicated in Figure 5 (Phase 1) and include the following:

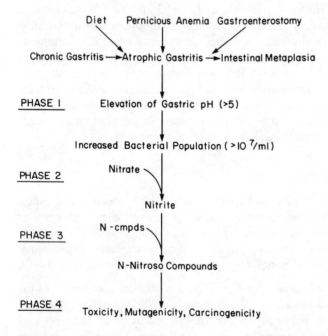

Figure 5
Model for gastric cancer etiology

1. Antrectomy followed by surgical reestablishment of GI tract continuity (e.g., Billroth I and II) (Langhans et al. 1981). In these cases the loss of gastric glands is accompanied by a subsequent reflux of bile into the stomach which causes irritation of the mucosa and elevation of the gastric pH. The remaining gastric stump is often found to have focal intestinal metaplasia (Domellof et al. 1977).
2. Pernicious anemia is associated with autoimmune loss of parietal cells, decreased secretion of hydrochloric acid, and, ultimately, complete gastric atrophy (Correa 1980).
3. Dietary factors are suggested primarily by the results of the epidemiological studies described elsewhere in this discussion. Injury to the gastric mucosa could be caused by excessive intake of salty foods (Sato et al. 1959), consumption of very hard foods (e.g., coarsely ground corn) (Correa 1980), or by other unknown factors that lead to loss of surface epithelial cells and exposure of gastric pits. Previously protected gastric stem cells could thus become more easily accessible to putative carcinogens. This is a largely untapped area and could be the subject of more extensive research.

In Phase 2 of the model elevation of gastric pH above 5 leads to rapid growth of bacteria, many of which have nitrate reductase activity. The source of the bacteria is mainly swallowed saliva or duodenal reflux. Due to the rich nature of alkalized gastric juice as a microbiological growth medium, coupled with a large inoculum and an aerobic environment, growth of bacteria is very rapid. Therefore, cycling of pH above and below pH 5 will be followed by cycling of bacterial growth in phase with pH.

The reduction of nitrate to nitrite in Phase 3 will be determined by the presence of a suitable microflora and the availability of nitrate. The extent of nitrite accumulation will be determined by the concentrations of nitrate-reducing bacteria and nitrate and by the absence or presence of factors which lead to nitrite destruction (Lintas et al. 1982). Nitrite has been shown to be stable in gastric juice samples from individuals with chronic atrophic gastritis and intestinal metaplasia, but unstable in that of normal individuals (Tannenbaum et al. 1981). The reaction of nitrite with nitrogen compounds to form carcinogenic N-nitroso compounds is the final phase (4). For gastric cancer this would most likely be a nitrosamide, since these types of compounds and not nitrosamines have been shown experimentally to cause gastric cancer in rats and guinea pigs (Magee et al. 1976; Magee et al. 1980).

A key problem for this model is how nitrite could accumulate and react in the gastric environment, when the condition favoring the first process is a high pH and the condition favoring the second is a low pH. Two possible situations may explain this apparent paradox:

1. The conditions in the gastric lumen alternate between periods of high pH and low pH; this leads first to nitrite accumulation and then to reaction. Since atrophy of gastric glands and intestinal metaplasia occur primarily in the

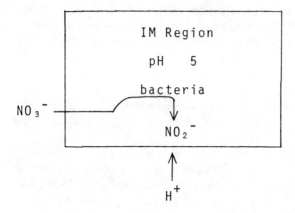

Normal Gastric Mucosa

Figure 6
Scheme illustrating the manner in which a nitrosating agent could be formed at the border of normal and intestinalized gastric regions.

antrum, intact parietal cells in the fundus can still be stimulated to secrete acid (Correa 1980).
2. Focal intestinal metaplasia is embedded in a normal area of the gastric mucosa. The pH in the intestinalized region is sufficiently high to permit growth of bacteria and formation of nitrite. At the border of the normal and metaplastic regions, a gradient will occur for both nitrite and pH, as shown in Figure 6. The most favorable condition for the formation of N-nitroso compounds will be at the boundary between the normal and the metaplastic regions, since this area will have the highest concentration of nitrite and the lowest pH.

Thus, each phase in the model is essential in order for continuity to the next to be possible. Nitrate per se cannot be of etiologic significance to gastric cancer unless there is a substantial nitrate-reducing population in the stomach. Even if there was the potential for nitrite formation, it would be theoretically possible to block N-nitrosation, e.g., through the use of blocking agents such as ascorbic acid or α-tocopherol (Tannenbaum and Mergens 1980). Future research will bring about either further substantiation or destruction of this hypothetical model. In the interim it would be possible to proceed with an intervention program based upon the characteristics of the model, particularly by introducing blocking agents into the diet of high-risk groups.

ACKNOWLEDGMENT

The authors would like to thank Ms. Olga V. Woodworth for her assistance in the preparation of this manuscript. This research was supported by PHS Grant Number 1-PO1-CA26731-03, awarded by the National Cancer Institute, DHHS.

REFERENCES

Abe, M., N. Ohuchi, and H. Sokano. 1974. Enzyme histo- and biochemistry of intestinalized gastric mucosa. *Acta Histochem. Cytochem.* 7:282.

Bell, B., T.P. Almy, and M. Lipkin. 1967. Cell proliferation kinetics in the gastrointestinal tract of man. III. Cell renewal in esophagus, stomach, and jejunum of a patient with treated pernicious anemia. *J. Natl. Cancer Inst.* 38:615.

Bonne, C. 1935. Cancer in Java and Sumatra. *Am. J. Cancer* 25:811.

Chatterjee, D. 1976. Idiopathic chronic gastritis. *Surg. Gynecol. Obstet.* 143:986.

Chang, W.W.L. 1978. Histogenesis of sym. 1-2 DMN-induced neoplasms of the colon in the mouse. *J. Natl. Cancer Inst.* 60:1405.

Clemmeson, J. and A. Nielsen. 1951. The social distribution of cancer in Copenhagen, 1943-1947. *Br. J. Cancer* 5:159.

Correa, P. 1980. The epidemiology and pathogenesis of chronic gastritis: Three etiologic entities. *Front. Gastrointest. Res.* 6:98.

Correa, P. and S.R. Tannenbaum. 1981. The microecology of gastric cancer. *ACS Symp. Ser.* 174:319.

Correa, P., W. Haenszel, C. Cuello, S. Tannenbaum, and M. Archer. 1975. A model for gastric cancer epidemiology. *Lancet* ii:58.

Correa, P., C. Cuello, E. Duque, L.C. Burbano, F.T. Garcia, O. Bolanos, C. Brown, and W. Haenszel. 1976. Gastric cancer in Colombia. III. Natural history of precursor lesions. *J. Natl. Cancer Inst.* 57:1027.

Cuello, C., P. Correa, G. Zarama, J. Lopez, J. Murray, and G. Gordillo. 1979. Histopathology of gastric dysplasias. *Am. J. Surg. Pathol.* 3:491.

Cuello, C., P. Correa, W. Haenszel, G. Gordillo, C. Brown, M. Archer, and S. Tannenbaum. 1976. Gastric cancer in Colombia. I. Cancer risk and suspect environmental agents. *J. Natl. Cancer Inst.* 57:1015.

Deschner, E. and M. Lipkin. 1975. Proliferative patterns in colonic mucosa of polyposis families. *Cancer* 35:413.

Deschner, E.E., S.J. Winawer, and M. Lipkin. 1972. Patterns of nucleic acid and protein synthesis in normal human gastric mucosa and atrophic gastritis. *J. Natl. Cancer Inst.* 48:1567.

Deschner, E.E., K. Tamura, and S.P. Bralow. 1979. Sequential histopathology and cell kinetic changes in rat pyloric mucosa during gastric carcinogenesis induced by MNNG. *J. Natl. Cancer Inst.* 63:171.

Doll, R. 1956. Environmental factors in the aetiology of cancer of the stomach. *Gastroenterologia* 86:320.

Domellof, S., S. Eriksson, and K.G. Janunger. 1977. Carcinoma and possible precancerous changes of the gastric stump after Billroth II resection. *Gastroenterology* 73:462.

Dorn, H.F. and S.J. Cutler. 1959. Morbidity from cancer in the United States, Part II. *Publ. Health Monogr.*, Government Printing Office, Washington, D.C.

Everson, T. 1969. Carcinoma of the stomach. In *Cancer of the digestive tract, clinical management* (eds., T.C. Everson and W.H. Cole) Appleton Century-Crofts, New York.

Fugimoto, S., K. Kawai, T. Hattori, and S. Fujita. 1979. Tritiated thymidine autoradiographic study on origin and renewal of gastrin cells in pyloric area of hamsters. *Gastroenterology* 76:1136.

Fujita, S. and T. Hattori. 1977. Cell proliferation, differentiation, and migration in the gastric mucosa: A study on the background of carcinogenesis. In *Pathophysiology of carcinogenesis in digestive organs.* (eds., E. Farber et al.). p. 21, University Park Press, Baltimore.

Furihata, C., K. Kodama, and T. Matsushima. 1981. Induction of changes in the pepsinogen content and the pepsinogen isoenzyme pattern of the pyloric mucosa of the rat stomach by short-term administration of stomach carcinogens. *J. Natl. Cancer Inst.* 67:1101.

Furihata, C., K. Sosajima, S. Kazama, K. Koguru, T. Kawachi, T. Sugimura, M. Tatematsu, and M. Takahashi. 1975. Changes in pepsinogen isozymes in stomach carcinogenesis induced in rats by MNNG. *J. Natl. Cancer Inst.* 55: 925.

Guiss, L.W. and Stewart, F.W. 1943. Chronic atrophic gastritis and cancer of the stomach. *Arch. Surg.* 10:505.

Haenszel, W.M. 1958. Variation in incidence of and mortality from stomach cancer with particular reference to the United States. *J. Natl. Cancer Inst.* 21:213.

_____. 1961. Cancer mortality incidence among the foreign-born in the United States. *J. Natl. Cancer Inst.* 26:37.

Haenszel, W. and P. Correa. 1975. Developments in the epidemiology of stomach cancer over the past decade. *Cancer Res.* 35:3452.

Haenszel, W.M., M. Kurihara, M. Segi, and R.K.C. Lee. 1972. Stomach cancer among Japanese in Hawaii. *J. Natl. Cancer Inst.* 49:969.

Haenszel, W., M. Kurihara, F.B. Locke, K. Shimuzu, and S. Mitsuo. 1976. Stomach cancer in Japan. *J. Natl. Cancer Inst.* 56:265.

Hartman, P. 1982. Nitrates and nitrites: Ingestion, pharmacodynamics, and toxicology. In *Chemical mutagens* (eds., F.J. de Serres and A. Hollaender), vol. 7, p. 211. Plenum Publishing Co., New York.

Hasegawa, I., Y. Matsumira, and S. Tojo. 1976. Cellular kinetics and histological changes in experimental cancer of the uterine cervix. *Cancer Res.* 36:359.

Hattori, T. and S. Fujita. 1976. Tritiated thymidine autoradiographic study on cellular migration in the gastric gland of the golden hamster. *Cell Tissue Res.* 172:171.

Johnson, L.R. 1981. Regulation of gastrointestinal growth. In *Physiology of the gastrointestinal tract* (ed. L.R. Johnson), p. 169. Raven Press, New York.

Langhans, P., R.A. Heger, J. Hohenstein, and H. Bunte. 1981. Operation-sequel carcinoma—an experimental study. *Hepato-Gastroenterology* 28:34.

Lawson, H.H. 1970. The origin of chief and parietal cells in regenerating gastric mucosa. *Br. J. Surg.* **57**:139.

Lehy, T. and G. Willems. 1976. Population kinetics of antral gastrin cells in the mouse. *Gastroenterology* **71**:614.

Lev, R. 1965. The mucin histochemistry of normal and neoplastic gastric mucosa. *Lab. Invest.* **14**:2080.

Lintas, C., A. Clark, J. Fox, S.R. Tannenbaum, and P.M. Newberne. 1982. In vivo stability of nitrite and nitrosamine formation in the dog stomach: Effect of nitrite and amine concentration and of ascorbic acid. *Carcinogenesis* **3**:161.

Logan, W. 1976. Cancers of the alimentary tract: International mortality trends. *WHO Chron.* **30**:413.

Magee, P.N., R. Montesano, and R. Preussmann. 1976. N-Nitroso compounds and related carcinogens. *ACS Monogr.* **173**:491.

Matsukura, N., M. Itabashi, T. Kawachi, T. Hirota, and T. Sugimura. 1980. Sequential studies on the histopathogenesis of gastric carcinoma in rats by a weak gastric carcinogen, N-propyl-N'-nitro-N-nitrosoguanidine. *J. Cancer Res. Clin. Oncol.* **98**:153.

Ming, S.C. 1982. Histochemistry of intestinal metaplasia of the stomach. *Intestinal metaplasia and stomach cancer.* (Abstract), U.S.–Japan Cooperative Cancer Research Program Conference, Shimoda, Japan.

Morson, B.C. 1955. Intestinal metaplasia of the gastric mucosa. *Br. J. Cancer* **9**:365.

Nakahara, K. 1978. Special features of intestinal metaplasia and its relation to early gastric carcinoma in man: Observation by a method in which leucine aminopeptidase activity is used. *J. Natl. Cancer Inst.* **61**:693.

Ragins, H., F. Wincze, and S.M. Liv. 1968. The origin of gastric parietal cells in the mouse. *Anat. Rec.* **162**:99.

Robbins, S.L. 1974. *Pathological basis of disease.* W.B. Saunders Co., Philadelphia, Pennsylvania.

Sato, T., T. Fukuyama, T. Suzuki, and J. Takayanagi. 1959. Studies on the causation of gastric cancer. 2. The relation between gastric cancer mortality rate and salted food intake in several places in Japan. *Bull. Inst. Publ. Health.* **8**:187.

Siurala, M., K. Varis, and M. Wiljasala. 1966. Studies of patients with atrophic gastritis: A 10 to 15 year follow-up. *Scand. J. Gastroenterol.* **1**:40.

Slaga, T.J. 1980. Antiinflammatory steroids: Potent inhibitors of tumor promotion. In *Carcinogenesis: A comprehensive survey* (ed. T.J. Slaga), Vol. 5, p. 111. Raven Press, New York.

Spicer, S.S. 1965. Diamine methods for differentiating mucosubstances histochemically. *J. Histochem. Cytochem.* **13**:211.

Stocks, P. 1947. Regional and local differences in cancer death rates, Studies on medical and population subjects, No. 1, General Register Office, HMSO, London.

Tannenbaum, S., M. Archer, J. Wishnok, P. Correa, C. Cuello, and W. Haenszel. 1977. Nitrate and the etiology of gastric cancer. *Cold Spring Harbor Symp. Quant Biol.* **4**:1609.

Tannenbaum, S.R. and W. Mergens. 1980. Reaction of nitrite with vitamins C and E. *Ann. N.Y. Acad. Sci.* **355**:267.

Tannenbaum, S.R., D. Moran, K.R. Falchuk, P. Correa, and C. Cuello. 1981. Nitrite stability and nitrosation potential in human gastric juice. *Cancer Lett.* **14**:131.

Torgersen, O. and M. Peterson. 1956. The epidemiology of gastric cancer in Oslo: Material, diagnosis, and mobility of population. Some sources of error. *Br. J. Cancer* **10**:292.

U. S. Department of Health and Human Services. 1981. Surveillance, epidemiology, and end results: Incidence and mortality data, 1973-1977. *NCI Monogr.* **57**.

Weisburger, J.H., H. Marquardt, N. Hirota, H. Mori, and G.M. Williams. 1980. Induction of cancer of the glandular stomach in rats by an extract of nitrite-treated fish. *J. Natl. Cancer Inst.* **64**:163.

Willems, G., P. Galand, and Y. Vansteenkiste. 1972. Cell population kinetics of zymogen and parietal cells in the stomachs of mice. *Z. Zellforsch. Mikrosk. Anat.* **134**:505.

Winawer, S.J. and M. Lipkin. 1969. Cell proliferation kinetics in the gastrointestinal tract of man. IV. Cell renewal in the intestinalized gastric mucosa. *J. Natl. Cancer Inst.* **42**:9.

Wynder, E., J. Kmet, N. Dungal, and M. Segi. 1963. An epidemiological investigation of gastric cancer. *Cancer* **16**:1461.

On the Factors Associated with

Esophageal and Gastric Cancer in Man

JOHN H. WEISBURGER AND CLARA L. HORN
Naylor Dana Institute for Disease Prevention
American Health Foundation
Valhalla, New York 10595

There have been considerable advances in achieving an understanding of the mechanisms of carcinogenesis. The causation and development of cancer involves a series of steps. Multidisciplinary approaches and various lines of evidence have provided a sound scientific basis for a somatic mutation being a first event in the overall carcinogenic process. Changes in the genetic material can arise through a direct attack by radiation, chemicals, or viruses. Radiation or chemicals can damage the genetic material at a number of loci along the DNA chain which are then converted to permanent alterations by the mispairing of bases and transposition of codons during replication of the damaged regions. In the case of viruses, specific polymerases operate to insert viral codons into DNA sequences, or, through reverse transcriptase, into RNA sequences, hence yielding an abnormal DNA containing new information. Another mechanism is the faulty operation of DNA polymerase during DNA synthesis, which results in an inaccurate transcription of the parent DNA segment to produce abnormal DNA. Certain carcinogenic metal ions may have this effect. Abnormal DNA can also ensue through the errors introduced by specific DNA polymerases concerned with DNA repair, especially during postreplicative DNA synthesis. The infidelity of DNA polymerases may lead to further abnormalities in the DNA produced during the replication of early tumor cells, and thus, may represent the means whereby tumor cells progress to less differentiated, more malignant cancer types during their growth and development.

A cell containing abnormal DNA stemming from any of the above mechanisms is only the first element of a series of steps eventually yielding an invasive malignant neoplasm. An important factor is the ability of an abnormal cell population to achieve a selective growth advantage in the presence of surrounding normal cells. The cell duplication process is highly dependent on a number of endogenous and exogenous controlling elements that operate by incompletely known or epigenetic mechanisms. Agents that act as promoters or inhibitors of growth are two such elements that may either enhance or retard the expression of preexisting latent neoplastic cells.

This study is dedicated to the founder of the American Health Foundation, Dr. Ernst L. Wynder, on the occasion of the tenth anniversary of the Naylor Dana Institute for Disease Prevention.

It is important to emphasize that promoters do not lead to the production of an invasive cancer from a normal cell in the absence of an antecedent gene change. Thus, in exploring the causes of any specific human cancer, consideration must be given both to the agents leading to an abnormal genome and any other agents possibly involved in the growth and development of the resulting abnormal neoplastic cells, and their further progression to neoplasia.

Chemical carcinogens have been classified into two broad categories: genotoxic carcinogens and epigenetic agents. The latter include promoters. These two categories in turn are comprised of eight classes of compounds (Weisburger and Williams 1981). This classification is an important aid in understanding the carcinogenic mechanisms for each type of cancer by dissecting the complex causes of the diverse types of cancer and arriving at a delineation of the role of each agent—genotoxic carcinogen, cocarcinogen, or promoter—in the overall carcinogenic process for each kind of cancer. This aspect applies to the nutritionally linked cancers, which are some of the major types of human cancer in the world, including esophageal and gastric cancer discussed here.

GENOTOXIC CARCINOGENS FOR UPPER GASTROINTESTINAL TRACT CANCER

Nitrosamines as Possible Human Carcinogens

Certain tobacco-specific nitrosamines, such as nitrosonornicotine, comprise a substantial portion of the genotoxic carcinogens in tobacco smoke and in tobacco chews (see Hoffmann et al., this volume). The specific association of these kinds of carcinogens with cancer at sites related to the use of tobacco, such as cancers of the lung, pancreas, kidney, urinary bladder, and also, in the presence of heavy alcohol intake, cancers of the oral cavity and esophagus, remains to be fully documented. It is reasonable to assume, however, that these carcinogens play a role in the development of cancer in these target organs that accounts for a substantial portion of the cancers in various countries (Table 1).

In countries, such as Eastern Iran, Southern Soviet Union, and Central China, cancer of the esophagus is seen in people who do not appear to smoke and drink heavily. Despite extensive cooperative efforts between investigators in Iran and the International Agency for Research on Cancer, the etiology of esophageal cancer in Iran remains obscure. Nitrosamines have been suspected as etiologic factors but, as yet, have not been found. Nonetheless, the nutritional intake is poor in terms of green and yellow vegetables, fruits, and other vitamin C- and E-containing foods which act as antidotes to nitrite, and thus, through this association, the endogenous formation of nitrosamines cannot be ruled out. This appears to be true since recent data from China, the easternmost extension of the belt of esophageal cancer incidence, suggest that nitrosamines are present in that environment.

Table 1
Comparison of High- and Low-Risk Dietary Factors for Cancer in Specific Organs

Organ	Population lower risk	Dietary factors lower risk	Population higher risk	Dietary factors higher risk
Esophagus	USA, Utah; Rural Norway	Low alcohol and smoking habits	France, Calvados, Normandy	Extensive alcohol and smoking.
Esophagus	Idem	Idem	USA—lower socio-economic groups	Alcohol and smoking
Esophagus	Idem	Idem	Eastern Iran, Southern Soviet Union	Low micronutrient vitamin C intake
Esophagus	Idem	Idem	Central China	Dietary carcinogen? low vitamin C intake.
Stomach	USA	Fresh fruit, salad, vitamin C, and vitamin E	Japan, Chile, Columbia	Salted, pickled foods, geochemical and water nitrate, low vitamin C and vitamin E.

Nitrosamides as Possible Human Carcinogens

Sugimura administered the mutagen N-methyl-N'-nitro-N-nitrosoguanidine (MNNG), a water-soluble, rather polar substance, to rats in drinking water, and discovered that this agent was not only a powerful carcinogen but reliably induced cancer in the glandular stomach, accurately mimicking the human disease. A study of the pathogenesis showed that MNNG induced not only the invasive neoplasm but also the antecedent and accompanying lesions, such as gastritis and intestinalization of the gastric epithelium, as also seen in humans (see Charnley et al., this volume).

S. Mirvish (this volume) and I (Weisburger 1981) linked Sugimura's gastric cancer model to the development of hypotheses concerning factors associated with the occurrence of human gastric cancer and to a consideration of the underlying mechanisms. Gastric cancer was one of the major types of cancer in the United States, but its incidence and mortality have decreased sharply since 1950. The concepts presented account for this decline.

Gastric cancer remains one of the major cancers in Japan, the mountainous regions of central and western Latin America, northern and eastern Europe, and Iceland, but even there, there is a beginning indication of a decline. There is a north-south gradient, or south-north gradient in the southern hemisphere, with a larger incidence occurring in more frigid or mountainous zones (Table 1).

Foods eaten by high-risk people include dried, salted, pickled, or smoked fish, or other pickled foods. Also, there usually is a variable intake of fresh fruits and vegetables, i.e., a seasonal low consumption of such foods during winter and spring. The geochemistry often involves an elevated nitrate content in the soil and, thus, foods and water rich in nitrate.

We have suggested that an alkylnitrosoureido type of compound, such as the one developed by Sugimura (Sugimura and Kawachi 1978), which induces glandular gastric cancer in animal models, may be involved in human gastric carcinogenesis, and Mirvish (1981) has proposed a similar scheme. We believe such compounds arise in pickled or smoked foods, although it is also possible that these chemicals form in the achlorhydric stomach as visualized by P. Correa and by S. Tannenbaum (see Charnley et al., this volume).

EXPERIMENTAL MODEL

A mackerel, *Sanma hiraki* is eaten in a region of Japan at high risk for gastric cancer. Homogenates of this fish were "pickled" in the laboratory by treatment with nitrite at pH 3 yielding a direct-acting mutagen for *Salmonella typhimurium* TA 100 with properties similar to those of the prototype MNNG. The formation of this mutagen could be completely blocked by vitamin C. Mirvish (1981) discovered that the formation of nitroso compounds could be inhibited by vitamin C, and Mergens and Newmark (1981) noted that vitamin E also has such properties. The fish, *Sanma, Aji,* and *Iwashi,* yielded more mutagenic activity than other species of fish, but it is important to note that several kinds of meat failed to produce such direct-acting mutagens. We also found that similar pickling of beans, as eaten in high-risk Latin America, or of borscht, as consumed in eastern Europe, led to mutagenic activity. Yano (1981) noted alkylating activity towards 4-(p-nitrobenzyl)pyridine in nitrite-treated or smoked fish.

The active mutagenic principle, from the reaction of nitrite and *Sanma*, was not only carcinogenic but specifically induced glandular stomach cancer in rats. Since the formation of the mutagen can be blocked by vitamin C, it would seem that the formation of glandular stomach cancer may also be so inhibited. Thus, treatment of fish of a type eaten in Japan, a region at high risk for gastric cancer, with nitrite at pH 3 yielded not only an extract with mutagenic activity, but one which induced cancer in the glandular stomach. Glandular stomach cancer is rare in rats, and the control group had no neoplastic lesions in their stomachs. Also, a high incidence of epithelial hyperplasia or intestinalization of glandular stomach cancer was observed only in the experimental group. Thus, the neoplastic lesions in the glandular stomach were, no doubt, due to the treatment administered. As is true for rats given MNNG, we also noted tumors in the small intestine and in the pancreas (Weisburger et al. 1980).

The structure of the mutagen responsible for carcinogenesis is not yet known and is being investigated. It is clear from the fact of the inhibition of the substance's formation by vitamin C, and from its production of cancer in the glandular stomach, similar to alkylnitrosoureido compounds, that we are dealing with this kind of compound. However, in contrast to compounds such as methylnitrosourea, we noted that the mutagenic activity was rather stable at pH 3 and even at higher pH values. Nonetheless, Mirvish et al. (1980) have evidence that Bonito fish contains some nitrosatable alkylureas. Perhaps nitroso derivatives of Maillard type products in fish and other foods deserve consideration.

Since migrants maintain their risk for gastric cancer when changing residence from high-risk to low-risk regions, it may be that the nature of the carcinogens operating in man is similar to what we have identified through mutagen and carcinogen bioassays. With such compounds, exposure throughout life is not required in order to yield eventual stomach cancer. It follows that for effective gastric cancer prevention, exposure to agents causing this disease must be minimized or avoided from the earliest age. In turn, this means that foods providing the necessary vitamin C, such as fresh fruits, vegetables, and salads, or supplementary vitamin C, ought to be consumed with every meal.

Salt has a promoting effect in gastric carcinogenesis, although in some areas of the world it may also lead to mucosal damage, gastritis, rise in stomach pH, bacterial overgrowth, and thence to another source of nitrite through bacterial reduction of nitrate in the stomach. In the MNNG model, however, the antecedent precancerous lesions occur with or without salt, and thus we believe that heavy salt use augments the risk through promotion, rather than causes gastric cancer. Nonetheless, lowering salt intake would not only reduce the risk of gastric cancer, but would also lower the occurrence of hypertension and stroke that is associated with salt in genetically sensitive individuals (Joossens and Geboers 1981).

SUMMARY

If the concepts and facts presented are correct, a major kind of human cancer in many regions of the world, cancer of the stomach, is due to a type of nitroso compound, a nitrosoureido derivative. Similarly, esophageal cancer may be due to a nitrosamine. It is quite certain that the formation of such compounds can be blocked by vitamins C and E, as well as by some other nitrite-trapping agents such as gallates. Thus, the primary prevention of cancers of the upper GI tract caused by nitroso compounds can be achieved through an adequate intake of such harmless inhibitors with every meal from infancy onwards, and through the avoidance of highly salted, pickled foods.

ACKNOWLEDGMENTS

Research described was supported in part by USPHS grant CA-29602 from the National Cancer Institute.

REFERENCES

Joossens, J.B. and J. Goeboers. 1981. Nutrition and gastric cancer. *Nutr. Cancer* **2**:250.

Mergens, W.J. and H.L. Newmark. 1981. Blocking nitrosation reactions in vivo. *ACS Monogr.* **174**:193.

Mirvish, S.S. 1981. Inhibition of the formation of carcinogenic N-nitroso compounds by ascorbic acid and other compounds. In *Cancer: Achievements, challenges, and prospects for the 1980s* (eds. J.H. Burchenal and H.F. Oettgen), vol. 1, p. 557. Grune and Stratton, New York.

Mirvish, S.S., K. Karlowski, D.A. Cairnes, J.P. Sams, R. Abraham, and J. Nielsen. 1980. Identification of alkylureas after nitrosation-denitrosation of a bonito fish product, crab, lobster and bacon. *J. Agric. Food Chem.* **28**: 1175.

Sugimura, T. and T. Kawachi. 1978. Experimental stomach carcinogenesis. In *Gastrointestinal tract cancer* (eds. M. Lipkin and R. Good), p. 327. Plenum Press, New York.

Weisburger, J.H. 1981. N-Nitroso compounds: Diet and cancer trends. An approach to the prevention of gastric cancer. *ACS Monogr.* **174**:305.

Weisburger, J.H. and G.M. Williams. 1981. Carcinogen testing: Current problems and new approaches. *Science* **214**:401.

Weisburger, J.H., E.L. Wynder, with C. Horn. 1982. Nutritional factors and etiologic mechanisms in the causation of gastrointestinal cancers. *Cancer* **50**:11.

Weisburger, J.H., H. Marquardt, N. Hirota, H. Mori, and G.M. Williams. 1980. Induction of cancer of the glandular stomach in rats by an extract of nitrite-treated fish. *J. Natl. Cancer Inst.* **64**:163.

Yano, K. 1981. Alkylating activity of processed fish products treated with sodium nitrite in simulated gastric juice. *Gann.* **72**:451.

SESSION VII:

DOSE RESPONSE RELATION- SHIPS IN NITROSAMINE CARCINOGENESIS

Lung Tumorigenesis in
Strain A Mice by Low Doses
of Dimethylnitrosamine

LUCY M. ANDERSON,* KATHLEEN VAN HAVERE,
AND JOHN M. BUDINGER
Walker Laboratory
Memorial Sloan-Kettering Cancer Center
Rye, New York 10580

The widespread occurrence of low ppb levels of nitrosamines in a variety of human contact sources (Fine et al. 1977a; Fine 1980) and in human blood (Fine et al. 1977b; Lakritz et al. 1980; Yamamoto et al. 1980; Tannenbaum 1980) raises the question of whether chronic cellular exposure to such small amounts might contribute significantly to human cancer risk. Tests of low-dose effects of nitrosamines in several laboratories have employed the rat, with liver tumors as the endpoint. Diethylnitrosamine (NDEA) in the drinking water at a dosage of 0.075 mg/kg/day (equivalent to 0.75 ppm in the diet) induced liver tumors in a high percentage of treated rats at 2-3 years of age (Druckrey et al. 1963; Preussmann 1972, 1980). This carcinogen at a dose of 0.45 ppm in the drinking water resulted in significant occurrence of liver carcinomas and upper gastrointestinal tract neoplasms after 60 weeks or more of treatment, and liver nodules after 30 weeks of treatment (Lijinsky et al. 1981). Dimethyl-nitrosamine (NDMA) incorporated in the diet caused a small number of liver tumors after a 2-year exposure of rats to 2 ppm (Terracini et al. 1967) or 1 ppm (Arai et al. 1979); in the latter experiment, no tumors occurred after treatment with 0.1 ppm NDMA. A preliminary summary of unpublished data (Crampton 1980) indicated that 132 ppb NDMA or NDEA given to rats for 800-900 days caused an increase in tumor incidence, and that hyperplastic nodules were observed in livers of rats given 32 ppb NDMA. The results of these several experiments confirm that nitrosamines are highly potent carcinogens, but leave open the question of whether tumorigenesis may occur with the chronic 10-50 ppb level doses incurred by the human population.

As a low-dose carcinogenesis bioassay model, the rat has the advantage of very low rate of occurrence of spontaneous tumors of the liver and gastro-intestinal tract. However, the extensive treatment periods required, and the long latencies of the tumors, as well as uncertainties in diagnosis of many liver

*Present Address: Laboratory of Comparative Carcinogenesis, Perinatal Carcino-genesis Section, National Cancer Institute, Fort Detrick, Frederick, Maryland 20205

nodules as neoplastic, limit the practical usefulness of this model. It seemed worthwhile to develop an additional model system for low-dose nitrosamine tumorigenesis studies, employing the mouse. The primary lung tumor of the strain A mouse was chosen as the endpoint because of its several advantages: quantitative sensitivity to initiation, reproducibility, short latency, and ease of definitive gross and histopathologic diagnosis. Also, mice are less expensive than rats in terms of space and maintenance costs. A limitation of this model is a fairly high rate of spontaneous occurrence of the primary lung tumors; but this is not necessarily an impediment as long as adequate numbers of control mice are included with each experiment. The usefulness of the mouse lung tumor as a bioassay system has been extensively discussed and documented by Shimkin and Stoner (1975).

In a preliminary experiment (Anderson et al. 1979) we combined the genetic susceptibility of the strain A mouse to lung tumorigenesis with the known special responsiveness of fetal and newborn mouse lungs to carcinogenic stimuli (Heston and Steffee 1957; Toth 1968) in order to obtain a model system of maximum quantitative sensitivity. Female strain A mice were given 10 ppb NDMA in their drinking water for 4 weeks before mating. Treatment was continued throughout pregnancy and lactation and the postnatal life of the offspring until these were 22 weeks old. Control mice were maintained in parallel and were found to have a spontaneous lung tumor rate of 4% in males and 10% in females (8% for all mice). Of the NDMA-treated mice, 32% of the males, 17% of the females, and 23% of the total number had a lung tumor. This increase was of statistical significance for the males and for all mice. These results indicated that early-life treatment of strain A mice with a dose of NDMA approaching possible human exposure levels may have a significant tumorigenic effect.

This report presents the results of two additional experiments assessing the effects of low doses of NDMA on lung tumorigenesis in strain A mice. Both experiments employed semipurified diets, to reduce the possibility of the nitrosamine contamination sometimes observed with commercial laboratory chows Kann et al. 1977; Edwards et al. 1979). These experiments included: 1) exposure of mice to 10 ppb NDMA throughout early life, in duplication of the initial experiment; 2) exposure of mice to 10 ppb NDMA from preconception until 16 months of age, to determine whether cumulative tumorigenic effects would occur; and 3) treatment of mice with five doses of NDMA between 10 ppb and 1000 ppb NDMA, from weaning (4 weeks of age), for a total of 16 weeks. The rationale for the exposure period of the latter experiment was that mice might have a particularly high sensitivity to the tumorigenic effect of NDMA immediately after weaning; they would be consuming the NDMA-containing water directly, and would still be growing, with a possible increased susceptibility to carcinogenesis conferred by cell proliferation. It might also be noted that the 16-week exposure period is standard for carcinogenicity bioassays employing strain A mice (Shimkin and Stoner 1975).

The results of these experiments confirm the usefulness of the strain A lung tumorigenesis system as a model for investigation of low-dose effects of nitrosamines. Unequivocal tumorigenic effects were seen with 500 ppb NDMA administered for 16 weeks. In addition, in both experiments male mice treated with 10 ppb NDMA experienced a small increase in lung tumor incidence, compared with controls, providing tentative confirmation of the positive effect already demonstrated (Anderson et al. 1979).

METHODS

Strain A mice (Jackson Laboratories, Bar Harbor, ME) were maintained in plastic cages with hardwood shavings as bedding, in a room at $25 \pm 1°C$, 40-60% humidity, and a fluorescent light-dark cycle of 14/10 hours. NDMA (Aldrich Chemical Co.) was stored at $-15°C$. NDMA-drinking water solutions were prepared in reagent grade water (rH_2O, Milli-Q2, Millipore Corp., Bedford, MA) by dilution from a 10 ppm stock solution. The latter was prepared fresh every 3-6 weeks and stored wrapped in foil at $4°C$; under such conditions 10 ppm NDMA can be kept without loss for at least several months. All water bottles and sipper tubes were rinsed with rH_2O prior to filling. Bottles, cages, and mixing vessels were brightly color-coded according to treatment. Water bottles on the animal cages were shielded from room lighting with aluminum foil.

At termination the mice were weighed and then killed with CO_2 or by decapitation, all organs were inspected, and the lobes of the lungs were separated in 0.9% saline and examined for tumors. After fixation in Bouin's solution, all lungs were examined twice under a dissecting microscope. Most primary lung tumors were diagnosed with certainty by gross inspection after fixation. Questionable nodules were processed histologically (5μ sections, hematoxylin and eosin staining).

In Experiment 1, the mice were fed Normal Protein Diet (ICN Pharmaceuticals, Inc.) which was ascertained by the ThermoElectron Corp. to be free of nitrosamines (< 1 ppb). Adult strain A females (6-12 weeks of age) were treated with 10 ppb NDMA in the drinking water for 4 weeks prior to mating. Treatment was continued until conception and during pregnancy and lactation. The progeny were weaned and housed 1-4 per cage and NDMA treatment continued until they were 22 weeks old. Control mice, given rH_2O, were bred and maintained in parallel. Fresh water solutions were prepared three times per week.

In Experiment 2, the mice were fed the AIN-76 semipurified diet (ICN Pharmaceuticals, Inc.) which contains choline and methionine, and 5% fiber, which are lacking in the Normal Protein Diet, and 5% instead of 10% oil. Special precautions were taken to minimize intercurrent disease. All materials were autoclaved before first use and the mice were housed and handled separately from all other mice. Cages were rinsed with deionized water after washing. Mice were housed 12-13 per large cage, and cages for different dose groups were placed at random on the rack. The NDMA doses were 10, 50, 100, 500, and 1000 ppb.

These drinking water solutions were diluted fresh daily, including weekends and holidays. Group sizes and approximate daily and total doses are given in Table 1. Treatment was begun when the mice were 4 weeks of age, and was continued for 15½ weeks. Weight gain and water consumption were measured periodically and were the same for all groups. The mice were killed during the last half of week 16.

RESULTS

Experiment 1

The strain A mice fed the Normal Protein Diet displayed an unusually high percentage of control mice with lung tumors at 22 weeks, 15% for the females and 13% for the males (Table 2), compared with the expected value of about 5% (Shimkin and Stoner 1975) and the values in our previous experiments, 4% (δ) and 10% ($\circ$) (Anderson et al. 1979). However, at 16 months the percentages of control mice with tumor, 52% for the females and 63% for the males, is similar to the 67.5% value reported by Shimkin and Stoner (1975).

At 22 weeks, NDMA-treated males experienced an approximate 50% increase in the percentage of mice with tumor and average number of tumors per mouse, compared with controls, whereas NDMA-treated females had fewer tumors than controls. None of these differences are of statistical significance (logistic regression analysis carried out by the Biostatistics Laboratory of the Sloan-Kettering Institute).

At 16 months, the NDMA-treated females slightly exceeded controls with regard to the percentage of mice with tumor and average number of tumors per mouse, but this difference was not of statistical significance. The values for average number of tumors per mouse were similar to that expected for mice of this age (1.09 tumors) (Shimkin and Stoner 1975).

Experiment 2

Treatment of strain A mice for 16 weeks starting at weaning with 500 or 1000 ppb NDMA in the drinking water had a clear and significant effect on lung-tumor incidence (Table 3). There was a three- to fourfold increase in the percentage of mice (males plus females) with tumor in both groups, compared to controls. The largest effect was seen among the males exposed to 500 ppb NDMA, who showed an eightfold increase in tumor incidence relative to control males. 1000 ppb NDMA did not have a larger effect than 500 ppb.

The mice exposed to 10, 50, or 100 ppb NDMA had overall a slightly higher tumor incidence than the controls. Only the 50 ppb females and the 100 ppb males did not exceed the controls. When males and females were considered together, the highest tumor incidence occurred in the 10 ppb group, the next lowest in the 50 ppb group, and the lowest after treatment with 100 ppb. A

Table 1
Experiment 2. Lung Tumorigenesis in Strain A Mice Exposed to 10 ppb NDMA Postweaning (Group Compositions and Doses)

NDMA concentration (ppb)	NDMA dose daily (µg/mouse)	NDMA dose daily (µg/kg)	NDMA dose total (µg/mouse)	NDMA dose total (µg/kg)	Number females initial	Number females final	Number males initial	Number males final
0	–	–	–	–	36	36	25	25
10	0.03	1.2	3.24	130	38	38	25	25
50	0.15	6	16.2	650	26	26	25	25
100	0.3	12	32.4	1,300	25	24	25	24
500	1.5	60	162	6,500	25	22	25	23
1000	3.0	120	324	13,000	25	24	25	25

Dose levels have been estimated based on 3 ml water consumed daily by a 25g mouse and are only approximate, assuming no NDMA loss during each 24-hr period. Total dose is that consumed over 108 days.

535

Table 2

Experiment 1. Lung Tumorigenesis in Strain A Mice Exposed to 10 ppb NDMA During Early Life

Exposure time	Sex	Number mice with tumor total number tumors		Total number tumors	Number tumors Number mice
Preconception	♀	E[a]	3/53 (5.7%)	4	0.08
to		C[b]	8/54 (15%)	9	0.17
22 weeks	♂	E	14/61 (23%)	16	0.26
		C	7/52 (13%)	9	0.17
Preconception	♀	E	27/36 (75%)	43	1.19
to		C	15/29 (52%)	21	0.72
16 months	♂	E	21/31 (68%)	29	0.94
		C	24/38 (63%)	37	0.97

Female mice were exposed to 10 ppb NDMA or rH_2O for 4 wk before mating, and exposure of the progeny was continued until they were 22 wk or 16 mo. The mice were fed a semisynthetic Normal Protein Diet; the waters were freshly prepared 3 times/week. There are no significant differences between the values within each endpoint group (logistic regression analysis).

[a]E = NDMA-treated
[b]C = controls

Table 3

Experiment 2. Lung Tumor Incidences in Strain A Mice Exposed to Five NDMA Doses after Weaning

NDMA concentration (ppb)	Number tumor bearers[a]/Total number mice		
	female	male	total
0	4/36 (11.1)[b]	2/25 (8)	6/61 (9.8)
10	6/38 (15.8)	5/25 (20)	11/63 (17.5)
50	3/26 (11.5)	4/25 (16)	7/51 (13.7)
100	4/24 (16.7)	2/24 (8.3)	6/48 (12.5)
500	6/22 (27.3)	10/23[d] (43.5)	16/45[c] (35.6)
1000	7/24 (29.2)	7/25 (28)	14/49[d] (28.6)

[a]Each tumor bearer had one tumor except for: 2 tumors in 1 control male, in 1 50 ppb dose group male, in 1 100 ppb dose group female, in 1 female and 2 males in the 500 ppb dose group (plus a male with 5 tumors in this group), and in 1 female and 1 male in the 1000 ppb dose group.
[b]Percentage
[c,d]Significantly greater than corresponding control value, χ^2 test, [c]$p < 0.01$, [d]$p < 0.05$

linear plot of these three values versus dose revealed a straight line with negative slope. However, none of these three low-dose groups, or all three considered together, differed significantly from the control group by the Fisher Exact Test. With this test p = .298 for the 10 ppb group versus controls.

As in Experiment 1, the percentage of tumor-bearing control mice, 9.8%, was higher than expected, 2.9% at 5 months of age (Shimkin and Stoner 1975).

DISCUSSION

The usefulness of the strain A mouse lung tumor as a model for investigating low-dose effects of nitrosamines (Anderson et al. 1979) is further demonstrated by the results presented here from Experiment 2. A tumorigenic effect of 500 ppb NDMA in the drinking water was clearly shown after an experiment time of 16 weeks and a total dose of about 160 μg/mouse, with total group sizes of 50-60 mice. This dose is somewhat lower than the suggested minimal amount needed for an unequivocal carcinogenic effect of NDMA in rat liver (Arai et al. 1979; Preussmann 1980). Of special interest is the fact that the approximate total dose of NDMA received by each mouse in the 500 ppb dose group in our experiment, about 6.5 mg/kg, is roughly comparable to the total dose of NDEA/kg received over 30 weeks as a 450 ppb solution by the Fischer rats in the experiments of Lijinsky et al. (1981). The latter treatment resulted, at the end of the lifetime of the rats, in neoplastic or preneoplastic lesions in 30% of the livers. This value compares favorably with the 35.6% tumor bearers among all mice given 500 ppb NDMA in our experiment. These comparative considerations might suggest that NDMA (the more prevalent environmental contaminant) is at least as potent a carcinogen as NDEA, and that rat liver and mouse lung, though biologically diverse test systems, can give quantitatively similar dose-response results with nitrosamines.

An important difference in the mouse lung and rat liver assay systems is that the mouse lung tumors were counted 16 weeks after the start of treatment, whereas rat liver tumorigenesis experiments such as that of Lijinsky et al. (1981) require the life of the animal, up to 130 weeks. The practical advantages of the short endpoint of the lung-tumor model are obvious. However, it must be noted that the lack of latency in the strain A mouse lung tumor (Jones and Grendon 1975) contrasts with the inverse relation between dose and latency characteristic of rat liver tumors (Druckrey et al. 1967) and perhaps of some or many types of human cancer. The strain A lung tumor might be regarded as a specialized model giving immediate expression to first-step initiation events in carcinogenesis.

The effects of 1000 ppb NDMA in Experiment 2 were no greater or possibly less than those of 500 ppb. This situation could indicate that the dose-response curve is quite flat in this region, or might reflect operation of other factors, such as higher toxicity to neoplastic cells or greater induction of DNA repair enzymes at the higher dose (Montesano et al. 1980). Similar lack of expected dose-responsiveness has occurred in other nitrosamine assays (Cardesa et al. 1974; Ii et al. 1976; Preussmann et al. 1977).

The results with environmental-level doses of NDMA (10-100 ppb) from Experiments 1 and 2 provide tentative confirmation of our initial finding, that 10 ppb NDMA is tumorigenic in strain A mouse lung if given during the sensitive early-life period. This effect was partly obscured by an elevation in control tumor incidence, which was probably attributable to acceleration of growth of the first-appearing spontaneous tumors by the calorie density and nutritional excellence of the semipurified diets. Larger group sizes and (or) shorter end-points in time may permit circumvention of this limitation in future experiments and statistically sound confirmation of the 10 ppb effect. Nevertheless, the fact that at this dose an increase in tumor incidence of similar magnitude occurred in the male mice in three separate assays supports the contention that the effect is real and potentially measurable. A tumorigenic effect of 10 ppb NDMA should in fact not be surprising. Another type of carcinogen, aflatoxin B_1 was found to be tumorigenic at a dose of 1 ppb in food (Wogan et al. 1974). NDMA doses as low as 1-50 μg/kg resulted in alkylation of the DNA of liver and other organs after oral administration to rats (Diaz Gomez et al. 1977; Pegg and Hui 1978; Pegg and Perry 1981).

In Experiment 2 there was a decrease in measured total tumor incidence as the dose was increased from 10 ppb to 50 ppb and 100 ppb; these three values plotted against dose closely fit a straight line with negative slope. More dose points and larger group sizes will be required to determine if this phenomenon is real. While such a dose-response relationship would be anomalous, it is not beyond explanation, when factors such as carcinogen metabolism and induction of repair of methylated DNA are considered. It is a possibility of sufficient potential importance to indicate further study.

No cumulative effects of 10 ppb NDMA were seen over 16 months of treatment in Experiment 1; any excess of tumors induced by NDMA during early life were obscured by the large number of spontaneous tumors that had appeared by this time. It seems that lung tumorigenesis by low doses of NDMA may be most readily observed after early life treatment. A comparison of the results obtained in the three assays carried out thus far indicates that tumors are induced both pre- and post-weaning by a low dose of NDMA in the drinking water, although further investigation will be required for more accurate assignment of proportions of tumors originating during various ontogenetic stages.

ACKNOWLEDGMENTS

This work was supported by National Cancer Institute Grants CA-22509 and CA-08748.

REFERENCES

Anderson, L.M., L.J. Priest, and J.M. Budinger. 1979. Lung tumorigenesis in mice after chronic exposure in early life to a low dose of dimethylnitrosamine. *J. Natl. Cancer Inst.* **62**:1553.

Arai, M., Y. Aoki, K. Nakanishi, Y. Miyata, T. Mori, and N. Ito. 1979. Long-term experiment of maximal non-carcinogenic dose of dimethylnitrosamine for carcinogenesis in rats. *Gann* **70**:549.

Cardesa, A., P. Pour, J. Althoff, and U. Mohr. 1974. Comparative studies of neoplastic response to a single dose of nitroso compounds. 4. The effect of dimethyl- and diethyl-nitrosamine in Swiss mice. *Z. Krebsforsch.* **81**: 229.

Crampton, R.F. 1980. Carcinogenic dose-related response to nitrosamines. *Oncology* **37**:251.

Diaz Gomez, M.I., P.F. Swann, and P.N. Magee. 1977. The absorption and metabolism in rats of small oral doses of dimethylnitrosamine. *Biochem. J.* **164**:497.

Druckrey, H., R. Preussmann, S. Ivankovic, and D. Schmähl. 1967. Organotrope carcinogene Wirkungen bei 65 verschiedenen N-Nitroso-Verbindungen an BD-Ratten. *Z. Krebsforsch.* **69**:103.

Druckrey, H., A. Schildbach, D. Schmähl, R. Preussmann, and S. Ivankovic. 1963. Quantitative Analyse der carcinogenen Wirkung von Diathylnitrosamin. *Arzneim. Forsch.* **13**:842.

Edwards, G.S., J.G. Fox, P. Policastro, U. Goff, M.H. Wolf, and D.H. Fine. 1979. Volatile nitrosamine contamination of laboratory animal diets. *Cancer Res.* **39**:1857.

Fine, D.H. 1980. Exposure assessment to preformed environmental N-nitroso compounds from the point of view of our own studies. *Oncology* **37**: 199.

Fine, D.H., D.P. Rounbehler, T. Fan, and R. Ross. 1977a. Human exposure to N-nitroso compounds in the environment. *Cold Spring Harbor Conf Cell Proliferation* **4**:293.

Fine, D.H., R. Ross, D.P. Rounbehler, A. Silvergleid, and L. Song. 1977b. Formation *in vivo* of volatile N-nitrosamines in man after ingestion of cooked bacon and spinach. *Nature* **265**:753.

Heston, W.E. and C.H. Steffee. 1957. Development of tumors in fetal and adult lung transplants. *J. Natl. Cancer Inst.* **18**:779.

Ii, Y., A. Cardesa, K. Patil, J. Althoff, and P. Pour. 1976. Comparative studies of neoplastic response to a single dose of nitroso compounds. 5. The effect of dimethylnitrosamine in Swiss, ASW/SN and A-strain mice. *Z. Krebsforsch.* **86**:165.

Jones, H.B. and A. Grendon. 1975. Environmental factors in the origin of cancer and estimation of the possible hazard to man. *Food Cosmet. Toxicol.* **13**: 251.

Kann, J., B. Spiegelhalder, G. Eisenbrand, and P. Preussmann. 1977. Occurrence of volatile N-nitrosamines in animal diets. *Z. Krebsforsch.* **90**:321.

Lakritz, L., M.L. Simenhoff, S.R. Dunn, and W. Fiddler. 1980. N-Nitrosodimethylamine in human blood. *Food Cosmet. Toxicol.* **18**:77.

Lijinsky, W., M.D. Reuber, and C.W. Riggs. 1981. Dose response studies of carcinogenesis in rats by nitrosodiethylamine. *Cancer Res.* **41**:4997.

Montesano, R., H. Brésil, G. Planche-Marcel, G.P. Margison, and A.E. Pegg. 1980. Effect of chronic treatment of rats with dimethylnitrosamine on the removal of O^6-methylguanine from DNA. *Cancer Res.* **40**:452.

Pegg, A.E. and G. Hui. 1978. Formation and subsequent removal of O^6-methylguanine from deoxyribonucleic acid in rat liver and kidney after small doses of dimethylnitrosamine. *Biochem. J.* **173**:739.

Pegg, A.E. and W. Perry. 1981. Alkylation of nucleic acids and metabolism of small doses of dimethylnitrosamine in the rat. *Cancer Res.* **41**:3128.

Preussmann, R. 1972. On the significance of N-nitroso compounds as carcinogens and on problems related to their chemical analysis. *IARC Sci. Publ.* **3**:6.

_____. 1980. Dose-response studies and 'no-effect-levels' of N-nitroso compounds. *Oncology* **37**:243.

Preussmann, R., D. Schmähl, and G. Eisenbrand. 1977. Carcinogenicity of N-nitrosopyrrolidine: Dose-response study in rats. *Z. Krebsforsch.* **90**:161.

Shimkin, M.B. and G.D. Stoner. 1975. Lung tumors in mice: Application to carcinogenesis bioassay. *Adv. Cancer Res.* **21**:2.

Tannenbaum, S.R. 1980. A model for estimation of human exposure to endogenous N-nitrosodimethylamine. *Oncology* **37**:232.

Terracini, B., P.N. Magee, and J.M. Barnes. 1967. Hepatic pathology in rats on low dietary levels of dimethylnitrosamine. *Br. J. Cancer* **21**:559.

Toth, B. 1968. Critical review of experiments in chemical carcinogenesis using newborn animals. *Cancer Res.* **28**:727.

Wogan, G.N., S. Paglialunga, and P.M. Newberne. 1974. Carcinogenic effects of low dietary levels of aflatoxin B_1 in rats. *Food Cosmet. Toxicol.* **12**:681.

Yamamoto, M., T. Yamada, and A. Tanimura. 1980. Volatile nitrosamines in human blood before and after ingestion of a meal containing high concentrations of nitrate and secondary amines. *Food Cosmet. Toxicol.* **18**:297.

COMMENTS

GRASSO: Did you find multiple tumors in your treated animals?

ANDERSON: Yes. Most of the groups had one mouse with two tumors. At the 500 ppb dose, which resulted in the highest percent mice with tumors, there were three mice with two tumors and one mouse with five tumors.

GRASSO: Did you find that there was any difference in the histology between your controls and the ones that are induced? Were the ones induced with NDMA more malignant?

ANDERSON: I haven't analyzed them in the second experiment. In experiment 1, I looked at about half of them, simply scoring papillary versus nonpapillary, and I did not see a difference.

HOFFMANN: What was the source of your protein in the synthetic diet?

ANDERSON: Casein.

HOFFMANN: There is an NIH diet on the market which has 10 ppb NDMA.

ANDERSON: That is why I started using the semisynthetic diets.

HOFFMANN: Yes, but that is an NIH semisynthetic diet, which has about 10 ppb.

ANDERSON: I sent a sample of the Normal Protein Diet to Thermal Electron, and they did not reveal any nitrosamines at their level of detection at that time.

PREUSSMANN: That is astonishing.

CONNEY: We have used the newborn mouse model for identifying ultimate carcinogenic metabolites of polycyclic aromatic hydrocarbons. We do it in a little different way. We use the Swiss-Webster mouse and inject these animals on day one of life, on day eight of life we double the dose, and on day 15 of life we double that dose. That has been a very useful model for polycyclic hydrocarbons. At between 20 and 30 weeks of life, we usually kill the animals, and we find pulmonary tumors that are formed. Usually we obtain excellent dose-response curves, particularly when we express the data as pulmonary tumors per mouse. I think it is important to count the number of pulmonary tumors and then to express the data as tumors per mouse, as well as expressing it as percent tumors.

ANDERSON: These are two different ways of presenting mouse lung tumor data. For some purposes, the value percent mice with tumor is more useful than average tumors per mouse. This is particularly true with low doses, as in our experiments. There were so few animals in these experiments having more than one tumor that it seemed more revealing to talk about percent mice with tumor. One of the attractive features of this model is that one can go all the way from a very low dose, with which only a few mice out of the whole population develop tumors, up to a huge dose, where the parameter measured is average number of tumors per mouse. It is quite nicely quantitatively dose-responsive, as you have found.

CONNEY: Our modification of the system simplifies it very much, in that you only treat with carcinogen on three occasions, and then wait for tumor development.

ANDERSON: It would be very useful to try that with these lower doses, and see how the effects of three acute treatments compares with chronic daily exposure.

ARCHER: I just wondered if you have made any analytical determinations on the NDMA in water. Did you just make it up and assume it was 10 ppb?

ANDERSON: No. Again, I sent a few samples to Thermal Electron at an early stage in order to make sure that the concentration was actually what it was supposed to be and to determine what the decay rate in the water was.

ARCHER: But you didn't see any decay?

ANDERSON: Yes. That is why in the most recent experiment the water was changed 7 days a week. When the water bottle has been on a cage for 3 days half of the NDMA is lost.

CASTONGUAY: Did you look at other sites, especially liver and nasal area?

ANDERSON: We did what I would call a limited necropsy, in which we looked at the abdominal and thoracic organs, and I would have seen anything striking in the liver. Dissecting into the nasal cavity or opening of the stomach were not done.

MIRVISH: Did you check water consumption in different groups?

ANDERSON: Yes. It was the same.

A Sensitive Short-term In Vivo Bioassay for
N-Nitroso Carcinogenesis in Mouse Liver

STANLEY GOLDFARB, THOMAS D. PUGH, AND HIROFUMI KOEN
Department of Pathology
University of Wisconsin
School of Medicine
Madison, Wisconsin 57306

The development of reliable, short-term in vivo bioassays to measure carcinogen potency, to replace currently recommended lifetime tests (Page 1977) could be of great value to speed up the testing of the large number of potentially dangerous agents accumulating in our environment, and to reduce the staggering cost of the studies. The problem is of particular urgency in assessing the relative carcinogenicity of N-nitroso compounds, which range from noncarcinogenic (e.g., N-nitrosoproline) to highly carcinogenic (e.g., N-nitrosodiethylamine [NDEA]). In order to be useful for an assay system, an animal model with a broad range of sensitivity and low spontaneous incidence of neoplasms is particularly desirable. In addition, the early lesions being quantitated should not undergo spontaneous regression, and should be demonstrated to be precursors of the fully autonomous later-appearing neoplasms. Furthermore, the early lesions should be readily identified and easily counted while still microscopic.

The infant mouse liver tumor model appeared potentially useful for this purpose, since single injections of a broad range of carcinogens in B6C3 F_1 infant mice induced metastasizing trabecular hepatocellular carcinomas after one year (Vesselinovitch et al. 1978). Since the biologic and morphologic characteristics of the lesions preceding the development of these neoplasms has not been described in detail (Moore et al. 1981), we decided to characterize the precursor lesions induced by NDEA and determine whether their quantitation would be useful for an in vivo bioassay system. Preliminary reports characterizing the early lesions (Goldfarb et al. 1980; Goldfarb et al. 1981) and describing a method for their quantitation (Pugh et al. 1982) have appeared.

MATERIALS AND METHODS

Male B6C3 F_1 mice were injected i.p. with 30 μl of saline, or with 5 μg/g body weight of NDEA in the same volume of saline, when they were 15 days of age. Groups of mice were killed at 3 days, and after 1, 2, 4, 10, 20, 28, 36, and 44 weeks following injection. Mice killed at 4 weeks and later were injected i.p.

with 0.6 μCi of (methyl-^{3}H) thymidine (New England Nuclear, Boston, MA; specific activity, 7.6 Ci/mmole) in six divided doses at six hourly intervals beginning 36 hours prior to sacrifice.

Representative blocks of liver were fixed in formalin, cut at 5 μm, and stained with hematoxylin and eosin or with periodic acid Schiff stain, with or without prior incubation in diastase. Sections were also stained with toluidine blue, either with or without prior RNAase digestion, to evaluate their RNA content. Additionally, frozen samples were cut on the cryostat and stained for alkaline phosphatase, ATPase, glucose-6-phosphatase, and γ-glutamyl transpeptidase. Other sections were stained for neutral lipid with oil red 0.

Autoradiograms were prepared from paraffin sections of livers from mice killed at 20, 28, and 36 weeks. Thymidine labeling indices were determined in all focal hepatocellular lesions and in background hepatocytes. Labeling indices were based on the evaluation of all hepatocytes in focal lesions having transectional diameters less than 700 μm. However, to avoid counting in areas that might have suffered ischemic injury, only cells in the peripheral 250 μm in transections with radii larger than 700 μm were evaluated. The areas of transections of focal hepatic lesions and of liver sections were determined by computer assisted planimetry (Goldfarb and Pugh 1982). In some livers, the exact volumes of individual foci and their size distributions were determined in serially sectioned blocks of livers. The volumes of 26 foci from blocks of livers from 3 mice killed at 10, 20, and 28 weeks were also evaluated. Since the relationship of a sphere to its radius is described mathematically and graphically, it was thus possible to assess the degree of sphericity of the foci by comparing the largest cross-sectional areas of the foci with the equatorial plane areas of perfect spheres having the same volumes as the foci.

RESULTS

Body and Liver Weights in Control and Experimental Animals

Major increases in body and liver weights in control and experimental animals occurred prior to the tenth week after injection. The mean body weights of both groups of animals increased to 25 gm at 20 weeks after NDEA, and was essentially unchanged throughout the remainder of the study. In control animals, the mean liver weight had reached about 90% of its maximum by 10 weeks and it, too, remained quite constant at about 1.25 gm at 20 weeks and later (Fig. 1). The weights of the livers were similar in control and experimental animals until 28 weeks after carcinogen treatment. After that time, due to enlargement of neoplasms, the livers of carcinogen-treated mice underwent marked increases in weight. They were 26% heavier than controls by 36 weeks, and twice the mean control weight by 44 weeks.

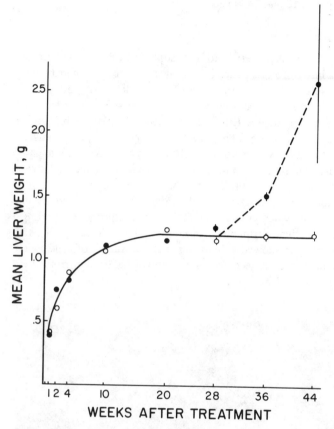

Figure 1
Mean liver weight at sacrifice of control mice (o) and mice injected with NDEA (•). Mean ±
S.E.M. are shown at 28, 36, and 44 weeks after injection.

Hepatic Changes During the First 4 Weeks

Lipid accumulation was prominent in central and midzonal areas of hepatic
lobules by 3 days after NDEA injection, but these changes had completely re-
gressed after an additional 4 days. At no time were fatty changes observed in
control mice. All other histochemical studies revealed no differences between
control and experimental animals. At 4 weeks after injection, livers from control
and experimental animals were indistinguishable.

Hepatic Changes Between 10 and 44 Weeks

Morphological Features

Distinctive collections of cells, referred to as basophilic hepatic foci, were the only alterations in addition to late-appearing (44 weeks) trabecular hepatocellular carcinomas that were identified in the livers of mice killed during this period. At 10 weeks after injection, the foci were infrequent, very small, and composed entirely of basophilic hepatocytes (Fig. 2). However, after that time, focal hepatic lesions were more numerous and showed a progressive increase in size. On randomly cut sections, the vast majority of these also contained only hepatocytes. However, when cut serially, some of the larger foci contained relatively small well-delineated aggregates of proliferated bile ductules in addition to the hepatocytes. Invariably, these clusters of proliferated ductules were connected to interlobular bile ducts which entered the foci in association with "feeding" portal vein branches at their peripheries. In addition to their basophilia, the hepatocytes within the foci showed a characteristic "crowding" of cells which resulted from their high nuclear to cytoplasmic ratios (Fig. 2), and from their

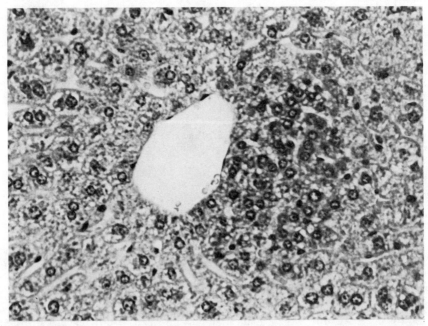

Figure 2
Tiny basophilic hepatic focus adjacent to a terminal hepatic vein. The high nuclear to cytoplasmic ratio results in a "crowded" appearance. The mouse was killed 10 wk after injection of NDEA. H&E x380.

growing in sheets. Because of the "crowding" of cells within basophilic foci, it was often difficult to determine the thickness of hepatic plates. When discernible, however, they were predominantly one to two cells in thickness (Fig. 3).

Infiltration into small hepatic veins was a prominent characteristic of the basophilic foci (Fig. 4). Although present in only 5% of foci from mice sacrificed at 10 weeks, it was very common at 20 weeks and later. In fact, in one serially sectioned block of liver from a 20-week mouse, 9 of 45 identified foci were found to infiltrate the hepatic veins. In contrast, portal veins were not invaded. The preferential invasion of hepatic veins was of particular interest, since smaller foci often seemed to be located closer to the terminal hepatic veins than to the portal vein branches (as shown in Fig. 1).

A few grossly visible nodules, with the histologic features of foci, and measuring up to 2 mm in diameter, were first noted in mice sacrificed at 36 weeks after injection. By 44 weeks, these had become more frequent, showed further enlargement, and, in a few instances, manifested more marked cytologic atypia, mitoses, and further thickening of hepatic plates (4-5 cells) characteristic of trabecular carcinomas (Fig. 5). It was noteworthy that none of the livers

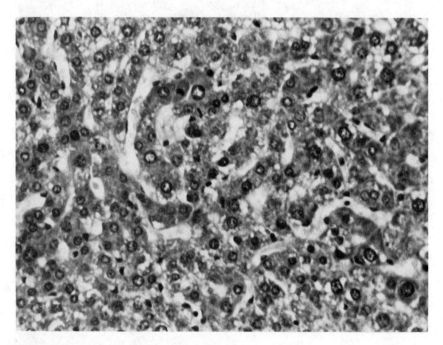

Figure 3
Hepatocytes in the center of a basophilic hepatic focus showing one cell thick plates. The mouse was killed 20 weeks after NDEA injection. H&E x380.

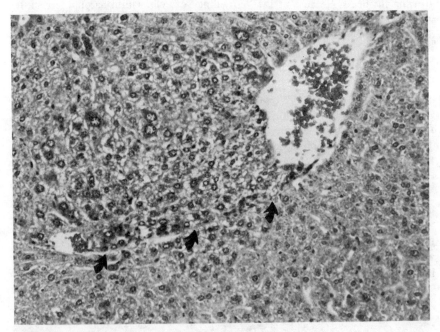

Figure 4
Basophilic hepatic focus that has infiltrated a small hepatic vein branch. A tumor thrombus
(→ → →) fills approximately one-half of the lumen. The mouse was killed 20 weeks after
NDEA injection. H&E x195.

from control mice killed up to 44 weeks after injection contained any neoplasms.

Histochemical Features of Hepatocytes in Basophilic Foci

The cytoplasmic basophilia in the foci resulted from accumulation of RNA,
since it was totally eradicated by incubation with RNAase prior to staining
with toluidine blue. An additional histochemical alteration, seen in all basophilic
foci, was a generally uniform deficiency of glucose-6-phosphatase. The distribution of the other enzyme histochemical activities were no different from
controls.

Nuclear to Cytoplasmic Ratios of Hepatocytes in Basophilic Foci

The nuclear to cytoplasmic ratios in foci from livers of mice injected with NDEA
10 or 20 weeks earlier, were consistently and significantly increased when this
parameter was compared to adjacent background hepatocytes or to hepatocytes

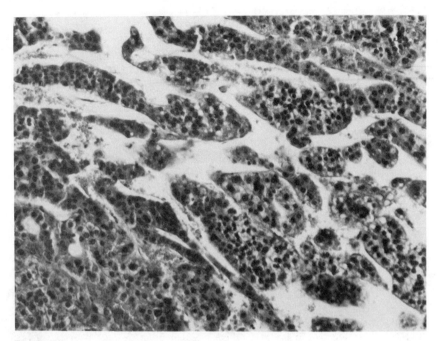

Figure 5
Trabecular hepatocellular carcinoma showing papillary features and marked anaplasia in a mouse that was killed 44 weeks after NDEA injection. H&E x195.

from control livers (Table 1). At each sacrifice time, the ratios were about two times higher in the foci than in the comparable control tissue.

Shape of Basophilic Foci

A particularly good correlation (r = .99) was demonstrated between the maximal cross sectional areas of foci, presumed to be through their equatorial planes, and the volumes of the foci (as shown in Fig. 6). Since the line depicting this experimentally derived relationship was very close to and almost parallel to the line showing the correlation between spheres and their largest cross-sectional areas, it appeared reasonable to conclude that most foci had almost spherical shapes.

Quantitation of Size, Number, and Volumes of the
Basophilic Hepatic Foci

In order to compare the number and sizes of basophilic hepatic foci at different sacrifice times, serially sectioned blocks of liver from mice were compared. For this study it was sufficient to identify and determine the largest cross-sectional

Table 1
Nuclear to Cytoplasmic Ratios of Hepatocytes in Basophilic Hepatocellular Foci, Background Areas, and Control Livers

Weeks after NDEA injection	Number of experimental mice	N/C Ratios		
		foci	background areas	control areas
10	3	0.115 ± 0.042 (6)[a,b,c,d]	0.055 ± 0.011 (6)	0.054 ± 0.013 (16)
20	8	0.140 ± 0.048 (40)	0.070 ± 0.017 (16)[e]	0.068 ± 0.016 (16)

Background areas represent normal appearing hepatocytes in livers that also contained basophilic hepatocellular foci.
[a] Number in parentheses = number of hepatocellular foci or number of microscopic fields of normal hepatocytes.
[b] Mean ± SEM for this and subsequent charts.
[c] Differences between N/C ratios in 10-wk foci v. background areas. p < .01 Student's t-test for this and subsequent charts.
[d] Differences between N/C ratios in 10-wk foci v. control areas. p < .002.
[e] Differences between labeling indices in 20-wk foci v. background areas and between 20-wk foci and control areas. p < .002.

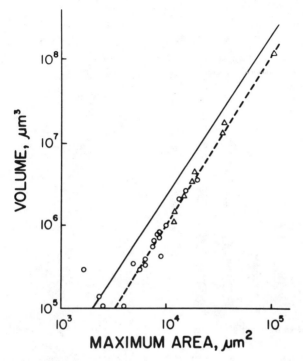

Figure 6
Plot depicting the correlation between the maximal cross sectional areas and volumes of individual foci. The data were derived from serial section reconstructions. (△) depict data from mice killed 20 wk after NDEA injection; (○) similar data from mice killed at 10 wk after injection; (————) relationship between the volumes of perfect spheres and the areas of circular profiles through their equatorial planes. The correlation coefficient (r) = 0.99.

area of the foci, since this parameter provides a close approximation of the foci volumes (see above). This was accomplished by first identifying all foci and then, for each, determining the five or six largest cross-sectional areas planimetrically. The single largest transection was then readily selected. Data for two of the livers, one at 20 weeks and one at 28 weeks post-carcinogen injection, are indicated in Figure 7 and Table 2. As noted, the two mice, selected for comparison, had almost identical total numbers of foci, but the 28-week mouse liver had three times more foci (12% of the total) in the four largest size classes than the 20-week mouse liver (4% of the total). This small increase in the absolute number of larger foci resulted in a very great increase (sevenfold) in the aggregate volume of all the foci. The effect of these larger foci on the total number of transections is also apparent in Figure 7. Clearly, the larger foci generated more profiles in the tissue sections. Thus, despite a similar number of foci, the liver from the 28-week old mouse contained almost twice as many transections as that from the 20-week mouse.

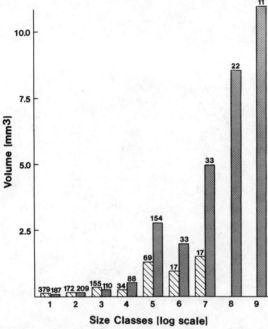

Figure 7

Histogram of foci size distribution in two mice killed at 20 and 28 weeks. The size classes denote the largest cross-sectional areas of the foci and increase exponentially through nine size ranges. For example, size class one includes all foci having largest cross-sectional areas between 5,000-10,000 μm^2 and size class two includes all foci between 10,000-20,000 μm^2, etc. The largest size class, nine, includes all foci whose largest cross sectional areas measure between 1.28 and 2.56 mm^2. The numbers above the bars refer to the number of foci in the particular size class, while the height of the bar indicates the total volume contribution of all foci in that size class. The data is summarized in Table 2.

Table 2

Comparison of the Total Number of Foci, Profiles, and Their Aggregate Volumes in Livers of Two Mice Killed at 20 and 28 Weeks

	20 weeks	28 weeks
Total number of foci/cm^3	845	846
Foci profiles/cm^2	8.9	16
Total volume of foci (mm^3/cm^3)	4.5	31

Summary of data shown in Figure 7.

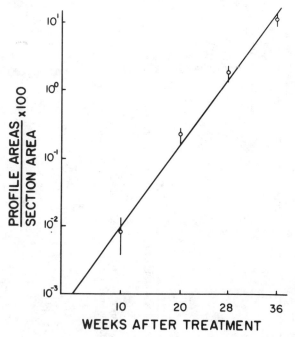

Figure 8
Percentage of section areas occupied by profiles of hepatocellular foci in sections from livers of mice injected with NDEA. The plotted data points are means ± S.E.M. for groups of 8 mice at each sacrifice time. The correlation coefficient (r) = 0.99.

The effect of the progressively increasing number of larger foci on the total volume of the tumor may be deduced from Figure 8, which depicts an exponential increase with time in the fraction: $\dfrac{\text{profile areas}}{\text{section areas}}$ since the liver weights showed only slight increase between 10 and 36 weeks, and since the ratios between areas are proportional to the ratios between volumes (Delesse 1848), it follows that, in aggregate, the foci volumes also showed exponential increases during the interval under study.

Labeling Indices of Foci

As further measure of growth rate, the ^{3}H-TdR labeling indices were determined for most of the foci at 20 weeks, and for a comparable number of randomly selected foci at 20 and 36 weeks after NDEA injection. The cumulative data (Table 3) demonstrated a 10- to 80-fold increase in mean labeling indices in the foci when compared to normal appearing (background) areas within the experimental livers. The mean labeling index was 1.6% after 20 weeks, and underwent

Table 3
3H-dT Labeling Indices in Livers of Mice at Intervals after NDEA Injection

Weeks after injection	Number of mice	Types of sampled areas	Number of foci or areas[a]	Labeling indices
20	6	foci	28	1.62 ± 0.35[b,c,d]
		background	154	0.08 ± 0.03
28	8	foci	34	3.73 ± 0.39[e]
		background	427	0.32 ± 0.03
36	8	foci	49	3.22 ± 0.27[f]
		background	383	0.04 ± 0.01

[a]Background areas were randomly sampled fields (62,500 μm^2) of normal appearing hepatocytes from the experimental livers. Each field contained approximately 100 cells.
[b]Mean ± SEM
[c]Difference between labeling indices in 20 v. 28-wk mice and 20 v. 36-wk mice. $p < .002$, Student's t-test.
[d,e,f]Differences between labeling indices in foci and their comparable background areas; $p < .0001$, Student's t-test.

a further increase to 3.7% at 28 weeks. The labeling indices remained at this high rate (3.2%) in mice sacrificed at 36 weeks after injection. The increase in labeled cells was not restricted to foci from particular livers since it was documented, to a similar degree, in foci from all livers. The presence of mitoses in some of the foci in mice killed at 20 weeks, appeared to correlate with the increase in the mean labeling index that occurred at that time.

DISCUSSION

This report documents the early homogeneous appearance and progressive changes in foci of hepatocytes that appeared after a single injection of diethyl-nitrosamine in infant mice. The smallest foci, first noted at 10 weeks following carcinogen treatment, were composed of hepatocytes showing high nuclear to cytoplasmic ratios, diminished or absent glucose-6-phosphatase activity, and increased cytoplasmic RNA. In many organs, an increase in nuclear to cytoplasmic ratio is generally considered a feature of premalignant and malignant cells (Koss 1979), and in rat liver, the loss of glucose-6-phosphatase activity characterizes a subset of putative premalignant hepatocellular islands (Goldfarb and Zak 1961; Gossner and Friedrich-Freksa 1964; Pugh and Goldfarb 1978). More significantly, the malignant and premalignant character of the early foci is supported by the finding that some of them were found to invade terminal hepatic veins as early as 10 weeks following injection of NDEA. Indeed, the early invasive character of the foci appears to correlate quite well with the late appearance, in high incidence, of pulmonary metastases (Vesselinovitch 1980; Vesselinovitch et al. 1980).

After 10 weeks, the focal lesions continued to enlarge, became more anaplastic, and further increased their already high thymidine labeling indices. Since tumor progression is accompanied by a process of selection in which the most rapidly replicating cells overgrow those that divide less frequently (Nowell 1976), one would expect to see a progressive increase with time in the growth rates of tumors. However, to our knowledge, the present report of a doubling of ^{3}H-TdR labeling indices between 20 and 28 is the first example of its kind, suggesting a spontaneous increase in growth rate in primary experimental hepatic neoplasms. In summary, the temporal evidence for tumor progression is compelling, and it appears that the seemingly uniform early basophilic foci developed into trabecular hepatocellular carcinomas by a stepwise or sequential process similar to that suggested for diverse neoplasms (Farber and Cameron 1980).

During the course of this study, the aggregate volume of the focal lesions increased exponentially in a fashion consistent with the early growth phase of autonomous neoplasms (Steel 1977). Of course, the observed aggregate tumor doubling time of 2.5 weeks is only an average of the growth rates of all the focal lesions. In fact, the effect of only a few large foci was evident in the serial section study of two livers from mice killed at 20 and 28 weeks. In both cases, the foci were spread through a very broad range of sizes and only about 10%-

15% of them accounted for approximately 90% of the tumor volume. The two mice had almost identical numbers of foci, but a small fraction of the total were considerably larger in the older mouse. This resulted in a sevenfold greater aggregate tumor volume, and clearly indicates that future kinetic analyses will require an accurate assessment of the size distributions of foci.

In our most recent studies, in collaboration with mathematicians and statisticians at the University of Wisconsin, our group developed and evaluated a mathematical-stereologic method which permits the accurate estimation of the number of microscopic neoplasms from the numbers and sizes of their transections (Pugh et al. 1982). The new method employs the following mathematical formula:

$$N_3^\epsilon = \frac{1}{\pi A} \sum_{x_i > \epsilon} \frac{1}{\sqrt{x_i^2 - \epsilon^2}} \qquad (1)$$

in which:

N_3^ϵ = expected number of foci (of size larger than ϵ)/cm^3

$x_i,...,x_n$ = radii of observed foci transections

ϵ = radius of foci transections above which profiles are reliably recognized

A = total tissue slice area

This formula differs from others that have recently been employed for this type of extrapolation, in that it takes into consideration the inability of the observer to reproducibly recognize foci that are smaller than a certain size (ϵ). In our laboratory, we have found ϵ to be only 38.5 μm. The method was tested on actual transection data after reconstructing over 700 foci from their serial sections in 17 livers. We have also tested the new method by Monte Carlo computer simulations of the actual data at 20 and 28 weeks (D. Nychka et al., in prep.). In the studies, we compared the estimates using the formula with two other methods that do not take cognizance of the lower limit of observation (Moore et al. 1981; Scherer et al. 1972). We found the new method provided a far better estimate of the number of foci than either of the other estimators. The use of this formula to extrapolate three-dimensional estimates from two-dimensional data is particularly important for the development of a short term in vivo bioassay, since the fraction of the foci in size classes close to the lower limit of observation is greatest at early sacrifice times. These distributions increase the tendency of the previously employed methods to underestimate the number of foci (T.D. Pugh et al., unpubl. results; D. Nychka et al., in prep.).

Although we have not yet completed dose response studies with NDEA preliminary results suggest a close to linear response for the total number of foci, with little change in size distribution between 1.25 to 5 μg NDEA/g body weight. Tests of other N-nitroso compounds are also incomplete. However, since two additional members of this group—ethylnitrosourea and N-nitrosodimethylamine—are reported to induce hepatocellular carcinomas after one year in this same mouse model (Vesselinovitch 1969; Kyriazis and Vesselinovitch 1973), there is every reason to believe that the foci will also be induced by many *N*-nitroso compounds. In summary, it now appears most likely that measurement of the number and size of foci transections in mouse liver after only 10-20 weeks, when analyzed with the newly developed mathematical method, will provide accurate estimates of many hundreds of foci per liver, and thus greatly improve the ability to estimate carcinogenic potency of *N*-nitroso compounds in this species in relatively short periods of time.

ACKNOWLEDGMENTS

Supported by NIH grants CA15664 and CA25522.

We thank Dr. Stan D. Vesslinovitch, and his associate, Dr. N. Mihailovich, of the Departments of Radiology and Pathology at the University of Chicago, for providing us with the treated and control mice used in this study.

The superb technical assistance of Mrs. Donna Pearce is also gratefully acknowledged.

REFERENCES

Delesse, A. 1848. Procédé méchanique pour déterminer la composition des roches. *Ann. Mines* **13**:379.

Farber, E. and R. Cameron. 1980. The sequential analysis of cancer development. *Adv. Cancer Res.* **31**:125.

Goldfarb, S. and F.G. Zak. 1961. Role of injury and hyperplasia in the induction of hepatocellular carcinoma. *J. Am. Med. Assoc.* **178**:729.

Goldfarb, S. and T.D. Pugh. 1982. The origin and significance of hyperplastic hepatocellular islands and nodules in hepatic carcinogenesis. *J. Am. Coll. Toxicol.* **1**:119.

Goldfarb, S., S.D. Vesselinovitch, T.D. Pugh, N. Mihailovich, H. Koen, and Y.Z. He. 1980. Remarkable uniformity of premalignant and malignant hepatocellular foci after single dose injection of diethylnitrosamine (DEN) in infant mice. *Gastroenterology* **79**:1021.

———. 1981. Progression during early stages of mouse hepatocarcinogenesis in mice injected with diethylnitrosamine during infancy. *Proc. Am. Assoc. Cancer Res.* **22**:124.

Gossner, W. and H. Freidrich-Freksa. 1964. Histochemische untersuchungen uber die glucose-6-phosphatase in der rattenleber wahrend der kanzerisierung durch nitrosamine. *Z. Naturforsch.* **19B**:862.

Koss, L.G. 1979. *Diagnostic cytology and its histopathologic bases,* 3rd ed., vol. 1, p. 76. Lippincott, Philadelphia, Pennsylvania.

Kyriazis, A.P. and S.D. Vesselinovitch. 1973. Transplantability and biologic behavior of mouse liver tumors induced by ethylnitrosourea. *Cancer Res.* **33**:332.

Moore, M.P., N.R. Drinkwater, E.C. Miller, J.A. Miller, and H.C. Pitot. 1981.

Quantitative analysis of the time-dependent development of glucose-6-phosphatase-deficient foci in the livers of mice treated neonatally with diethylnitrosamine. *Cancer Res.* **41**:1585.

Nowell, P.C. 1976. The clonal evolution of tumor cell populations. *Science* **194**: 23.

Page, N.P. 1977. Concepts of a bioassay program in environmental carcinogenesis. In *Advances in modern toxicology*, vol. 3, p. 87. Hemisphere Publishing, Washington, D.C.

Pugh, T.D. and S. Goldfarb. 1978. Quantitative histochemical and autoradiographic studies of hepatocarcinogenesis in rats fed 2-acetylaminofluorene followed by phenobarbital. *Cancer Res.* **38**:4450.

Pugh, T.D., J. King, H. Koen, Y. He, D. Nychka, S. Vesselinovitch, J. Chover, G. Wahba, and S. Goldfarb. 1982. An improved method for quantitating neoplastic foci during hepatocarcinogenesis. *Proc. Am. Assoc. Cancer Res.* **23**:105.

Scherer, E., M. Hoffmann, P. Emmelot, and M. Friedrich-Freksa. 1972. Quantitative study on foci of altered cells induced in the rat by a single dose of diethylnitrosamine and partial hepatectomy. *J. Natl. Cancer Inst.* **49**:93.

Steel, G.G. 1977. *Growth kinetics of tumours*, p. 13. Clarendon Press, Oxford, England.

Vesselinovitch, S.D. 1969. The sex-dependent difference in the development of liver tumors in mice administered dimethylnitrosamine. *Cancer Res.* **29**:1024.

_____. 1980. Infant mouse as a sensitive bioassay system for carcinogenicity of N-nitroso compounds. *IARC Sci. Publ.* **31**:645.

Vesselinovitch, S.D., H. Mihailovich, and K.V. Rao. 1978. Morphology and metastatic nature of induced hepatic nodular lesions in C57BL x C3H F$_1$ mice. *Cancer Res.* **28**:2003.

_____. 1980. Dose dependent rate of induction of hepatocellular carcinoma following single administration of diethylnitrosamine. *Proc. Am. Assoc. Cancer Res.* **21**:101.

COMMENTS

TANNENBAUM: Is this conceivably a way that one could do a carcinogenicity study in several months instead of years?

GOLDFARB: Well, that is precisely the point. I tried to stress that one should take advantage of tumor multiplicity data. In this model one can use a small number of animals and induce a large number of lesions. It is therefore possible to accurately quantitate the relative carcinogenicity of different compounds in a very short time.

KIMBROUGH: Aren't these lesions similar to those induced in rats? In the rat, carcinogens induce basophilic as well as acidophilic foci. I don't know whether one sees both types of lesions in the mouse. But I wonder whether you feel that it is only the basophilic lesions which give rise to the trabecular carcinomas. Second, do any of the basophilic lesions regress?

GOLDFARB: I don't think that the basophilic foci in this mouse model are either histologically or biologically similar to the rat enzyme-altered foci. Most rat foci are eosinophilic and many of them regress, especially if the rats are not maintained on a promoter, like phenobarbital. In contrast, in this mouse model, the kinetics suggest progressive growth. Their spheroidal shapes also suggest irreversibility. I feel that there is a continuum from the basophilic foci to the trabecular carcinomas. I think these foci have a distinctly different biology than the enzyme-altered foci in the rat models.

KIMBROUGH: Have you actually shown that there is this progression?

GOLDFARB: Of course this is difficult to prove. But the exponential growth characteristics of the early lesions strongly suggest that they are autonomous, irreversible lesions. Also, their spherical shapes favor this conclusion. They don't seem to undergo the remodeling that has been well described by Farber's group.

Dose-response Studies with Nitrosamines
and Species Differences

WILLIAM LIJINSKY
Chemical Carcinogenesis Program
NCI-Frederick Cancer Research Facility
Frederick, Maryland 21701

N-nitroso compounds are among the most potent groups of carcinogens. Combined with this, the likelihood that people are exposed to them makes them excellent candidates for attempts at carcinogenic risk extrapolation. A dose-response study is a solid starting point for such an extrapolation and the first dose-response study on a large scale was conducted by Druckrey and his colleagues with nitrosodiethylamine (NDEA) more than 15 years ago (Druckrey et al. 1963). A great deal of fundamental information about nitrosamine carcinogenesis emerged from that study, including a semiquantitative relationship between dose received by an animal and its time of death with tumors, $dt^n =$ constant, with n being approximately 2.3 in this case.

We undertook similar studies with a number of nitrosamines which are very potent carcinogens, including NDEA, administering each compound in controlled doses in drinking water. Our results with NDEA (Lijinsky et al. 1981) were very similar to those reported by Druckrey, although the doses we used covered a different range. The total dose received by each animal ranged from approximately 1 mg-200 mg. At the two higher doses most of the animals died with both liver tumors and tumors of the upper gastrointestinal tract, while at lower doses tumors of the upper GI tract were common and liver tumors few (Table 1). At the highest dose there was considerable liver toxicity and a large number of hemangioendothelial sarcomas, as well as hepatocellular carcinomas. At 40% of that dose there were many hepatocellular carcinomas, but few hemangioendothelial sarcomas. The average time of death of the rats given the highest concentrations of NDEA, 113, 45, 18, and 7 mg per liter for 30 weeks or less, could be plotted against total dose per animal, even though the cause of death was liver tumors at the highest dose and esophageal tumors at the lower doses. In the groups of rats receiving the other doses of NDEA, there was no noticeable effect on survival, the pattern of mortality being very similar to that of the untreated controls. However, the higher the dose in these latter groups, the larger the proportion of animals with induced tumors. Almost all F344 rats die with tumors, but in the absence of carcinogen treatment these are mainly

Table 1
Tumors Induced by NDEA in Various Doses to Rats (♀)

Concentration in water (mg/liter)	Duration of treatment (weeks)	Total dose (mg)	Number of rats	Number of rats with tumors						
				Upper gastrointestinal tract				Liver		
				total	esophagus	forestomach	tongue/pharynx	total	hepato-carcinoma	angio-sarcoma
113	17	192	20	19	18	3	0	19	18	18
45	22	98	20	19	19	2	0	10	10	2
18	30	54	12	12	12	0	0	1	1	0
7	30	21	20	16	16	1	0	1	1	0
2.8	30	8.4	20	18	18	6	7	5	5	0
1.1	30	3.3	20	11	4	4	3	5	5	0
1.1	60	6.6	20	19	18	2	8	3	3	0
0.45	30	1.4	20	2	1	1	0	1	1	0
0.45	60	2.7	20	6	3	2	2	6	6	0
0.45	104	4.7	20	14	13	5	2	4	4	0
0	—	—	20	0	0	0	0	1	1	0

tumors of the endocrine and reproductive systems. The induction of tumors of the upper GI tract and of the liver by low doses of NDEA does not seem to affect the incidence of the "spontaneous" tumors. In the NDEA study, the lowest concentration administered was 0.45 ppm. Of the animals given this dose for 30 weeks (a total of 1.35 mg), 2 developed upper GI tract tumors, an incidence of 10% not in itself statistically significant. However, of the rats given the same dose for 60 weeks (a total of 2.7 mg), 6 developed tumors of the upper GI tract plus some with liver tumors, and 14 of those given the same dose for 104 weeks had tumors of the upper GI tract, after a total dose of 4.7 mg. This bespeaks a very great potency of NDEA.

Similar studies with nitroso-1,2,3,6-tetrahydropyridine (NTHP) and dinitrosohomopiperazine (DNHP) yielded similar results, although neither of these compounds was as potent as NDEA. In each case the total dose received by the animals in the higher dose groups could be plotted against average time of death with tumors. At the lower doses, again, there was little difference in mortality from the untreated rats, but in this range higher doses led to increased numbers of animals with tumors. NTHP was similar to NDEA in that liver tumors, mostly hemangioendothelial tumors, were seen at the highest dose, but mainly tumors of the upper GI tract at lower doses, with few liver tumors. On the other hand, although the pattern of mortality was the same, DNHP induced almost exclusively upper GI tract tumors. It is notable that the slope of the line (Fig. 1) for DNHP resembled that for NDEA very closely, but that for NTHP was different, although in its carcinogenic action NDEA resembled NTHP more than DNHP.

Two additional nitrosamines with which similar dose-response studies were carried out were nitrosomethyl-2-phenylethylamine (Lijinsky et al. 1982a) and nitrosoheptamethyleneimine (Lijinsky et al. 1982b). Both produced tumors in Fischer rats mainly in the upper GI tract (esophagus and forestomach). The experiments were carried out in much the same way as with NDEA, both the concentration in drinking water and the length of treatment being varied, the animals being allowed to die naturally. The general character of the results was similar to the aforementioned studies, the higher doses leading to accelerated death compared with untreated animals. At lower doses, mortality was similar to that of untreated animals, but the number of animals with induced tumors increased with increasing total dose. At the lower doses in all of the studies, there was not much difference in effect between treatments with a given dose for 6 months and treatment with approximately half that dose for 1 year. However, in neither of these last two studies was it possible to relate total dose linearly to average time of death with tumors over any part of the dose-response curve. This suggests either that the proportionality found with the first three compounds is an accident, or that the kinetics of metabolism and activation of the compounds related to carcinogenesis are in some cases different. Unfortunately, we do not know the mechanism of carcinogenesis by any nitrosamine, and it is quite conceivable that the mechanisms differ considerably

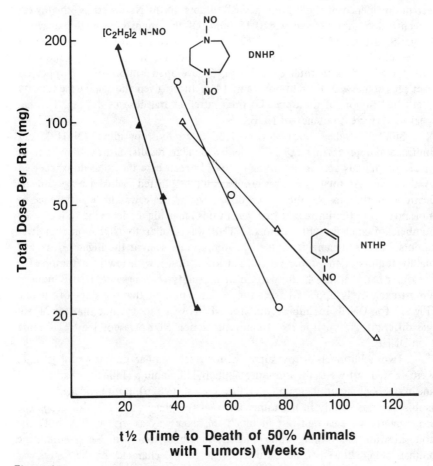

Figure 1
Relation of median time to death from tumors with total dose of nitrosamine per rat (female F344): (▲) NDEA; (○) DNHP; (△) NTHP.

between one nitrosamine and another. It is certainly possible that the proportion of a given dose activated to the proximate carcinogenic agent is very different between one nitrosamine and another, and perhaps even between different doses, so that quantification of the response might be difficult outside a narrow dose range. One fact that emerges from these studies is that a number of nitrosamines evoke a measurable carcinogenic response after administration of doses totaling only a few milligrams per rat, illustrating the great potency of many members of this class of carcinogens.

Another matter of concern in our efforts to extrapolate carcinogenic risks to man from data in animals is the extent to which responses vary from one species to another. Among nitrosamines we seldom find what is common with other classes of carcinogen, namely susceptible species and resistant species. Instead we find marked differences in the type of tumor elicited between one species and another. There is sometimes also a difference in susceptibility, or in the responsiveness of the species to a given dose or dose regimen. Examples abound in the work of many laboratories, although most nitrosamine studies have been in rats, because they seem to be more susceptible to many nitrosamines than mice. It is notable that the most common site for tumor induction by nitrosamines in rats is the esophagus, whereas esophageal tumors are seldom seen in hamsters and never in guinea pigs following treatment with nitrosamines. The liver, as well as the lung, are common sites for tumor induction in rats but in hamsters the same nitrosamines often induce tumors of the trachea and of the nasal cavity. These responses are not always exclusive and there are nitrosamines that induce the same type of tumor, for example several bladder carcinogens, in rats, hamsters, and other species.

It is reasonable to assume that the differences in response are related to differences in metabolism and activation in different species and this is an area of very active investigation. It is important because metabolism of some of these compounds in human tissue, as has been investigated by Harris, Autrup and others (Harris et al. 1977; Harris et al., this volume), might indicate the risk of exposure of humans to them. However, we must be cautious in interpreting the results of these studies, because it is possible that the main routes of metabolism, easily elucidated in some cases, might not be relevant to carcinogenesis, while minor pathways, difficult to unravel, might be the important ones in carcinogenesis. We have done experiments with nitroso-2,6-dimethylmorpholine, which induces esophageal tumors in rats, tumors of the liver and pancreas in hamsters, and hemangioendothelial tumors of the liver in guinea pigs, and have found only minor differences in the major metabolites between the 3 species, but some quantitative differences and marked differences in the rate of metabolism of the parent compound (Underwood and Lijinsky 1982). It has not yet been possible for us to use these results to define those metabolic pathways that are related to carcinogenesis, although our studies with deuterium-labeled compound (Lijinsky et al. 1980b; Rao et al. 1981) and with the *cis* and *trans* isomers (Lijinsky and Reuber 1980, 1981; Rao et al. 1981) indicate that the pathways of activation are profoundly different between the rat on one hand and hamsters and guinea pigs on the other.

It is possible that the differences in response evoked by nitrosamines in several species are in part due to particular susceptibilities of certain types of cell in a given species to neoplastic transformation. This might help to explain why a number of nitrosamines have induced ductal carcinomas of the pancreas in Syrian hamsters, whereas this tumor has not been seen in rats treated with more than 200 *N*-nitroso compounds. We have examined the carcinogenic action in

Syrian hamsters of a number of N-nitroso compounds which have formed part of an extensive structure-activity investigation in rats. As far as possible similar doses were given to both rats and hamsters. The treatment of rats was mainly with solutions of the compound in drinking water, by which the dose could be measured and the exposure of the animals was slow and steady. This procedure was not practical for hamsters, because they tended to be much less tidy, and hamsters were all given the nitroso compounds in concentrated solution by gavage. There was, therefore, some difference in the rate at which the compound was delivered to the two species, but the total dose per unit body weight was similar.

The compounds for which fairly complete results are available are mainly those of interest because they include the type of nitrosamine that has been found to induce pancreatic carcinomas in Syrian hamsters. The three related compounds nitrosobis-(2-hydroxypropyl)-amine (BHP), nitrosobis-(2-oxopropyl)-amine (BOP) and nitroso(hydroxypropyl)(oxopropyl)-amine (HPOP) have been extensively studied by Pour and his associates (Pour et al. 1979). They proposed that both BHP and BOP were converted metabolically to HPOP, which was the proximate carcinogen for the pancreas of the Syrian hamster. This was based partly on the fact that BHP was considerably less potent than BOP, and partly on the finding that both BHP and BOP were converted to some extent into HPOP which was found in the blood of the animals by Gingell and his colleagues (Gingell et al. 1976). Similarly, the cyclic compound nitroso-2,6-dimethylmorpholine was also partly metabolized to HPOP in hamsters, and the former compound, also, is a pancreatic carcinogen in the hamster (Reznik et al. 1978). The extent of conversion of all of these nitrosamines to HPOP was very small, of the order of 1% of the dose measured in the blood (Gingell et al. 1976). HPOP is also found in the urine of rats, hamsters and guinea pigs treated with nitrosodimethylmorpholine (Underwood and Lijinsky 1982). A comparison of the results of administering these four nitrosamines to rats and hamsters (Table 2) shows that BOP is more effective in inducing pancreas tumors in hamsters than either BHP (which is comparatively weak) or HPOP. Nitrosodimethylmorpholine is less effective in the hamster than BOP and a little less effective than HPOP. These nitrosamines, except BHP, induce liver tumors in the hamster in addition to tumors of the pancreatic ducts, but the liver tumors induced by nitrosodimethylmorpholine are hemangioendothelial sarcomas, while those from BOP and HPOP are hepatocellular carcinomas and cholangiocarcinomas. This suggests that the pathways of activation of nitrosodimethylmorpholine or of BHP do not involve conversion to HPOP, but rather that all might have certain pathways in common converging on the pancreas.

The contrast with the rat in the case of these four nitrosamines is very marked. There are no pancreas tumors induced in rats by any of them. Nitroso-dimethylmorpholine is by far the most potent carcinogen among them in the rat, and gives rise to esophageal tumors, as does the much less potent BHP. In contrast, BOP induced only liver tumors, both hepatocellular carcinomas and

Table 2
N-Nitroso Compounds: Comparative Carcinogenesis in F344 Rats and Syrian Hamsters

Compound	Dose rate mg/week	Duration (weeks)	Total dose mg/kg	Principal Tumors		Median week of death with tumor
				rat	hamster	
N-Nitroso-Bis-(oxopropyl)amine	5.5	50	1100	liver carcinoma liver sarcoma lung		61
	2.4	24	600		liver carcinoma cholangiocarcinoma pancreas	25
Bis-(hydroxypropyl)-amine	22	42	3700	esophagus		42
	20	32	6000		pancreas lung	32
Hydroxypropyl-oxopropylamine	5.5	40	900	liver carcinoma esophagus lung		41
	6	21	1200		liver carcinoma cholangiocarcinoma pancreas	27
2,6-Dimethyl-morpholine	2	30	240	esophagus		30
	6	30	1500		liver sarcoma pancreas lung	34

hemangioendothelial sarcomas. In rats HPOP induced both hepatocellular carcinomas and esophageal carcinomas, and appeared to be somewhat more potent than BOP. It is not unreasonable to assume, therefore, that HPOP might be an intermediate metabolite in activation of BOP in the rat (except that BOP never induces esophageal tumors), but it is almost certainly not the main carcinogenic metabolite formed from nitrosodimethylmorpholine in the rat. These contrasting results suggest that the proposed pathways of carcinogenesis for these related compounds are not correct, and that a more likely explanation is that all of them can be metabolized to carcinogenic intermediates, perhaps common ones, which are yet unknown.

A further illustration of the same problem of simplifying the probable pathways of carcinogenic activation too much is a comparison of the action of nitrosomethyloxopropylamine (MOP), nitrosomethyl-2-hydroxypropylamine (MHP) and nitrosoethanol-2-hydroxypropylamine in rats and hamsters. MOP has been suggested by Pour et al. (1980) as a further proximate carcinogen formed from BOP in the hamster, which can be expected to be more potent than BOP. However, in our studies (Table 3) MOP, at approximately one third the dose of BOP given, failed to induce pancreas tumors in hamsters, although it was very effective in inducing liver tumors, including hemangiosarcoma which was a tumor not induced by BOP in hamsters. On the other hand, MHP, which can be considered in the same relationship to MOP as BHP is to BOP, is approximately as potent a carcinogen as MOP and induces pancreatic tumors in hamsters as well as three types of liver tumor. The very much weaker nitrosoethanol-2-hydroxypropylamine induced pancreatic tumors and cholangiocarcinomas in hamsters, suggesting that the 2-hydroxypropyl moiety is involved in this activity, but that the presence of the 2-hydroxyethyl group on the nitrogen atom reduces the effectiveness, possibly through easier excretion of the unchanged compound.

In the rat nitrosoethanol-2-hydroxypropylamine is also a rather weak carcinogen, again possibly because of the ease of excretion. Nevertheless, the influence of alternative activation of the two alkyl chains is illustrated by the induction of both liver tumors and esophageal tumors, after a fairly long latent period, whereas MOP and MHP both induce mainly esophageal tumors in the rat. The difference in potency between MOP and MHP is not very large, with MHP possibly a little weaker. It is known that in rats MOP is reduced to MHP which is excreted in the urine, at least to some extent (Singer et al. 1981). Again these results do not suggest that we can yet deduce a chain of reactions by which these compounds are converted to proximate carcinogenic forms, or whether formation of a specific alkylating moiety is involved. It is almost certain that conversion of one of these carcinogenic nitrosamines to the other is not part of the mechanism of carcinogenesis, but that each undergoes individual pathways of activation. These might, however, end with formation of a few common active species.

Table 3
N-Nitroso Compounds: Comparative Carcinogenesis in F344 Rats and Syrian Hamsters

Compound	Dose rate mg/week	Duration (weeks)	Total dose mg/kg	Principal Tumors rat	Principal Tumors hamster	Median week of death with tumor
N-Nitroso-Methyl-oxopropylamine	2.5	30	300	esophagus		40
	1	22	200		liver sarcoma cholangiocarcinoma	26
Methyl-hydroxypropylamine	10	22	900	esophagus lung		29
	2	18	350		liver carcinoma liver sarcoma cholangiocarcinoma pancreas lung	22
Ethanol-hydroxypropylamine	20	50	4000	liver carcinoma liver sarcoma esophagus		59
	18	29	5000		cholangiocarcinoma pancreas lung	35

In the case of nitrosamides, the formation of the active carcinogenic species, assumed to be an alkylating agent, is probably direct, since these compounds require no metabolic activation and are directly acting carcinogens in mouse skin, for example. Nevertheless, comparing the carcinogenic action of nitroso-2-hydroxyethylurea in the rat and hamster (Table 4), sharp differences are seen, even though the compound would be expected to act through spontaneous formation of a 2-hydroxyethylating agent, analogous to the methylating agent derived from nitrosomethylurea. Nitrosohydroxyethylurea induced tumors in a wide range of organs in rats; frequently tumors of several types were present in one animal. The lung and forestomach were the most common sites, followed by colon, bone, bladder, glandular stomach, and duodenum. Tumors of these sites are rarely, if ever, seen in untreated control rats of this strain. After a somewhat higher total dose administered to Syrian hamsters the animals died earlier, but the tumor spectrum induced by nitrosohydroxyethylurea was very much narrower than in rats. Tumors of the forestomach were found commonly in both rats and hamsters. Possibly this is a consequence of administering the compound by gavage. In addition, there were hemangiosarcomas of the liver and spleen, two organs that were unaffected by nitrosohydroxyethylurea in the rat.

Similar striking differences were seen between the rat and hamster in response to two nitrosotrialkylureas, which are much more stable than nitrosomonoalkylureas and almost certainly need metabolic activation to exert their carcinogenic action. Nitrosotriethylurea gave rise mainly to breast carcinomas, with a small number of brain tumors, when given to female rats (Lijinsky et al. 1980a). In contrast, nitrosomethyldiethylurea administered to female rats did not induce breast tumors, but instead gave rise to tumors of the brain and spinal cord in high incidence (Lijinsky et al. 1980a). The effect on survival in hamsters given very similar doses of the two nitrosotrialkylureas was very similar to that in rats, half of the animals being dead at 6 months. However, the tumor spectrum in the hamsters was entirely different from that in the rats. The principal tumors induced by both compounds were in the forestomach and the spleen, the latter being hemangiosarcomas. Surprisingly, in addition, nitrosomethyldiethylurea also caused a few hamsters to develop hepatocellular carcinomas and ductal adenocarcinomas of the pancreas.

These results suggest that the characteristics of the animal species is perhaps as large a factor in the type of tumor induced by a carcinogen, and in its effectiveness, as the chemical nature of the carcinogen. Thus far our observations of interspecies differences in the metabolism of nitrosamines, which have been limited to very few compounds, indicate that there are only small differences in gross metabolism. This leads us to conclude that minor pathways of metabolism are responsible for the events leading to induction of tumors, and that great care must be taken in interpreting the results of comparative metabolism studies in animals and man before attempting to assess the risk of exposure of humans to a proven carcinogen in animals.

Table 4
N-Nitroso Compounds: Comparative Carcinogenesis in F344 Rats and Syrian Hamsters

Compound	Dose rate mg/week	Duration (weeks)	Total dose mg/kg	Principal Tumors — rat	Principal Tumors — hamster	Median week of death with tumor
N-Nitrosotriethylurea	16.5	31	2000	breast	forestomach	33
	9	25	2000		spleen sarcoma	30
Methyldiethylurea	15	33	2000	brain spinal cord		32
	8	25	1800		forestomach spleen sarcoma pancreas liver	29
Hydroxyethylurea	5.6	30	420	lung, forestomach colon, bone, bladder, glandular stomach, duodenum		49
	2.8	22	600		liver sarcoma spleen sarcoma forestomach	24

ACKNOWLEDGMENTS

This work was supported by Contract No. NO1-CO-75380, with the National Cancer Institute, NIH, Bethesda, Maryland 20205.

REFERENCES

Druckrey, H., A. Schildbach, D. Schmähl, R. Preussmann, and S. Ivankovic. 1963. Quantitativ analyse der carcinogen en Wirkung von Diäthylnitrosamin. *Arzneimittel-Forsch.* **13**:841.

Gingell, R., L. Wallcave, D. Nagel, R. Kupper, and P. Pour. 1976. Common metabolites of N-nitroso-2,6-dimethylmorpholine and N-nitrosobis(2-oxopropyl)amine in the Syrian hamster. *Cancer Lett.* **2**:47.

Harris, C.C., H. Autrup, G. Stoner, E. McDowell, B. Trump, and P. Schafer. 1977. Metabolism of acyclic and cyclic N-nitrosamines in cultured human bronchi. *J. Natl. Cancer Inst.* **59**:1401.

Lijinsky, W. and M.D. Reuber. 1980. Comparison of carcinogenesis by two isomers of nitroso-2,6-dimethylmorpholine. *Carcinogenesis* **1**:501.

———. 1981. Comparative carcinogenicity of two isomers of dimethylnitrosomorpholine in guinea pigs. *Cancer Lett.* **14**:7.

Lijinsky, W., M.D. Reuber, and B.-N. Blackwell. 1980a. Carcinogenicity of nitrosotrialkylureas in Fischer rats. *J. Natl. Cancer Inst.* **65**:451.

Lijinsky, W., M.D. Reuber, and C.W. Riggs. 1981. Dose-response studies in rats with nitrosodiethylamine. *Cancer Res.* **41**:4997.

Lijinsky, W., J.E. Saavedra, M.D. Reuber, and B.-N. Blackwell. (1980b). The effect of deuterium labeling on the carcinogenicity of nitroso-2,6-dimethylmorpholine in rats. *Cancer Lett.* **10**:325.

Lijinsky, W., M.D. Reuber, T.S. Davies, and C.W. Riggs. 1982b. Dose-response studies with nitrosoheptamethyleneimine and its α-deuterium-labeled derivative in F344 rats. *J. Natl. Cancer Inst.* (in press).

Lijinsky, W., M.D. Reuber, T.S. Davies, J.E. Saavedra, and C.W. Riggs. 1982a. Dose-response studies in carcinogenesis by nitrosomethyl-2-phenylethylamine in rats and the effect of deuterium. *Food Cosmet Toxicol.* **20**: 393.

Pour, P., R. Gingell, R. Langenbach, D. Nagel, C. Grandjean, T. Lawson, and S. Salmasi. 1980. Carcinogenicity of N-nitrosomethyl(2-oxopropyl)-amine in Syrian hamsters. *Cancer Res.* **40**:3585.

Pour, P., L. Wallcave, R. Gingell, D. Nagel, T. Lawson, S. Salmasi, and S. Tines. 1979. Carcinogenic effect of N-nitroso(2-hydroxypropyl)-(2-oxopropyl)-amine, a postulated proximate pancreatic carcinogen in Syrian hamsters. *Cancer Res.* **39**:3828.

Rao, M.S., D.G. Scarpelli, and W. Lijinsky. 1981. Carcinogenesis in Syrian hamsters by N-nitroso-2,6-dimethylmorpholine, its cis and trans isomers, and the effect of deuterium labeling. *Carcinogenesis* **2**:731.

Reznik, G., U. Mohr, and W. Lijinsky. 1978. Carcinogenic effect of N-nitroso-2,6-dimethylmorpholine in Syrian golden hamsters. *J. Natl. Cancer Inst.* **60**:371.

Singer, G.M., W. Lijinsky, L. Buettner, and G.A. McClusky. 1981. Relationship of rat urinary metabolites of N-Nitrosomethyl-N-alkylamine to bladder carcinogenesis. *Cancer Res.* **41**:4942.

Underwood, B. and W. Lijinsky. 1982. Comparative metabolism of 2,6-dimethyl-nitrosomorpholine in rats, hamsters and guinea pigs. *Cancer Res.* **42**:54.

COMMENTS

PREUSSMANN: To me, this is very fascinating. I think these nitrosamine carcinogenesis studies are still full of wonders. As you said, we always must
keep in mind not to extrapolate organ-specific effects to other species.

REED: Can you reverse the final conclusion that you have drawn, namely
that you shouldn't extrapolate from animal to man, and say that things
which may not be in animals in fact do appear in man?

LIJINSKY: Yes. Man is another experimental animal, as far as I am concerned.
He is being experimented with all the time.

HOFFMANN: Or we didn't find the right animal. You have to find the right
model.

LIJINSKY: Of course.

HARTMAN: I think Guttenplan has shown that one nitrosamine is recirculated
in saliva. I am not sure whether it is diethylnitrosamine or not. But if that
is true, at low oral dose you might expect liver tumors. But if you exceed
first pass, then recirculation would be in saliva, and you would just have it
plastered on the esophagus. Therefore it might just be a positional effect.
    Have you looked at the rat and the hamster to see if there is any
recirculation of any of these esophageal-specific agents through saliva?

LIJINSKY: We can find them in the blood even half an hour later.

HARTMAN: Do you mean after IV injection?

LIJINSKY: I don't use IV injection. I always use oral administration. I like to
administer my compound in the same manner to all animals. I think that
the compounds are very rapidly distributed in the blood and they get
everywhere, whichever route of administration you use.

PREUSSMANN: But it is clear from some other studies that carcinogenesis in
the esophagus is certainly not a local effect. It can be affected by systemic
administration.

LIJINSKY: Subcutaneous injection will give you esophageal carcinogenesis.

PREUSSMANN: Subcutaneous or intravenous injection of several nitroso compounds selectively always induce esophageal cancer. It is not only an oral
administration.

HARTMAN: That is where you put it, but that may not be where the organism is distributing it. I am just asking the question as to whether this has been looked at.

PREUSSMANN: I don't think it has been looked at.

PEGG: I agree entirely with your comments and conclusions. But I must say that, in view of the results that Peter Swann was showing with first-pass effects, it is a bit dangerous to compare a compound which you put in the drinking water with rats, which drink small amounts many times in the day, and to give one large amount by gavage into the stomach. That is a weakness which could lead to a difference in distribution of the compound.

LIJINSKY: It could indeed. And, in fact, the reason I discussed my findings with nitrosohydroxyethylurea is because in both instances when the compound was given by gavage at the same rate to both rats and hamsters it showed a vast difference in effect, nevertheless. Of course, your comment is very valid.

CONNEY: One trivial point experimentally, but important, I think, conceptually is that there are differences in absorption between chemicals and in the ways the compounds are given.

LIJINSKY: Absolutely.

CONNEY: If one could measure blood levels and try to relate dose with blood level, I think that one could have a more accurate assessment of dose response kinds of studies.

LIJINSKY: There is also the possibility that rates of excretion of unchanged compounds differ, as Rudolf showed with nitrosodiethanolamine. The dose delivered to the liver cells is probably only a small proportion of the dose you administer, and yet is very, very effective, because you get lots of liver tumors, even though 70 or 80% of it is excreted unchanged. Both pharmacodynamics and kinetics are a very important part of this. But you can't do everything. I like to get the biological results first and then go back to study metabolism and distribution and things like that.

PREUSSMANN: I think it is quite evident that a comparative pharmacokinetics of different nitroso compounds is a field which needs much more work. We have so many data on structure-activity relationships, and we have many, many data on the final interaction of the activated species with biopolymers, but this area in between, we really don't know much about it.

HECHT: Could you just briefly indicate the differences between your assay and Pour's on this methyloxopropyl compound?

LIJINSKY: He used higher doses than I used. I think he gave it subcutaneously. I am not sure what the route was but they were definitely higher doses. We did get 100% liver tumors.

ARCHER: I think Pour normally uses the subcutaneous route.

HECHT: Didn't he find exclusively pancreatic tumors?

LIJINSKY: No. He got liver tumors, too. And we did, of course, look for pancreas tumors but there were none there.

AFTERWORD

PETER N. MAGEE
Fels Research Institute
Temple University School of Medicine
Philadelphia, Pennsylvania 19140

It seems reasonable to draw the following conclusions from the results presented at this Conference and from the discussions that followed their presentation:

(1) Human cells and organs in culture can be transformed to malignancy by nitrosamines.

(2) Human beings poisoned by dimethylnitrosamine (NDMA) show closely similar acute, subacute, and chronic pathological changes to those observed after treatment of experimental animals with the same compound. In one subject, chronically exposed to NDMA, pathological changes in the liver were described as preneoplastic.

(3) Human cells in organ culture and human liver slices in vitro are capable of metabolism of NDMA to yield methylating intermediates which react with nucleic acids. Liver DNA is methylated in human subjects poisoned with NDMA, the pattern of base methylation being similar to that characteristic for strongly carcinogenic methylating agents as observed in experimental animals.

(4) Very carefully controlled measurements, using high resolution mass spectrometry, have confirmed the presence of NDMA in the blood plasma of some human subjects. The concentrations of NDMA in the plasma samples were considerably less than those reported previously, however. Prior administration of ethanol was shown to reduce the rate of clearance of NDMA from the circulating blood of rabbits and NDMA could be detected in the blood in human subjects after consumption of alcohol although it was not detected by the same methods in subjects who had not taken alcohol. These findings suggest that nitrosamines formed endogenously in the stomach may reach extra hepatic organs in greater concentrations when their metabolism in the liver is inhibited by alcohol consumption.

(5) Measurements of the metabolic production of molecular nitrogen from ^{14}N-labeled nitrosamines suggest that the formation of alkylating intermediates is the main metabolic pathway of the nitrosamines if these intermediates are assumed to be formed in quantities equivalent to the molecular nitrogen produced. These findings support the idea that the molecular mecha-

nisms of the biological actions of the *N*-nitroso compounds are mediated by their alkylating metabolic products.

(6) Very sensitive and reliable analytical methods for nitrosamines are now available and their use has confirmed the presence of nitrosamines in some foods and in tobacco smoke. Tobacco specific nitrosamines are metabolized by pathways leading to the formation of alkylating intermediates.

(7) The formation of carcinogenic nitroso compounds from amine precursors and nitrites in the stomach and elsewhere in experimental animals is well established and the simultaneous administration of these compounds results in the induction of the tumors characteristic of the nitrosamine formed. Such endogenous nitrosation reactions have been shown to occur in human subjects, as exemplified by the formation of the noncarcinogenic compound *N*-nitroso-proline. This important finding indicates that the endogenous formation of carcinogenic nitroso compounds could also occur in human beings exposed to appropriate nitrosatable amines.

(8) Enzyme mediated DNA repair processes for removal of alkyl groups introduced by nitrosamines are recognized. The enzyme responsible for transfer of the methyl group from O^6-methylguanines in DNA to sulfhydryl groups on the enzyme protein is present in human liver where it is more active than in rat liver. These enzyme systems may provide defense mechanisms against the induction of cancer by nitroso compounds in man and other species.

(9) Epidemiological studies on the possible role of nitrosamines in human cancer are difficult to plan and to carry out. There is some evidence suggesting that nitrosamines or other nitroso compounds may be involved in the causation of human bilharzial bladder cancer, nasopharyngeal cancer in Hong Kong, esophageal cancer in Northern China and gastric cancer in several parts of the world.

(10) From the limited data available from dose-response studies it is clear that several of the nitrosamines are very potent carcinogens which, under some conditions, can increase the incidence of tumors in experimental animals at dietary levels in the parts per billion range.

Conclusion

None of the information presented at this Conference provides unequivocal evidence that nitrosamines are involved in the causation of human cancer or that they are carcinogenic for man. Nevertheless, taken as a whole, the accumulated data do suggest that the possibility of such a role for these powerful and versatile carcinogens should not be excluded and that further research is warranted.

NAME INDEX

SUBJECT INDEX

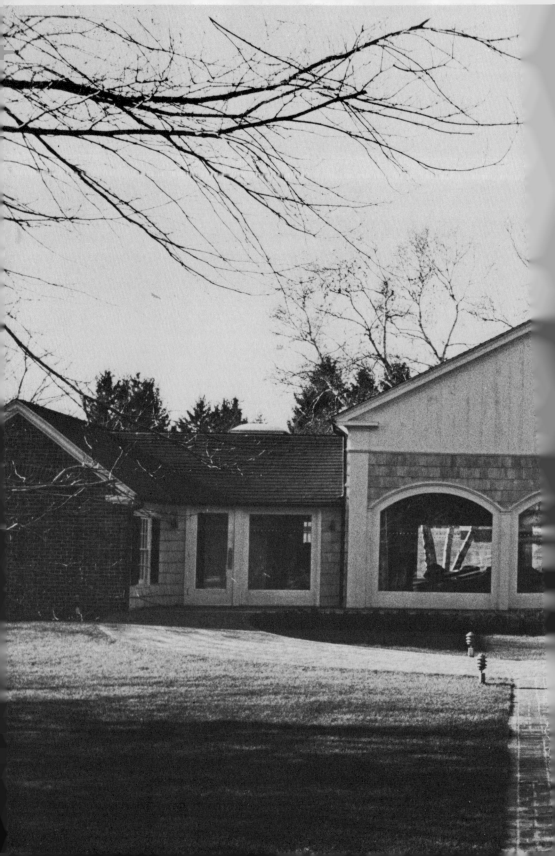